HANDBOOK OF EXPERIMENTAL EXISTENTIAL PSYCHOLOGY

Handbook of Experimental Existential Psychology

Edited by

JEFF GREENBERG
SANDER L. KOOLE
TOM PYSZCZYNSKI

THE GUILFORD PRESS
NEW YORK   LONDON

© 2004 The Guilford Press
A Division of Guilford Publications, Inc.
72 Spring Street, New York, NY 10012
www.guilford.com

Lyrics from "Roadhouse Blues"
Words and Music by The Doors
Copyright © 1970 Doors Music Co.
Copyright renewed
All rights reserved Used by permission

Printed in the United States of America

This book is printed on acid-free paper.

Last digit is print number: 9 8 7 6 5 4 3 2

Library of Congress Cataloging-in-Publication Data

Handbook of experimental existential psychology / edited by Jeff Greenberg,
Sander L. Koole, Tom Pyszczynski.
    p. cm.
  Includes bibliographical references and index.
  ISBN 1-59385-040-9 (hardcover : alk. paper)
 1. Existential psychology. 2. Psychology, Experimental. I. Greenberg,
Jeff, 1954– II. Koole, Sander Leon, 1971– III. Pyszczynski, Thomas A., 1954–
  BF204.5.H34 2004
  150.19′2—dc22

                                                              2004007991

*In memory of our esteemed colleague Victor Florian,
a paragon of courage both as a pioneer
of experimental existential psychology
and as a human being*

About the Editors

Jeff Greenberg is Professor of Psychology at the University of Arizona and associate editor of the *Journal of Personality and Social Psychology*. He received his PhD from the University of Kansas in 1982. Dr. Greenberg has published many articles and chapters, focused primarily on understanding self-esteem, prejudice, and depression. In collaboration with Tom Pyszczynski and Sheldon Solomon, he developed terror management theory, a broad theoretical framework that explores the role of existential fears in diverse aspects of human behavior. He is coauthor of the books *Hanging on and Letting Go: Understanding the Onset, Progression, and Remission of Depression* (1992) and *In the Wake of 9/11: The Psychology of Terror* (2003) and coeditor of *Motivational Analyses of Social Behavior* (2004).

Sander L. Koole is Associate Professor of Psychology at the Free University in Amsterdam. He received his PhD in social psychology from the University of Nijmegen in 2000. Dr. Koole has published articles and chapters on self-affirmation, implicit self-esteem, terror management processes, and affect regulation. In collaboration with Julius Kuhl and other colleagues, his recent work has focused on personality systems interactions theory, an integrative perspective that seeks to understand the functional mechanisms that underlie human motivation and personality processes. Together with Constantine Sedikides, he was guest editor of a special issue of *Social Cognition* on *The Art and Science of Self-Defense* (2004).

Tom Pyszczynski is Professor of Psychology at the University of Colorado at Colorado Springs. He received his PhD in social psychology from the University of Kansas in 1980. In collaboration with Jeff Greenberg and Sheldon Solomon, Dr. Pyszczynski developed terror management theory. His recent research has focused on applications of terror management theory to questions about the need for self-esteem, prejudice and intergroup conflict, unconscious processes, anxiety, and ambivalence regarding the human body. He is coauthor of the books *In the Wake of 9/11: The Psychology of Terror* and *Hanging on and Letting Go: Understanding the Onset, Progression, and Remission of Depression*.

Contributors

Sara Algoe, MA, Department of Psychology, University of Virginia, Charlottesville, Virginia

Jamie Arndt, PhD, Department of Psychological Sciences, University of Missouri, Columbia, Missouri

Denise Baden, PhD, School of Psychology, University of Southampton, Southampton, United Kingdom

John A. Bargh, PhD, Department of Psychology, Yale University, New Haven, Connecticut

C. Daniel Batson, PhD, Department of Psychology, University of Kansas, Lawrence, Kansas

Roy F. Baumeister, PhD, Department of Psychology, Florida State University, Tallahassee, Florida

W. Keith Campbell, PhD, Department of Psychology, University of Georgia, Athens, Georgia

Trevor I. Case, PhD, Department of Psychology, University of Auckland, Auckland, New Zealand

Emanuele Castano, PhD, Graduate Faculty of Political and Social Science, New School University, New York, New York

Alison Cook, MA, Department of Psychological Sciences, University of Missouri, Columbia, Missouri

Mark Dechesne, PhD, Department of Social and Organisational Psychology, University of Groningen, Groningen, The Netherlands

Edward L. Deci, PhD, Department of Clinical and Social Sciences in Psychology, University of Rochester, Rochester, New York

Gráinne Fitzsimons, MA, Department of Psychology, New York University, New York, New York

Victor Florian, PhD (deceased), Department of Psychology, Bar-Ilan University, Ramat Gan, Israel

Jamie L. Goldenberg, PhD, Department of Psychology, University of California, Davis, California

Jeff Greenberg, PhD, Department of Psychology, University of Arizona, Tucson, Arizona

Jonathan Haidt, PhD, Department of Psychology, University of Virginia, Charlottesville, Virginia

Michael J. Halloran, PhD, School of Psychological Science, LaTrobe University, Melbourne, Australia

Christopher D. Henry, MA, Department of Psychology, University of Georgia, Athens, Georgia

Gilad Hirschberger, PhD, Department of Psychology, Bar-Ilan University, Ramat Gan, Israel

Ronnie Janoff-Bulman, PhD, Department of Psychology, University of Massachusetts, Amherst, Massachusetts

John T. Jost, PhD, Department of Psychology, New York University, New York, New York

Tim Kasser, PhD, Department of Psychology, Knox College, Galesburg, Illinois

Aaron C. Kay, MA, Department of Psychology, Stanford University, Stanford, California

Sander L. Koole, PhD, Department of Psychology, Free University, Amsterdam, The Netherlands

Arie W. Kruglanski, PhD, Department of Psychology, University of Maryland, College Park, Maryland

Julius Kuhl, PhD, Department of Personality Psychology, University of Osnabruck, Osnabruck, Germany

Mark J. Landau, MS, Department of Psychology, University of Arizona, Tucson, Arizona

Anson E. Long, BS, Department of Psychology, Pennsylvania State University, University Park, Pennsylvania

Leonard L. Martin, PhD, Department of Psychology, University of Georgia, Athens, Georgia

Debra J. Mashek, PhD, Department of Psychology, George Mason University, Fairfax, Virginia

Ian McGregor, PhD, Department of Psychology, York University, Toronto, Canada

Mario Mikulincer, PhD, Department of Psychology, Bar-Ilan University, Ramat Gan, Israel

Michael W. Morris, PhD, Graduate School of Business, Columbia University, New York, New York

Maria-Paola Paladino, PhD, Department of Sociology, Università degli Studi di Trento, Trento, Italy

Elizabeth C. Pinel, PhD, Department of Psychology, Pennsylvania State University, University Park, Pennsylvania

Tom Pyszczynski, PhD, Department of Psychology, University of Colorado, Colorado Springs, Colorado

Tomi-Ann Roberts, PhD, Department of Psychology, Colorado College, Colorado Springs, Colorado

Clay Routledge, MA, Department of Psychological Sciences, University of Missouri, Columbia, Missouri

Richard M. Ryan, PhD, Department of Clinical and Social Sciences in Psychology, University of Rochester, Rochester, New York

Michael B. Salzman, PhD, Department of Counselor Education, University of Hawaii at Manoa, Honolulu, Hawaii

Constantine Sedikides, PhD, School of Psychology, University of Southampton, Southampton, United Kingdom

Kennon M. Sheldon, PhD, Department of Psychological Sciences, University of Missouri, Columbia, Missouri

Sheldon Solomon, PhD, Department of Psychology, Skidmore College, Saratoga Springs, New York

E. L. Stocks, MA, Department of Psychology, University of Kansas, Lawrence, Kansas

June Price Tangney, PhD, Department of Psychology, George Mason University, Fairfax, Virginia

Orit Taubman - Ben-Ari, PhD, School of Social Work, Bar-Ilan University, Ramat Gan, Israel

Agnes E. van den Berg, PhD, Alterra Green World Research Institute, Wageningen, The Netherlands

Kees van den Bos, PhD, Department of Social and Organizational Psychology, Utrecht University, Utrecht, The Netherlands

Renate Vida-Grim, PhD, Department of Psychology, University of Trieste, Trieste, Italy

Kathleen D. Vohs, PhD, Sauder School of Business, University of British Columbia, Vancouver, British Columbia

Robert A. Wicklund, PhD, Department of Psychology, University of Trieste, Trieste, Italy

Tim Wildschut, PhD, School of Psychology, University of Southampton, Southampton, United Kingdom

Kipling D. Williams, PhD, Department of Psychology, Macquarie University, Sydney, Australia

Darren J. Yopyk, BA, Department of Psychology, University of Massachusetts, Amherst, Massachusetts

Maia J Young, PhD, Graduate School of Business, Stanford University, Stanford, California

Vincent Yzerbyt, PhD, Department of Psychology, Catholic University of Louvain, Louvain la Neuve, Belgium

Acknowledgments

$\mathbf{W}$e would like to thank a number of individuals and organizations for the support and contributions necessary to make this book "a reality," an enjoyable and rewarding contribution to our own individual realities, and, we hope, a positive contribution to the realities of our readers. We thank Editor-in-Chief Seymour Weingarten and The Guilford Press, who made the leap of faith to back this project. Editorial and Contracts Administrator Carolyn Graham, Production Editor Craig Thomas, Art Director Paul Gordon, and a number of other professionals behind the scenes at Guilford did an excellent job of making this an enjoyable experience for us and of turning a collection of documents into an impressive handbook.

Sincere thanks to each of the contributing authors for being interested, timely, and responsive, as well as for the quality of their efforts; obviously an edited volume can only be as good as the work of its contributing authors. We would also like to thank the Free University Amsterdam for hosting the First International Conference on Experimental Existential Psychology, the Netherlands Organization for Scientific Research (NWO) and the European Association of Experimental Social Psychology (EAESP) for helping to fund this meeting, and Gün Semin for his support and advice. Additional thanks to The Doors for allowing us to quote some of their lyrics, and to Ingrid K. Olson, Danny Sugerman, Kerry Humpherys, Maria Jackson, and Randall Wixen for helping us gain permission to do so.

On a final, personal note, we would like to thank our wives, Liz Greenberg, Agnes van den Berg, and Wendy Matuszewski, whose unwavering support helped us focus our energies on doing our best as editors.

JEFF GREENBERG
SANDER L. KOOLE
TOM PYSZCZYNSKI

Contents

PART V. FREEDOM AND THE WILL

PART VI. POSTMORTEM

Well, I woke up this morning, I got myself a beer
Well, I woke up this morning, and I got myself a beer
The future's uncertain, and the end is always near

Let it roll, baby, roll
Let it roll, baby, roll
Let it roll, all night long

—THE DOORS

Part I

Introduction

Chapter 1

Experimental Existential Psychology

Exploring the Human Confrontation with Reality

TOM PYSZCZYNSKI
JEFF GREENBERG
SANDER L. KOOLE

WHAT IS EXPERIMENTAL EXISTENTIAL PSYCHOLOGY?

> When we look for answers to the questions we have been discussing, we find, curiously enough, that every answer seems to somehow impoverish the problem. Every answer sells us short; it does not do justice to the depth of the question but transforms it from a dynamic human concern into a simplistic, lifeless, inert line of words. . . . The only way of resolving—in contrast to solving—the questions is to transform them by means of deeper and wider dimensions of consciousness. The problems must be embraced in their full meaning, the antimonies resolved even with their contradictions.
>
> The microcosm of consciousness is where the macrocosm of the universe is known. It is the fearful joy, the blessing, and the curse of man that he can be conscious of himself and his world.
>   —ROLLO MAY, *Love and Will* (1969, pp. 307–308, 324)

For most of the relatively short history of scientific psychology the mere idea of an experimental existential psychology would have been considered oxymoronic—in fact, such a juxtaposition of experimental and existential psychology was probably never even considered at all. Although experimental psychology has flourished for well over 100 years, and existential ideas have made their way into the theories of clinically oriented theorists and thera-

3

pists for most of the 20th century, these two approaches have traditionally been thought of as opposite ends of the very broad and typically finely demarcated field of psychology. Experimental psychologists applied rigorous research methods to relatively simple phenomena, usually with the intention of discovering the most basic building blocks of human behavior. Existential psychologists, on the other hand, speculated about the human confrontation with very abstract questions regarding the nature of existence and the meaning of life—ideas that typically are considered far too abstruse and intractable to be fruitfully addressed by the scientific method. For the most part, experimentalists and existentialists acknowledged the existence of each other only when pointing to the fundamental absurdity of what the other was trying to accomplish. Indeed, Irvin Yalom, a prominent existential psychotherapist whose work has been a major source of inspiration for our attempts to develop an experimental existential psychology, commented that in psychological research, "the precision of the result is directly proportional to the triviality of the variables studied. A strange type of science!" (1980, p. 24).

Yalom's critical comments were written in the later 1970s, which was precisely when two of the authors of this chapter were engaged in doctoral study in social psychology. Although Yalom was commenting on the state of affairs in the field of psychotherapy research, we had very similar feelings about the work that was then dominating the study of social psychology. The "cognitive revolution" had captured the imagination of most of the field, and a movement was afoot to explain virtually all human behavior as resulting from the basically rational but sometimes biased workings of the "human information processing system." The motivational theorizing that had flourished throughout most of the history of social psychology was being replaced by analyses that attempted to explain behavior by specifying the information-processing sequences through which external events led to inferences or conclusions, which were then assumed to rather directly determine human action. Conceptualizations of the impact of needs, desires, and emotions seemed to be rather rapidly receding from social psychological discourse, and consideration of how people come to grips with the really big issues in life was virtually nonexistent. Like Yalom, we felt disenchanted and had the sense that something very basic and important was missing from the social psychological thinking of the time. To paraphrase Rollo May (1953), the field of psychology seemed intent on making molehills out of mountains.

Certainly we are not suggesting that cognitive analyses are unimportant, uninformative, or unnecessary for a comprehensive and well-rounded psychology. Just as all behavior has physiological and biochemical underpinnings, so too is cognitive activity of some sort involved in virtually everything people do. But the social cognitivists' attempt to explain human behavior by relying solely on information-processing analyses was just as short-sighted as the behaviorists' attempt to deny the importance of higher-level cognitive processes in human functioning. Important pieces of the human puzzle were being systematically left out of psychology's explanations for why people do the things they do. Just as the behaviorists had rejected internal cognitive processes from their explanations because such processes could not be directly observed, most other experimental psychologists continued to ignore the impact of existential issues because they seemed beyond the realm of empirical research. In the years since then, the incompleteness of a purely cognitive approach has been recognized by theorists in virtually all areas of psychology. The content of psychological journals has changed radically over the last 20 years or so, and current theorizing incorporates a wider range of influences than ever, with a growing emphasis on broad integrative theorizing.

Yes, a lot has changed in psychology over the past few decades. Somewhat ironically, many of these changes were inspired by the hard-core social cognitive paradigm that dominated the field of social psychology from the mid 1970s through the late 1980s. Cognitive psychology provided psychologists of all stripes with a new set of conceptual tools to think about the workings of the mind. Furthermore, cognitive psychology provided a wide range of new research methods and technologies to enable us to assess and indirectly observe mental processes that had for decades been assumed to be hidden from view and thus beyond the realm of scientific analysis. The old behaviorist doctrine that mental events could not be studied scientifically because they could not be observed had disintegrated in response to the advances coming out of cognitive laboratories. Just as important, we believe, the massive popularity of purely cognitive explanations for human behavior, and the resulting sense that something very important was being left out of mainstream theorizing, provided an impetus to spur theorists to look back to the classic psychological theories and bring motivational, emotional, unconscious, and psychodynamic processes back into their analyses. Theories of the self have flourished, and out of this renewed interest in the abstract sense of identity, meaning, value, and purpose that the study of the self required, a trend toward consideration of existential issues in modern psychological theorizing and research has gradually emerged. This growing trend led to the First International Conference on Experimental Existential Psychology in August 2001 in Amsterdam. This *Handbook* was inspired by the success of that conference and ideally serves as a worthy representation of what are currently the best, most mature contemporary psychological theories and research programs addressing existential questions.

WHAT IS EXISTENTIALISM?

Philosopher William Barrett (1959, p. 126) defined existentialism as "a philosophy that confronts the human situation *in its totality* to ask what the basic conditions of human existence are and how man can establish his own meaning out of these conditions." Existential thinking is both old and new. One of the oldest known written documents, *The Gilgamesh Epic,* recounts the existential crisis brought on in the protagonist by the death of his friend, Enkidu:

> Now what sleep is this that has taken hold of thee? Thou has become dark and canst not hear me. When I die shall I not be like unto Enkidu? Sorrow enters my heart, I am afraid of death. (Heidel, 1946, pp. 63–64)

Consideration of existential issues can also be found in the work of the great thinkers of the Western classic era, such as Homer, Plato, Socrates, and Seneca, and continued through the work of theologians such as Augustine and Aquinas. Existential issues were also explored in the blossoming arts and humanities of the European Renaissance, for example by writers such as Cervantes, Dante, Milton, Shakespeare, and Swift. The arts became even more focused on these matters in the romantic period of the 19th century, for example in the poetry of Byron, Shelley, and Keats; the novels of Balzac, Dostoyevsky, Hugo, and Tolstoy; and the music of Beethoven, Brahms, Bruckner, and Tchaikovsky. And, of course, this issue has become even more dominant in art since then, as can be seen, for example, in the plays of Beckett, O'Neill, and Ionesco; the classical music of Mahler and Cage; the rock music of John Lennon and The Doors; and the surrealist paintings of Dalí, Ernst, Tanguy, and many others. One could even say that virtually everyone who is widely considered a "great artist" explored existential issues in his or her work in one form or another. Indeed, the expression of deep existential concerns may be the underlying commonality of all great artistic creation.

An explicit, focused consideration of existential issues came to full fruition of course in the Existentialist school of philosophy, which built on the philosophical line of thought of Descartes, Kant, and Hegel and blossomed in the writings of Kierkegaard, Nietzsche, Heidegger, Sartre, Marcel, Camus, Jaspers, Unamuno, Ortega y Gasset, Buber, Tillich, and others. Although approaching existential questions from very diverse perspectives and sometimes drawing dramatically different conclusions, all these thinkers addressed the questions of what it means to be a human being, how we humans relate to the physical and metaphysical world that surrounds us, and how we can find meaning given the realities of life and death. Most important, they considered the implications of how ordinary humans struggle with these questions for what happens in their daily lives. Thus, existential issues were not conceived of as material for the abstruse musings of philosophers and intellectuals but, rather, as pressing issues with enormous impact on the lives of us all.

THE TRADITION OF EXISTENTIAL PSYCHOLOGY

Within the field of psychology, a loosely defined existentialist movement began to emerge, initially as a reaction to orthodox Freudian theory. In Europe, theorists such as Ludwig Binswanger, Medard Boss, and Viktor Frankl argued for the importance of basing our analyses of human behavior in the phenomenological world of the subject. As Binswanger put it, "There is not one space and time only, but as many spaces and times as there are subjects" (1956, p. 196). Otto Rank was perhaps the first theorist to incorporate existentialist concepts into a broad theoretical conception of human behavior, with his theorizing of the role of the twin fears of life and death in the development of the self in the child and the ongoing influence of these forces across the lifespan. Indeed, Rank's work anticipated many of the themes to be found in later existential psychological work, in his analysis of art and creativity, the soul, the fears of life and death, and the will. Similar existentialist leanings can be found in Karen Horney's emphasis on our conception of the future as a critical determinant of behavior, Erich Fromm's analysis of the pursuit and avoidance of freedom, Carl Rogers's emphasis on authenticity, Abraham Maslow's thinking regarding self-actualization, and more recently in the writings of R. D. Laing, Ernest Becker, Robert Jay Lifton, and Irvin Yalom.

In his classic text on existential psychotherapy, Irvin Yalom (1980) described existential thought as focused on human confrontation with the fundamentals of existence. He viewed existential psychology as rooted in Freudian psychodynamics, in the sense that it explored the motivational consequences of important human conflicts, but argued that the fundamental conflicts of concern to existentialists are very different from those emphasized by Freud: "neither a conflict with suppressed instinctual strivings nor one with internalized significant adults, but *instead a conflict that flows from the individual's confrontation with the givens of existence*" (Yalom, 1980, p. 8, emphasis in original). In other words, existential psychology attempts to explain how ordinary humans come to terms with the basic facts of life with which we all must contend. But what are these basic "givens of existence"?

Yalom delineated four basic concerns that he believes exert enormous influence on all people's lives: death, freedom, existential isolation, and meaninglessness. These are deep, potentially terrifying issues, and consequently, people typically avoid direct confrontation with them. Indeed, many people claim that they *never* think about such things. Nonetheless, Yalom argued that these basic concerns are ubiquitous and influential regardless of whether we realize it or not. The inevitability of death is a simple fact of life of which we are all aware; the inevitability of death in an animal that desperately wants to live produces a conflict that simply cannot be brushed aside. The concern with freedom reflects the conflict between a desire for self-determination and the sense of groundlessness and ambiguity that results when one realizes that much of what happens in one's life is really up to oneself—that there are few if any absolute rules to live by. By existential isolation, Yalom referred to "a fundamental isolation . . . from both creatures and world. . . . No matter how close each of us becomes to another, there remains a final, unbridgeable gap; each of us enters existence alone and must depart from it alone" (1980, p. 9). Existential isolation is the inevitable consequence of the very personal, subjective, and individual nature of human experience that can never be fully shared with another being. The problem of meaninglessness is the result of the first three basic concerns: In a world where the only true certainty is death, where meaning and value are subjective human creations rather than absolute truths, and where one can never fully share one's experiences with others, what meaning does life have? The very real possibility that human life is utterly devoid of meaning lurks just beneath the surface of our efforts to cling to whatever meaning we can find or create. According to Yalom, the crisis of meaninglessness "stems from the dilemma of a meaning-seeking creature who is thrown into a universe that has no meaning" (1980, p. 9).

THE PRIMARY THEMES OF EXPERIMENTAL
EXISTENTIAL PSYCHOLOGY

One or more of the four basic existential issues delineated by Yalom are addressed in various ways by virtually all the authors of the chapters of this volume. However, Yalom acknowledged that these four concerns by no means constituted an exhaustive list, and indeed, a wide range of additional existential concerns are also currently being actively explored by the new wave of experimental existential psychologists. Included among these are questions of how we humans fit into the physical universe, how we relate to nature, and how we come to grips with the physical nature of our own bodies—questions about beauty, spirituality, and nostalgia, and questions about the role of existential concerns in intrapersonal, interpersonal, and intergroup conflict. Of course, there are undoubtedly many other important ways in which people's confrontations with the basic givens of human existence influence their lives, and we hope that this volume will spark interest in further exploration of such issues.

To attempt to capture the main themes of the wide-ranging experimental existential work appearing in this volume, based largely on Yalom's four ultimate concerns, we have organized the *Handbook* into four sections: Existential Realities, Systems of Meaning and Value, The Human Connection, and Freedom and the Will. Part II, Existential Realities, focuses on the psychological confrontation with death, trauma, the body, and nature. Part III, Systems of Meaning and Value, focuses on the human quest for meaning, identity, and significance, utilizing perspectives such as terror management theory, lay epistemics, uncertainty management, and systems justification in the context of examining culture, morality, justice, identity maintenance, nostalgia, and religion. Part IV, The Human Connection, highlights the interpersonal dimensions of experimental existential psychology, dealing with attachment, social identity, shared subjective experience, ostracism, perspective taking, and shame and guilt as intrinsically social existential phenomena. Finally, Part V, Freedom and the Will, explores the possibilities of human freedom, utilizing contributions from self-determination theory, automaticity research, and German will psychology.

EXPERIMENTAL EXISTENTIAL PSYCHOLOGY
AND MODERN SOCIAL PSYCHOLOGY

A case could be made that, even though they may not have realized it, social psychologists have been concerned with existential issues in one way or another all along. Classic social psychological topics such as attitudes, values, morality, the impact of the group on the individual, causal attribution, decision making and choice, cognitive dissonance, and reactance all touch on the human attempt to find meaning in an ambiguous world and find values to orient one's life around. Fritz Heider focused his entire career on exploring the human quest to understand the causal structure of the world in which we live. This work played a major role in inspiring the cognitive revolution in social psychology and its influence continues to be felt across the field even to this day. But whereas Heider focused on the way the "man in the street" comes to understand the behavior of those around him, the existentialist focus is on how this same "man in the street" grapples, whether consciously or unconsciously, with even more basic questions about life itself.

Similarly, Leon Festinger's social comparison theory (1954) focused on how people rely on social reality to understand and evaluate themselves, and his cognitive dissonance theory (Festinger, 1957) explored how people grapple with the inconsistencies in their lives. Later work in the dissonance tradition by Brehm and Cohen (1962), Aronson (1968), and many others explored the role of free choice, responsibility, and hypocrisy. Brehm's (1956) classic analysis of the dilemma that results from making choices is remarkably similar to that discussed by Fromm (1941) and other existentially oriented thinkers: The very act of choosing a given course of action limits one's freedom to pursue other courses of action, and thus sets a series of intricate conflict-reducing processes in motion. Melvin Lerner (1980) inspired the empirical study of the human quest for justice and the exploration of how people respond to injustice with his seminal "just world" hypothesis and the research that followed from it. Stanley Milgram's (1963) classic studies of obedience explored the startling readiness of people to cede responsibility to authority figures and the potentially lethal consequences of such surrender of control. In a similar vein, Zimbardo, Banks, Haney, and Jaffe (1973) explored the loss of self and control over one's actions that result from immersion in social roles and the deindividuating consequences of immersion in groups.

Perhaps the one construct that pervades all existential concerns is that of self-awareness. Ernest Becker (1962) argued that self-awareness is the most important feature that distinguishes human beings from other animals and that it is this capacity for self-awareness that sets the stage for the existential terror that led to the development of culture and humankind as we know it today. Of course, social psychologists were introduced to the notion of self-awareness by Shelley Duval and Robert Wicklund's (1972) highly influential objective self-awareness theory. Although the experimental study of the self within social psychology, which set the stage for the emergence of the experimental existential perspective, emerged from a variety of divergent and related lines of inquiry that were being explored in the early 1970s, we believe that Duval and Wicklund's seminal work on self-awareness was a landmark contribution that signaled the emergence of the self as a central and indispensable focus of social psychological inquiry.

In retrospect, it seems that the 1950s and 1960s were a time at which social psychologists were heavily immersed in the exploration of existential issues. Indeed, this exciting period of intellectual fomentation inspired many contemporary social psychologists to enter the field. We believe, however, that a more explicit acknowledgment of the importance of existential issues and the confrontation with the basic realities of human existence will add an important new dimension to the study of these classic issues. An existential perspective focuses not so much on *what* we know or *how* we know but, rather, on *that* we know. It has the potential to provide a new look, from a different perspective, at the issues that have captured psychologists' imaginations for the past century.

OF OUR OWN MAKING: CONFINEMENT AND LIBERATION

How *do* people cope with their understanding of their place in the universe? Often, this amounts to the study of how people shield themselves from their knowledge of their mortality, their uncertainty, their isolation, and their deficits in meaning. Although confrontation with the fundamental dilemmas of human existence can be terrifying, can lead to a great deal of self-deception, can instigate hostility and hatred, and can undermine our freedom, it also has the potential to be inspiring and liberating and provide the impetus for a better way of being. This was the hope of many existential thinkers and the impetus for the emergence of the existentially inspired humanistic movement in psychology. In fact, many of those currently pursuing an experimental existential agenda are committed to these very same ideals, of acquiring the understanding that might provide the key to a freer, more open, and less defensive way of being. Our hope is that, by bringing existential issues back to the forefront of social psychological discourse, this volume will reinvigorate our discipline and inspire new decades of debate and discovery directed toward greater authenticity and benevolence in human affairs.

REFERENCES

Aronson, E. (1968). Dissonance theory: Progress and problems. In R. P. Abelson, E. Aronson, W. J. McGuire, T. M. Newcomb, M. J. Rosenbaum, & P. H. Tannebaum (Eds.), *Theories of cognitive consistency: A sourcebook* (pp. 5–27). Chicago: Rand-McNally.

Barrett, W. (1959, November 21). What is existentialism? *Saturday Evening Post*, pp. 45, 126, 129–130.

Becker, E. (1962). *The birth and death of meaning*. New York: Free Press.

Binswanger, L. (1956). Existential analysis and psychotherapy. In F. Fromm-Reichman & J. Moreno (Eds.), *Progress in psychotherapy* (pp. 196–229). New York: Grune & Stratton.

Brehm, J. W. (1956). Post-decision changes in desirability of alternatives. *Journal of Abnormal and Social Psychology, 52*, 384–389.

Brehm, J. W., & Cohen, A. R. (1962). *Explorations in cognitive dissonance*. New York: Wiley.

Duval. S., & Wicklund, R. W. (1972). *A theory of objective self-awareness*. New York: Academic Press.

Festinger, L. (1954). A theory of social comparison processes. *Human Relations, 7*, 117–140.

Festinger, L. (1957). *A theory of cognitive dissonance*. Evanston, IL: Row, Peterson.

Fromm, E. (1941). *Escape from freedom*. New York: Holt.

Heidel, A. (Trans.). (1946). *The Gilgamesh epic and Old Testament parallels*. Chicago: University of Chicago Press.

Lerner, M. J. (1980). *The belief in a just world: A fundamental delusion*. New York: Plenum Press.

May, R. (1953). *Man's search for himself*. New York: Delta.

May, R. (1969). *Love and will*. New York: Norton.

Milgram, S. (1963). Behavioral study of obedience. *Journal of Abnormal and Social Psychology, 67*, 371–378.

Yalom, I. (1980). *Existential psychotherapy*. New York: Basic Books.

Zimbardo, P., Banks, W. C., & Haney, C., & Jaffe, D. (1973, April 8). The mind is a formidable jailer: A Pirandellian prison. *New York Times Magazine*, pp. 38–60.

Part II

Existential Realities

Chapter 2

The Cultural Animal

*Twenty Years of Terror Management
Theory and Research*

SHELDON SOLOMON
JEFF GREENBERG
TOM PYSZCZYNSKI

We are very pleased to be part of the diverse and rapidly proliferating group of psychologists applying experimental methods to existential psychological questions who present their fine work in this volume. We would like to claim that we prophetically envisioned a fruitful experimental existential psychology when we started developing terror management theory (TMT) back in the early 1980s, but in truth, such a happy prospect was quite unfathomable to us at the time. As graduate students of Jack Brehm at the University of Kansas in the late 1970s, we were enamored with the rigorous scientific methods of academic psychology but disenchanted by the narrow, superficial, and often artificial questions to which these potentially powerful experimental methods were being applied.

Our impression at the time was that the field of social psychology was more oriented toward understanding the minute cognitive details of laboratory phenomena than toward making sense of the forces that underlie human social behavior. Although questions of how cognitive processes unfolded were receiving intense scrutiny, questions of why people behave the way they do seemed to have fallen by the wayside. We were persuaded by Jack Brehm's insistence on the fundamental importance of broad theories in general, and theories framed in motivational terms in particular, for experimental social psychology. Accordingly, we vowed to be on the lookout for broader perspectives that would provide insights into what people were actually doing in their daily lives. Then shortly after completing our graduate studies, in 1983 we quite accidentally stumbled on what struck us as the most compelling book to emerge from the existential psychodynamic tradition in the 20th century, Ernest Becker's 1973 Pulitzer Prize winner, *The Denial of Death*. Becker—in books such as

13

The Birth and Death of Meaning (1962/1971), *Beyond Alienation* (1967), *The Structure of Evil* (1968), *Angel in Armor* (1969), and *Escape from Evil* (1975), in addition to *The Denial of Death*—ambitiously strove to integrate and synthesize a wide range of theories and findings across a host of disciplines (most notably, the work of Søren Kierkegaard, Charles Darwin, William James, Sigmund Freud, Otto Rank, Gregory Zilboorg, Norman Brown, and Robert Jay Lifton) into a cogent account of the motivational underpinnings of human behavior.

Becker's examination of human affairs had generally fallen between the academic cracks: rejected by psychoanalysts for straying from Freud's orthodox emphasis on sexuality; rejected by anthropologists and philosophers as tainted and intellectually compromised by crossing traditional disciplinary boundaries and incorporating ideas that were alien to them; and rejected, dismissed, or entirely ignored by proponents of mainstream psychology (especially adherents of the newly emerging cognitive science) as beyond the purview of modern empirical science. But we saw in his work answers to two very basic questions that we felt were not adequately addressed by social psychologists at the time.

1. *Why are people so intensely concerned with their self-esteem?* Indeed, when TMT was originally gestated, although self-esteem was one of the oldest (William James noted its importance in his 1890 classic *Principles of Psychology*) and most common constructs in social psychological discourse, there had been no serious efforts by experimental social psychologists to define what self-esteem is, how it is acquired and maintained, what psychological function it serves, and how it does so.
2. *Why do people cling so tenaciously to their own cultural beliefs and have such a difficult time coexisting with others different than themselves?* In the early 1980s, there were only the beginnings of a dawning awareness among social psychologists of the importance of culture as a defining human characteristic.

For the most part, prevailing social psychological conceptions of human behavior viewed human beings as either social animals (e.g., Aronson, 1972) or complex information-processing machines. Whereas this first important and indisputable insight surely differentiates human beings from bacteria and rose bushes, it did little to inform our understanding of vast differences between the behavior of human beings and other very social creatures such as ants, termites, bees, and chimps. While the second insight drew attention to the important role that cognitive processes play in many human activities, it virtually ignored humankind's animal nature and the urgency of the motivational forces that impinge upon us. And neither metaphor (humans as social animals or information processors) granted any explanatory power to the specific systems of meaning and value—which is what cultures are—in which people live their lives. As Julian Jaynes (1976, p. 9) forcefully observed: "Culture . . . is different from anything else we know of in the universe. That is a fact. It is as if all life evolved to a certain point, and then in ourselves turned at a right angle and simply exploded in a different direction." Only human beings exist ensconced in a humanly constructed symbolic conception of reality that is subjectively experienced as an absolute representation of reality by the average enculturated individual. Accordingly, a comprehensive understanding of the human estate requires the explicit recognition that we are *cultural animals* and consequent efforts to define what culture is, how it is acquired and maintained, what psychological function it serves, and how it does so.[1]

We distilled Becker's answers to these two fundamental questions down to a simple but potentially powerful analysis of human behavior. At first, our colleagues did not quite share our enthusiasm for this TMT. Indeed, during our first presentation of the theory at the Society for Experimental Social Psychology (SESP) meeting in 1984, well-known psychologists jostled each other vigorously to escape as the talk unfolded. Most of those who stayed seemed to be wondering what any of this had to do with the discipline of social psychology. Although in our minds the theory did not emerge from a conceptual and intellectual vacuum, it certainly seemed that way to most psychologists back then. The *American Psychologist* rejected our first formal presentation of TMT with a one-line review: "I have no doubt that these ideas are of absolutely no interest to any psychologist, alive or dead." We had been hoping that at least the dead might have shown some interest.

But if we learned anything from our graduate training it was persistence; so we insisted that the editors of the *American Psychologist*, a journal that continually claims to seek broad perspectives, explain why these ideas were not worthy of publication. Leonard Eron eventually informed us that although terror management theory was interesting and may even have merit, it would never gain credibility in the field without empirical support. Interestingly, we really had no intention of pursuing research on Becker's ideas; to us they stood on their own because they helped explain much of what we already knew about human behavior. We continue to believe (see, e.g., Greenberg, Solomon, Pyszczynski, & Steinberg, 1988)—as Festinger (1980), among others, did—that dismissing theoretical ideas as unworthy of consideration until empirically validated retards scientific progress. However, it dawned on us that designing experiments to empirically assess the validity of hypotheses derived from social psychological theories was the one thing we could actually do. And so in the mid-1980s we began to test hypotheses derived from the theory, an endeavor that (to our pleasant surprise) continues to keep us busy, along with former and current students, and independent researchers around the world. In this way, we inadvertently became part of a trend toward examining existential ideas empirically; and this *Handbook* is a gratifying testament to the prevalence of this approach and to how much things have changed since those early days.

TERROR MANAGEMENT THEORY

You have all the fears of mortals and all the desires of immortals.
—Seneca, *On the Shortness of Life* (AD 49/1951, p. 295)

Following Darwin, TMT asserts that human beings, like all forms of life, are the products of evolution by natural selection, having acquired over extremely long periods (either gradually or in abrupt "punctuated" moments; Gould, 2002) adaptations that rendered individual members of their species able to successfully compete for resources necessary to survive and reproduce in their respective environmental niches. Specific adaptations differ radically across species and include morphological, functional, biochemical, behavioral, and psychological affectations (e.g., eagles' keen eyesight, bats' prodigious auditory feats, peacocks' courtship rituals, and chimps' use of deception to advance their gustatory and sexual interests).

What then is the particular nature of human evolutionary adaptations that render us different from any other species? Human beings are not especially formidable from a purely physical perspective as isolated individuals; we are not especially large, our senses (especially olfactory and auditory) are not keen; we are slow and have impoverished claws and teeth for meat-eating predators. But we are highly social, vastly intelligent creatures. These attributes fostered cooperation and division of labor and led to the invention of tools, agriculture, cooking, houses, and a host of other very useful habits and devices that allowed our ancestral forebears to rapidly multiply from a small band of hominids in a single neighborhood in Africa to the huge populations of *Homo sapiens* that currently occupy almost every habitable inch of the planet.

Surely one of the important aspects of human intelligence is self-awareness: We are alive and we know that we are alive; and this sense of "self" enables us to reflect on the past and ponder the future and, in so doing, function effectively in the present. But as Kierkegaard (1844/1957) noted, although knowing one is alive is tremendously uplifting and provides humans the potential for unbridled awe and joy, we are also perpetually troubled by the concurrent realization that all living things, ourselves included, ultimately die, and that death can occur for reasons that can never be anticipated or controlled. Human beings are thus, by virtue of the awareness of death and their relative helplessness and vulnerability to ultimate annihilation, in constant danger of being incapacitated by overwhelming terror. And this potential for terror is omnipresent in part because, as Rank (1941/1958) insisted, we are uncomfortable as corporeal creatures: fornicating, defecating, urinating, vomiting, flatulent, exfoliating pieces of meat. As such, we are destined, like ears of corn, to wither and die, but only if we are lucky enough to have dodged a predator's grasp, an enemy's lunge, or the benignly indifferent (to human concerns) battering of a tidal wave or earthquake. Becker (1973, p. 26) neatly summed up this uniquely human existential dilemma by observing:

> Man . . . is a creator with a mind that soars out to speculate about atoms and infinity. . . . Yet at the same time, as the Eastern sages also knew, man is a worm and food for worms.

Homo sapiens solved this existential quandary by developing cultural worldviews: humanly constructed beliefs about reality shared by individuals in a group that serves to reduce the potentially overwhelming terror resulting from the awareness of death. Culture reduces anxiety by providing its constituents with a sense that they are valuable members of a meaningful universe. Meaning is derived from cultural worldviews that offer an account of the origin of the universe, prescriptions of appropriate conduct, and guarantees of safety and security to those who adhere to such instructions—in this life and beyond, in the form of symbolic and/or literal immortality (see Lifton [1979] for an extended discussion of different modes of literal and symbolic immortality). For example, Alfonso Ortiz, a Tewa Indian from New Mexico spoke most eloquently (1991, p. 7) about the psychological needs served by cultural constructions:

> A Tewa is interested in our own story of our origin, for it holds all that we need to know about our people, and how one should live as a human. The story defines our society. It tells me who I am, where I came from, the boundaries of my world, what kind of order exists within it; how suffering, evil, and death came into this world; and what is likely to happen to me when I die.

Symbolic immortality can be obtained by perceiving oneself as part of a culture that endures beyond one's lifetime, or by creating visible testaments to one's existence in the form of great works of art or science, impressive buildings or monuments, amassing great fortunes or vast properties, and having children. Literal immortality is procured via the various afterlives promised by almost all organized religions, be it the familiar heaven of devout Christians (e.g., based on a 1994 poll, Panati [1996] reported that 77% of the American public believe that heaven exists and that 76% feel that they have an excellent chance of residing there some day. Heaven is peaceful place, free of stress, and with ample leisure time—according to 91% of those who believe in its existence, and over 70% believe that in heaven they will be in God's eternal presence, meet up with family and friends, and be surrounded by humor and frequent laughter), the opulent and sensual paradise awaiting the denizens of Islam (males at least: "the Islamic Heaven physically resembles the Garden of Eden, though it is no longer populated with only one man and one woman. There are many available young maidens in this male-oriented Paradise, which brims with an abundance of fresh figs, dates, and sweet libations" [Panati, 1996, pp. 446–447]), or the ethereal existence promised in perpetuity to Hindus and Buddhists in the form of Nirvana.

All cultural worldviews thus provide their constituents with a sense of enduring meaning and a basis for perceiving oneself to be a person of worth within the world of meaning to which one subscribes. By meeting or exceeding individually internalized standards of value, norms, and social roles derived from the culture, people qualify for death transcendence and hence can maintain psychological equanimity despite their knowledge of their own mortality. For TMT, *self-esteem* consists of the belief that one is a person of value in a world of meaning, and the primary function of self-esteem is to buffer anxiety, especially anxiety engendered by the uniquely human awareness of death.

From this theoretical perspective, the *need* for self-esteem is universal (Goldschmidt [1990] referred to this psychological imperative as "affect hunger"), in that people everywhere need to feel that life has meaning and that they are valuable participants in the cultural drama to which they subscribe. However, self-esteem is ultimately a culturally based construction in that it is derived from adhering to the individual's internalized conception of the standards of value that are prescribed by the culture. One implication of this analysis is that attributes and behaviors that confer self-esteem can vary greatly between cultures. Pastoral herders derive feelings of self-worth by the number of cattle in their possession; traditional Japanese women by their gracious hospitality; Samurai warriors by their courage and ferocity; American males by the size of their penis and bank accounts; American women by the extent to which their figure approximates the shape of a piece of linguini.

Two cultures may even prescribe entirely opposite standards of value. Indeed, the same behavior that confers great self-regard in one culture may be grounds for ostracism or even capital punishment in another. For example, adolescent Sambian boys in New Guinea (Herdt, 1982) perform oral sex on the male elders of the tribe as a normal rite of passage into adulthood; to not do so would be considered an abhorrent abomination. However, when the Taliban were in power in Afghanistan, homosexual activity was an unambiguously capital crime. Men caught in homosexual acts were "propped against any convenient old wall, which was then toppled onto them by a tank" (reported in Eckholm, 2001).[2]

To summarize, TMT proposes that the juxtaposition of a biological inclination toward self-preservation common to all life forms[3] with the uniquely human awareness that this desire will be ultimately thwarted, and could be at any time, gives rise to potentially debilitating terror. This terror is managed by the construction and maintenance of cultural worldviews. These worldviews consist of humanly constructed beliefs about reality shared by individuals in groups that provide a sense that one is a person of value in a world of meaning. Psychological equanimity thus depends on maintaining faith in an individualized version of the cultural worldview and perceiving oneself to be meeting or exceeding the standards of value prescribed by the social role that one inhabits in the context of that worldview. Given that all cultural worldviews are fragile human constructions that can never be unequivocally confirmed, and none of them are likely to be literally true, TMT posits (following Festinger, 1954) that social consensus is an utterly essential means to sustain culturally constructed beliefs.

Because so many of the meaning- and value-conferring aspects of the worldview are ultimately fictional, the existence of other people with different beliefs is fundamentally threatening. Acknowledging the validity of an alternative conception of reality would undermine the confidence with which people subscribe to their own points of view, and so doing would expose them to the unmitigated terror of death that their cultural worldviews were erected to mollify. People consequently react to those who are different by derogating them, convincing them to dispose of their cultural worldviews and convert to one's own (e.g., religious or political proselytizing), absorbing important aspects of "alien" worldviews into mainstream culture in ways that divest them of their threatening character (e.g., the 1960s radical antiwar, anti-corporate capitalism rock stars singing Budweiser beer jingles on television), or obliterating them entirely to demonstrate that one's own cultural worldview is indeed superior after all. From this perspective, humankind's long and sordid history of violent inhumanity to other humans is thus understood as (at least in part) the result of a fundamental inability to tolerate those who do not share our death-denying cultural constructions.

Human Awareness of Mortality and the Evolution of Culture

How did our primate ancestors evolve into the highly intelligent, self-aware, meaning-seeking, symbol-trafficking, death-denying species we are today? Evolutionary theorists (see, e.g., Donald, 1991) agree that our lineage diverged from other primates between 4.5 and 6 million years ago, and the first major evolutionary innovation leading to the eventual emergence of humankind was the upright bipedalism of the Australopithecines some 3.5 million years ago (Kingdon, 2003). Australopithecines, like the famous fossil remnant Lucy, walked upright, but had small brains and used no tools. However, walking upright freed the hands for direct exploration and manipulation of the physical environment, and subsequent primitive tool use fostered selection pressure leading to consequent alterations in brain size, structure, and function. Simultaneously, bipedalism caused the constriction of the birth canal, resulting in the necessity of bearing young that are dramatically more immature and helplessly dependent than other primates. This in turn required a radical alteration in protohuman family and social structure: Our ancestors now needed to live in larger groups to survive and provide a richer diet for mothers and their infants.

The complex cognitive demands of social interaction in large groups in turn led to the gradual emergence of self-reflective consciousness (Humphrey, 1984). In the process of trying to figure out what others were thinking and feeling in order to better predict and control their behavior, our forebearers became aware of their own existence and, consequently, the inevitability of death. Uniquely human awareness of mortality was thus a by-product of self-consciousness, which otherwise provides human beings with remarkable adaptive advantages (Deacon, 1997). However, conscious creatures oriented toward survival in a threatening world but now encumbered with the awareness of mortality might be overwhelmed by debilitating terror to the point of cognitive and behavioral paralysis, in which case self-consciousness would no longer confer an adaptive benefit. At this point evolutionary advantages emerged for those who developed and adopted cultural worldviews that could compellingly assuage the anxiety engendered by the uniquely human problem of death. Archeological evidence, theory and research from evolutionary psychology, anthropology, and cognitive neuroscience converge in support of the assertion that humans "solved" the problems associated with the realization of their mortality by the creation of uniquely human cultural affectations, including art, language, religion, agriculture, and economics (see Solomon, Greenberg, Schimel, Arndt, & Pyszczynski, 2003, for a detailed exposition of how the awareness of mortality directly influenced the evolution of culture).

The Humanizing Spells: The Incredible Journey from Biological Creature to Cultural Being

Besides supplying a plausible account of the evolution of cultural worldviews, it is also incumbent upon TMT to provide a developmental account of how human infants acquire cultural worldviews and how self-esteem attains its anxiety-buffering properties in the context of those worldviews. Following Bowlby's (1969) classic work on the formation of infant attachments, TMT starts with the profound immaturity of the human infant at birth and the consequent proneness to anxiety that results in response to threat and/or unmet physiological and/or psychological needs. Bowlby asserted that abject terror was the psychological impetus for the formation of infant attachments, and that babies were comforted by direct physical contact with, and affection from, their seemingly larger-than-life and omniscient parents. Early in life, parents (ideally) generally provide care and affection for their young charges in an unconditional fashion; babies are changed when they are wet, fed when they are hungry, and covered when they are cold.

But over the course of development, parental affection becomes increasingly contingent upon engaging in certain behaviors and refraining from others in the context of the socialization process in order to adhere to cultural dictates and/or to keep the child alive. There is nothing lethal from a biological perspective when American children eat worms, but most suburban parents frown on this activity, and all parents are justly concerned when their children try to touch the pretty flames emanating from the fireplace or campfire. Consequently, socialization requires that parents actively modify their children's behavior long before babies are intellectually and emotionally able to understand the basis for such restrictions of their freedom. This behavior modification is accomplished by conditional dispensation of affection. When children behave appropriately (e.g., by keeping their food on their plates rather than throwing it at their pets) they are rewarded with the unmitigated enthusiasm of their parental ancestors and feel good and safe as a result. Inappropriate behavior (e.g., flushing the healthy family goldfish down the toilet to watch it swim in circles) results in parental disapprobation, causing bad feelings and associated insecurity implicitly or explicitly connected to the prospect of parental abandonment. Very early in life, then, children come to equate being good with being safe and being bad with anxiety and insecurity (cf. Sullivan, 1953).

This immature and inchoate sense of good = safe and bad = unsafe is then transferred from personal relationships to the culture at large when children begin to become aware of the inevitability of death and realize that their parents are also mortal and ultimately unable to provide them with safety and security in perpetuity (see Yalom [1980] for an excellent discussion of the early and pervasive effects of children's death anxiety). At this point, children embark on the lifelong quest for psychological equanimity via the acquisition and maintenance of self-esteem by perceiving themselves as satisfying the standards of value associated with the social roles they inhabit in the context of their cultural worldviews. As

Geza Roheim (1943, p. 31) put it: "The caressing and praise received from his parents is transformed into praise from his countrymen. Fame and praise are socialized equivalents of love."

Summary of Terror Management Theory

TMT posits that humans share with all forms of life a biological predisposition to continue existence, or at least to avoid premature termination of life. However, the highly developed intellectual abilities that make humans aware of their vulnerabilities and inevitable death create the potential for paralyzing terror. Cultural worldviews manage the terror associated with this awareness of death primarily through the cultural mechanism of self-esteem, which consists of the belief that one is a valuable contributor to a meaningful universe. Effective terror management thus requires (1) faith in a meaningful conception of reality (*the cultural worldview*) and (2) belief that one is meeting the standards of value prescribed by that worldview (*self-esteem*). Because of the protection from the potential for terror that these psychological structures provide, people are motivated to maintain faith in their cultural worldviews and satisfy the standards of value associated with their worldviews.

IS IT TRUE?: EMPIRICAL ASSESSMENTS OF TERROR MANAGEMENT THEORY

Self-Esteem as Anxiety Buffer Hypothesis

We began our efforts to empirically assess TMT by deriving two general hypotheses from it. The first was the *self-esteem as anxiety buffer hypothesis,* which stated that if self-esteem functions to buffer anxiety, then raising self-esteem (or dispositionally high self-esteem) should reduce anxiety in response to subsequent threats. In support of this proposition, we demonstrated that momentarily elevating self-esteem (by false personality feedback or false feedback on a supposed IQ test) reduced self-reported anxiety in response to graphic video footage of an autopsy and an electrocution and reduced physiological arousal (assessed by skin conductance) in response to anticipation of electrical shocks (relative to appropriate control groups in all studies; Greenberg et al., 1992a). We also demonstrated that momentarily elevated or dispositionally high self-esteem reduced vulnerability denying defensive distortions (Greenberg et al., 1993). Specifically, participants in neutral self-esteem control conditions rated themselves as more or less emotional when these proclivities were described as being associated with longevity; this tendency was eliminated when self-esteem was high. Convergent empirical evidence thus supports a central tenet of TMT regarding the anxiety-buffering qualities of self-esteem.

Mortality Salience Hypothesis

A concurrent line of research tested derivatives of the general *mortality salience* hypothesis: If cultural worldviews and self-esteem provide beliefs about the nature of reality that function to assuage anxiety associated with the awareness of death, then asking people to ponder their own mortality ("mortality salience"; MS) should increase the need for the protection provided by such beliefs. The first hypotheses we tested were based on the notion that MS should result in vigorous agreement with and affection for those who uphold or share our beliefs (or are similar to us) and equally vigorous hostility and disdain for those who challenge or do not share our beliefs (i.e., are different from us). "Worldview defense" is our term for exaggerated evaluations of similar and different others following MS. In a typical study, participants were told we were investigating the relationship between personality attributes and interpersonal judgments. After completing a few standard personality assessments to sustain the cover story, participants in MS conditions were asked to respond to the following open-ended questions: "Please briefly describe the emotions that the thought of your own death arouse in you."; "Jot down, as specifically as you can, what you think will happen to *you* as you physically die." Participants in control conditions in initial studies completed parallel questions about benign topics (e.g., eating a meal or watching television). Afterward, participants rated target individuals who upheld or violated cherished aspects of participants' worldviews.

For example, Greenberg et al. (1990, Study 1) had Christian participants evaluate Christian and Jewish targets (very similar demographically except for religious affiliation) after an MS or control induction. Although there were no differences in evaluation of the targets in the control condition, MS participants reported a greater fondness for the Christian target and more adverse reactions to the Jewish target. An additional study replicated and extended this finding by showing that after an MS induction, American participants increased their affection for a pro-American author and increased their disdain for an anti-American author. Other research showed that MS leads to positive reactions to those who exemplify the values of the worldview and negative reactions to those who violate them (e.g., Mikulincer & Florian, 1997; Rosenblatt, Greenberg, Solomon, Pyszczynski, & Lyon, 1989). This work also demonstrated that MS effects are not the result of anxiety or negative mood; specifically, asking participants to ponder their demise does not typically engender negative affect or self-reported anxiety, and covarying out self-reported mood does not eliminate MS effects. Rosenblatt et al. (1989) also demonstrated that MS effects are not caused by self-awareness or physiological arousal, and that they are quite precisely directed at worldview threatening or bolstering targets (e.g., in Rosenblatt et al., 1989, Study 2, only participants morally opposed to prostitution prescribed a higher bond for an alleged prostitute after an MS induction, but doing so did not adversely affect participants' ratings of the experimenter, which one would predict if MS effects were nonspecific in nature).

Additional research established that MS effects can be obtained using a variety of operationalizations of MS (death anxiety scales [e.g., Rosenblatt et al., 1989, Study 6; Mikulincer & Florian, 1997]; gory automobile accident footage [Nelson, Moore, Olivetti, & Scott, 1997]; proximity to a funeral home [e.g., Pyszczynski et al., 1996]; and subliminal death primes [e.g., Arndt, Greenberg, Pyszczynski, & Solomon, 1997a]) and are quite specific to reminders of death (see Greenberg et al., 1995b; Greenberg, Solomon, & Pyszczynski, 1997, specifically, section titled "What's Death Got to Do With It?", pp. 97–99). Asking participants to ponder their next important exam, cultural values, speaking in public, general anxieties, worries after college, meaninglessness, failure, being paralyzed in a car crash, being socially excluded, and dental pain or physical pain, or making them self-aware, does not produce the same effects engendered by the MS induction.

Behavioral effects of MS have been obtained in addition to the attitudinal effects described previously. For example, Greenberg, Simon, Porteus, Pyszczynski, and Solomon (1995c) found that participants took longer and felt more uncomfortable using cherished cultural icons in a blasphemous fashion (i.e., sifting colored dye through an American flag and using a crucifix as a hammer) after an MS induction. Ochsmann and Mathy (1994) showed that following an MS induction, German participants sat closer to a German confederate and further away from a Turkish confederate. And McGregor et al. (1998) demonstrated that MS increased physical aggression (assessed by the amount of hot sauce administered to a fellow participant known to dislike spicy food in the context of a supposed study of consumer taste preferences) toward those who attack one's political orientation. Recently, Jonas, Greenberg, and Frey (2003) demonstrated that MS leads people to donate more money to charity, particularly charities that benefit one's ingroup.

Theoretically predicted MS effects have been now been found in over 160 published studies. Although this work began in our labs in collaboration with our students, the study of terror management processes is an enterprise now shared among independent researchers in at least 11 different countries (e.g., Canada, Germany, Israel, Italy, Japan, China, Korea, The Netherlands, United Kingdom, and the United States, and in a recent study of Australian Aborigines [Halloran, 2001]), many of whom are contributors to this *Handbook*. Subtle reminders of mortality have been shown to influence a wide range of human thoughts, feelings, and activities, including those concerning national identity (e.g., Castano, Yzerbyt, & Paladino, Chapter 19, this volume), aggression (McGregor et al., 1998), stereotyping (Schimel et al., 1999), creativity and guilt (e.g., Arndt et al., 1999), religion (Jonas & Fischer, 2003), disgust and feelings about sex and the body (Goldenberg, Pyszczynski, McCoy, Greenberg, & Solomon, 1999; Goldenberg & Roberts, Chapter 5, this volume), romantic relationships (Mikulincer, Florian, & Hirshberger, Chapter 18, this volume), psychopathology (Strachan et al., 2003), structuring of the social world (Landau, Johns, et al., in press; also see Dechesne & Kruglanski, Chapter 16, this volume), conformity to norms (e.g., Greenberg et al., 1995c; Jonas et al., 2003), self-structuring (Landau, Johns, et al., in press), art (Landau, Solomon, Greenberg, & Pyszczynski, 2003), and nature (Koole & Van den Berg, Chapter 6, this volume).

Self-Esteem and Mortality Salience

After obtaining independent support for the self-esteem anxiety buffer hypothesis and the MS hypothesis, subsequent research has investigated the relationship between self-esteem and MS. If self-esteem serves to buffer anxiety, then worldview defense following MS should be significantly reduced (or eliminated) in individuals who have high self-esteem (dispositional or situationally induced). This hypothesis was confirmed in a series of studies by Harmon-Jones et al. (1997) and more recently by Arndt and Greenberg (1999). Also consistent with this idea is work showing that other self-esteem–related psychological resources, such as hardiness (Florian, Mikulincer, & Hirschberger, 2001) and secure attachment styles (Mikulincer, Florian, & Hirschberger, 2003) reduce the effects of MS, and that deficits in such resources, such as neuroticism (Goldenberg, Pyszczynski, McCoy, Greenberg, & Solomon, 1999) and depression (Simon, Greenberg, Harmon-Jones, & Solomon, 1996), increase MS effects.

Recently, another central derivative of the general MS hypothesis has been assessed. If self-esteem serves to buffer anxiety associated with the awareness of death, then an MS induction should increase efforts to procure self-esteem. Greenberg, Simon, Pyszczynski, Solomon, and Chatel (1992b) provided preliminary evidence suggesting that mortality salience increases self-esteem striving by demonstrating that MS led liberals, who are committed to the value of tolerance, to respond more favorably to someone who challenged their worldviews. Taubman - Ben-Ari, Florian, and Mikulincer (1999) subsequently provided direct behavioral evidence for this proposition by showing that MS increased risky driving behavior (both self-reports and on a driving simulator) among Israeli soldiers who valued their driving ability as a source of self-esteem. Taubman - Ben-Ari et al. (1999) also hypothesized that after MS, a boost to self-esteem would eliminate the need to demonstrate driving skill through risky driving, and that is precisely what they found.

Another set of studies to establish that MS intensifies self-esteem striving was based on the idea that MS will increase or decrease identification with entities that impinge positively or negatively upon self-esteem. Goldenberg, McCoy, Pyszczynski, Greenberg, and Solomon (2000) showed that MS increased identification with one's body as an important aspect of self among those high in body self-esteem and decreased monitoring of one's physical appearance among those low in body self-esteem who nonetheless put high value on their physical attractiveness. And a series of recent experiments has demonstrated that MS leads people to alter their levels of identification with their own ingroups (gender, ethnic, and school affiliation) to protect and enhance self-esteem (Arndt, Greenberg, & Cook, 2002; Dechesne, Greenberg, Arndt, & Schimel, 2000; Dechesne, Janssen, & van Knippenberg, 2000). MS is also been known to influence a variety of other behaviors likely to bolster self-esteem: Kasser and Sheldon (2000) demonstrated that MS increased participants' desire to amass wealth and possessions; Jonas, Schimel, Greenberg, and Pyszczynski (2002) found that MS increased generosity toward favored charities; Simon et al. (1997b) showed that MS increases perceived social consensus if people are accused of being deviants but decreases perceived social consensus if they are accused of being conformists; Arndt, Schimel, and Goldenberg (2003) established that MS increased fitness intentions for individuals who valued personal fitness; and Peters, Greenberg, Williams, and Scneidr (2003) found that MS increased strength output on a hand dynamometer for individuals who valued physical strength.

Recent research has also shown that MS leads to self-esteem bolstering in the form of a self-serving bias. Specifically, Mikulincer and Florian (2002) found that MS increased the self-serving attributional bias and Dechesne et al. (2003) showed that MS leads to increased belief in the validity of positive information about the self, whether it came from horoscopes or personality tests. Interestingly, in another series of studies, Dechesne et al. (2003) found that convincing individuals that there is scientific evidence of consciousness after death eliminated the tendency of MS to increase these self-serving biases. This provides particularly direct evidence that self-esteem serves to quell concerns about death as the end of existence.

The Psychodynamics of Terror Management

We recently proposed a dual process theory to explicate the nature of the cognitive processes that underlie cultural worldview defense in response to mortality salience (Pyszczynski, Greenberg, & Solomon, 1999, p. 835):

> Distinct defensive responses are activated by thoughts of death that are conscious and those that are on the fringes of consciousness (highly accessible but not in current focal attention). Proximal defenses entail the suppression of death-related thoughts or pushing the problem of death into the distant future by denying one's vulnerability to various risk factors. These defenses are rational, threat-focused, and are activated when thoughts of death are in current conscious attention. Distal terror management defenses entail maintaining self-esteem and faith in one's cultural worldview and serve to control the potential for anxiety resulting from awareness of the inevitability of death. These defenses are experiential, not related to the problem of death in any semantic or rational way, and are increasingly activated as the accessibility of death-related thoughts increases, up to the point at which such thoughts enter consciousness and proximal threat-focused defenses are initiated.

In support of this dual process conception, Greenberg, Simon, Arndt, Pyszczynski, & Solomon (2000) demonstrated that immediately after an MS induction, people engage in proximal defenses (vulnerability-denying defensive distortions) but do not show evidence of distal defense (exaggerated regard and disdain for similar and dissimilar others respectively); as expected, distal defense was obtained after a delay but proximal defenses were not. In addition, defense of the cultural worldview does not occur when mortality is *highly* salient, or when people are forced to keep thoughts of death in consciousness following our typical subtle MS manipulation (Greenberg, Pyszczynski, Solomon, Simon, & Breus, 1994), or when they are asked to behave "rationally" (Simon et al., 1997a). We also showed that the accessibility of death-related thoughts is low immediately following MS as a result of an active suppression of such thoughts, and that a delayed increase in the accessibility of death-related thoughts (presumably from relaxation of the suppression) is responsible for the delayed appearance of cultural worldview defense (Arndt, Greenberg, Solomon, Pyszczynski, & Simon, 1997b). Heightened accessibility of death-related thoughts has been shown to covary with worldview defense following MS (Arndt et al., 1997a; Arndt et al., 1997b), and cultural worldview defense serves to keep levels of death-thought accessibility low (Arndt et al., 1997b; Harmon-Jones et al., 1997). Arndt, Cook, and Routledge (Chapter 3, this volume) provide a detailed overview of this body of work along with some fascinating new developments that have enhanced our understanding of the cognitive processes that underlie terror management phenomena.

Summary of Research on Terror Management Theory

In sum, there is now a substantial empirical literature that unequivocally supports the central tenets of TMT: (1) self-esteem reduces anxiety in response to threatening circumstances; (2) reminders of death engender exaggerated need for the anxiety-buffering properties of cultural worldviews, which is in turn reflected by increased regard for worldview bolstering people and behaviors, as well as increased disdain for worldview threatening people and behaviors; (3) momentarily elevated or dispositionally high self-esteem reduces or eliminates worldview defenses following MS; (4) MS instigates efforts to bolster self-esteem; and (5) MS effects are instigated by heightened accessibility of implicit death thoughts and the function of terror management processes is to reduce the accessibility of such thoughts.

CURRENT ISSUES, FUTURE DIRECTIONS

Although we believe that TMT provides a coherent and comprehensive (although by no means complete) explanation for a very broad range of human social behaviors and has been supported by a wide range of converging studies, many theoretical and empirical issues still remain to be resolved. Here we briefly note some important ongoing concerns.

Where's the Terror?

From the outset of the TMT research program, the reminders of mortality we have employed have failed to generate much affect, whether measured through self-report or through physiological indicators. And although this has troubled certain critics of the theory (e.g., Muraven & Baumeister, 1997), from Rosenblatt et al. (1989) on, we have argued that this not at all problematic for the TMT, because the theory is precisely about how we cope with our knowledge of mortality without perpetual anxiety. But then how does MS intensify worldview defense without arousing anxiety?

Erdelyi's (1974) cognitive analysis of psychological defense provides the basis for an answer. He argued that because the brain is clearly a multistage processing system that involves conscious as well as unconscious monitoring of stimuli, defensive reactions can be instigated by the informational value of stimuli prior to the arousal of affect. If the defense decreases the threat posed by the stimulus, the experience of anxiety can be averted. As we noted in Greenberg et al. (1995b, p. 431):

> . . . reminders of one's mortality signal the potential for experiencing a good deal of distress . . . people avoid the subjective experience of distress by increasing their commitment to the cultural worldview and the pursuit of a positive self-image within the context of this framework.

Recently we found the first direct empirical evidence supporting this assertion. Greenberg et al. (2003) told half of their participants they would be drinking an herbal beverage that blocks anxiety for 1 hour, while the other half were told they would be drinking an herbal beverage that enhances memory. Then, after the typical MS manipulation, the American participants evaluated pro and anti-American essays to assess worldview defense. In support of the role of potential for anxiety in MS effects, MS increased pro-U.S. bias in the memory enhancer condition but not in the anxiety-blocker condition. This study clearly shows that it is the potential to experience affect rather than the actual subjective experience of affect that mediates MS effects.

The Psychodynamics of Terror Management Revisited

As Arndt, Cook, and Routledge (Chapter 3, this volume) make clear, considerable progress has been made in understanding the cognitive processes generating MS effects. However, additional questions remain. One issue concerns the particular ways in which a given individual will bolster terror management defenses after a reminder of mortality. Arndt et al. (2002) recently demonstrated that reminders of mortality increase the spontaneous accessibility of particular aspects of people's worldviews. Further efforts are needed to explore situational and individual difference variables (recent work suggests that both gender and need for structure may be particularly important) that contribute to these effects, and the implications of these effects for the use of particular defenses, for the structure of worldviews and the centrality of particular aspects of worldviews, and for the memory structures that underlie them.

A second fundamental set of questions surrounds the operation of terror management processes independent of recent activation of death-related thoughts, as produced by an induction of MS. Although MS has been a tremendously valuable tool for exploring TMT-based hypotheses, the theory posits that because the knowledge of mortality is always with us, terror management is an ongoing process, even when death is far from consciousness. Thus, from the perspective of the theory, although currently salient reminders of mortality intensify terror management processes, they are not the only factors that initiate it.

TMT was originally designed to explain why people so vigorously defend their self-esteem when it is threatened and why they so often react negatively to different others—behaviors that clearly occur on an ongoing basis in the absence of explicit reminders of mortality. According to the theory, these propensities exist because self-esteem and the cultural worldview serve an ongoing terror management function. Thus threats to either psychological construct should arouse defense even in the absence of an explicit reminder of death. Are such defenses necessarily mediated by increased death accessibility? TMT as originally formulated is mute on this process-level point; however, this is not likely to always be the case.

If a psychological entity serves an important function for the individual, then threats will provoke defense of that entity, but it may not be necessary for thoughts of the underlying function to be brought close to consciousness for this to occur. For example, if a small child tugs at another child's security blanket, the tugged-upon child is likely to lash out and cling harder to the blanket, but probably without thoughts or feelings of insecurity that might occur if the blanket were actually gone. Or an adult male may lash out at someone who scratches his new Lexus, without cognitive mediation by thoughts of how the scratch affects his self-image. In other words, we often defend entities that we care about when these entities are threatened because of the functions they serve (e.g., providing security from other threats), without necessarily having those functions brought to mind. Of course, one can ask, if death-thought accessibility does not always mediate worldview and self-esteem defenses, how can one know whether it is attributable to terror management concerns? Perhaps in any particular instance one cannot, but the logic we have used is that if the defense of these constructs occurs because they serve a terror management function, then bringing to mind that underlying function should intensify defense of that structure, precisely what MS research has shown.

On the other hand, if the threat to the protecting structure is sufficiently strong, or the individual's structures are fragile to begin with, then increased death-thought accessibility is likely to increase and motivate defense. Indeed, research suggests that contemplating loss of a close romantic relationship (Mikulincer, Florian, & Hirschberger, Chapter 18, this volume), a threat of temporal discontinuity (Chaudhary, Tison, & Solomon 2002) and threats of creatureliness, particularly for neurotic individuals (Goldenberg et al., 2000), can increase death-thought acccessibility. Of course, further research is needed to delineate the conditions under which death-thought accessibility does and does not play a role in worldview and self-esteem defense.

Terror Management and Social Connections

Clearly social connections are important to people. From its outset (Greenberg, Pyszczynski, & Solomon, 1986), TMT has emphasized the importance of other people to validate the individual's worldview and self-worth. Thus, we believe TMT provides some important insights into social relationships and group identifications. Although others have posited that people have a gregariousness instinct (McDougall, 1908), or a need to belong (e.g., Maslow, 1968; Baumeister & Leary, 1995), we believe that TMT has significant advantages over theories that simply posit a broad desire for social connections. Even a casual glance at social relations in daily life, or over the course of history, shows that social relationships are quite complex: People do not always want to belong or want social connections, people vary greatly in their sociability, power relations between people differ substantially, and people make very clear distinctions between those whose presence they seek and those whose presence they try to avoid or even stamp out. TMT suggests that understanding an individual's or a group's social relationships requires examining the pertinent worldviews and bases of self-worth of the parties involved.

Although we are skeptical that theories based on a broad need to belong provide much explanatory or heuristic value, we do believe that attachment theory is of great value in understanding social relations in general and terror management in particular. Indeed, Mikulincer, Florian, and colleagues developed an impressive research program highlighting connections between the theories (Mikulincer, Florian, & Hirshberger, 2003; Chapter 18, this volume). Based on this work, they proposed and provided evidence to support their claim that close relationships serve a terror management function independent of their roles in validating the two original components (cultural worldview and self-esteem) of terror management.[4]

Terror Management and Other Motives

Research has established links between TMT and a number of other motivational theories, including dissonance (Jonas et al., 2003), cognitive-experiential self theory (Simon, et al., 1997a), optimal distinctiveness theory (Simon et al., 1997b), social identity theory (e.g., Castano, Yzerbyt, & Paladino, Chapter 19, this volume; Harmon-Jones, Greenberg, & Solomon, 1995), and system justification theory (Jost, Fitzsimons, & Kay, Chapter 17, this volume). Theoretical analyses in need of research have also been offered regarding the relationship between TMT and growth or approach-oriented motivation (e.g., Greenberg, Pyszczynski, & Solomon, 1995a; Pyszczynski, Greenberg, Solomon, Arndt, & Schimel, in press). As Florian and Mikulincer (Chapter 4, this volume) argue, death is a complex phenomenon, and so additional connections are quite likely.

One recent development has been work on how people cope with another basic existential reality, uncertainty in life (see, e.g., McGregor, Zanna, Holmes, & Spencer, 2001, McGregor, Chapter 12, this volume; Van den Bos, 2001, Chapter 11, this volume). These theorists have proposed and provided some evidence suggesting that death-related concerns and MS effects may have to do with the uncertainties death arouses. However, it seems unlikely to us that the primary threat of reminders of the certain inevitability of something that threatens to eliminate an organism's existence is its contribution to uncertainty (we also believe it is unlikely an uncertainty-based explanation can account for the empirical work noted previously examining conditions that increase or decrease death-thought accessibility, and the latter's role in worldview defense). Would death be any less frightening if you knew for sure that it would come next Tuesday at 5:15 P.M., and that your hopes for an afterlife are illusory?[5]

Practical Implications of Terror Management Theory

Becker (1971, 1973, 1975) struggled with the practical implications of his analysis in the final chapters of each of his last three books. Terror management, although perhaps necessary, is neither inherently bad nor inherently good; it depends on the values of the individual's worldview and the paths to self-esteem it prescribes. As we have proposed elsewhere (e.g., Pyszczynski, Solomon, & Greenberg, 2003; Solomon, Greenberg, & Pyszczynski, 1991b), TMT implies that worldviews can be evaluated based on the extent to which they offer compelling meaning and widely attainable bases of self-worth with minimal costs to individuals both within and outside the culture. We argue that the best worldviews are ones that value tolerance of different others, that are flexible and open to modifications, and that offer paths to self-esteem minimally likely to encourage hurting others. Rigid, fundamentalist worldviews, whether Christian, Islamic, fascist, communist, religious, or secular, are model opposites of such ideals. Similarly, for people having problems functioning in their lives, TMT suggests we should look to ways in which their worldviews and strivings for self-worth are not working for them and seek ways that they could construct more compelling and attainable versions of these psychological resources.

In addition to better bases of terror management, perhaps there are ways to get beyond the need for terror management at all, to fully face mortality and vitiate the need for defense. In fact, Janof-Bulman and Yopyk (Chapter 8, this volume) and Martin, Campbell, and Henry (Chapter 27, this volume) discuss theory and evidence regarding the possibility that serious confrontations with mortality can have positive, liberating effects, facilitating real growth and life satisfaction (see also Yalom, 1980). Research is needed to better understand these hopeful possibilities and the individual predispositions and conditions under which these effects, rather than intensified defensiveness, are likely to occur.

CONCLUSION

> Our ability, unlike the other animals, to conceptualize our own end creates tremendous psychic strains within us; whether we like to admit it or not, in each man's chest a tiny ferret of fear at this ultimate knowledge gnaws away at his ego and his sense of purpose. We're fortunate, in a way, that our body, and the fulfillment of its needs and functions, plays such an imperative role in our lives; this physical shell creates a buffer between us and the mind-paralyzing realization that only a few years of existence separate birth from death. . . . The most terrifying fact about the universe is not that it is hostile but that it is indifferent; but if we can come to terms with this indifference and accept the challenges of life within the boundaries of death—however mutable man may be able to make them—our existence as a species can have genuine meaning.
> —STANLEY KUBRICK, interview in *Playboy Magazine* (1968;
> cited in Phillips, 2001, pp. 72–73)

Terror management theory proposes that the uniquely human awareness of mortality is a ubiquitous concern that plays an important role in virtually all forms of human behavior and underlies the development and maintenance of culture and self-esteem as the primary means by which the fear of death is ameliorated. Although existential psychodynamic accounts of human behavior have historically been repudiated by academic psychologists on the grounds that they cannot be empirically tested, TMT stands in stark contradistinction to this claim. A substantial body of empirical evidence now supports the basic tenets of TMT. TMT has attracted the interest and engaged the efforts of scholars in a variety of disciplines throughout the world and has generated research on a range of topics far beyond the original scope of the theory. We are gratified by the cumulative progress to date and excited about the provocative prospects ahead, as exploration of the psychological consequences of the uniquely human dilemma continues.

ACKNOWLEDGMENT

The authors share equal responsibility for this work, which was generously supported by grants from the National Science Foundation and the Ernest Becker Foundation.

NOTES

1. Subsequent to the original formulation of TMT in Greenberg et al. (1986), prominent theorists from a number of disciplines have also argued that a theoretical account of culture—humanly created and transmitted beliefs about the nature of reality manifested through uniquely human institutions such as religion, art, and science—is a central problem in the study of mind (see, e.g., Mithen, 1996; Pinker, 1997; Tooby & Cosmides, 1992; Wilson, 1998).

2. Sadly, homosexuals in the United States often suffer the same fate. For example, in 1998, Aaron McKinney and Russell Henderson lured University of Wyoming student Matthew Shepard from a Laramie bar, lashed him to a fence, bludgeoned his head with a gun, and left him to die because he was gay.

3. Some critics of TMT (see, e.g., Batson & Stocks, Chapter 9, this volume) have objected to our reference to an overarching drive or instinct for self-preservation. Indeed, TMT is sometimes dismissed in an *a priori* fashion (e.g., Buss, 1997; Pelham, 1997) by claims that the theory must be wrong because of our "antiquated" view of evolution as serving individuals (via a problematic self-preservation instinct) rather than genes, and because we fail to posit domain-specific reactions to particular adaptive challenges as demanded by the canonical formulations of modern evolutionary theory (e.g., Tooby & Cosmides, 1992). As we pointed out in Solomon, Greenberg, and Pyszczynski (1991a), the central tenets of TMT remain unchanged regardless of where one stands on the issue of the appropriate unit of selection (genes, individuals, and/or groups) for natural selection and/or the status of a "self-preservation instinct." In addition, it should be noted that the notion that all evolutionary adaptations must be domain-specific responses to specific selection pressures has fallen on hard times of late on theoretical and empirical grounds (e.g., Karmiloff-Smith, 1992; Mithen, 1996). We agree with these and other like-minded theorists who argue that some important and uniquely human evolutionary adaptations are general in character in that they that operate across multiple domains that are completely encapsulated and thus precluded from influencing each other in higher primates.

4. Mikulincer et al.'s proposed revision of TMT may very well be right, but we believe further confirmation is required to definitively determine if this is the case. Although the evidence of a terror management role of close relationships is extensive and compelling, we are not yet completely convinced that self-esteem concerns have been entirely ruled out in the empirical work as the underlying factor.

5. Clearly, the relationship between death and uncertainty warrants continued conceptual consideration and empirical investigation. Along the latter lines, two recent studies found that one of McGregor et al.'s (2001) uncertainty inductions (temporal discontinuity) increases death-thought accessibility (Chaudhary et al., 2002) and other recent studies have shown that Van den Bos's (2001) uncertainty induction has different effects than MS (Landau, Solomon, Greenberg, & Pyszczynski, 2003; Martens, Greenberg, & Schimel, 2003).

REFERENCES

Arndt, J., & Greenberg, J. (1999). The effects of a self-esteem boost and mortality salience on responses to boost relevant and irrelevant worldview threats. *Personality and Social Psychology Bulletin, 25,* 1331–1341.

Arndt, J., Greenberg, J., & Cook, A. (2002). Mortality salience and the spreading activation of worldview-relevant constructs: Exploring the cognitive architecture of terror. *Journal of Experimental Psychology: General, 131,* 307–324.

Arndt, J., Greenberg, J., Pyszczynski, T., & Solomon, S. (1997a). Subliminal presentation of death reminders leads to increased defense of the cultural worldview. *Psychological Science, 8,* 379–385.

Arndt, J., Greenberg, J., Solomon, S., Pyszczynski, T., Schimel, J., & Nerham, N. (1999). Creativity and terror management: The effects of creative activity on guilt and social projection following mortality salience. *Journal of Personality and Social Psychology, 77,* 19–32.

Arndt, J., Greenberg, J., Solomon, S., Pyszczynski, T., & Simon, L. (1997b). Suppression, accessibility of death-related thoughts, and cultural worldview defense: Exploring the psychodynamics of terror management. *Journal of Personality and Social Psychology, 73,* 5–18.

Arndt, J., Schimel, J., & Goldenberg, J. L. (2003). Death can be good for your health: Fitness intentions as a proximal and distal defense against mortality salience. *Journal of Applied Social Psychology, 33,* 1726–1746.

Aronson, E. (1972). *The social animal.* San Francisco, CA: Freeman.

Baumeister, R. F., & Leary, M. R. (1995). The need to belong: Desire for interpersonal attachments as a fundamental human motivation. *Psychological Bulletin, 117,* 497–529.

Becker, E. (1962). *The birth and death of meaning.* New York: Free Press.

Becker, E. (1967). *Beyond alienation: A philosophy of education for the crisis of democracy.* New York: George Braziller.

Becker, E. (1968). *The structure of evil.* New York: George Braziller.

Becker, E. (1969). *Angel in armor.* New York: Free Press.

Becker, E. (1971). *The birth and death of meaning: An interdisciplinary perspective on the problem of man* (2nd ed.). New York: Free Press.

Becker, E. (1973). *The denial of death.* New York: Free Press.

Becker, E. (1975). *Escape from evil.* New York: Free Press.

Bowlby, J. (1969). *Attachment and loss: Vol 1. Attachment.* New York: Basic Books.

Buss, D. M. (1997). Human social motivation in evolutionary perspective: Grounding terror management theory. *Psychological Inquiry, 8,* 22–25.

Chaudary, N., Tison, J., & Solomon, S. (2002). *What's death got to do with it?: The role of psychological uncertainty on implicit death thoughts.* Paper presented at the annual meeting of the American Psychological Society, New Orleans.

Deacon, T. (1997). *The symbolic species: The co-evolution of language and the brain.* New York: Norton.

Dechesne, M., Greenberg, J., Arndt, J., & Schimel, J. (2000). Terror management and the vicissitudes of sports fan affiliation: The effects of mortality salience on optimism and fan identification. *European Journal of Social Psychology, 30,* 813–835.

Dechesne, M., Janssen, J., van Knippenberg, A. (2000). Derogation and distancing as terror management strategies: The moderating role of need for closure and permeability of group boundaries. *Journal of Personality and Social Psychology, 79,* 923–932.

Dechesne, M., Pyszczynski, T., Arndt, J., Ransom, S., Sheldon, K., van Knippenberg, A., & Janssen, J. (2003). Literal and symbolic immortality: The effect of evidence of literal immortality on self-esteem striving in response to mortality salience. *Journal of Personality and Social Psychology, 84,* 722–737.

Donald, M. (1991). *Origins of the modern mind: Three stages in the evolution of culture and cognition.* Cambridge, MA: Harvard University Press.

Eckholm, E. (2001, December 26). Taliban justice: Stadium was scene of gory punishment. *New York Times,* p. B1.

Erdelyi, M. H. (1974). A new look at the new look: Perceptual defense and vigilance. *Psychological Review, 81,* 1–25.

Festinger, L. (1954). A theory of social comparison processes. *Human Relationships, 1,* 117–140.

Festinger, L. (1980). Looking backward. In L. Festinger (Ed.) *Retrospectives on social psychology* (pp. 247–254). London: Oxford University Press.

Florian, V., Mikulincer, M., & Hirschberger, G. (2001). An existentialist view on mortality salience effects: Personal hardiness, death-thought accessibility, and cultural worldview defense. *British Journal of Social Psychology, 40,* 437–453.

Goldenberg, J., McCoy, S. K., Pyszczynski, T., Greenberg, J., & Solomon, S. (2000). The body as a source of self-esteem: The effect of mortality salience on identification with one's body, interest in sex, and appearance monitoring. *Journal of Personality and Social Psychology, 79,* 118–130

Goldenberg, J. L., Pyszczynski, T. McCoy, S. K., Greenberg, J., & Solomon, S. (1999). Death, sex, and neuroticism: Why is sex such a problem? *Journal of Personality and Social Psychology, 77,* 1173–1187.

Goldschimidt, W. R. (1990). *The human career: The self in the symbolic world*. New York: Blackwell.

Gould, S. J. (2002). *The structure of evolutionary theory*. Cambridge, MA: Belknap Press of Harvard University Press.

Greenberg, J., Arndt, J., Simon, L., Pyszczynski, T., & Solomon, S. (2000). Proximal and distal defenses in response to reminders of one's mortality: Evidence of a temporal sequence. *Personality and Social Psychology Bulletin, 26,* 91–99.

Greenberg, J., Martens, A., Jonas, E., Eisenstadt, D., Pyszczynski, T., & Solomon, S. (2003). Psychological defense in anticipation of anxiety: Eliminating the potential for anxiety eliminates the effect of mortality salience on worldview defense. *Psychological Science, 14,* 516–519.

Greenberg, J., Pyszczynski, T., & Solomon, S. (1995a). Toward a dual motive depth psychology of self and social behavior. In M. Kernis (Ed.) *Self, efficacy, and agency*. New York: Plenum Press.

Greenberg, J., Pyszczynski, T., & Solomon, S. (1986). The causes and consequences of a need for self-esteem: A terror management theory. In R. F. Baumeister (Ed.), *Public self and private self* (pp. 189–212). New York: Springer-Verlag.

Greenberg, J., Pyszczynski, T., Solomon, S., Pinel, E., Simon, L., & Jordan, K. (1993). Effects of self-esteem on vulnerability-denying defensive distortions: Further evidence of an anxiety-buffering function of self-esteem. *Journal of Experimental Social Psychology, 29,* 229–251.

Greenberg, J., Pyszczynski, T., Solomon, S., Rosenblatt, A., Veeder, M., Kirkland, S., & Lyon, D. (1990). Evidence for terror management theory II: The effects of mortality salience on reactions to those who threaten or bolster the cultural worldview. *Journal of Personality and Social Psychology, 58,* 308–318.

Greenberg, J., Pyszczynski, T., Solomon, S., Simon, L., & Breus, M. (1994). Role of consciousness and accessibility of death-related thoughts in mortality salience effects. *Journal of Personality and Social Psychology, 67,* 627–637.

Greenberg, J., Simon, L., Harmon-Jones, E., Solomon, S., Pyszczynski, T., & Lyon, D. (1995b). Testing alternative explanations for mortality salience effects: Terror management, value accessibility, or worrisome thoughts? *European Journal of Social Psychology, 25,* 417–433.

Greenberg, J., Simon, L., Porteus, J., Pyszczynski, T., & Solomon, S. (1995c). Evidence of a terror management function of cultural icons: The effects of mortality salience on the inappropriate use of cherished cultural symbols. *Personality and Social Psychology Bulletin, 21,* 1221–1228.

Greenberg, J., Simon, L., Pyszczynski, T., Solomon, S., & Chatel, D. (1992b). Terror management and tolerance: Does mortality salience always intensify negative reactions to others who threaten one's worldview? *Journal of Personality and Social Psychology, 63,* 212–220.

Greenberg, J., Solomon, S., & Pyszczynski, T. (1997). Terror management theory of self-esteem and cultural worldviews: Empirical assessments and conceptual refinements. In Mark Zanna (Ed.), *Advances in experimental social psychology* (Vol. 29, pp. 61–139), Orlando, FL: Academic Press.

Greenberg, J., Solomon, S., Pyszczynski, T., Rosenblatt, A., Burling, J., Lyon, D., & Simon, L. (1992a). Assessing the terror management analysis of self-esteem: Converging evidence of an anxiety-buffering function. *Journal of Personality and Social Psychology, 63,* 913–922.

Greenberg, J., Solomon, S., Pyszczynski, T., & Steinberg, L. (1988). A reaction to Greenwald, Pratkanis, Leippe, and Baumgardner (1986): Under what conditions does research obstruct theory progress? *Psychological Review, 95,* 566–571.

Halloran, M. (2001). *Cultural validation and social context: The effect of mortality salience on endorsement of the multiple worldviews of Aboriginal and Anglo-Australians in contexts defined by social identities*. Paper presented at the First International Conference on Experimental Existential Psychology: Finding Meaning in the Human Condition. Free University, Amsterdam, The Netherlands.

Harmon-Jones, E., Greenberg, J., & Solomon, S. (1995). The effects of mortality salience on intergroup discrimination in a minimal-group paradigm. *European Journal of Social Psychology, 25,* 781–785.

Harmon-Jones, E., Simon, L., Greenberg, J., Pyszczynski, T., Solomon, S., & McGregor, H. (1997). Terror management theory and self-esteem: Evidence that increased self-esteem reduces mortality salience effects. *Journal of Personality and Social Psychology, 72,* 24–36.

Herdt, G. (1982). *Rituals of manhood*. Berkeley: University of California Press.

Humphrey, N. (1984). *Consciousness regained*. Oxford, UK: Oxford University Press.

James, W. (1890). *Principles of psychology*. New York: Henry Holt.

Jaynes, J. (1976). *The origin of consciousness in the breakdown of the bicameral mind*. Boston: Houghton Mifflin.

Jonas, E., & Fischer, P. (2003). *Terror management and religion—Do religious beliefs prevent worldview defense following mortality salience?* Unpublished manuscript, Ludwig-Maximilians-Universität, München, Germany.

Jonas, E., Greenberg, J., & Frey, D. (2003). Connecting terror management and dissonance theories: Evidence that mortality salience increases the preference for supportive information after decisions. *Personality and Social Psychology Bulletin, 9,* 1181–1189.

Jonas, E., Schimel, J., Greenberg, J., & Pyszczynski, T. (2002). The Scrooge effect: Evidence that mortality salience increases prosocial attitudes and behavior. *Personality and Social Psychology Bulletin, 28,* p. 1342–1353.

Karmiloff-Smith, A. (1992). *Beyond modularity*. Cambridge, MA: MIT Press.

Kasser, T., & Sheldon, K. M. (2000). Of wealth and death: Materialism, mortality salience, and consumption behavior. *Psychological Science, 11,* 348–351.

Kierkegaard, S. (1957). *The concept of dread* (W. Lowrie, Trans.). Princeton, NJ: Princeton University Press. (Original work published 1844)

Kingdon, J. (2003). *Lowly origin: Where, when and why our ancestors first stood up*. Princeton, NJ: Princeton University Press.

Landau, M. J., Johns, M., Greenberg, J., Pyszczynski, T., Goldenberg, J., & Solomon, S. (in press). A function of form: Terror management and structuring the social world. *Journal of Personality and Social Psychology*.

Landau, M. J., Solomon, S., Greenberg, J., & Pyszczynski, T. (2003). *Death, art, meaning, and structure*. Unpublished manuscript, University of Arizona.

Lifton, R. J. (1979). *The broken connection: On death and continuity of life*. New York: Simon and Schuster.

Martens, A., Greenberg, J., & Schimel, J. (2003). *Distancing form the elderly in response to mortality salience*. Unpublished manuscript, University of Arizona.

Maslow, A. (1968). *Toward a psychology of being*. New York: Van Nostrand.

McDougall, W. (1908). *Introduction to social psychology*. London: Methuen.

McGregor, H. A., Lieberman, J. D., Greenberg, J., Solomon, S., Simon, L., Arndt, J., & Pyszczynski, T. (1998). Terror management and aggression: Evidence that mortality salience motivates aggression against worldview-threatening others. *Journal of Personality and Social Psychology, 74,* 590–605.

McGregor, I., Zanna, M. P., Holmes, J. G., & Spencer, S. J., (2001). Compensatory conviction in the face of personal uncertainty: Going to extremes and being oneself. *Journal of Personality and Social Psychology, 80,* 472–488.

Mikulincer, M., & Florian, V. (1997). Fear of death and the judgment of social transgressions: A multidimensional test of terror management theory. *Journal of Personality and Social Psychology, 73,* 369–380.

Mikulincer, M., & Florian, V. (2002). The effects of mortality salience on self-serving attributions—Evidence for the function of self-esteem as a terror management mechanism. *Basic and Applied Social Psychology, 24,* 261–271.

Mikulincer, M., Florian, V., & Hirschberger, G. (2003). The existential function of close relationships: Introducing death into the science of love. *Personality and Social Psychology Review, 7,* 20–40.

Mithen, S. (1996). *The prehistory of the mind: The cognitive origins of art, religion and science*. London: Thames and Hudson.

Muraven, M., & Baumeister, R. F. (1997). Suicide, sex, terror, paralysis, and other pitfalls of reductionist self-preservation theory. *Psychological Inquiry, 8,* 36–39.

Nelson, L. J., Moore, D. L., Olivetti, J., & Scott, T. (1997). General and personal mortality salience and nationalistic bias. *Personality and Social Psychology Bulletin, 23,* 884–892.

Ochsmann, R., & Mathy, M. (1994). *Depreciating of and distancing from foreigners: Effects of mortality salience*. Unpublished manuscript, Universität Mainz, Mainz, Germany.

Ortiz, A. (1991). Origins: Through Tewa eyes. *National Geographic, 180,* 4–13.

Panati, C. (1996). *Sacred origins of profound things: The stories behind the rites and rituals of the world's religions.* New York: Penguin Books.

Pelham, B. W. (1997). Human motivation has multiple roots. *Psychological Inquiry, 8,* 44–47.

Peters, H. J., Greenberg, J., Williams, J., & Scneidr, N. R. (2003). *Applying terror management theory to performance: Can reminding individuals of their mortality increase strength output?* Unpublished manuscript, University of Arizona.

Phillips, G. D. (Ed.). (2001). *Stanley Kubrick: Interviews.* Jackson, MS: University Press of Mississippi.

Pinker, S. (1997). *How the mind works.* New York: Norton.

Pyszczynski, T., Greenberg, J., & Solomon, S. (1999). A dual process model of defense against conscious and unconscious death-related thoughts: An extension of terror management theory. *Psychological Review, 106,* 835–845.

Pyszczynski, T., Greenberg, J., & Solomon, S., Arndt, J., & Schimel, J. (in press). Why do people need self-esteem? A theoretical and empirical review. *Psychological Bulletin.*

Pyszczynski, T., Solomon, S., & Greenberg, J. (2003). *In the wake of 9/11: The psychology of terror.* Washington, DC: American Psychological Association.

Pyszczynski, T., Wicklund, R., Floresku, S., Gauch, G., Koch, H., Solomon, S., & Greenberg, J. (1996). Whistling in the dark: Exaggerated consensus estimates in response to incidental reminders of mortality. *Psychological Science, 7,* 332–336.

Rank, O. (1958). *Beyond psychology.* New York: Dover Books. (Original work published 1941)

Roheim, G. (1943). *The origin and function of culture* (Nervous and Mental Disease Monograph No. 69.) New York: Nervous and Mental Disease Monographs.

Rosenblatt, A., Greenberg, J., Solomon, S., Pyszczynski, T., & Lyon, D. (1989). Evidence for terror management theory. I: The effects of mortality salience on reactions to those who violate or uphold cultural values. *Journal of Personality and Social Psychology, 57,* 681–690.

Seneca. (1951). On the shortness of life. In J. W. Basore (Trans.), *Moral essays* (Vol. II). Cambridge, MA: Harvard University Press. (Original work published AD 49)

Schimel, J., Simon, L., Greenberg, J., Pyszczynski, T., Solomon, S., Waxmonsky, J., & Arndt, J. (1999). Stereotypes and terror management: Evidence that mortality salience enhances stereotypic thinking and preferences. *Journal of Personality and Social Psychology, 77,* 905–926.

Simon, L., Greenberg, J., Arndt, J., Pyszczynski, T., Clement, R., & Solomon, S. (1997b). Perceived consensus, uniqueness, and terror management: Compensatory responses to threats to inclusion and distinctiveness following mortality salience. *Personality and Social Psychology Bulletin, 23,* 1055–1065.

Simon, L., Greenberg, J., Harmon-Jones, E., & Solomon, S. (1996). Mild depression, mortality salience, and defense of the worldview: Evidence of intensified terror management in the mildly depressed. *Personality and Social Psychology Bulletin, 22,* 81–90.

Simon, L., Greenberg, J., Harmon-Jones, E., Solomon, S., Pyszczynski, T., Arndt, J., & Abend, T. (1997a). Terror management and cognitive-experiential self-theory: Evidence that terror management occurs in the experiential system. *Journal of Personality and Social Psychology, 72,* 1132–1146.

Solomon, S., Greenberg, J., & Pyszczynski, T. (1991a). A terror management theory of social behavior: The psychological functions of self-esteem and cultural worldviews. In M. Zanna (Ed.), *Advances in experimental social psychology* (Vol. 24, pp. 91–159). Orlando, FL: Academic Press.

Solomon, S., Greenberg, J., & Pyszczynski, T. (1991b). A terror management theory of self-esteem. In C. R. Snyder & D. Forsyth (Eds.), *Handbook of social and clinical psychology: The health perspective* (pp. 21–40). New York: Pergamon Press.

Solomon, S., Greenberg, J., Schimel, J., Arndt, J., & Pyszczynski, T. (2003). Human awareness of death and the evolution of culture. In M. Schaller & C. Crandal (Eds.), *The psychological foundations of culture.* Mahwah, NJ: Erlbaum.

Strachan, E. D., Schimel, J., Greenberg, J., Solomon, S., Pyszczynski, T., & Arndt, J. (2003). *The effects of mortality salience on fear reactions in spider phobia and compulsive behavior: Terror mismanagement.* Manuscript under review.

Sullivan, H. S. (1953). *The interpersonal theory of psychiatry.* New York: Norton.

Taubman - Ben-Ari, O., Florian, V., & Mikulincer, M. (1999). The impact of mortality salience on reckless driving: A test of terror management mechanisms. *Journal of Personality and Social Psychology, 76,* 35–45.

Tooby, J., & Cosmides, L. (1992). The psychological foundations of culture. In J. H. Barkow, L. Cosmides, & J. Tooby (Eds.), *The adapted mind.* New York: Oxford University Press.

Van den Bos, K., (2001). Uncertainty management: The influence of uncertainty salience on reactions to perceived procedural fairness. *Journal of Personality and Social Psychology 80,* 931–941.

Yalom, I. (1980). *Existential psychotherapy.* New York: Basic Books

Wilson, E. O. (1998). *Conscilience: The unity of knowledge.* New York: Knopf.

Chapter 3

The Blueprint of Terror Management

Understanding the Cognitive Architecture of Psychological Defense against the Awareness of Death

JAMIE ARNDT
ALISON COOK
CLAY ROUTLEDGE

One of the core issues of existential psychology has long been how the human organism fashions a world of meaning in a reality of inevitable despair. As Otto Rank, Ernest Becker, Norman Brown, and many others have articulated, it is the despair of inevitable mortality that poses a unique psychological problem for a species with a biological proclivity for self-preservation. Terror management theory (TMT; see Solomon, Greenberg, & Pyszczynski, Chapter 2, this volume) advances an explanation of how people manage the concerns that the awareness of death engenders. Whereas Solomon et al. (Chapter 2, this volume) revealed the breadth and roots of the theory, here we focus the lens to elucidate the cognitive processes by which conscious and unconscious awareness of death influence human social behavior.

The juxtaposition of cognitive and existential perspectives may in some ways seem to be the proverbial odd couple of psychological theorizing. However, owing in part to the recognition that cognitive and motivational accounts of social phenomena often represent different but complementary levels of analysis, and to the recent mainstream acceptance of unconscious processes, it is now possible to articulate an understanding of the cognitive dynamics through which existential motivations influence human social behavior. We begin with a very brief overview of TMT and research and then consider a developmental perspective of how the awareness of death and the consequent investment in a world of symbolic meaning weave themselves into the human cognitive landscape. Finally, the majority of the chapter is then devoted to reviewing different directions of research that culminate in a model of the cognitive architecture of terror management processes.

A COGNITIVE PERSPECTIVE ON TERROR MANAGEMENT THEORY

Terror Management Theory and Research on Cultural Worldview Defense

Because TMT (Greenberg, Pyszczynski, & Solomon, 1986) and its main hypotheses are covered in Chapter 2, we offer only a brief refresher here. The theory builds from a tradition of existential and psychodynamic perspectives (e.g., Becker, 1973) to posit the uniquely human capacity to be aware of the inevitability of one's mortality is juxtaposed with biological instincts aimed at self-preservation, and creates the potential for extreme anxiety or terror. Consider, moreover, that the profound developmental immaturity of the human infant—a twitching blob of protoplasm incapable of even rolling over by itself let alone ordering an espresso—further exposes an unparalleled capacity for anxiety. The human situation only becomes more precarious as the child comes to grapple with the ability to think temporally and self-reflectively. Most important from the perspective of TMT, the child becomes aware of his or her own inevitable mortality.

People, however, are usually not plagued by the anxiety this awareness might be expected to engender. This of course makes a good deal of sense given our relatively productive functioning. We have after all been able to overcome anxiety to invent Slinkies, rubber-band balls, and Shoe-goo. The original articulation of TMT focused on how people manage the unconscious resonance of death-related thought by identifying with cultural beliefs and ideologies (cultural worldviews) that prescribe not only a meaningful and enduring conception of reality but also avenues through which the individual can obtain and maintain a sense of self-esteem within that meaning system (Solomon, Greenberg, & Pyszczynski, 1991).

In support of this initial reasoning, over 150 studies to date have found that after being primed with thoughts of their mortality (mortality salience; MS), participants show enhanced favorability to that which validates their worldview and increased negativity toward that which threatens it (worldview defense). As but a few examples, these responses include reactions to those who transgress legal or cultural morals, one's patriotic identification, as well as a range of social affiliations (see Greenberg, Solomon, & Pyszczynski, 1997). Interestingly, reminders of death produce these effects on social judgment and behavior without creating, or being mediated by, self-reported negative affect, or even subtle physiological signs of anxiety (e.g., skin conductance, Rosenblatt, Greenberg, Solomon, Pyszczynski, & Lyon, 1989; facial electromyography, Arndt, Allen, & Greenberg, 2001). How then do reminders of death lead to such trenchant investment in symbolic conceptions of meaning if not by evoking feelings of fear and anxiety? Although the (null) findings regarding affect are quite consistent with even the earliest articulations of the theory (Solomon et al., 1991; but see also Greenberg et al., 2003), it was in part in response to this question that research began to look for answers using contemporary methods from cognitive psychology (Pyszczynski, Greenberg, & Solomon, 1999).

Integrating Existential and Cognitive Perspectives

Although the notion of a cognitive existential perspective may sound as strange as a garlic-flavored gummy bear, juxtaposing the two has yielded provocative insights. Considered broadly, cognitive psychology developed with a focus on understanding the mental structures and strategies involved with human thinking and processing of information. Soon after the cognitive revolution in psychology began to pick up steam in the late 1950s, social psychologists recognized that a number of its information processing constructs could be of tremendous value in understanding human social behavior (Kunda, 1999). Over the years, researchers have therefore adopted many of the methods developed in cognitive science research to illuminate the nature and processes involved with human social inference and interaction. Recently, terror management researchers have extended and applied these methods in the service of unveiling the mechanics of people's existential experience.

One of the most notable contributions of cognitive psychology for ultimately understanding existential processes was the conceptualization of mental representations as linked via associative networks (e.g., Collins & Loftus, 1975), with such connections often forming and being manifested outside conscious awareness (see, e.g., Bargh, 1996; Kihlstrom, 1987). Although there are important differences in the specific models that have been proposed over the years, the basic premise is that through any number of both conscious and unconscious means (e.g., conditioning, learning, and semantic relatedness), information is stored in the mind within a web of connected ideas or cognitions. What follows is that certain ideas can activate—or prime—other ideas, heightening their availability in working memory and their consequent influence on information processing (e.g., mentioning hunger may lead one to perceive a triangle as a piece of pizza). To the extent that one can consider existential processes at this cognitive level of analysis, a framework can be adapted to understand how it is that thoughts of death would lead to the powerful effects that they do. As we will see, the instantiation and operation of an associated network of defense surrounding thoughts of death can operate both similarly and quite a bit differently than many other types of information processing.

The Association between Unconscious Terror and Symbolic Value

The abstractions of meaning and value by which people manage unconscious death-related fear are introduced to the child through the process of socialization. From the beginning of the child's life, the parents provide the sustenance, warmth, and comfort that are critical for the child's survival. Thus, the love and protection of the apparently omnipotent parents provide the essential feelings of security to the child. But as the child grows, this love and protection become more and more dependent on the child's meeting the parental standards of goodness. This then establishes a critical foundation whereby the child learns the connection between the amelioration of anxiety and the sense of value derived from a symbolic world.

Eventually, however, children learn that their parents are incapable of ultimately protecting them from the many forces and realities that threaten their existence. The child realizes, for example, that maybe his or her father is not stronger than Superman, is likely not as good a baseball player as Barry Bonds, or can't save the goldfish from its fate of being flushed down the toilet. Concurrently, as the awareness of death crystallizes into an undeniable inevitability, the basis of security and meaning is transferred to the culture, and also broadened to include a range of personally meaningful social affiliations. Yet, as Led Zeppelin reminds us, "the song remains the same." The association between death-related cognitive constructs and symbolic value only now operates on a grander stage. In both cases, a link is forged between thoughts of death and the thoughts that are indicative of meaning and value. As spreading activation models in cognitive psychology explain (e.g., McNamara, 1992), such repeated pairing forms the basis for, and strengthens the associations between, different cognitive elements. Knowledge of one's mortality thus comes to occupy a prominent and deeply rooted position within a larger network of knowledge structures that function as self-protective beliefs. The question then becomes, How does this death-related network operate?

THE ARCHITECTURE OF DUAL DEFENSES
AGAINST DEATH-RELATED THOUGHT

Based on accumulating research, the processes of psychological defense within the death-related network are hypothesized to unfold as depicted in Figure 3.1. In brief, because of its motivational importance, knowledge of mortality is considered a central construct in people's cognitive networks that can be activated by a variety of situations. This activation, building from the notion of dual-process models that have become widespread in cognitive and social cognition research, is then thought to progress through two systems of defense.

Although there are a number of variations, dual-process models tend to share the view that people can process information in ways that reflect logically based deliberations, or more intuitive and experiential reactions (Chaiken & Trope, 1999; Epstein, 1994). In the present context, when conscious, thoughts of death are posited to instigate proximal or direct defenses: relatively rational strategies that minimize threat and ultimately facilitate the removal of death-related thoughts from current focal attention. This then results in initially low levels of death-thought accessibility, or how much death remains in a person's focal attention. When the accessibility of death thoughts later increases outside awareness, the symbolic system is engaged and activates beliefs that serve the self-protective goal of imbuing the world with a sense of meaning and value. With the elevated accessibility of these beliefs, unconscious death thoughts trigger distal or symbolic defenses—experiential, indirect strategies to bolster faith in the cultural worldview. Consistent with this reasoning, studies show that symbolic worldview investments (e.g., prejudice toward those who disparage one's central beliefs) found after MS do not occur when participants are induced to process information in a rational mode but are quite robust when participants are induced to process information in a more experiential, intuitive manner (Simon et al., 1997).

Beyond the mechanisms through which these different classes of defense manifest themselves, this model also integrates cognitive and existential insights by specifying a critical function that symbolic defenses serve for the individual. Specifically, the successful engagement of symbolic defenses then restores relative psychological equanimity in part by reducing the heightened accessibility of death-related thoughts that instigated the response. In the sections that follow, we review the research that has both tested and led to each facet of this model.

The Provocation of Death-Related Thought

Facing the initial challenge of how to operationalize reminders of mortality, Rosenblatt et al. (1989) devised the MS questionnaire; two open-ended questions in response to which people write about the thoughts associated with their own death (see also Solomon et al., Chap-

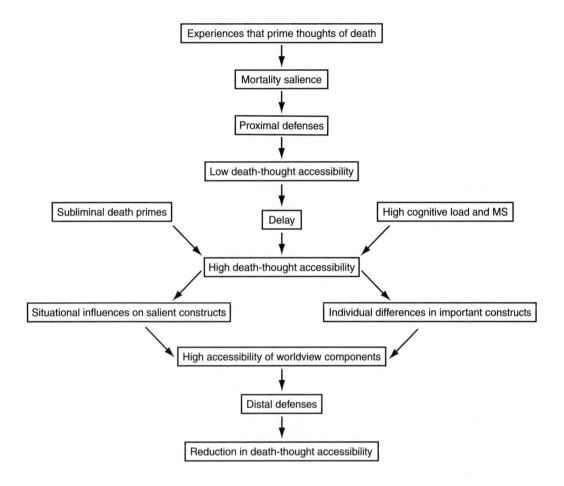

FIGURE 3.1. The cognitive architecture of terror management.

ter 2, this volume). However, similar to other associative models, other stimuli may also function to activate death-related cognition. The array of alternative operationalizations of MS in TMT research (e.g., viewing fatal accident footage; Nelson, Moore, Olivetti, & Scott, 1997) attests in part to the multitude of ways this can occur. Moreover, because of death's motivational significance, activation of death thoughts has been hypothesized to occur in response to unconscious and also very subtle reminders of death, to emanate from failures in the psychological anxiety buffers that serve to keep unconscious concern with mortality at bay, and to form relatively quickly—even at an implicit level—when people are confronted with particularly tragic situations.

To examine these ideas, researchers needed some way to measure the extent to which death-related thoughts are on peoples' mind, even in the absence of peoples' awareness of this activation. In 1994, Greenberg and colleagues adapted measures that had previously been used in cognitive research for such a purpose (e.g., Tulving, Schacter, & Stark, 1982). Participants were given a list of word fragments and asked to complete them with the first word that came to mind. Amidst a number of filler fragments, some of the fragments (e.g.,

COFF __ __) could be completed with a neutral word (e.g., coffee) or with a word related to death (e.g., coffin). The reasoning behind such measures is that the more fragments a participant completes with, in this case, death-related words, the more death is inferred to be cognitively accessible and influencing his or her perception of the fragment stimuli.

Unconscious and Subtle Provocations of Death-Related Thought

Over the past few decades, research has firmly established that stimuli presented below conscious thresholds of awareness can serve to activate related constructs (see, e.g., Bargh, 1996). It is not surprising therefore that a number of experiments have demonstrated that subliminal exposure to the word "death" or "dead" can increase the accessibility of death-related thought. Specifically, in a series of studies by Arndt, Greenberg, Pyszczynski, and Solomon (1997a), participants completed a computer task wherein they made judgments about whether two words (e.g., "sneaker" and "fajita" or "rose" and "flower") were related. In between these two words, which were each presented for approximately 350 milliseconds, participants were exposed to presentations of the word "death" or a control word (e.g., "pain") for 29 milliseconds. Participants reported being unable to see the prime word and, in a separate study, could not accurately guess which word had been presented beyond that which would be expected by chance even when told that it would be one of two possibilities ("dead" or "pain"). Yet the results of these studies indicate that such subliminal primes can indeed increase death-thought accessibility.

In addition, a number of other studies point to the subtlety with which exposure to certain stimuli can elicit death-related concerns. For example, in a series of field studies, Pyszczynski et al. (1996) interviewed pedestrians either 100 yards before they walked by a funeral parlor or when they were right in front of a funeral parlor. When participants were interviewed right in front of the funeral parlor they displayed evaluative reactions that conceptually parallel peoples' responses to more explicit reminders of death. Such findings highlight the sensitivity of people's perceptual systems to death-related stimuli and indicate that even relatively mundane exposure to death-related themes (e.g., watching television or reading the newspaper) are sufficient to render thoughts of death more accessible in memory. However, it need not only be stimuli that bear an obvious connection to death that serve to elicit death-related concerns. Rather, a number of situations—most notably those that signify a breakdown in the effective functioning of the structures designed to protect people from the awareness of mortality—can elevate death-related thought.

Breakdowns in Anxiety Buffers and Death-Related Thought

To the extent that anxiety-buffering constructs offer protection from the accessibility of death-related thoughts, undermining these constructs should also increase death-thought accessibility. The hypothesis that many of the beliefs in which people invest function to insulate their minds from thoughts about death has and continues to be explored in a number of different ways. For example, Goldenberg, Pyszczynski, McCoy, Greenberg, and Solomon (1999) argued that certain individuals, particularly those high in neuroticism, are unable to successfully divorce sexual activity from biological behavior that places people in the same organismic category as other animalistic life forms. Because such individuals conceive of sex as primarily biological copulation, having them think about sex also serves to activate and increase the accessibility of concerns about the physical and ultimately mortal nature of human existence. On the other hand, people low in neuroticism have more successfully separated human sex from animal mating by integrating the act of sex into a romanticized worldview of societal prescriptions about love and its expression through intimate behavior, and thus do not show such effects. Notably, subsequent studies show that this heightened death-thought accessibility from priming sex can be reduced in high neurotics by also priming thoughts about love. Using the trait of neuroticism to represent the failed filtration of physical sex through a meaningful lens of romanticized love demonstrates how other constructs, namely, sex, potentially serve as reminders of mortality. Similarly, when people's sense of symbolic value is compromised by leading them to think of their animal nature, the salience of disgust can also increase the accessibility of death-related thoughts (Cox, Pyszczynski, & Goldenberg, 2003).

Mikulincer, Florian, Birnbaum, and Malishkevich, (2002) expose an anxiety-buffer breakdown of a different type when they contend that, like worldviews and self-esteem, close relationships function as anxiety-buffering mechanisms. As with Goldenberg et al. (1999), this research indicates that compromising the strength of romantic relationships—by, for example, having participants think about problems in their romantic relationships—increases the accessibility of death-related constructs. Thus, studies to date indicate that the mechanisms that typically minimize death-thought accessibility can be compromised dispositionally (e.g. neuroticism) or situationally (e.g., priming relationship problems).

The Sensitivity of Death-Thought Associations

Although implicit learning may often take time and considerable experience to develop, as Rozin, Millman, and Nemeroff's (1986) laws of contagion explicate, certain associations that involve evolutionary significant threats to survival or stimuli with extensive negative connotations can form very quickly and with only minimal exposure. To the extent that concern with mortality is a hot button within people's cognitive networks, this button should be very "easy to light up" following exposure to particularly tragic circumstances. With the tragic events in the United States on September 11, 2001, we were presented with a situation that enabled us to test this hypothesis. Specifically, in light of the power of the terrorist attack on the World Trade Center, frequently thereafter "WTC" in the media, and the infamy of the date "9/11," we reasoned that even unconscious presentations of these stimuli should elicit elevated death-thought accessibility. And indeed, in November 2001, Arndt, Pyszczynski, and Cook (2003) found that participants exposed to subliminal primes of "911" or "WTC" showed increased levels of death-thought accessibility relative to participants exposed to the digits "573" (the area code in Columbia, Missouri, where the study took place—which thus controlled for some sense of familiarity with the prime). Whereas "911" may also be associated with emergencies, it seems safe to assume that the letters "WTC" had little psychological significance to people prior to September 11, and yet such stimuli still had sufficient impact to elevate death-thought accessibility outside conscious awareness.

As alluded to earlier, however, circumstances need not be tragic to activate thoughts of death. Consider the effects, for example, of seeing one's reflection in the mirror. According to classic theory and research on self-awareness (Duval & Wicklund, 1972), a mirror can be a particularly potent stimulus that serves to increase self-focused attention. From a TMT perspective, it is the uniquely human capacity to be self-aware and reflect on ourselves as objects of attention that reveals to us our vulnerability and mortality—to know that we exist is also to know that one day we will not exist. Self-awareness, then, by facilitating the realization of the inevitability of death, is a potential catalyst for the experience of existential terror (Arndt, Greenberg, Simon, Pysczynski, & Solomon, 1998; Pyszczynski, Greenberg, Solomon, & Hamilton, 1990). Consistent with this idea, Silvia (2001) has found that elevating self-awareness can also increase the accessibility of death-related thought.

Summary

An increasing amount of recent research points to a number of different ways that death-related thought can be activated. These ways include the obvious cases of asking people to think about death but extend to priming from outside conscious awareness either death-related constructs or constructs that have a particularly powerful connection to thoughts of death, as well as puncturing the psychological buffers that typically keep mortality concerns at bay. The flavor of these different research examples attest to the ubiquity with which people encounter stimuli—from the tragic to the mundane—that permeate daily life and activate concerns relevant to the awareness of mortality. Next we turn to considering the way in which people both passively and actively deal with this inescapable facet of human experience.

Reactions to Conscious Thoughts of Death: Proximal/Direct Defense

When vulnerabilities to mortality become conscious, it becomes necessary to try to at least pseudo-rationally diffuse the threat. We use the term "pseudorationally" because the strategies that people use may not "objectively" reduce vulnerability to mortality; what is at stake is that the individual is able to convince him- or herself of this vulnerability reduction using the logically derived deductions that tend to dominate conscious thought (Epstein, 1994; Pyszczynski & Greenberg, 1987). The first indication that participants were using some form of defense in response to the explicit provocation of mortality concerns came from studies by Greenberg, Pyszczynski, Solomon, Simon, and Breus (1994). In this research it was found that immediately after contemplating mortality, death-thought accessibility (as well as worldview defense) was low but increased when participants were confronted with a delay or distraction (e.g., completing an innocuous word-search puzzle). This suggested that participants were engaging some form of psychological defense to reduce conscious concerns with death. Next we review some of the routes these defenses may take.

The Avoidance of Self-Awareness when Mortality Is Salient

One of the more obvious responses that people have at their disposal is to simply remove themselves from the situation that does or threatens to activate death-related concerns. As suggested previously, the prospect of mortality becomes a psychological problem when paired with the capacity for self-reflective thought (cf. Duval & Wicklund, 1972). Because of this relationship between self-awareness and the awareness of death, when mortality is salient people should be motivated to avoid circumstances that engender self-focused attention. Arndt et al. (1998) have found that this is in fact the case. Immediately after being asked to contemplate their own mortality, participants were more prone to avoid situations and stimuli that tend to focus attention on themselves (e.g., sitting in a room with a mirror, or writing shorter essays that necessitated the use of self-reflective words). Although these studies show that participants will avoid self-awareness when thoughts of mortality are conscious, there are clearly circumstances in which people are unable to simply exit the situations that are threatening to raise existential concerns.

The Suppression of Conscious Death-Related Thought

Another prolific way in which people avoid thinking of unwanted thoughts is to try to suppress those thoughts (e.g., Wegner, 1992). Based on the dynamics explicated by Wegner's theory of the ironic processes of mental control, this would explain why death-thought accessibility is initially low following an explicit contemplation of mortality; a possibility that Arndt et al. (1997b) sought to test empirically. Drawing further from Wegner's research on thought suppression, Arndt et al. (1997b) hypothesized that if such an effortful suppression process is employed in response to MS, because suppression requires the availability of sufficient processing resources, denying participants the resources needed to perform this suppression should reveal high levels of death-thought accessibility immediately following the contemplation of one's mortality. This was in fact the case. When participants were told to rehearse an 11-digit number, a standard manipulation of cognitive load (e.g., Gilbert & Hixon, 1991) that deprives subjects of mental resources, they were presumably less effective in their suppression efforts and consequently evidenced an immediate increase in the accessibility of death-related thought after MS, an effect that was absent when participants were not deprived of processing resources.

Research by Cook, Arndt, and Goldenberg (2003) also speaks to the suppression of death-related thought; however, these studies concern the suppression of death cognitions provoked by thoughts of cancer. Based on the death-thought activation sequence reviewed earlier, Cook et al. (2003) reasoned that if primes related to tragic events can increase death-thought accessibility, explicitly thinking of a topic related to death, such as cancer, would result in similar effects. However, Cook et al. found that after thinking about either death, cancer, or a control topic of dental pain, only participants asked to think about death showed increased death-thought accessibility. Death-thought accessibility was as low for participants primed to think about cancer as for the control participants. Because this pattern contradicts the expectations of basic priming effects, Cook et al. hypothesized that thinking about cancer may be particularly threatening to people and may arouse an especially robust suppression effort, therefore leading to low death accessibility even after a delay. Two subsequent studies supported this reasoning: One study showed that under high cognitive load, cancer prime participants evidenced increased death-thought accessibility; the other showed that when female participants were led to believe that they were especially vulnerable to breast cancer (and therefore would be in greater need of suppression), they showed lower levels of death-thought accessibility than female participants led to believe they were not vulnerable to breast cancer. Taken together, these findings indicate that after MS or the salience of threatening topics connected to death, participants suppress death-related thoughts. However, suppression is not the only recourse that people have to consciously diffuse the threat of death, and such strategies may be often augmented by other cognitive and motivational biases.

The Denial of Vulnerability as Proximal Defense

Another way that people may try to deal with the conscious awareness of death is to deny that it is going to happen to them. Of course, few of us maintain the belief that we will physically transcend death, but many of us do engage in cognitive bias by which we maintain that death is around somebody else's corner, not ours. This is equivalent to what Steven Chaplin (2000) refers to as the "not me, not now" response and entails denying vulnerability to those risk factors that may be associated with an early demise (see also, e.g., Croyle &

Hunt, 1991). However, because conscious thoughts of death are posited to provoke direct efforts to minimize the threat posed by the awareness of mortality, these defenses should be unnecessary once the problem of death is no longer conscious. If this is indeed the case, then biased evaluation of health threats should occur immediately following MS but not after a delay and distraction, whereas the symbolic defenses of bolstering one's worldview should only appear when a delay and distraction follow reminders of death.

This is precisely what was found in a study by Greenberg, Arndt, Simon, Pyszczynski, and Solomon (2000). Participants biased self-reports of emotionality to deny vulnerability to a short life expectancy when this assessment immediately followed an explicit MS treatment; however, they did not do so after a delay. Conversely, subsequent to this delay, MS led to increased pro-American bias. This growing body of evidence thus supports the notion that unconscious concerns with mortality engender symbolic responses that affirm the beliefs providing meaning and self-esteem. Conscious death thoughts, in contrast, lead to attempts to either suppress the threat or rationally reduce one's perceived vulnerability.

Adaptive Proximal Defenses to Conscious Death Thought

Biases in perceptions of vulnerability need not always proceed along maladaptive health trajectories (Arndt, Goldenberg, Solomon, Greenberg, & Pyszczynski, 2000). Just as the person may say "I know I smoke, but I'm too young to get lung cancer," a person may also opt to pursue strategies of vulnerability denial in response to conscious thoughts of death that actually have proactive beneficial effects on physical health. Arndt, Schimel, and Goldenberg (2003) examined, for example, how standards and goals that underlie fitness behaviors may function as either direct or symbolic defenses. As a direct defense, an individual may advocate exercising regularly to lower his or her risk for health problems. However, individuals may also exercise in order to enhance self-esteem when fitness-oriented pursuits are an important contingency of self-worth (cf. Crocker & Wolfe, 2001). In line with these reasons for fitness, Arndt et al. (2003) found that increased fitness intentions are reported as a direct defense in response to conscious reminders of mortality independent of whether fitness is esteem relevant for the individual. In contrast, when fitness is relevant to an individual's sense of self-esteem, there is an increase in fitness intentions in response to unconscious thoughts of mortality. This suggests a manifestation of the symbolic defense of attending to self-esteem needs.

Conceptually similar results have been recently obtained in a study by Routledge, Arndt, and Goldenberg (in press). When sun-tan/protection lotion preferences were assessed immediately after MS (vs. a control topic), participants said they would purchase products with higher sun-protection factors. However, when preferences were assessed after a delay, participants reminded of death indicated they were less likely to purchase products that were geared toward sun protection, suggesting that here MS influenced not their rational concern with health but the self-esteem-relevant concern with physical appearance.

Summary

As depicted in the top boxes of Figure 3.1, different lines of research suggest that when thoughts of mortality are conscious, people respond by attempting to remove those thoughts from focal attention. These responses include such reactions as avoiding self-focused attention, suppressing death thoughts, or engaging in cognitive and motivational biases to reduce perceived vulnerability. Whereas most cognitive research has focused on more passive information processing, these effects speak to the very active role that the mind can take in managing conscious death-related concerns. Moreover, in contrast to much of the pioneering work on thought suppression conducted by Wegner and colleagues wherein participants were instructed to avoid thinking about a particular topic, reminders of death offer convergent insights with a scenario of self-initiated and naturally occurring thought suppression.

Reactions to Unconscious Death-Related Thought: Distal/Symbolic Defenses

Although many people may be inclined to think of the responses considered previously as the primary ways that people react to thoughts of death, this is in fact only the tip of the iceberg. Indeed, the focus of TMT has been to unveil how death-related thought operates at an unconscious level to exert a powerful effect on symbolic modes of social behavior. In this way thoughts of death also reflect what Wegner and Smart (1997) refer to as "deep cognitive activation," a state in which thoughts are unconscious but still highly accessible. In the sections that follow, we revisit some of these same studies reviewed earlier but here with a focus on the conditions that explicate the nature of distal defenses (e.g., self-esteem striving and prejudicial or aggressive response to those who threaten one's symbolic beliefs). We also consider studies that point to the strong convergence between those conditions that both elevate death-thought accessibility outside focal attention and increase these symbolic modes of defense.

The Role of Death-Theme Accessibility in Distal Defense

Recall that in Greenberg et al. (1994), death-thought accessibility was immediately low following an explicit MS manipulation but increased after a delay. Notably, these were the same conditions under which Greenberg et al. also observed an increase in worldview defense (i.e., pro-American bias). In addition, participants did not manifest worldview defense after MS when they were forced to keep death-related cognitions in focal attention by completing a death word-search puzzle or when they were asked to engage in a much more in-depth, deeper contemplation of their mortality. That is, participants only showed the heightened affirmation of symbolic beliefs after death-related thought was allowed to fade from focal attention.

The findings of Arndt et al. (1997b) offer a convergent picture. When participants were prevented from suppressing death-related thought immediately after an explicit MS manipulation by rehearsing a cognitive load, both death-thought accessibility and worldview defense increased immediately. However, as in Greenberg et al., under conditions of low cognitive load, MS participants only responded with elevated death accessibility and worldview defense when a delay intervened between the salience induction and assessment of the dependent variables. A number of other studies similarly point to the role of death-theme accessibility in distal defense reactions. For example, just as the experiential mode facilitated an MS-induced elevation of pro-American bias, it also facilitated a delayed increase in death-theme accessibility whereas a rational mode of processing did not (Simon et al., 1997; see also Harmon-Jones et al., 1997).

Using a Delay and Distraction to Elucidate Distal Defense

To the extent that distal defenses occur in response to the deep activation of death-related thought, distal defenses should primarily emerge when participants have been distracted from the subject of death. Evidence of this temporal sequence has been found in a number of studies to date. The first direct assessment of this possibility was provided by the Greenberg et al. (2000) study. In that research, participants were found to engage a proximal defense (i.e., deny vulnerability) immediately after MS but not after a delay. In contrast, participants were found to engage a distal defense (i.e., pro-American bias) after a delay but not immediately.

Recently, studies have conceptually replicated this finding with measures that adopt a more idiographic approach to what constitutes a given individual's standards for self-esteem. In Arndt et al. (2003), whereas relevance of fitness to self-esteem had no effect on the tendency for MS to increase exercise intentions when they were assessed immediately (and thus presumably as a form of proximal defense), when a delay followed MS, only those participants for whom fitness was relevant to self-esteem increased their intentions to exercise. A similar effect occurred in Routledge et al. (in press). Recall that here participants tended to endorse safe sun-product choices immediately after MS, but after a delay, participants for whom physical appearance was important to their self-esteem lowered their endorsement of safe sun products; a response that would presumably lead to a more attractive and tan appearance. Thus, what we see from studies using the delay paradigm is that when reactions are assessed immediately, reminders of death instigate defenses that are at least pseudorationally connected to the threat. However, when assessed following a distraction, reminders of death instigate more symbolically oriented investments in domains of meaning and self-worth.

The Effects of Subliminal Death Primes on Distal Defense

A number of studies thus indirectly suggest that it is the unconscious elevation of death-theme accessibility that produces distal defense effects. Arndt et al. (1997a) examined this notion more directly. Using the subliminal priming procedure previously described, American participants were exposed to presentations of either the word "death" (or in other studies, "dead") or "field" (in other studies "pain") for very brief exposure durations (43 milliseconds or 28 milliseconds). Not only did participants presented with the subliminal death primes show evidence of a semantic priming effect (more death-word completions) but they also showed elevated pro-American bias (see also, e.g., Arndt et al., 2001; Dechesne, Janssen, & van Knippenberg, 2000). In addition, when exposure durations of the critical prime were slowed down to be consciously identifiable (e.g., 428 milliseconds), the immediate increase in worldview defense did not occur.

It is important to note here that whereas the typical explicit MS treatment engenders its effects on worldview defense only after a delay, these studies that bypass conscious consideration of death with subliminal primes elicited the worldview defense effect immediately after the presentation. This suggests that it is indeed the nonconscious elevation in death-thought accessibility that drives the emergence of distal defense—a finding that significantly extends what were previously considered to be the boundaries of unconscious activation. That is, as Freud and many classic existential theorists suggest, the unconscious is capable of more than mere semantic or rudimentary connections (cf. Greenwald, 1992).

Summary

This chorus of findings converges to suggest that it is the unconscious concern with death that triggers MS effects on symbolic domains of judgment. Thus, whereas an explicit induction of MS requires a delay for such effects to emerge and thus the opportunity for participants to initially suppress death thoughts, unconscious provocations have no need of such procedures. Notably, the delayed effect of explicit treatments can be circumvented by introducing a cognitive load task that impairs suppression efforts and therefore leads to immediate increases in death-thought accessibility. Taken together, then, distal defense reactions wherein people increase their investment in domains of meaning appear to occur in response to the nonconscious activation of death-related thought.

The Spreading Activation of Unconscious Death Thought to Symbolic Value Constructs

One unavoidable aspect of these studies measuring symbolic worldview defense is that participants must defend in response to confrontation with some kind of target. As a result, however, we do not know how accessible death-related thought spontaneously progresses to implicate other constructs. Recent research has begun to address these issues. Recall the ideas that during childhood, and indeed throughout life, though for brief moments persons may experience a glimmer of dread as they realize they may be but a bug soon to go splat on a windshield, elaborate cultural constructs are there to provide the comfort and security that we are valued people with identities, histories, goals, and futures. Thus, intimations of death become associated in memory with aspects of the security-providing internalized worldview, particularly aspects central to providing meaning and bases of self-worth. To the extent that knowledge of mortality occupies a prominent and deeply rooted position within a network of knowledge structures that function as self-protective beliefs, spreading activation and related models (e.g., McKoon & Ratcliff, 1992; McNamara, 1992) should predict that when death is activated, accessibility should spontaneously spread to other interconnected concepts, which, from the perspective of TMT, would be those constructs that function to provide meaning and value.

In an initial effort to assess this hypothesis, Arndt, Greenberg, and Cook (2002) had male and female American students complete either a typical MS questionnaire or parallel questions about dental pain and then, following a delay, complete a word-fragment measure of worldview accessibility. The measure of accessibility initially considered what previous research suggested was a robust element of the worldview: nationalism (e.g., fragments such as F __ __ G, which could be completed with *flag* or *frog*). Participants who thought about death did indeed evidence enhanced accessibility of nationalistic themes. However, perhaps even more interesting was an unexpected gender-by-salience interaction, such that this effect of MS increasing nationalistic bias was in fact only evident for male participants.

There are of course individual differences in what constitutes an important security-providing belief (Greenberg et al., 1997). Although the TMT literature had not previously uncovered gender differences, other research suggests that patriotism is often a stronger identification for men than for women (e.g., Geary, 1998), and to the extent death-related thought triggers the more vital self-protective beliefs, it is reasonable that it would motivate spreading to nationalistic beliefs for men but not women. One question then becomes, What aspects of women's protective beliefs might be spontaneously activated by thoughts of MS? Insight here is provided by evolutionary, cultural, and sociological perspectives that suggest, for women, romantic relationships form one of the primary avenues for meaning and value. Indeed, Rank (e.g., 1941/1958) wrote extensively about the "romantic solution" to human's existential plight (see also, e.g., Goldenberg & Roberts, Chapter 5, this volume; Mikulincer, Florian, & Hirschberger, Chapter 18, this volume). Consistent with this analysis, using an expanded measure of worldview accessibility that also included fragments that could be completed with romantic words (e.g., __ OVER as *lover* or *cover*), a second study found that MS increased the accessibility of nationalistic themes for men and romantic themes for women.

To the extent that the increased accessibility of worldview relevant domains represents the vehicle that people then use to engage in distal (or symbolic) defenses, worldview accessibility effects should map onto the conditions under which worldview defenses occur: namely, in response to the nonconscious accessibility of death-related thought. This appears to be the case. Additional studies from that research provide converging evidence that unconscious but accessible thoughts of death trigger the heightened accessibility of constructs that reflect important domains of value and meaning.

However, an interesting question emerges when considering these findings in light of prior TMT research. On the one hand, females have consistently responded to MS with increased pro-American bias. On the other hand, these studies indicate that women do not respond to MS with spontaneous increases in patriotic accessibility as do men. This is because, although the most central, security-providing aspects of the worldview are what spontaneously becomes accessible following MS, other aspects of the worldview may also become accessible and be defended when those aspects are made salient. And in every study on worldview defense, the to-be-defended element of the worldview (e.g., nationalistic pride) is made salient in confrontation with, for example, a validating or threatening essay or a vignette of some particular transgression. Thus, whereas a variety of beliefs can be used for existential protection, the belief that is used toward this end depends not only on individual differences in what constitutes an individual's "preferred" route of defense but also via situational factors that render some beliefs more accessible than others. In support of this reasoning, when America is made salient prior to MS, reminders of death increase the accessibility of nationalistic thoughts in American women. These results thus add a key piece to the process model of MS effects and suggest that both individual differences in what constitutes a domain of value, as well as situational factors, exert an influence on the constructs that are spontaneously activated by death-related thought.

The Reduction of Death-Thought Accessibility by Worldview Defense

The developmental perspective on TMT suggests that people "learn" that faith and identification with symbolic worldviews assuage the potential for terror engendered by unconscious concerns with mortality. How does this occur? When such a question is put into the dynamic cognitive perspective we have been describing, one possibility that emerges is that cultural worldview and self-esteem defenses serve their terror management function by reducing that which causes their manifestation. Thus, to the extent that accessible nonconscious death-related thought spreads to activate worldview constructs which are then evaluatively defended, such defense then serves to reduce the accessibility of death-related cognition.

To assess this proposition, Arndt et al. (1997b, Study 3) reminded participants of their mortality, or not, and then confronted them with essays that praised or attacked the United States. However, only some of the participants were allowed to respond evaluatively toward the authors, whereas others had to answer nonjudgmental questions (e.g., estimating the number of words in the essay). Among those participants who were given the opportunity to evaluate the essays, participants reminded of mortality showed more bias than did participants not reminded of mortality. Most important, those MS participants who were allowed to defend their worldview showed lower death-thought accessibility (equivalent to levels in control conditions) than did those MS participants who were not allowed to defend their worldview. This study thus provided one of the first demonstrations of how worldview defense serves its psychological function. Recently, Mikulincer and Florian (2002) have pro-vided similar evidence with regard to self-esteem strivings. Specifically, this research found that those participants who were reminded of their mortality and given the opportunity to express a self-serving attributional bias showed reduced death-thought accessibility relative to those who were not given such an opportunity.

However, one issue these studies did not address is whether the opportunity to defend the worldview or bolster self-esteem actually reduced levels of death-thought accessibility or simply gave participants the cognitive resources to resuppress these cognitions. Greenberg, Arndt, Schimel, Pyszczynski, and Solomon (2001) thus replicated Study 3 of Arndt et al. (1997b) but placed half the participants under high cognitive load after evaluating the essays and half under low cognitive load. If participants are simply resuppressing death-related thought, then introducing cognitive load should disrupt the suppression effort and lead to high death-thought accessibility even after worldview defense. However, the results revealed no effect of load, suggesting that worldview defense is in fact reducing death-thought accessibility. Notably, though, the opportunity for worldview defense will only reduce death-thought accessibility when the person takes advantage of it. For example, Mikulincer and Florian (2000, Study 3) found that whereas people with an avoidant attach-ment style responded to MS with increased severity rating to moral transgressors, those with a secure attachment did not. Accordingly, whereas avoidant participants then showed de-creased death-thought accessibility relative to those avoidant participants who were re-minded of their death but did not have the opportunity to respond defensively, securely attached participants did not show a significant decrease.

CONCLUSION

> Let sanguine healthy-mindedness do its best with its strange power of living in the moment and ignoring and forgetting, still the evil background is there to be thought of, and the skull will grin in at the banquet.
>
> —WILLIAM JAMES, *The Varieties of Religious Experience* (1902, p. 158)

In the last decade or so, psychological research has made substantial progress toward under-standing facets of human social behavior through a juxtaposition of cognitive and motiva-tional perspectives, an examination of unconscious processes, and an empirical scrutiny of existential pressures. This chapter summarizes research that has uniquely built from each of these domains to advance a heuristic model of the cognitive architecture of how people defensively respond to the awareness of death (see Figure 3.1). By virtue of its motivational significance, the TMT analysis argues that the awareness of death, as the quote from William James conveys, is an ever-present shadow that looms beneath our everyday func-tioning. In this light, thoughts of death can be activated by a number of situations and sce-narios, whether they are associated events or dispositional and situational breakdowns in the protective mechanisms that keep conscious concern with death at bay. When such thoughts become conscious, it initiates proximal defenses (e.g., suppression and vulnerabil-ity denial) that pseudorationally ameliorate the need for further attention to death-related concerns. With death-related cognition now accessible but outside current focal attention, this activation spreads to constructs that are associated with the individuals' culturally pre-scribed investments in meaning and esteem. To the extent that such investments become ac-tivated by thoughts of death, they are then defended in the face of stimuli that impinge upon those beliefs. These worldview defensive responses in turn function in part to reduce the heightened accessibility of death-related thought that led to the reaction.

Taken together, this model has implications for understanding a number of domains concerning the management of existential fears as well as unconscious cognitive processes more generally. On this latter note, for example, Bargh and Chartrand (1999) posit that goals operate in the same way and have the same effects whether they are activated consciously or unconsciously. Although parallels between conscious and unconscious activation exist for certain types of goals, there are clearly situations—such as the deeply rooted goals people have about protecting themselves from the awareness of death—in which this does not appear to be the case. Rather, at least in the domain of terror management, there are critical differences that emanate from conscious versus unconscious activation, and understanding these distinctions can yield important insights.

These insights may give us an important understanding of a multifaceted range of human social behaviors. Previous TMT research has been directed toward diverse areas such as prejudice, aggression, altruism, creativity, legal judgments, and health behaviors, and the more finely tuned analysis offered in this chapter can potentially enrich each of these applications. It is also important to consider that reminders of death can potentially engage multiple motivational responses. People's worldviews inevitably contain a variety of beliefs and values, some of which may be dissonant with one another and brought into conflict in particular situations. In addition, although the research on which we have focused has used worldview and self-esteem investments as the vehicles to investigate the cognitive dynamics of responses to death-related thought, emerging research directions highlight that a number of other domains, such as close relationships (e.g., Mikulincer & Florian, 2000), generalized belongingness (Wisman & Koole, 2003), and creativity (e.g., Arndt, Greenberg, Solomon, Pyszczynski, & Schimel, 1999), can be affected by MS and serve important terror management functions. How then can we understand when and for whom the awareness of death will lead to which types of responses? Considering the cognitive architecture of death-related thought may help to provide insight into these questions by allowing us to trace the cognitive activation that follows reminders of death in different contexts and for different individuals. In so doing, the model facilitates a better understanding of how existential needs affect core social behaviors that characterize the human experience.

ACKNOWLEDGMENT

Preparation of this chapter was supported in part by NCI Grant No. R01 CA96581-01.

REFERENCES

Arndt, J., Allen, J. J. B, & Greenberg, J. (2001). Traces of terror: Subliminal death primes and facial electromyographic indices of affect. *Motivation and Emotion, 25,* 253–277.

Arndt, J., Goldenberg, J., Solomon, S., Greenberg, J., & Pyszczynski, T. (2000). Death can be hazardous to your health: Adaptive and ironic consequences of defenses against the terror of death. In J. Masling & P. Duberstain (Eds.), *Psychoanalytic perspectives on sickness and health* (Vol. 9, pp. 201–257). Washington DC: American Psychological Association.

Arndt, J., Greenberg, J., & Cook, A. (2002). Mortality salience and the spreading activation of worldview-relevant constructs: Exploring the cognitive architecture of terror management. *Journal of Experimental Psychology: General, 131,* 307–324.

Arndt, J., Greenberg, J., Pyszczynski, T., & Solomon, S. (1997a). Subliminal exposure to death-related stimuli increases defense of the cultural worldview. *Psychological Science, 8,* 379–385.

Arndt, J., Greenberg, J., Simon, L., Pyszczynski, T., & Solomon, S. (1998). Terror management and self-awareness: Evidence that mortality salience provokes avoidance of the self-focused state. *Personality and Social Psychological Bulletin, 24,* 1216–1227.

Arndt, J., Greenberg, J., Solomon, S., Pyszczynski, T., & Schimel, J. (1999). Creativity and terror management: The effects of creative activity on guilt and social projection following mortality salience. *Journal of Personality and Social Psychology, 77,* 19–32.

Arndt, J., Greenberg, J., Solomon, S., Pyszczynski, T., & Simon, L. (1997b). Suppression, accessibility of death-related thoughts, and cultural worldview defense: Exploring the psychodynamics of terror management. *Journal of Personality and Social Psychology, 73,* 5–18.

Arndt, J., Pyszczynski, T., & Cook, A. (2003). *Subliminal tragedy and death-thought accessibility.* Manuscript in progress, University of Missouri, Columbia.

Arndt, J., Schimel, J., & Goldenberg, J. L. (2003). Death can be good for your health: Fitness intentions as a proximal and distal defense against mortality salience. *Journal of Applied Social Psychology, 33,* 1726–1746.

Bargh, J. A. (1996). Automaticity in social psychology. In E. T. Higgins & A. W. Kruglanski (Eds.), *Social psychology: Handbook of basic principles* (pp. 169–183). New York: Guilford Press.

Bargh, J. A., & Chartrand, T. L. (1999). The unbearable automaticity of being. *American Psychologist, 54,* 462–479.

Becker, E. (1973). *The denial of death.* New York: Free Press.

Chaiken, S., & Trope, Y. (1999). *Dual-process theories in social psychology.* New York: Guilford Press.

Chaplin, S. (2000). *The psychology of time and death.* Ashland, OH: Sonnet Press.

Collins, A. M., & Loftus, E. F. (1975). A spreading-activation theory of semantic processing. *Psychological Review, 82,* 407–428.

Cook, A., Arndt, J., & Goldenberg, J. L. (2003). *The suppression of death-related thought as a function of cancer salience and perceived vulnerability.* Manuscript under review, University of Missouri, Columbia.

Cox, C. R., Pyszczynski, T., & Goldenberg, J. L. (2003). *Disgust, creatureliness, and the accessibility of death-related thoughts.* Manuscript under review, University of Colorado at Colorado Springs.

Crocker, J., & Wolfe, C. (2001). Contingencies of worth. *Psychological Review, 108,* 593–623.

Croyle, R. T., & Hunt, J. R. (1991). Coping with health threat: Social influence processes in reactions to medical test results. *Journal of Personality and Social Psychology, 60,* 382–389.

Dechesne, M., Janssen, J., & van Knippenberg, A. (2000). Defense and distancing as terror management strategies: The moderating role of need for structure and permeability of group boundaries. *Journal of Personality and Social Psychology, 79,* 923–932.

Duval, S., & Wicklund, R. A. (1972). *A theory of objective-self-awareness.* New York: Academic Press.

Epstein, S. (1994). Integration of the cognitive and psychodynamic unconscious. *American Psychologist, 49,* 709–724.

Geary, D. C. (1998). *Male, female: The evolution of human sex differences.* Washington, DC: American Psychiatric Association Press.

Gilbert, D. T., & Hixon, J. G. (1991). The trouble of thinking: Activation and application of stereotypic beliefs. *Journal of Personality and Social Psychology, 60,* 509–517.

Goldenberg, J. L., Pyszczynski, T., McCoy, S. K., Greenberg, J., & Solomon, S. (1999). Death, sex, love, and neuroticism: Why is sex such a problem? *Journal of Personality and Social Psychology, 77,* 1173–1187

Greenberg, J., Arndt, J., Schimel, J., Pyszczynski, T., & Solomon, S. (2001). Clarifying the function of mortality salience-induced worldview defense: Renewed suppression or reduced accessibility of death-related thoughts? *Journal of Experimental Social Psychology, 37,* 70–76.

Greenberg, J., Arndt, J., Simon, L., Pyszczynski, T., & Solomon, S. (2000). Proximal and distal defenses in response to reminders of one's mortality: Evidence of a temporal sequence. *Personality and Social Psychology Bulletin, 26,* 91–99.

Greenberg, J., Martens, A., Jonas, E., Eisenstadt, D., Pyszczynski, T., & Solomon, S. (2003). Psychological defense in anticipation of anxiety: Eliminating the potential for anxiety eliminates the effects of mortality salience on worldview defense. *Psychological Science, 14*(5), 1516–1519.

Greenberg, J., Pyszczynski, T., & Solomon, S. (1986). The causes and consequences of a need for self-esteem: A terror management theory. In R. F. Baumeister (Ed.), *Public self and private self* (pp. 189–212). New York: Springer-Verlag.

Greenberg, J., Pyszczynski, T., Solomon, S., Simon, L., & Breus, M. (1994). Role of consciousness and accessibility of death-related thoughts in mortality salience effects. *Journal of Personality and Social Psychology, 67*, 627–637.

Greenberg, J., Solomon, S., & Pyszczynski, T. (1997). Terror management theory of self-esteem and social behavior: Empirical assessments and conceptual refinements. In M. P. Zanna (Ed.) *Advances in experimental social psychology* (Vol. 29, pp. 61–139). New York: Academic Press.

Greenwald, A. G. (1992). New Look 3: Unconscious cognition reclaimed. *American Psychologist, 47*, 766–779.

Harmon-Jones, E., Simon, L., Greenberg, J., Pyszczynski, T., Solomon, S., & McGregor, H. (1997). Terror management theory and self-esteem: Evidence that increased self-esteem reduces mortality salience effects. *Journal of Personality and Social Psychology, 72*, 24–36.

James, W. (1978). *The varieties of religious experience.* Garden City, NY: Image Books. (Original work published in 1902)

Kihlstrom, J. F. (1987). The cognitive unconscious. *Science, 237*, 1445–1452.

Kunda, Z. (1999). *Social cognition: Making sense of people.* Cambridge, MA: MIT Press.

McKoon, G., & Ratcliff, R. (1992). Spreading activation versus compound cue accounts of priming: Mediated priming revisited. *Journal of Experimental Psychology: Learning, Memory, and Cognition, 18*, 1155–1172.

McNamara, T. P. (1992). Priming and constraints it places on theories of memory and retrieval. *Psychological Review, 99*, 650–662.

Mikulincer, M., & Florian, V. (2000). Exploring individual differences in reactions to mortality salience: Does attachment style regulate terror management mechanisms? *Journal of Personality and Social Psychology, 79*, 260–273.

Mikulincer, M., & Florian, V. (2002). The effect of mortality salience on self-serving attributions: Evidence for the function of self-esteem as a terror management mechanism. *Basic and Applied Social Psychology, 24*, 261–271.

Mikulincer, M., Florian, V., Birnbaum, G., & Malishkevich, S. (2002). The death-anxiety buffering function of close relationships: Exploring the effects of separation reminders on death-thought accessibility. *Personality and Social Psychology Bulletin, 28*, 287–299.

Nelson, L. J., Moore, D. L., Olivetti, J., & Scott, T. (1997). General and personal mortality salience and nationalistic bias. *Personality and Social Psychology Bulletin, 23*, 884–892.

Pyszczynski, T., & Greenberg, J. (1987). Toward an integration of cognitive and motivational perspectives on social inference: A biased hypothesis-testing model. In L. Berkowitz (Ed.) *Advances in experimental social psychology* (Vol. 20, pp. 294–340). San Diego, CA: Academic Press.

Pyszczynski, T., Greenberg, J., & Solomon, S. (1999). A dual-process model of defense against conscious and unconscious death-related thoughts: An extension of terror management theory. *Psychological Review, 106*, 835–845.

Pyszczynski, T., Greenberg, J., Solomon, S., & Hamilton, J. (1990). A terror management analysis of self-awareness and anxiety: The hierarchy of terror. *Anxiety Research, 2*, 177–195.

Pyszczynski, T., Wicklund, R. A., Floresky, S., Gauch, G., Koch, S., Solomon, S., et al. (1996). Whistling in the dark: Exaggerated estimates of social consensus in response to incidental reminders of mortality. *Psychological Science, 7*, 332–336.

Rank, O. (1958). *Beyond psychology.* New York: Dover. (Original work published 1941)

Rosenblatt, A., Greenberg, J., Solomon, S., Pyszczynski, T., & Lyon, D. (1989). Evidence for terror management theory I: The effects of mortality salience on reactions to those who violate or uphold cultural values. *Journal of Personality and Social Psychology, 57*, 681–690.

Routledge, C., Arndt, J., & Goldenberg, J. L. (in press). A time to tan: Proximal and distal effects of mortality salience on intentions to sun-tan. *Personality and Social Psychology Bulletin.*

Rozin, P., Millman, L., & Nemeroff, C. (1986). Operation of the law of sympathetic magic in disgust and other domains. *Journal of Personality and Social Psychology, 50,* 703–721.

Silvia, P. J. (2001). Nothing of the opposite: Intersecting terror management and objective self-awareness. *European Journal of Personality, 15,* 73–82.

Simon, L., Greenberg, J., Harmon-Jones, E., Solomon, S., Pyszczynski, T., Arndt, J., et al. (1997). Cognitive-experiential self-theory and terror management theory: Evidence that terror management occurs in the experiential system. *Journal of Personality and Social Psychology, 72,* 1132–1146.

Solomon, S., Greenberg, J., & Pyszczynski, T. (1991). A terror management theory of social behavior: The psychological functions of self-esteem and cultural worldviews. In M. P. Zanna (Ed.), *Advances in experimental social psychology* (Vol. 24, pp. 93–159). New York: Academic Press.

Tulving, E., Schacter, D. L., & Stark, H. A. (1982). Priming effects in word-fragment completion are independent of recognition memory. *Journal of Experimental Psychology: Learning, Memory, and Cognition, 8,* 336–342.

Wegner, D. M. (1992). You can't always think what you want: Problems in the suppression of unwanted thoughts. In M. P. Zanna (Ed.), *Advances in experimental social psychology* (Vol. 25, pp. 193–225). San Diego, CA: Academic Press.

Wegner, D. M., & Smart, L. (1997). Deep cognitive activation: A new approach to the unconscious. *Journal of Consulting and Clinical Psychology, 65,* 984–995.

Wisman, A., & Koole, S. L. (2003). Hiding in the crowd: Can mortality salience promote affiliation with others who oppose one's worldview? *Journal of Personality and Social Psychology, 84,* 511–526.

Chapter 4

A Multifaceted Perspective on the Existential Meanings, Manifestations, and Consequences of the Fear of Personal Death

VICTOR FLORIAN
MARIO MIKULINCER

Since the initial writings of Freud on Eros and Thanatos, psychologists have attempted to understand the existential meanings that people give to their life and death. One topic that has received theoretical and empirical attention is the existential terror of personal death. In particular, Florian and his colleagues have developed and empirically validated a multifaceted theoretical framework for assessing and analyzing the multidimensional meanings, manifestations, and psychological consequences of the fear of personal death. This framework is constructed around the answers to three major questions. First, what is terrifying about personal death? This question concerns the existential meanings people attach to their own mortality, with death being conceptualized as having intrapersonal, interpersonal, and transpersonal consequences. Second, how is fear of personal death manifested and expressed? This question concerns both conscious and unconscious manifestations of the fear of death. Third, how is the phenomenon of death conceptualized? This question refers to both the formal understanding of death as a natural, universal phenomenon and the subjective meanings of the concept of death.

In this chapter, we explain Florian's multifaceted perspective on the fear of personal death, state the major theoretical propositions, and summarize empirical findings concerning the three major aspects of this fear. We review two bodies of empirical findings: (1) studies conducted by Florian and his colleagues on the contribution of cultural, social, demographic, and personal factors to individual variations in the meanings and expressions of the fear of death as well as the subjective concept of death; and (2) recent findings from our laboratory that have refined terror management theory (TMT; Greenberg, Solomon, & Pyszczynski, 1997) and highlighted the important role of the three components of the fear of death in regulating the activation of cultural anxiety-buffer mechanisms. We integrate Florian's multifaceted approach to fear of death with research on terror management. The integration enriches and extends both TMT and the psychology of death and dying.

WHAT IS TERRIFYING ABOUT DEATH?

In the first 25 years of death anxiety research, from the mid-1950s through the late 1970s, researchers conceptualized the fear of death in a simplistic, unidimensional manner. Initial attempts to assess death anxiety focused on the extent of such anxiety (e.g., Cameron, 1968; Durlak, 1973; Lester, 1971; Templer, 1970) and were limited to unidimensional measures of fear of death. Although these measures contained items assessing a broad range of death-related concerns (e.g., concern over loss of bodily integrity and fear of a painful death), the diverse worries were simply averaged to yield a single death anxiety score. As a result, these measures failed to tap qualitative differences in the concerns that death-related thoughts can elicit and thus were not able to represent the complexities of a person's fear of death. Moreover, this simplistic conceptualization, combined with imprecision in measurement, led to confusion and ambiguities about the causes, correlates, and consequences of the fear of personal death and revealed the need for a multidimensional conceptualization of death anxiety (e.g., Kastenbaum & Costa, 1977; Pollak, 1979).

In a preliminary contribution to the multidimensional study of death anxiety, Collett and Lester (1969) claimed that fear of death is organized around two basic dimensions. The first dimension distinguishes between two types of fear: fear of death itself and fear of the process of dying. The second dimension distinguishes between two possible objects of death anxiety: fear of one's own death and fear of other people's deaths. This conceptualization was further supported by Durlak (1972) and Nelson and Nelson (1975), who clearly showed that fear of one's own death can be distinguished from other categories of fear of death and can be considered a separate psychological entity. Unfortunately, this early two-dimensional approach failed to consider that the fear of personal death is also a psychologically complex phenomenon. In fact, people can be afraid of their personal death for different reasons, and these individual differences can be extremely important for understanding the meanings and consequences of death anxiety.

The need to investigate fear of personal death using a multidimensional approach led several scholars to propose specific components of this fear and specific meanings attached to it (e.g., Hoelter, 1979; Kastenbaum & Aisenberg, 1972; Minton & Spilka, 1976; Murphy, 1959). For example, Murphy (1959) suggested seven possible death-related concerns: (1) fear of death as the end of life, (2) fear of losing consciousness, (3) fear of loneliness, (4) fear of the unknown, (5) fear of retribution, (6) fear of consequences of death for loved others, and (7) fear of failure. Accordingly, Hoelter (1979) proposed that a person can be afraid of his or her own death due to concerns about decay, dissection, cremation, and isolation of the body; concerns about the failure to accomplish important life goals or to have significant experiences; worries about the impact of death to significant others; and worries about the mystery surrounding what will happen in the hereafter.

Based on a comparative content analysis of these multidimensional suggestions, Florian and his colleagues (Florian, 1979; Florian & Har-Even, 1983; Florian & Kravetz, 1983; Florian, Kravetz, & Frankel, 1984) proposed a theoretical model comprising three dimensions of the fear of personal death. These dimensions refer to the intrapersonal, interpersonal, and transpersonal meanings that people can attach to their own death. The intrapersonal dimension includes all the meanings related to the consequences of death for one's own mind and body, such as failure to accomplish important life goals and decomposition of the body. The interpersonal dimension includes all the meanings related to the possible impact of death on one's interpersonal life, such as the cessation of close relationships, failure to care for loved others, and the possibility of being forgotten. The transpersonal dimension includes all the meanings related to the hereafter and the transcendental nature of one's existence, such as uncertainty about what to expect in the hereafter and the possibility of punishment in the hereafter. In this way, fear of death may reflect concerns about the impact of death on intrapersonal or interpersonal areas of life or worries related to the transcendental nature of the self.

To tap the three theoretical dimensions of the fear of personal death, Florian and Kravetz (1983) constructed a 31-item self-report scale—the Fear of Personal Death Scale (FPDS)—and administered it to a sample of 178 young Israeli adults. In this scale, respondents are asked to rate the personal relevance of various reasons for being afraid of death rather than indicating the extent of the fear per se. As such, the FPDS is an attributional measure of the sources of fear and worry when reflecting on one's mortality. Ratings are made on 7-point Likert scales reflecting the degree of agreement or disagreement with each of the 31 items.

Florian and Kravetz (1983) factor-analyzed respondents' ratings and found that the 31 items were grouped into six main factors reflecting intrapersonal, interpersonal, and transpersonal meanings of one's death. The intrapersonal meanings were captured by two factors: fear of loss of self-fulfillment (e.g., "death frightens me because my life will not have been properly used") and fear of self-annihilation (e.g., "I am afraid of death because of the decomposition of my body"). The interpersonal meanings were also conveyed by two factors: fear of loss of social identity (e.g., "death frightens me because my absence will not be felt") and fear of consequences of death to family and friends (e.g., "I'm afraid of my death because my family will still need me when I'm gone"). The transpersonal meanings were conveyed by two factors: fear of the transcendental consequences of death (e.g., "Death frightens me because of the uncertainty of any sort of existence after death") and fear of punishment in the hereafter (e.g., "I am afraid of death because of the expected punishment in the next world"). Several studies have replicated this six-factor structure across different ethnic and religious groups and have shown that the FPDS factors have good test–retest reliability and internal consistency (e.g., Florian & Har-Even, 1983; Florian & Mikulincer, 1992; Florian & Snowden, 1989).

Florian's (1979) three-dimensional conceptualization is extremely helpful for understanding individual variations in the fear of personal death and dissipating confusions and ambiguities stemming from a simplistic, unidimensional conceptualization of this important form of fear. Specifically, individual variations in the fear of personal death cannot be appropriately analyzed through a unidimensional lens in which people vary in the intensity of a global, nonspecific fear. Rather, these variations must be mapped in terms of the major dimensions of the fear of personal death. There are important individual variations that can be observed in the intensity of the intrapersonal, interpersonal, and transpersonal aspects of the fear of death.

Florian and his colleagues have applied this multidimensional approach to the analysis of the cultural, personal, and contextual factors that are theoretically expected to affect a person's death-related concerns. In four independent studies, Florian and his colleagues

(Florian & Har-Even, 1983; Florian & Kravetz, 1983; Florian et al., 1984; Florian & Mikulincer, 1992) examined the contribution of a person's religious beliefs to the three dimensions of the fear of personal death. Early theoretical writings suggested that active commitment to religious beliefs and practice can reduce the intensity of death anxiety, because this commitment entails a promise of symbolic immortality (e.g., Feifel & Branscomb, 1973; Schulz, 1978). Accordingly, early studies found an inverse association between religiosity and fear of death (e.g., Feifel, 1977; Feifel & Nagy, 1981; Templer, 1972). However, Florian and his colleagues revealed a more complex picture of the possible psychological benefits and costs of religious beliefs. Whereas religious people report less intense intrapersonal foci of death fear (self-annihilation, loss of self-fulfillment) than do nonreligious persons, they report more intense fears related to punishment in the hereafter and consequences of death to their family and friends. That is, religious beliefs seem to act as a symbolic shield that protects people from the consequences of death to the body and the self but tend to intensify worries about the hereafter and their inability to protect their loved ones after death.

In their study of the effects of death-risk experiences on the fear of personal death, Florian and Mikulincer (1992) further emphasized the importance of a multidimensional approach for understanding the protective effects of commitment to religious beliefs. In this study, Israeli soldiers who differed in their actual exposure to recent death-risk experiences (being involved in dangerous and threatening military activities during the previous 3 months) completed the FPDS and a measure of religious beliefs. Findings revealed that exposure to death-risk experiences by itself had no significant impact on the various dimensions of the fear of personal death. Such exposure did, however, affect some of the fear-of-death dimensions in interaction with a participant's commitment to religious beliefs. Exposure to death-risk experiences was associated with higher levels of fear of personal death due to loss of self-fulfillment, self-annihilation, and loss of social identity only among non-religious people. Religious individuals' fears of the intrapersonal and interpersonal consequences of death were not significantly affected by exposure to death-risk experiences. That is, religiosity served as a defense against the personal and interpersonal consequences of death, particularly in circumstances that involved encounters with undeniably dangerous circumstances.

Studies have shown that other sociodemographic variables exhibit complex associations with the fear of personal death. For example, Florian and Snowden (1989) reported highly differentiated profiles of fear of personal death among American college students who came from diverse religious backgrounds (Catholics, Protestants, Jews, Buddhists). Specifically, whereas the Buddhist-affiliated group reported higher fear of the consequences of death to their family and friends than did the other groups, the Protestant-affiliated group scored higher on the fear of punishment in the hereafter. These findings imply that the diverse religious groups attached different meanings to their death and became afraid of death due to different reasons. Moreover, Florian and Har-Even (1983) found some gender differences in the three dimensions of fear of personal death. Whereas women reported more intense fears of death related to loss of social identity and self-annihilation than did men, men reported more intense fears related to the consequences of death to family and punishment in the hereafter. This pattern of findings can explain why early studies using unidimensional measures of fear of death consistently failed to reveal significant gender differences (e.g., Dickstein, 1972; Pollack, 1979; Templer, 1970).

At first sight, the finding that men report more fear of death related to the consequences of death to family than do women seems to run counter to the general tendency for women to be especially oriented toward nurturing and caring for their families. However, a detailed item analysis of this interpersonal death fear factor reveals that it entails worries about the inability to provide material resources and a sense of security for one's family after death, which seems to be more consistent with a masculine gender role. In most societies, men are expected to provide security to their families and provide the needed resource for raising off-spring and maintaining the welfare of family members. As a result, the observed finding implies that men seem to perceive death as a threat to their gender identity and to be especially anxious about the negative consequences that death has on the accomplishment of their gender-related tasks.

A person's history and current life circumstances also seem to contribute to his or her death-related concerns (Florian & Mikulincer, 1997a; Florian, Mikulincer, & Green, 1993; Mikulincer & Florian, 1995). For example, Florian et al. (1993) and Mikulincer and Florian (1995) found that the experience of recent stressful life events or personal losses (during the previous 3 years) was associated with more intense intrapersonal fears of death (e.g., loss of self-fulfillment) among middle-age men. Moreover, Mikulincer and Florian (1995) found that this fear was intensified by a person's reliance on emotion-focused coping strategies, such as rumination on worries and anxieties.

Along the same line of research, Florian and Mikulincer (1997a) found differential patterns of associations between early and recent losses of significant others and fear-of-death dimensions in a sample of young Israeli adults. On the one hand, the recent loss of a relationship partner (within the previous year) was associated with more intense fears of the intrapersonal and transpersonal consequences of death. On the other hand, loss of a parent during childhood was associated with more intense interpersonal fears of death (loss of social identity) in adulthood. This finding implies that early loss of a parent, which is a source of attachment insecurity and has negative long-term consequences for interpersonal functioning (Bowlby, 1973, 1980), may be generalized to fear of the interpersonal consequences of death. As Florian and Mikulincer (1997a) said, this attachment insecurity may become a major life motif that generalizes to a wide variety of situations, leading people to experience fear of death for the same reasons that they were distressed in the original attachment situation. Furthermore, this attachment security may prevent the use of close relationships as a means for managing the terror of death awareness, because commitment to these relationships can reactivate the pain caused by the loss of meaningful relationship partners and the consequent interpersonal death concern (see Mikulincer, Florian, & Hirschberger, Chapter 18, this volume, for a review).

Differential patterns of associations have also been found between personality traits and the three dimensions of the fear of personal death (Florian & Mikulincer, 1998a; Florian et al., 1993; Mikulincer, Florian, & Tolmacz, 1990). For example, Florian et al. (1993) reported complex associations between Minnesota Multiphasic Personality Inventory (MMPI) scales and FPDS scores in a middle-age sample. Whereas some MMPI scales (paranoia, psychasthenia, and schizophrenia) were associated with higher scores on all of the FPDS scales, implying a nonspecific association between signs of maladjustment and fear of death, other MMPI scales were associated only with specific FPDS scales. For example, the MMPI masculinity–femininity scale was associated with higher fear of the consequences of death for family and friends, and the MMPI defensiveness and social introversion scales were associated with higher fear of loss of social identity after death. In another study, Florian and Mikulincer (1998a) found that the sense of symbolic immortality (Lifton, 1979)—a transformational, constructive belief that although not solving the unsolvable problem of death, leads a person to invest in his or her children's care and to engage in creative, growth-oriented activities whose products will live on after the person dies—was associated with less intense fears of the intrapersonal and interpersonal consequences of death but made no protective contribution to the transpersonal fears of death.

Based on theoretical analyses highlighting the relevance of attachment theory to death anxiety (Kalish, 1985; McCarthy, 1981), Mikulincer et al. (1990) and Florian and Mikulincer (1998a) examined the contribution of a person's attachment style—relatively stable patterns of relational cognitions, emotions, and behavior (Hazan & Shaver, 1987)—to the three dimensions of the fear of personal death. Findings revealed theoretically coherent attachment-style differences. On the one hand, attachment-anxious persons (people who chronically worry about rejection and abandonment and possess negative mental models of the self in close relationships) tend to report relatively high levels of the fear of loss of social identity after death. On the other hand, attachment-avoidant persons (people who prefer emotional distance from relationship partners, possess negative mental models of others, and emphasize self-reliance) tend to report relatively high levels of fear of the unknown nature of the hereafter. These findings seem to be a direct reflection of a person's habitual attachment-related strategies of affect regulation (Mikulincer & Shaver, 2003). Anxious people habitually magnify worries about rejection and others' unavailability (Mikulincer & Shaver, 2003) and hence view death as yet another relational setting in which they may be abandoned and forgotten. Avoidant individuals habitually try to remain self-reliant in order to avoid the frustration of their attachment needs (Mikulincer & Shaver, 2003). They are therefore particularly afraid of the uncertain and unknown aspects of death that threaten their sense of control and mastery. That is, insecurely attached people fear death for the same reasons they are distressed in attachment contexts (e.g., rejection and loss of control).

Beyond clarifying the contribution of personal, cultural, and contextual factors to the fear of personal death, Florian's multidimensional approach also helps us understand the ways in which people cope with the terror of death awareness. According to TMT (Greenberg et al., 1997), reminding people of their own death (inducing mortality salience) increases the terror of death awareness and activates cognitive and behavioral efforts aimed at validating predominant cultural worldviews as a means of managing anxiety. Despite strong empirical support for this hypothesis (see Greenberg et al., 1997, for a review), Florian's multidimensional approach can elaborate and refine this simple causal pathway by incorporating the diverse components of fear of personal death into the equation. In fact, people differ in the meanings they attach to death, so the effects of mortality salience may depend on the extent to which death reminders increase awareness to the predominant component of death anxiety that characterizes a person. Moreover, the anxiety-buffering effect of cultural worldviews may also depend on the extent to which these worldviews touch on the basic concerns that underlie a person's fear of death.

Following this line of reasoning, Florian and Mikulincer (1997b) hypothesized that the activation of worldview defenses following a mortality salience induction is not as simple as TMT had suggested. Rather, such activation may depend on three factors: (1) a person's predominant fear of death (intrapersonal, interpersonal, transpersonal), (2) the specific component of the fear of death that is elicited by a death reminder, and (3) the specific component of this fear that is buffered by the validation of a cultural worldview. Specifically, mortality salience should heighten a person's efforts to validate a cultural worldview when this induction increases awareness of a person's predominant fear of death and defense of this worldview buffers the predominant fear of death. When death reminders increase awareness of components of fear of death that do not characterize a particular person, or the targeted cultural worldview does not touch on the concerns that underlie a person's predominant fear of death, death reminders should not heighten a person's efforts to validate this worldview. In such cases, terror management mechanisms should not be activated despite the induction of mortality salience.

To examine this complex hypothesis, Florian and Mikulincer (1997b, Study 2) designed an experiment in which they attempted to replicate a previously observed cultural worldview defense—the heightening of negative reactions to social transgressors following a mortality salience induction (Rosenblatt, Greenberg, Solomon, Pyszczynski, & Lyon, 1989). Unlike Rosenblatt et al. (1989), however, Florian and Mikulincer (1997b) assessed a person's predominant fear of death (intrapersonal, interpersonal), constructed specific death reminders that impinged upon either intrapersonal or interpersonal components of the fear of death, and constructed specific social transgressions that were relevant to either intrapersonal or interpersonal components of this fear. Specifically, participants completed the FPDS, and variations along the intrapersonal and interpersonal dimensions were assessed. Participants were then randomly divided into three conditions in which (1) intrapersonal components of death, (2) interpersonal components of death, or (3) a neutral theme (control condition) were made salient. Following a distracting task, participants rated the severity of social transgressions that were described as having either intrapersonal consequences on the body and self of the victim or interpersonal consequences on the social identity and family of the victims.

Florian and Mikulincer's (1997b) findings indicated that mortality salience led to higher severity ratings of social transgressions than did a control condition only (1) when people who were predominantly afraid of the intrapersonal consequences of death were exposed to a reminder of this specific fear and were asked to judge transgressions that have direct personal effects on the body and self of the victim and (2) when people who were predominantly afraid of the interpersonal consequences of death were exposed to a reminder of this specific fear and were asked to judge transgressions that have direct interpersonal repercussions on the social identity and family of the victim. These findings seem to imply that terror management mechanisms are mainly activated when there was a fit between the particular aspect of death that was made salient, the aspect of death that people most feared, and the type of judged transgression. Alternatively, they can also imply that people differ in their sensitivity to different aspects of the worldview that are used to provide protection and that the fit between this sensitivity and the contextual death reminders channel the direction in which people go to cope with death awareness.

Overall, the reviewed findings emphasize the importance of a multidimensional approach to the fear of death and the need to assess not only the intensity of a person's global and undifferentiated fear but also the diverse meanings he or she attaches to death. These meanings seem to determine a person's unique profile of death concerns and are crucial for delineating the contribution of cultural, personal, and contextual factors to the fear of personal death as well as explaining individual variations in the activation of terror management responses following death reminders.

HOW IS THE FEAR OF PERSONAL DEATH EXPRESSED?

Beyond advocating a multidimensional conceptualization of the fear of death, Thanatos psychology has emphasized the need for a multilevel conceptualization of this fear in order to delineate the expressions of death concerns at different levels of awareness (e.g., Kastenbaum, 2000; Neimeyer, 1997; Tomer, 2000). That is, people can express death concerns at different levels of awareness, and these concerns can differ when they are expressed in conscious self-reports or below the threshold of awareness. Furthermore, cultural, personal, and contextual factors can have different effects on conscious death concerns and unconscious expressions of these concerns, and this multilevel approach can be highly relevant for understanding the psychological effects of death reminders and the consequent activation of terror management mechanisms.

This multilevel approach is based on cognitive theories that have proposed that thoughts and concerns can be active and expressed at different levels of awareness (e.g., Wegner, 1994). A thought is "active" above the level of awareness if people can report that they are mentally occupied with the thought in question. That is, a thought is "active" if it is present in a person's stream of consciousness. A thought is "active" below the level of awareness if it is cognitively accessible—that is, ready to be used in information processing or physiologically accessible (i.e., is influencing autonomic, physiological activity). This definition implies that a thought can be brought to mind and can influence cognitive and physiological activities before one recognizes it in one's stream of consciousness (Wegner & Smart, 1997). In such cases, the extent to which a thought biases one's representations of the self and the world and one's interpretations of relevant stimuli, or influences plans, behaviors, or physiological responses, is indicative of the activation of that thought below the level of awareness.

The multilevel approach to fear of death is also based on Thanatos psychology and TMT explanations of the ways people defend against the fear of death (e.g., Greeenberg et al., 1997; Kastenbaum, 2000). These theories propose that the paralyzing terror produced by the awareness of one's mortality leads to the denial of death awareness and the repression of death-related thoughts. That is, denial and repression should be important defenses against the fear of personal death, even in people who typically use other defense mechanisms to cope with more mundane sources of fear and anxiety. As a result, the adoption of a single-level approach that focuses on the assessment of conscious death concerns can lead to faulty conclusions. Denial and repression can hold these concerns out of awareness, but the repressed material can still be active below the level of awareness and can unconsciously influence cognition, affect, and behavior. This account emphasizes the need to assess both conscious and unconscious manifestations of death concerns, because large discrepancies can exist between these manifestations. Some death concerns that cannot be found in a person's conscious self-reports may still appear below the level of awareness.

The multilevel approach has led to the development of a wide variety of implicit measures (see Kastenbaum, 2000; Neimeyer, 1997, for reviews). These measures include the assessment of physiological signs of autonomic arousal (e.g., galvanic skin responses and heart rate) following exposure to death-related stimuli (e.g., Alexander & Adlerstein, 1959); the use of the Stroop color-naming task to examine interference with the naming of the color in which death-related words are printed (e.g., Feifel & Branscomb, 1973; Feifel & Nagy, 1981); the use of word-completion tasks that assess the number of death-related words a person produces when confronted with ambiguous word fragments (e.g., Arndt, Greenberg, Pyszczynski, Solomon, & Simon, 1997; Greenberg, Pyszczynski, Solomon, Simon, & Breus, 1994; Mikulincer & Florian, 2000); and the content analysis of nightmares (e.g., Feldman & Hersen, 1967). With a few exceptions (e.g., Lester, 1968; Templer, 1971), most of the studies that have compared these measures to conscious self-reports of fear of death have uncovered stronger fear of death below the level of awareness than in conscious self-reports. These studies provide support for the defensive action of denial and repression.

Unfortunately, although these studies have embodied a multilevel approach to the study of death anxiety, most of them have assessed this fear of death in a simplistic, unidimensional manner. Not only do they fail to acknowledge that conscious fear of death is a multidimensional construct, but they also ignore that there are a wide variety of unconscious indicators of fear of death. To integrate the multidimensional and multilevel perspectives on fear of death, Florian and his colleagues (Florian et al. 1984; Mikulincer et al., 1990; Ungar, Florian, & Zernitsky-Shurka, 1990) have attempted to delineate the underlying dimensions that organize the unconscious indicators of death concerns and to examine associations between these dimensions and the dimensional structure of more conscious expressions of the fear of personal death.

For example, Florian et al. (1984) constructed a multidimensional scale for analyzing a person's responses to Thematic Apperception Task (TAT) cards that are known to elicit a relatively large percentage of death responses. Specifically, participants were asked to tell stories concerning the following four TAT cards: (1) 3BW—a boy reclining next to a gun-like object; (2) 8GF—two women huddled on a flight of stairs; (3) 15—a person in a cemetery; and (4) 5—a woman entering a room. Participants' stories were then content analyzed in order to examine the extent to which death-related thoughts were expressed in the stories, as well as the emotional and coping responses elicited by these thoughts. The content analysis yielded six highly reliable scales:

1. Centrality of death—the degree to which death plays a central role throughout the TAT stories.
2. Depression—the degree of unhappiness, helplessness, and apathy a person expresses in the TAT stories in response to death-related concerns.
3. Anxiety—the degree of discomfort, dismay, and apprehension a person expresses in the TAT stories in response to death-related concerns.
4. Aggression—the degree of anger, hostility, and aggression a person expresses in the TAT stories in response to death-related concerns.
5. Guilt—the degree of remorse, unconditional assumption of responsibility, and anger directed toward the self expressed in the TAT stories.
6. Denial—the degree to which the TAT stories include attempts to inhibit or limit the expression of death-related concerns and their accompanying emotions.

Florian et al. (1984) subjected the six scales to a multidimensional scale analysis and revealed that they were organized around two general dimensions. One dimension concerns the type of emotional reactions revealed in death concerns below the level of awareness. This dimension runs from internalization and projection of anger (guilt and aggression scales), at one end, to the expression of unhappiness and discomfort (anxiety and depression scales). The second dimension concerns the extent to which death concerns are freely expressed at the implicit, unconscious level. This dimension runs from attempts to limit and inhibit the expression of below-awareness death concerns (denial) to the identification and magnification of these concerns (death centrality). This two-dimensional structure suggests that implicit death concerns can be freely expressed or subjected to some degree of inhibition and that these concerns can elicit a sense of resentment and hostility or a sense of helplessness and vulnerability. Subsequent studies have replicated this two-dimensional structure of implicit expressions of fear of death (Mikulincer et al. 1990; Ungar et al., 1990).

This multidimensional analysis provides important information about individual differences in implicit expressions of the fear of death as well as the complex ways in which these expressions are related to conscious death concerns. For example, Florian et al. (1984) reported that commitment to religious beliefs was positively associated with the centrality of death, anxiety, and guilt in TAT stories, and that the association between conscious and unconscious death concerns was not straightforward and could not be entirely explained simply in terms of denial and repression. Specifically, for religious people there were positive associations between implicit expressions of fear of death (centrality of death, anxiety, and guilt) and conscious reports of the fear of punishment in the hereafter. At the same time, however, these people produced inverse associations between implicit expressions and conscious reports of intrapersonal and interpersonal fears of death. This pattern of findings implies that religious commitment is related to a heightened specific sensitivity to some aspects of death at different levels of awareness and to denial of conscious concerns about the intrapersonal and interpersonal consequences of death.

In their study of attachment-style differences in the fear of personal death, Mikulincer et al. (1990) also found that a multidimensional–multilevel approach was extremely useful for delineating the complex manifestations of insecure attachment orientations in conscious and unconscious death concerns. Whereas both attachment-anxious and attachment-avoidant individuals exhibited higher centrality of death and anxiety in their responses to death-eliciting TAT cards than did more securely attached individuals, the two insecure groups differed greatly in the observed association between conscious and unconscious death concerns. On the one hand, attachment-anxious persons showed a positive association between implicit expressions of fear of death and conscious reports of this fear. On the other hand, attachment-avoidant persons showed an inverse association between these two levels of awareness. These different patterns of association fit the way anxious and avoidant people generally deal with fears and threats (Mikulincer & Shaver, 2003). Whereas attachment-anxious persons tend to hyperactivate their fears and have free access to them at different levels of awareness, attachment-avoidant persons tend to repress their fears and prevent their intrusion into consciousness.

In a recent study, we examined the usefulness of a multidimensional–multilevel approach for delineating individual variations in the activation of terror management mechanisms following a mortality salience induction. Specifically, we asked whether a person's responses to death-eliciting TAT cards can moderate the effects of a mortality salience induction on the rated severity of social transgressions. In the first session of a two-session study, 60 Israeli undergraduates provided stories about four death-eliciting TAT cards (also used by Florian et al., 1984), and we computed their scores on the six scales described previously. In the second session, conducted some weeks later by another experimenter who was blind to participants' TAT scores, participants were randomly divided into two conditions: a mortality salience condition ($N = 30$), and a control condition in which physical pain was made salient ($N = 30$). This manipulation was based on the two open-ended questions used in Rosenblatt et al.'s (1989) study. Following a distracting task, all the participants rated the severity of 10 social transgressions (Florian & Mikulincer, 1997b).

The data were analyzed with two-step hierarchical regressions in which the rated severity of the transgressions (average rating across the 10 transgressions, alpha = .89) served as the dependent variable. In the first step, we examined the main effects of mortality salience (a dummy variable comparing mortality salience with physical pain salience) and each of the six TAT scales. In the second step, we examined interactions between mortality salience and each of the six TAT scales.

The findings revealed the moderating effects of implicit manifestations of fear of death. Significant effects were found for the mortality salience × centrality of death interaction, beta = .32, $p < .05$, and the mortality salience × anxiety interaction, beta = .35, $p < .05$. Examination of the significant interactions (using Aiken & West's, 1991, procedure) revealed that the regression for severity ratings predicted by mortality salience was significant when centrality of death was one standard deviation above the mean, beta = .49, $p < .01$, but not when this TAT score was one standard deviation below the mean, beta = .04. Moreover, mortality salience had a significant effect on severity ratings when TAT anxiety was one standard deviation above the mean, beta = .53, $p < .01$, but not when TAT anxiety was one standard deviation below the mean, beta = .06. That is, the induction of mortality sa-lience, as compared to the physical pain salience condition, led people to make more severe judgments of social transgressions mainly when they exhibited intense implicit expressions of death anxiety and the theme of death was central to their unconscious fantasies. When these implicit indicators of death concerns were not so intense, participants were less affected by death reminders and showed no observable terror management responses.

Overall, these findings highlight the importance of assessing and analyzing expressions of the fear of personal death that occur below the level of awareness. These expressions are complexly related to conscious death concerns and seem to regulate terror management re-sponses to heightened mortality salience.

HOW IS THE PHENOMENON OF DEATH CONCEPTUALIZED?

Beyond examining the multidimensional–multilevel manifestations of death concerns, Florian and his colleagues have devoted theoretical and empirical efforts to the study of how people conceptualize death, how these mental representations are affected by cultural and personal factors, and how they are related to death concerns and terror management re-sponses. These studies have shown that the subjective conceptualization of death is ex-tremely relevant for understanding variations in death concerns and the ways in which people attempt to manage these concerns.

The Formal Conceptualization of Death

From a formal, objective perspective, death is an irreversible outcome of natural processes, and a "mature" concept of death should include the recognition that death is an inevitable, universal, and irreversible phenomenon that can be caused by a wide variety of personal and environmental factors (Florian, 1985). However, this concept of death is the product of cog-nitive development. In a pioneering study, Nagy (1948) delineated three developmental stages. Children in the preschool years have a low understanding of the universality, irre-versibility, and inevitability of death. Children ages 5–9 tend to personify death and view it as avoidable but irreversible if one is not swift enough to avoid getting caught. Only at the third stage (ages 9–10) do children come to recognize death as a universal, inevitable, and irreversible phenomenon.

Following up Nagy's pioneering study, Florian (1985) examined the development of the concept of death from pre-kindergarten to first grade in a sample of Israeli children and once again found a gradual increase with age in the understanding the irreversibility and in-evitability of death. This finding has now been replicated in studies conducted in different Western countries (e.g., Smilansky, 1987; Speece & Brent, 1992; Wenestam & Wass, 1987). The critical stage in the development of the concept of death seems to be Piaget's (1955) stage of concrete operations (ages 7–11). At the beginning of this stage, children lack the cognitive ability to grasp the abstract concepts of universality, irreversibility, and inevitabil-ity of death. During the school years, children gradually acquire a realistic recognition of death as a natural, irreversible process that leads to the cessation of life (Speece & Brent, 1992).

Beyond this developmental process, Florian and Kravetz (1985) claimed that a child's physical and cultural environment influence his or her representation of death. In fact, cul-tures that emphasize ideas of divine purpose and reincarnation can inhibit the development of the view of death as an irreversible outcome of natural processes (Bowlby, 1980). In support of this view, Florian and Kravetz (1985) assessed beliefs about irreversibility, finality, causality, and inevitability of death in a sample of 10-year-old Israeli children and found that religion influenced the strength of these beliefs. Specifically, Moslem and Druze children received lower scores on scales measuring these beliefs about death than did their Jewish and Christian counterparts. This finding implies that religion and other related cultural and social factors, which influence the content and process of socialization, are also highly relevant for understanding the way people conceptualize death.

Individual variations in the development of the concept of death are also critical for delineating the psychological effects of death reminders. In fact, Solomon Greenberg, and Pyszczynski (1991) suggested that a person is terrified by death only when he or she is intelligent enough to know that death is inevitable. Following up this idea, Florian and Mikulincer (1998b) hypothesized that death reminders would activate terror management mechanisms only when the meaning of one's death is fully understood. Before reaching a mature understanding of death, the encounter with death may not necessarily lead to the experience of anxiety, and thereby to the activation of cultural anxiety buffers. Unable to fully conceptualize death, young children may not show clear and overt signs of fear of death. Only when children know that death is inevitable, universal, and irreversible (around ages 10–11), do they become afraid of death (Wenestam & Wass, 1997). At this stage, mortality salience should activate terror management mechanisms.

To examine this hypothesis, Florian and Mikulincer (1998b) exposed two theoretically relevant age groups of Israeli children (7-year-olds and 11-year-olds) to a mortality salience or neutral condition and then assessed the activation of a cultural anxiety buffer—ingroup favoritism and derogation of outgroup members (Greenberg et al., 1997). In addition, children completed the Death Concept Scale (Smilansky, 1987), which assessed beliefs about the irreversibility, universality, and inevitability of death.

We discovered that only 11-year-old children, who had a fairly mature concept of death, reacted to mortality salience in ways similar to those shown by adults in previous TMT studies (Greenberg et al., 1997). That is, mortality salience increased 11-year-old children's tendency to protect their cultural worldview by socially accepting an ingroup child and rejecting an outgroup child. Seven-year-old children, who were less certain about the irreversibility, universality, and inevitability of death, did not rate an ingroup child more positively when mortality was made salient. However, the findings did not imply that mortality salience had no effect among 7-year-olds. In fact, mortality salience led them to react more negatively to both ingroup and outgroup children. It seems that both age groups are affected by death reminders but that 7-years-olds, who had an immature concept of death, fail to activate the more adult-like form of worldview defense. Alternatively, the lack of differentiated reactions to the target groups might reflect that 7-year-old children do not have a mature concept of cultural worldviews or a well-defined need to preserve the ingroup value system.

Informal, Personal Conceptions of Death: Death Personified

The concept of death includes not only formal beliefs about its universality, irreversibility, and inevitability but also less formal, more metaphoric and associative representations. Often, death is conceptualized as a creature or person. Kastenbaum and Aisenberg (1972) claimed that these representations enable a person to imagine death in an idiosyncratic, subjective manner that helps him or her "come to terms" with mortality.

Kastenbaum and Aisenberg (1972) distinguished among four major types or portraits of death that people construe when asked how they perceive or imagine death. The first type is the "macabre" personification, visualized as physically repulsive and decaying. This personification is viewed as a bitter enemy of life and is sensed as being emotionally close to the person describing it. The second type is the "gentle comforter," visualized as wise, reassuring, quiet, powerful, sympathetic, and understanding. The third type is the "automaton," which has a human appearance but no emotions and does not establish a close relationship with the person describing it. The fourth type is the "gay deceiver," visualized as a few years older than the respondent, attractive, and sophisticated, and as promising pleasures but being deceptive. Kastenbaum and Aisenberg (1972) also claim that people differ in the sex they attribute to death, with some persons visualizing it as a man and others as a woman.

Some studies have found gender differences in the personification of death. For example, McClelland (1963) observed that women more than men tend to visualize death as a "gay seducer." Greenberger (1965) observed that more women than men assign a sexual meaning to death, libidinize death, and produce fantasies of illicit sexuality. Papageorgis (1966) failed to replicate these findings but found that men more than women used metaphors of death reflecting mutilation and injury. In his view, this finding supports psychoanalytic writings that symbolically equate fear of death with castration anxiety (Sarnoff & Cowin, 1959).

Following this line of research, Weller, Florian, and Tenenbaum (1988) examined individual differences in the extent to which the concept of death is personified with masculine and feminine attributes. They asked Israeli undergraduates to complete the Bem Sex-Role Inventory (Bem, 1974) and to rate the extent to which they use each of the feminine and masculine traits appearing in the inventory to describe death. The authors found that participants were more likely to use masculine than feminine traits for describing their death and that this pattern of response was stronger in women than in men. Specifically, participants considered death to have the following masculine traits: forceful, dominant, independent, decisive, and authoritative. The least salient attributes of death were feminine: cheerful, likable, and smiling. This pattern of findings fits the masculine personification of death characteristic of modern Western societies (e.g., the "Grim Reaper"; Kastenbaum, 2000).

In a recent study, we examined the possible effects of personifications of death on the activation of terror management mechanisms following death reminders. Specifically, we asked whether individual variations in the personification of death moderate the effects of a mortality salience induction on the rated severity of social transgressions. In the first session of a two-session study, 60 Israeli undergraduates provided open-ended descriptions of how they perceived or imagined death. Each participant's description was then content analyzed and assigned to one of Kastenbaum and Aisenberg's (1972) four categories: macabre, gentle comforter, automaton, and gay deceiver. Most of the participants' descriptions fit the macabre personification ($N = 35$). Eighteen participants' descriptions fit the gentle comforter personification, five participants described death as an automaton, and two personified death as a gay deceiver. Given this uneven distribution, we decided to focus on the two most frequently mentioned categories and to drop the seven participants who described death as an automaton or gay deceiver. That is, only the 53 participants who held macabre or gentle comforter personifications of death were invited to the second session of the study.

In the second session, conducted some weeks later by another experimenter who was blind to participants' death personifications, participants were randomly divided into two conditions: a mortality salience condition ($N = 27$) and a control condition in which dental pain was made salient (N = 26). This manipulation was based on the two open questions used in Rosenblatt et al.'s (1989) study. Following a distracting task, participants rated the severity of 10 transgressions (Florian & Mikulincer, 1997b).

The data were analyzed with a two-way analysis of variance, with mortality salience (yes, no) and death personification (macabre, gentle comforter) serving as the independent variables. The dependent variable was the rated severity of the transgressions (average rating across the 10 transgressions; alpha = .91). We obtained a significant interaction between mortality salience and death personification, F (1,49) = 4.54, p < .05. A test for simple main effects revealed that the mortality salience induction led to more severe ratings of social transgressions than the dental pain control condition only among persons who personified death in macabre terms (M = 5.76, SD = 0.75 vs. M = 4.64, SD = 0.77). This difference was not significant among persons who personified death as a gentle comforter (M = 4.84, SD = 0.87 for mortality salience, M = 4.73, SD = 0.95 for dental pain salience). That is, the activation of terror management mechanisms following death reminders seemed to depend on the visualization of death as repulsive and anxiety arousing. The visualization of death as reassuring and understanding may have some comforting and calming effect that makes less necessary the activation of cultural anxiety buffers in response to death reminders. Overall, these findings reveal the importance of death personifications to the activation of terror management mechanisms.

CONCLUSION

The theoretical and empirical work of Florian and his colleagues has radically changed the study of death anxiety from a simple, unidimensional approach to a complex, multifaceted approach organized around three meaning dimensions, expressed at multiple levels of awareness and cognitively represented in a wide variety of ways. Furthermore, this work has helped build a bridge between TMT and Thanatos psychology. On the one hand, Thanatos psychology focused mainly on the nature of the human fear of death as a dependent variable that might be influenced by other psychological and sociological factors but had not paid enough attention to the possible cognitive and behavioral implications of the encounter with death. On the other hand, TMT studies have focused mainly on the effects of death reminders, treated as independent variables that have important ramifications for a wide variety of social attitudes, cognitions, and behaviors. TMT researchers had largely overlooked the complex nature of the fear of death and the way the diverse facets of this fear can moderate the psychological effects of death reminders. The work by Florian and colleagues facilitates integration of these two main lines of scientific inquiry. It provides solid theoretical and empirical foundations for the assessment and understanding of the diverse facets of the fear of personal death as a dependent variable and at the same time reveals the roles played by these facets in regulating the activation of terror management mechanisms and moderating the psychological consequences of death reminders.

ACKNOWLEDGMENT

This chapter was completed near the time of Victor Florian's death. He contributed a great deal to the ideas and research summarized herein.

REFERENCES

Aiken, L. S., & West, S. G. (1991). *Multiple regressions: Testing and interpreting interactions.* Newbury Park, CA: Sage.

Alexander, I. E., & Adlerstein, A. N. (1959). Death and religion. In H. Feifel (Ed.), *The meaning of death* (pp. 97–123). New York: McGraw-Hill.

Arndt, J., Greenberg, J., Pyszczynski, T., Solomon, S., & Simon, L. (1997). Suppression, accessibility of death-related thoughts, and cultural worldview defense: Exploring the psychodynamics of terror management. *Journal of Personality and Social Psychology, 73,* 5–18.

Bem, S. L. (1974). The measurement of psychological androgyny. *Journal of Consulting and Clinical Psychology, 47,* 155–162.

Bowlby, J. (1973). *Attachment and loss: Separation, anxiety and anger.* New York: Basic Books.

Bowlby, J. (1980). *Attachment and loss: Sadness and depression.* New York: Basic Books.

Cameron, P. (1968). The imminence of death. *Journal of Consulting and Clinical Psychology, 32,* 479–481.

Collett, L. J., & Lester, D. (1969). The fear of death and the fear of dying. *Journal of Psychology, 72,* 179–181.

Dickstein, L. (1972). Death concern: Measurement and correlates. *Psychological Reports, 30,* 563–571.

Durlak, J. A. (1972). Measurement of the fear of death: An examination of some existing scales. *Journal of Clinical Psychology, 28,* 545–547.

Durlak, J. A. (1973). Relationship between various measures of death concern and fear of death. *Journal of Consulting and Clinical Psychology, 41,* 162–168.

Feifel, H. (1977). *New meanings of death.* New York: McGraw-Hill.

Feifel, H., & Branscomb, A. B. (1973). Who's afraid of death? *Journal of Abnormal Psychology, 81,* 282–288.

Feifel, H., & Nagy, V. T. (1981). Another look at fear of death. *Journal of Consulting and Clinical Psychology, 54,* 479–481.

Feldman, M. J., & Hersen, M. (1967). Attitudes toward death in nightmare subjects. *Journal of Abnormal Psychology, 72,* 421–425.

Florian, V. (1979). *Personal fear of death as expressed among religious and non-religious Jewish groups.* Unpublished doctoral dissertation, Bar-Ilan University, Ramat Gan, Israel.

Florian, V. (1985). Children's concept of death: An empirical study of a cognitive and environmental approach. *Death Studies, 9,* 133–141.

Florian, V., & Har-Even, D. (1983). Fear of personal death: The effects of sex and religious beliefs. *Omega, 14,* 83–91.

Florian, V., & Kravetz, S. (1983). Fear of personal death: attribution, structure, and relation to religious belief. *Journal of Personality and Social Psychology, 44,* 600–607.

Florian, V., & Kravetz, S. (1985). Children's concept of death. *Journal of Cross-Cultural Psychology, 16,* 174–189.

Florian, V., Kravetz, S., & Frankel, J. (1984). Aspects of fear of personal death, levels of awareness, and religious commitment. *Journal of Research in Personality, 18,* 289–304.

Florian, V., & Mikulincer, M. (1992). The impact of death-risk experiences and religiosity on the fear of personal death: The case of Israeli soldiers in Lebanon. *Omega, 26,* 101–111.

Florian, V., & Mikulincer, M. (1997a). Fear of personal death in adulthood: The impact of early and recent losses. *Death Studies, 21,* 1–24.

Florian, V., & Mikulincer, M. (1997b). Fear of death and the judgment of social transgressions: A multidimensional test of terror management theory. *Journal of Personality and Social Psychology, 73,* 369–380.

Florian, V., & Mikulincer, M. (1998a). Symbolic immortality and the management of the terror of death—The moderating role of attachment style. *Journal of Personality and Social Psychology, 74,* 725–734.

Florian, V., & Mikulincer, M. (1998b). Terror management in childhood: Does death conceptualization moderate the effects of mortality salience on acceptance of similar and different others? *Personality and Social Psychology Bulletin, 24*, 1104–1112.

Florian, V., Mikulincer, M., & Green, E. (1993). Fear of personal death and the MMPI profile of middle-age men: The moderating impact of personal losses. *Omega, 28*, 151–164.

Florian, V., & Snowden, L. (1989). Fear of personal death and positive life regard: A study of different ethnic and religious-affiliated American college students. *Journal of Cross-Cultural Psychology, 20*, 64–79.

Greenberg, J., Pyszczynski, T., & Solomon, S. (1997). Terror management theory of self-esteem and cultural worldviews: Empirical assessments and conceptual refinements. In P. M. Zanna (Ed.), *Advances in experimental social psychology* (Vol. 29, pp. 61–141). San Diego: Academic Press.

Greenberg, J., Pyszczynski, T., Solomon, S., Simon, L., & Breus, M. (1994). The role of consciousness and accessibility of death related thoughts in mortality salience effects. *Journal of Personality and Social Psychology, 67*, 627–637.

Greenberger, E. (1965). Fantasies of women confronting death. *Journal of Consulting Psychology, 29*, 252–260.

Hazan, C., & Shaver, P. R. (1987). Romantic love conceptualized as an attachment process. *Journal of Personality and Social Psychology, 52*, 511–524.

Hoelter, J. (1979). Multidimensional treatment of fear of death. *Journal of Consulting and Clinical Psychology, 47*, 996–999.

Kalish, R. A. (1985). *Death, grief, and caring relationships.* New York: Cole.

Kastenbaum, R. (2000). *The psychology of death* (3rd ed.). New York: Springer.

Kastenbaum, R., & Aisenberg, I. (1972). *The psychology of death.* New York: Springer.

Kastenbaum, R., & Costa, P. T. (1977). Psychological perspectives on death. *Annual Review of Psychology, 28*, 225–249.

Lester, D. (1968). The fear of death of those who have nightmares. *Journal of Psychology, 69*, 245–247.

Lester, D. (1971). Attitudes towards death today and thirty-five years ago. *Omega, 2*, 168–174.

Lifton, R. J. (1979). *The broken connection.* New York: Simon & Schuster.

McClelland, D. C. (1963). The harlequin complex. In R. White (Ed.), *The study of lives* (pp. 95–119). New York: Prentice-Hall.

McCarthy, J. (1981). *Death and anxiety.* New York: Academic Press.

Mikulincer, M., & Florian, V. (1995). Stress, coping, and fear of personal death: The case of middle-aged men facing early job retirement. *Death Studies, 19*, 413–431.

Mikulincer, M., & Florian, V. (2000). Exploring individual differences in reactions to mortality salience: Does attachment style regulate terror management mechanisms? *Journal of Personality and Social Psychology, 79*, 260–273.

Mikulincer, M., Florian, V., & Tolmacz, R. (1990). Attachment styles and fear of personal death: A case study of affect regulation. *Journal of Personality and Social Psychology, 58*, 273–280.

Mikulincer, M., & Shaver, P. R. (2003). The attachment behavioral system in adulthood: Activation, psychodynamics, and interpersonal processes. In M. P. Zanna (Ed.), *Advances in experimental social psychology* (Vol. 35, pp. 53–152). San Diego: Academic Press.

Minton, R., & Spilka, B. (1976). Perspectives on death in relation to powerlessness and form of personal religion. *Omega, 7*, 261–268.

Murphy, C. (1959). Discussion. In H. Feifel (Ed.), *The meaning of death* (pp. 129–138). New York: McGraw-Hill.

Nagy, M. (1948). The child's theories concerning death. *Journal of Genetic Psychology, 73*, 3–27.

Neimeyer, R. A. (1997). Death anxiety research: The state of the art. *Omega, 36*, 97–120.

Nelson, L. D., & Nelson, C. C. (1975). A factor analytic inquiry into the multidimensionality of death anxiety. *Omega, 6*, 171–178.

Papageorgis, G. (1966). On the ambivalence of death. The case of the missing harlequin. *Psychological Reports, 19*, 325–326.

Piaget, J. (1955). *The child's conception of the world.* Towota, NJ: Littlefield Adams.

Pollak, J. M. (1979). Correlates of death anxiety: A review of empirical studies. *Omega, 10*, 97–121.

Rosenblatt, A., Greenberg, J., Solomon, S., Pyszczynski, T., & Lyon, D. (1989). Evidence for terror management theory I: The effects of mortality salience on reactions to those who violate or uphold cultural values. *Journal of Personality and Social Psychology, 57*, 681–690.

Sarnoff, I., & Corwin, S. M. (1959). Castration anxiety and fear of death. *Journal of Personality, 27*, 374–385.

Schulz, R. (1978). *The psychology of death, dying, and bereavement.* Reading, MA: Addison-Wesley.

Smilansky, S. (1987). *On death: Helping children understand and cope.* New York: Peter Lang.

Solomon, S., Greenberg, J., & Pyszczynski, T. (1991). A terror management theory of social behavior: The psychological functions of self-esteem and cultural worldviews. In L. Berkowitz (Ed.), *Advances in experimental social psychology* (Vol. 24, pp. 93–159). New York: Academic Press.

Speece, M. W., & Brent, S. B. (1992). The acquisition of a mature understanding of three components of the concept of death. *Death Studies, 16*, 211–229.

Templer, D. I. (1970). The construction and validation of a death anxiety scale. *Journal of General Psychology, 82*, 165–174.

Templer, D. I. (1971). Relationship between verbalized and non-verbalized death anxiety. *Journal of Genetic Psychology, 119*, 211–214.

Templer, D. I. (1972). Death anxiety in religiously very involved persons. *Psychological Reports, 31*, 361–362.

Tomer, A. (2000). *Death attitudes and the older adult: Theories, concepts, and applications.* New York: Brunner-Routledge.

Ungar, L., Florian, V., & Zernitsky-Shurka, E. (1990). Aspects of fear of personal death, levels of awareness, and professional affiliation among dialysis unit staff members. *Omega, 21*, 51–67.

Wegner, D. M. (1994). Ironic processes of mental control. *Psychological Review, 101*, 34–52.

Wegner, D. M., & Smart, L. (1997). Deep cognitive activation: A new approach to the unconscious. *Journal of Consulting and Clinical Psychology, 65*, 984–995.

Weller, A., Florian, V., & Tenenbaum, R. (1988). The concept of death—"Masculine" and "feminine" attributes. *Omega, 19*, 253–263.

Wenestam, C. G., & Wass, H. (1987). Swedish and U.S. children's thinking about death: A qualitative study and cross-cultural comparison. *Death Studies, 11*, 99–121.

Chapter 5

The Beast within the Beauty

An Existential Perspective on the Objectification and Condemnation of Women

JAMIE L. GOLDENBERG
TOMI-ANN ROBERTS

> Every human being must wrestle with nature. But nature's burden falls more heavily on one sex.
>
> —CAMILLE PAGLIA, *Sexual Personae* (1990, p. 9)

> In women are incarnated disturbing mysteries of nature. . . . In woman dressed and adorned, nature is present but under restraint, by human will remolded and nearer to man's desire. A woman is rendered more desirable to the extent that nature is more . . . rigorously confined.
>
> —SIMONE DE BEAUVOIR, *The Second Sex* (1952, pp. 84, 179)

Throughout the history of the sexes, women have been perceived as inferior to men, but also have been elevated to the status of goddesses on earth. We suggest that these paradoxical biases often associated with women can be linked to an existential need to distance humanity from the natural world. The sources of discrimination against women are most commonly associated with their biological nature. For example, women are devalued for being more emotional than men, less rational, physically weaker, and at the mercy of their bodies' natural menstrual cycles and physical changes during pregnancy. On the flip side, when women are held in highest esteem they are typically stripped of their natural qualities—adorned, sanitized, deodorized, and denuded—becoming "objects" of beauty and even worship.

In this chapter we provide initial evidence for our proposition that women's "nature" plays a critical role in societal attitudes and behaviors toward women, and that these reactions to feminine nature are at least in part a result of existential concerns associated with the awareness of our vulnerability toward death. To explain why this connection between "man" and nature has disproportionately affected reactions toward women, we propose integration of an *existential perspective* that emphasizes threats associated with women's childbearing and menstruating bodies and with men's animalistic attraction to them, with a *feminist perspective* that emphasizes power inequities between men and women and men's greater influence on social and cultural mores. Finally, we discuss some implications of these dual reactions toward women, using objectification theory (Fredrickson & Roberts, 1997) to explain a number of negative consequences of the seemingly innocuous and sometimes even "benevolent" objectification of women.

AN EXISTENTIAL FRAMEWORK: I AM NOT AN ANIMAL!

Building on the groundwork laid by terror management theory (e.g., Greenberg, Pyszczynski, & Solomon, 1986; Solomon, Greenberg, & Pyszczynski, Chapter 2, this volume), Goldenberg, Pyszczynski, Greenberg, and Solomon (2000) recently argued that not only are human beings strongly motivated to avoid the frightening existential realization that they, like other animals, are material beings vulnerable to death but also that such a threat engenders specific difficulties with all that reminds us of our physical, animal nature. For if, as terror management theory suggests, human beings cope with the existential threat associated with the awareness of impending death through symbolic constructions of meaning (worldview) and value (self-esteem), then reminders of the physicality and "creatureliness" of human beings threatens the efficacy of these symbolic defenses against existential anxiety.

Countless philosophical, religious, and psychological perspectives have long viewed the physical and animal nature of humans as weaknesses to be controlled or transcended. Ancient Greek philosophers, such as Socrates, Plato, and Aristotle, extolled the virtues of intellectual over passionate life. Judeo-Christian theologians argued that the body was weak and prone to decay, whereas the soul was eternal; the capacity to exert the will over temptation was viewed as a primary difference that distinguished humans from animals. Some Eastern religions, such as Hinduism, have been more tolerant of sexual pleasure; however, in this case sexual ecstasy becomes a vehicle through which one may transcend the body and attain enlightenment. Freud too suggested that humans' fundamental psychological dynamic was the struggle to develop a workable compromise between our animal needs and the restraints placed on us by the culture and its agents. Others, such as Otto Rank, Ernest Becker, and Norman O. Brown have also suggested that humans struggle with recognition of their animal nature and have developed such abstract human constructs as the "soul" and "culture" in order to transcend this threat. In more contemporary empirical psychology, Rozin, Haidt, and colleagues (e.g., Haidt, Rozin, McCauley, & Imada, 1997; Rozin, Haidt, & McCauley, 1993) suggest that the emotion of disgust functions as an ideological response that dignifies humanity by allowing us to put ourselves above the animals that we deem as inferior.

In line with our premise that this threat is rooted in existential concerns, Goldenberg et al. (2001, Study 1) showed that when people are reminded of their mortality, they respond with greater disgust to body products and animals. Further, Goldenberg et al. (2001, Study 2) also found that death reminders cause people to like an essay that says humans are distinct from animals to a greater extent than a control condition, and also to like it substantially more than an essay that discussed the similarities between humans and animals. More recently, Cox, Pyszczynski, and Goldenberg (2002) have shown that the accessibility of death-related thoughts increases when people are reminded of their animal nature and then asked to answer questions about bodily products and functions. In addition, a handful of experiments have shown that such difficulty with one's own physicality even leads to distancing of physical sensation under certain conditions (Goldenberg, Hart, et al., 2004). Taken together, these findings provide empirical support for the proposition that people are threatened by their physical, animal nature, and further that existential concerns underlie these threats.

However, it is also clear, that we do not always respond to our physical selves with outright animosity; rather, very often reactions are marked with a great deal of ambivalence. We believe that the very physicalness of humanity can offer affirmation of life in addition to a reminder of death. For we feel alive through the experiences of our bodies and senses. But at the same time, this is the realm in which we are most vulnerable, because, at the very least, we are sure that death signifies the end of the physical body. For these reasons we suggest that there is an underlying *ambivalence* toward all that is physical or creaturely.

It follows that we respond to the threatening aspects of our physical nature with mechanisms of defense. On the one hand, we can distance from, deny, and devalue the aspects of our selves and others that are perceived as most creaturely. However, given that we are also drawn to the world of the physical, we suggest that we can ameliorate these threatening connotations by imbuing the threatening aspects of nature with symbolic and cultural meaning and value, so that they can be embraced with minimal threat. Thus although some aspects of our physicality are confined to private quarters, discussed only in euphemisms or as the brunt of jokes, other aspects are often viewed with more favorable reactions. It becomes apparent that negative and positive reactions to the physicality of humans are tied to a common source (i.e., existential terror) when we consider how the same behavior can be viewed with negative or with favorable attitudes as a function of existential factors. Several studies have illustrated such ambivalence in response to sex.

For example, Goldenberg, Cox, Pyszczynski, Greenberg, and Solomon (2002) demonstrated that when people were situationally induced to associate the physical aspects of sex with an animal act, by reading the essay described earlier in which people were reminded of their similarities to other animals, reminders of mortality decreased their reported appeal for the physical aspects of sex (Study 2). However, after reading the essay that described people as distinct from other species, reminders of death had no significant effect on the appeal of the physical aspects of sex (and even showed a trend toward increased appeal in this condition). Further, after the creaturely essay prime, thinking about physical sex increased the accessibility of death-related thoughts for participants, but the essay describing humans as unique did not (Study 1).

In this research, the more romantic aspects of sex were not distanced from at all, supporting the idea that symbolic meaning can ameliorate otherwise threatening aspects of our physical nature. This point was made more succinctly by Goldenberg, Pyszczynski, McCoy, Greenberg, and Solomon (1999, Study 3), who showed that while highly neurotic individuals showed heightened death-thought accessibility after contemplating the physical aspects of sex, when they were asked to think about love prior to thinking about physical sex, death was no longer highly accessible. Additional evidence that the physicality of sex is stripped of its threatening aspects when embedded in a symbolic context is illustrated by the finding that when people derive self-esteem from their physical body, then mortality reminders actually lead to greater interest in the physical aspects of sex (Goldenberg, McCoy, Pyszczynski, Greenberg, & Solomon, 2000).

We therefore maintain that there are two ways to defend against the threatening aspects of human physicality. First we can deny, conceal, and certainly devalue our more creaturely features, but, alternatively, we can also strip the threatening connotations of the physical body by imbuing those aspects of nature with symbolic, cultural meaning and value. It is in these two strategies of defense that we can better understand the duality of cultural reactions toward women and their bodies, which range, for example, from confinement to menstrual huts to the idealization of the female "nude" in both art and advertising.

THE BEAST

The perspective we have laid out thus far suggests that human beings have an inherent existential need to distance themselves from their animal nature, and further, that they do so by devaluing and denying their most creaturely aspects and also by transforming the physical by giving it symbolic, cultural meaning. However, as the opening quotes articulate, it is apparent that the burden of these reactions falls more heavily on women than on men. It is women, after all, for whom "nature's burden" appears to fall more heavily, and women whose nature must be more "rigorously confined."

Historically, conceptions of women's nature have emphasized women's connection to nature as a primary source of female inferiority (e.g., Gilmore, 2001; Tuana, 1993). Philosophical and religious perspectives have long emphasized the "mind" and the "soul" as the defining characteristics that elevate humans above the status of other mere physical animals. Women, in contrast to men, have been viewed as being ruled by their physical bodies, sensations, and emotions and therefore perceived as more distant from the Gods and closer to the status of the other animals. For example, Plato claimed that men who failed to exert rational control over their emotions were reincarnated as women, and continued loss of control resulted in reincarnation as an animal. Christian theologians argued that "original sin" occurred in the Garden of Eden because women's nature made them more susceptible to the passions of the body, rendering them incapable of higher human morality and reason (Weitz, 1998). In many texts of Buddhism, women are condemned because of their bodies as the polluted, not-quite-human sex (Sponberg, 1992), and Orthodox Jewish men thank God every day that they were not born with the body of a female (Gilmore, 2001).

In psychology, Freud's theory of psychosexual development suggests that women's inferiority stems from their incomplete formation of the superego, the part of the mind responsible for moral development and transcending one's hedonistic bodily needs. The boy, Freud argued, resolves his Oedipus complex out of fear of castration. The girl, on the other hand, has already been castrated and passes on to more sophisticated stages of development only if the wish for a penis is replaced by a wish for a baby. Freud went on to claim that woman's inferior moral development suffocates her ability to sublimate her instincts by investing in the collective culture. Existential theorists such as Brown (1959) and Becker (1973) suggested that the gender differences that Freud's penis-centered theory sought to explain could best be accounted for not out of the woman's desire for a penis but, rather, by both genders' fear of the mother's inherent creatureliness, as evidenced by menstruation, childbirth, and lactation.

In particular, women's weakness has explicitly been attributed to their role in reproduction. Plato wrote of the problems of hysteria and weakness caused in women by the "wandering uterus" searching for a fetus. More contemporary Western science too has purported that women's reproductive burden renders them the weaker sex. For instance, the prevailing medical opinion of the 19th and early 20th centuries suggested that women were built around, and mercilessly affected by their reproductive hormones. As Rudolf Virchow, a prominent medical doctor in the 1800s declared, "Woman is a pair of ovaries with a human being attached, whereas man is a human being furnished with testes" (quoted in Fausto-Sterling, 1992, p. 90). This view supported many a scientist's claim that women ought therefore to receive a different kind of education than men, if they ought to receive one at all. Many claimed that rigorous education of women would cause serious damage to their reproductive systems, and physicians even cited examples of women unable to bear children because they pursued an education fit for a man (Smith-Rosenberg & Rosenberg, 1973). Beyond the vulnerability of women's organs to damage from education, there also was (and still is in some circles) the belief that women's reproductive hormonal cycling simply rendered them more or less sick and unfit for hard intellectual work (Cayleff, 1992; Fausto-Sterling, 1992).

Women's menstruation in particular has not only been used to derogate their competence, but menstrual blood has long been feared, considered disgusting, and subject to cultural taboos and concealment norms. From the Bible to the Koran, injunctions against contact with women during menstruation illustrate the beliefs that women are polluting and that menstrual blood can have a contaminating effect. Many tribal cultures have intense fears of menstrual blood. The New Guinea Mae Enga, for example, believe that contacting a menstruating woman will "sicken a man and cause persistent vomiting, kill his blood so that it turns black, corrupt his vital juices so that his skin darkens and hangs in folds as his flesh wastes, permanently dull his wits, and eventually lead to a slow decline and death" (Delaney, Lupton, & Toth, 1988, p. 8). Respected medical doctors in the 19th century published work saying that a menstruating woman could spoil a ham and conducted studies in which they concluded that "menotoxins" in menstrual blood retard and kill plants (notably, these studies neglected to use control fluids, such as nonmenstrual blood). To avoid contamination from menstrual blood many non-Western cultures have required and still require women to remove themselves from the community, often by staying in menstrual huts for the duration of their menstrual periods.

Although contemporary Western women are not confined to menstrual huts, advertisers certainly market menstruation as a "hygienic crisis" that must be concealed and managed with products that enable women to avoid staining, soiling, odor, and humiliation (Havens & Swenson, 1988). Indeed, research shows that many contemporary women are anxious about being "discovered," and thus humiliated, through odor or staining their clothes (Kissling, 1996; Lee, 1994; Ussher, 1989). Lee (1994) has argued that staining is a visible emblem of women's contamination and supposed bodily inferiority, and it symbolizes a lapse in the culturally mandated responsibility of all women to conceal evidence of menstruation.

The findings from our own recent work in a laboratory setting illustrate the negative reactions that even contemporary Western people have to women's menstruation (Roberts, Goldenberg, Power, & Pyszczynski, 2002). In this study, both men and women exhibited negative reactions to a woman who inadvertently dropped a wrapped tampon out of her backpack. Not only was the woman viewed as less competent and less likable than when the same woman dropped a less "offensive" but equally feminine item—a hair barrette—from her bag, but the mere presence of the tampon also led participants to distance themselves physically from the woman. This indirect measure of distancing suggests a disgust reaction in which individuals avoid contact with contaminating entities. No wonder women heed the warnings of the advertisers! When others *find out*, indeed the consequences for women's social desirability are not favorable.

THE BEAUTY

However, just as there is a long tradition of belief claiming that women are closer to nature, there is also evidence of women being elevated above nature to the status of goddesses. Thus stereotypes about women are paradoxical, because they contain both negative and seemingly positive judgments. As Glick and Fiske (1996) have shown, women are simultaneously perceived as less competent and valuable than men but are also idealized in, for example, their roles as wives and mothers. On the one hand, as we have shown with respect to menstruation, women's reproductive and bodily functions are viewed with derision, but, on the other hand, other features of their bodies are revered as cultural symbols of beauty and male desire.

Our position in this chapter is that sexual objectification of women serves to strip women of their connection to nature. As we suggested at the outset, in addition to concealing and devaluing the more creaturely aspects of women's bodies, following from terror management theory, we suggest that the threat can also be diffused by symbolic drapery that transforms the threat. We would like to argue that objectifying women is one such form of drapery that enables a transformation of "natural" woman into "objects" of beauty and desire.

Objectification theory (Fredrickson & Roberts, 1997) argues that sexualized evaluation of women's bodies occurs in our culture with tremendous variety and yet monotonous similarity, both in interpersonal encounters via visual and verbal scrutiny and also in our interactions with the media, which seamlessly align viewers with a sexualizing gaze. Sexual objectification occurs when a woman's body, body parts, or sexual functions are separated from her person, or regarded as if they are capable of representing her (Bartky, 1990). Indeed, evolutionary psychologists have shown (Buss, 1989a) that men worldwide value physical appearance to a far greater extent than do women when selecting potential sexual partners. Of course, objectification occurs in obviously cruel and dehumanizing ways, when, for example, women's bodies are targeted for pornographic treatment or used in the sex trade industry. But the sexual objectification of women's bodies also occurs in a more seemingly benign, and many would argue even benevolent fashion, and is so widespread as to be part of the fabric of everyday life. Women's bodies and body parts are used as decorative, "beautifying" features all around us—to sell sports cars and beer, to adorn trucker's mud flaps, or to stand in a beaded gown and present prizes on a game show.

What we learn by scrutinizing these ubiquitous presentations of women is that women's bodies are acceptable and deemed "beautiful" only under certain conditions. For example, Wolf (1991) has shown that the images of the idealized female bodies to which we are exposed by the American media are invariably of youth, slimness, and whiteness, and these images are increasingly broadcast worldwide. In other cultures, such as the Karen of Upper Burma, the standard of feminine beauty involves an elongated neck with stacks of golden necklaces. Regardless of the particular features deemed essential by a culture for feminine beauty, we suggest that it is specifically when the more creaturely features and functions of women's bodies are actually or symbolically removed from the presentation, that the body is publicly acceptable and attractive.

Breasts provide a good example of the ambivalence with which we view women's bodies and the symbolic transformation that objectification achieves. In some cultures, large,
firm breasts are the standard of attractiveness, whereas in others, long, pendulous breasts
are considered the most desirable (Buss, 1994). But invariably, the "beautified breast" is an
object of sexual desire. In Western culture, when it comes to breasts—"cleavage is good;
nipples are a no-no" (Young, 1992, p. 220). This fits nicely with our position, for the nipples secrete milk and hence are reminders of our creaturely, mammalian nature. Of course,
we do not mean to imply that men are not aroused by women's nipples. They are! Indeed,
taboos in response to their creaturely aspects may be precisely the reason why nipples are so
sexually charged under some conditions (Bataille, 1957). But lactating nipples are certainly
not sexualized (outside, probably, of some fringe pornography). The sexualized breast and
the maternal breast are considered antithetical to one another (Stearns, 1999). By way of illustration, women who breastfeed in public are often judged as indecent (Ussher, 1989;
Yalom, 1997), but the Victoria's Secret fashion show airs on prime time television. By cover-
ing nipples with tassels or "X's," or by enhancing the other features of the bosom with
push-up bras, breasts are symbolically transformed via objectification into objects of
pleasure and sexual desire.

Female genitalia as well are considered desirable to the extent that they are transformed. Again, culturally specific standards hold here. Within our theoretical framework,
female circumcision and infibulation, still practiced in many African and Middle Eastern
nations, might be argued to be the most brutal means of objectification-as-existential-
protection. For by surgically removing the clitoris, the source of sexual arousal and satisfaction, a woman's animal pleasures are literally no longer available to her. In other cultures,
organs and tissue are not actually removed but merely altered. For example, the Nama of
Southwest Africa consider elongated labia majora to be beautiful, and thus the vulva is
enhanced by pulling and weighting it (Buss, 1994). In Western culture, many women undergo the regular application of hot wax to remove some or most of their public hair. Advertisements for vaginal deodorants and douches abound and imply moral failing on the part of
women who disregard this aspect of personal grooming. In Nairobi the word for vaginal
discharge translates to "dirt," and women there try to dry their vaginas, because a moist
vagina is considered disgusting (Angier, 2000). Indeed, unsanitized or ungroomed female
genitals are considered repellent and polluting in cultures worldwide, from "primitive" to
developed (Gilmore, 2001).

Beyond disgust and revulsion, there is also fear associated with the vagina. Psychologists have long noted man's view of the vagina as threatening, "uncanny" (as Freud, 1940,
called it), or even sinister (Hays, 1964). One symbolic expression of this fear is the
vagina-as-mouth, waiting to devour the male. The jawlike, cannibalistic vagina occurs as a
motif in folktales all over the world (Thompson, 1956), as well as in Freud's writings about
castration anxiety. Spiro (1997) writes of a verse from Buddhist holy text in which the
Buddha warns, "It is better for you, foolish man, that your male organ should enter the
mouth of a terrible poisonous snake than it should enter a woman" (p. 163).

In addition to such anthropological evidence, we have provided experimental evidence
that objectification of women's bodies serve as a defense against their more threatening
nature. In our tampon experiment, Roberts et al. (2002) found that not only were negative
reactions exhibited in response to the women who dropped the tampon, but when our participants were asked to describe their expectations for women's bodies in general, those who
had seen the confederate drop a tampon rather than a hair barrette were particularly likely
to rate women's physical appearance as especially important relative to health and function-

ing. Thus, the reaction to the tampon in this study generalized beyond the woman who dropped it to women in general, and took the form of viewing women in a more objectified light. That is, when reminded of women's more creaturely nature by the tampon, both men and women endorsed a less "physical," more appearance-oriented standard for women's bodies.

THE PRIZE AND PRICE OF SELF-OBJECTIFICATION

On first thought, it may seem surprising that the women participants in Roberts et al. (2002) responded to the tampon as did the men, by condemning and objectifying women. However, according to the position that we have provided, objectification of women serves an important existential function—it strips them of their creaturely connection and thus provides psychic protection from the threat of death. Thus, it is not surprising that women objectify other women, and in addition, it is also not surprising that women also objectify their own bodies, a phenomenon referred to as "self-objectification" and demonstrated by numerous studies (e.g., Fredrickson, Roberts, Noll, Quinn, & Twenge, 1998; Noll & Fredrickson, 1998). In other words, we suggest that women themselves participate willingly in the flight away from the corporeal, creaturely body.

This is not only because objectification of the body offers existential protection but because there are obvious and tangible rewards offered to women who conform to cultural standards for appropriate and desirable women's bodies. Women who are deemed attractive receive a host of positive interpersonal and even economic outcomes, relative to those considered more homely. As Unger (1979) has argued, physical beauty can function as a kind of currency for women. For example, physical attractiveness correlates more highly with popularity and marriage opportunities for women than for men (e.g., Berscheid, Dion, Walster, & Walster, 1971; Margolin & White, 1987). Obesity negatively affects women's, but not men's, social mobility (Snow & Harris, 1985; Wooley & Wooley, 1980). And, in general, women deemed unattractive in the workplace are described more negatively and are more likely to receive discriminatory treatment than are comparably unattractive men (Bar-Tal & Saxe, 1976; Fiske, Bersoff, Borgida, Deaux, & Heilman, 1991). Thus, it behooves women not only on an existential level but also on a very proximal, personal level to self-objectify; that is, to be evervigilant with respect to their own bodies' conformity to cultural standards of beauty.

Furthermore, we have demonstrated that revelation of the corporeal, creaturely, nonobjectified body "damns" women more than men. In a study in which a male or female experimenter excused him- or herself to either use the restroom or get some paperwork, results showed that participants rated the female experimenter more negatively in the bathroom condition than the control, but no differences were found for the male experimenter (Roberts & MacLane, 2002). Interestingly, neurotic individuals were found to be most reactive to the experimental manipulation. In popular culture, it is not uncommon to see males presented in urinal scenes in television sitcoms or movies. To imagine a similar scene of females talking to each other over the sound of urination seems preposterous. Instead, typically women's bathroom scenes are characterized by conversation while primping at the mirror.

However, as Fredrickson and Roberts (1997) have argued, objectification and self-objectification not only afford existential protection and social rewards but also come with a heavy psychological price. One set of consequences is to women's self-esteem, which result from their inability to attain the unrealistic standards for women's bodies. For example, although only a minority of girls and women in the United States are actually overweight, studies show that the overwhelming majority report feeling fat and ashamed of this "failure" (Silberstein, Striegel-Moore, & Rodin, 1987). In fact, over the past two decades, Western cultural standards for women's bodies have been getting thinner, and more unrealistic (Garner, Garfinkel, Schwartz, & Thompson, 1980), and are increasingly spread throughout the world via print, television, and film and even Internet media. As a result, women spend enormous amounts of time and money attempting to transform their physical bodies into idealized bodies through a mind-boggling array of methods, from makeup and fashion to dieting and even surgery (cf. Wolf, 1991).

We have conducted a number of experiments that illustrate that existential concerns in particular can fuel women's self-objectification practices and desire to attain cultural standards for their bodies. For example, in a series of experiments concerning societal expectations for women to be thin (Goldenberg, Arndt, & Brown, 2003), reminders of death lead women to restrict their consumption of a nutritious but fattening food, and women who were heavier than their peers were especially likely to deny themselves food when they were in a group context and social comparison was likely. A third experiment in this series demonstrated that women who were relatively higher in body-weight indeed became more aware of their failure to meet the cultural standards for thinness after being reminded of death, and that this perceived failure mediated the tendency to restrict food consumption. Findings in other domains, such as tanning intentions (Routledge, Arndt, & Goldenberg, in press), have shown a similar pattern of appearance striving in women, above and beyond concerns about health, when existential mortality concerns are salient.

Further, Fredrickson et al. (1998) demonstrated that, indeed, the emotional and behavioral consequences of self-objectification occur for women, but not men. In that study, experimentally induced self-objectification (trying on and evaluating swimwear compared to a sweater in the control condition) caused only women to experience shame about their bodies, which in turn predicted restrained eating. Finally, women in swimsuits demonstrated poorer performance on a concurrent cognitive task, illustrating that self-objectification occupies mental resources. No consequences were found for men.

In addition to the consequences that result from efforts and failures to attain objectified, idealized standards for women's bodies, there are consequences of denial and negative attitudes that women have in response to their own natural (non-objectified) physicality. For example, Roberts (2004) found that women who held a more self-objectified perspective on their own bodies also held more negative attitudes toward menstruation. The more women engaged in self-objectifying practices (e.g., chronic appearance monitoring), the more they endorsed extremely negative feelings about their menstrual periods—including disgust, contempt, embarrassment, and shame. In addition, Roberts, Gettman, Konik, and Fredrickson (2001) found that priming women with objectifying words (e.g., weight, attractive, and appearance) as opposed to words associated with health and functioning (e.g., fitness, stamina, and vitality) led them to rate the physical aspects of sex as less appealing, whereas no differences were found for men.

In sum, we argue that women themselves go to great lengths to conceal and control their bodies' more creaturely features and functions, and hence their association with nature, in order to live up to cultural beauty standards for the female body that provide protection from existential concerns. Doing so has potential health consequences as well as emotional and cognitive consequences for women, as Fredrickson et al. (1998) and others have demonstrated. More generally, social psychologists have demonstrated that striving to meet external standards to be accepted is in itself undermining to a person's autonomy and well-being (Crocker & Wolfe, 2001; Deci & Ryan, 1995; Schimel, Arndt, Pyszczynski, & Greenberg, 2001). We would argue that there are broader consequences on the cultural level as well. The body-altering practices of self-objectification, and the norms of secrecy and concealment that surround menstruation and other reproductive functions, which women tend to obey willingly and even enforce, serve the function of keeping women's *real,* corporeal bodies out of the public eye. This leaves the sanitized, deodorized, hairless, impossibly idealized images the media provide us with as the *only* women's bodies we encounter and accept. Thus, at least in Western culture, our existential concerns are in large measure allayed not by forcefully denying women's corporeal, physical bodies but by seemingly innocuous and widespread acceptance of an objectified definition of "normal."

WHY WOMEN?

An important question that has yet to be specifically addressed is, Why is it that women have been so disproportionately the target of both ends of this stick, both condemned for their base animal nature and worshiped for their goddess-like purity and beauty? We have suggested that both tendencies can be attributed to a core need for human beings to distance themselves from their physical, animal nature. But *why* are these dual reactions found to such a great extent in our attitudes toward women but so much less so in our responses to men?

Most feminist perspectives on this question emphasize real social and political power differences between the genders. Misogyny is the ideology behind patriarchy, the major form of inequality around the world. Men, who have the power to name, perhaps because of their greater physical size, cultivate prejudice against women in order to legitimize their oppression. Some feminist analyses of misogyny add anxiety to the equation (e.g., Ackley, 1992; Rogers, 1966) by arguing that men fear the potential power of women, who, freed from the restrictions placed on them by patriarchy, could become their masters.

Others have critiqued a purely feminist explanation for misogyny as insufficient on at least two grounds. For one, these reactions to women exist to some extent under all social, political, and economic systems; second, such explanations do not adequately explain the content of such attitudes toward women, nor do they explain the magnitude of feelings (Gilmore, 2001). In David Gilmore's (2001) recent anthropological treatise on misogyny he argues:

> Antiwoman feelings are usually driven by an irrational emotionality that is not the same as the simple expediency that characterizes political oppression or economic exploitation. Oppressing someone does not necessarily lead the oppressor to create a justifying ideology attributing pollution and magical danger to the oppressed. There must be some other, more visceral, more emotional element involved. (p. 181)

To shed light on the content of the negative attitudes toward women, Gilmore (2001) relies on some traditional psychoanalytic explanations. Most notably, the Freudian notion of castration anxiety is employed to explain the fears and taboos surrounding women's (bleeding) vaginas. We do not agree with such an argument but, rather, take a related position that is consistent with Becker's (1973) reconceptualization of such Freudian notions. Becker, arguing that Freud's own fear of death prevented him from realizing that the fears associated with sex and body were ultimately an expression of the fear of death, suggested that castration anxiety is not rooted in envy of the male penis, but rather any preference for male genitalia is by default a result of an inherent threat associated with the mother's body. For the mother's body represents sheer physicality and dependence. Hers is the body from which one was born, "between urine and feces" (Freud, 1961, p. 62), and hers is the body that secretes all manner of effluvia, disgusting and frightening, yet essential for life. Thus consistent with Becker, we believe that women's more obvious role in reproduction, and the existential threat associated with the physicality of related bodily processes, provides at least a partial explanation for the content and intensity of reactions to women.

Gilmore (2001) also suggests that another important factor in the magnitude of men's reactions toward women's bodies lies in men's dependence on women, starting in infancy and continuing into adulthood. While adult women can also be said to be equally, if not more, dependent on men, at least in the economic arena, one important difference concerns differences in sexual responsiveness. Disagreements about sexual access or availability are reportedly the most common source of conflict between men and women (Byers & Lewis, 1988). Evolutionary psychologists such as Buss (1989b) have shown that men worldwide condemn the "sexual withholding" of women, who, because of their greater need for investment from sexual partners, increase the value of sex by making it scarce. This "frustration–aggression" view (cf. Dollard, Miller, Mowrer, & Sears, 1939) of misogyny asserts that it is male sexual arousal, which is rarely fully satisfied, which fuels hostility toward women (i.e., the frustrating object). Although we believe that such an explanation does offer some explanatory value, we add to this position by suggesting that men's sexual arousal itself can pose an existential threat. For, if as terror management theory posits, we defend against anxiety associated with the awareness of death by creating a cultural system of meaning that allows us to feel more significant than mere animals, then as illustrated by Goldenberg et al. (e.g., 2001), animal desires have the ability to threaten the efficacy of this defense. Thus it makes sense that women, the objects of sexual arousal, would be degraded by men.

Some recent findings provide evidence that existential concerns fuel threats associated with women's sexuality. In one experiment, Landau, Goldenberg, et al. (2003) showed that after being primed with mortality reminders, men reported decreased attraction to a woman who was dressed in a sexually provocative manner but not to the same woman when she appeared more wholesome. While this finding points to a role of existential concerns in factors affecting men's attraction to women, it does not specify whether the nature of the threat concerns the explicit sexuality (i.e., physicality) of a seductive woman, or whether such difficulties stem also from threats associated with men's lust. However, in another experiment, Landau, Goldenberg, et al. (2003) showed that after being asked to think about a time when male participants had experienced lust, compared to excitement in response to a sporting event, mortality reminders led men to recommend more lenient penalties to a male who had aggressed against a woman but not to a male who had aggressed against another man. These findings suggest that male lust indeed poses an existential threat, and not only that, but male's defenses can include derogatory attitudes, and even aggression, toward women.

However, as we have emphasized throughout this chapter, attitudes toward women are obviously not wholly negative but also contain a seemingly benevolent component. It makes sense then that men would have two strategies of protection against the existential threat posed by women's bodies and men's reactions to them. One strategy is to condemn women for their ability to inspire animal-like lust. But a second strategy—raising "beautiful" (good) women to a higher, holier position—would also serve a similar function of protecting men from the threat associated with animalistic urges. For desiring a virginal, well-groomed, sanitized, deodorized, and goddess-like creature should not be so threatening. After all, there is no chance of contamination or pollution in interacting with such a creature.

This position fits with the findings of Glick and Fiske (e.g., 2001), who have observed that prejudice against women takes the form of both hostile sexism and also benevolent sexism (i.e., "characterizing women as pure creatures who ought to be protected, supported, and adored and whose love is necessary to make a man complete"; Glick & Fiske, 2001, p. 109). The primary reason offered for benevolent sexism is that men blend their hostile attitudes with benevolent ones to pacify women. Although we agree that sexism involves dual reactions toward women, our work leads us to differ somewhat in explanation for these dual reactions. In addition to pacifying women, we expect that such attitudes *protect men*. Men's physical, animal needs should be rendered less threatening if the object of these needs is construed as wholesome and pure. We particularly like Gilmore's summation: "'Woman' has the uncanny power to frustrate man's noble (but unrealistic) ideals, to subvert his lofty (hollow) ends, and to sully his (deluded) quest for spiritual perfection; but she also, and not coincidentally, provides him with the greatest pleasures of earthly life" (Gilmore, 2001, p. 183). Thus, we see why it is women who are targets of hostile and seemingly benevolent reactions, both of which are likely rooted in *men's power* to protect themselves from the threat of women.

CONCLUSION

In conclusion, we suggest that seemingly diametrically opposed attitudes toward women can be understood through an existential framework in which both tendencies are linked to a primary need to distance ourselves from the natural world. By considering existential threats associated with women's bodies and male desires along with traditional feminist explanations, we can better understand the content and intensity of negative attitudes toward women. However, it is important to emphasize that an existential perspective on its own is also insufficient, for although men do not play as obvious of a role in biological reproduction, their bodies are certainly not without creaturely aspects. For example, what about male ejaculation, which, like menstrual blood and mother's milk, is a bodily secretion with important reproductive involvement? Interestingly, unlike menstrual fluid, there is not a great stigma associated with this substance, and although few men we know of have tasted human breast *milk*, we view the fact that women swallow semen to be evidence that the male power to name plays an important role in reactions to human creatureliness, influencing which aspects are demeaning and which are a source of pride.

Our perspective additionally explains why objectification tends to co-occur with more obviously derogatory attitudes. Objectification-of-women-as-defense derives from terror management theory, which posits that human beings cope with the realization that they are dying animals by embedding themselves in a symbolic cultural framework. Objectification of women's bodies seems to exemplify this "exchange [of] a natural animal sense of our basic worth, for a contrived, symbolic one" (Becker, 1971, p. 71). Although a number of consequences result from this transformation, such as a host of emotional and cognitive difficulties for women stemming from the inability to achieve ideal standards for their bodies, we emphasize here that objectification serves an important existential function of rendering women (the objects of men desire) less threatening. Further, objectification not only protects men but seems to serve a similar function for women. In addition, the objectification of women's bodies indeed becomes a driving force of its own, because there are such clear societal rewards for women who successfully conceal the creaturely aspects of their bodies and conform to standards of ideal, contrived feminine embodiment.

The famous art historian John Berger (1972) has argued for a distinction between "naked" and "nude." According to his analysis, to be naked is to be oneself, without clothes. To be nude, in contrast, is to have one's naked body placed on display as an object. Furthermore, "the nude is condemned to never being naked" (p. 54). In locating an explanation for the objectification and condemnation of women in existential concerns, we do not mean to argue that such attitudes are therefore irreversible. Indeed, our hope is that in identifying these concerns as central to the practices of objectification, we can demystify women's "uncanny" bodies and enable a more accepting attitude toward their creaturely, corporeal, but life-giving features. It is our way of bringing the physical body—the naked body, if you will—out of the closet. In doing so, we hope that women might no longer be condemned to always being nude but could also enjoy the freedom and un-self-conscious joy of being naked.

REFERENCES

Ackley, K. A. (1992). *Misogyny in literature*. New York: Garland.

Angier, N. (2000). *Woman: An intimate geography*. New York: Anchor Books.

Bar-Tal, D., & Saxe, L. (1976). Physical attractiveness and its relationship to sex role stereotyping. *Sex Roles, 2*, 123–133.

Bartky, S. L. (1990). *Femininity and domination: Studies in the phenomenology of oppression*. New York: Routledge.

Bataille, G. (1957). *Eroticism: Death and sensuality*. San Francisco: City Lights Books.

Becker, E. (1971). *The birth and death of meaning* (2nd ed.) New York: Free Press.

Becker, E. (1973). *The denial of death*. New York: Free Press

Berger, J. (1972). *Ways of seeing*. London: British Broadcasting Company and Penguin Books.

Berscheid, E. Dion, K. L., Walster, E., & Walster, G. W. (1971). Physical attractiveness and dating choice: A test of the matching hypothesis. *Journal of Experimental Social Psychology, 7*, 173–189.

Brown, N. O. (1959). *Life against death: The psychoanalytical meaning of history*. Middletown, CT: Wesleyan Press

Buss, D. M. (1989a). Sex differences in human mate preferences: Evolutionary hypotheses tested in 37 cultures. *Behavioral and Brain Sciences, 12*, 1–49.

Buss, D. M. (1989b). Conflict between the sexes: Strategic interference and the evocation of anger and upset. *Journal of Personality and Social Psychology, 56*, 735–747.

Buss, D. M. (1994). *The evolution of desire: Strategies of human mating*. New York: Basic Books.

Byers, E. S., & Lewis, K. (1988). Dating couples' disagreements over desired level of sexual intimacy. *Journal of Sex Research, 24*, 15–29.

Cayleff, S. E. (1992). She was rendered incapacitated by menstrual difficulties: Historical perspectives on perceived intellectual and physiological impairment among menstruating women. In A. J. Dan., & L. L. Lewis (Eds.), *Menstrual health in women's lives* (pp. 229–235). Chicago: University of Illinois Press.

Cox, C. R., Pyszczynski, T., & Goldenberg, J. L. (2002). Understanding human ambivalence about sex: The effects of stripping sex of meaning. *Journal of Sex Research, 39*, 310–320.

Crocker, J., & Wolfe, C. T. (2001). Contingencies of self-worth. *Psychological Review, 108*, 593–623.

de Beauvoir, S. (1952). *The second sex* (H. M. Parshley, Trans.) New York: Knopf.

Deci, E. L., & Ryan, R. M. (1995). Human autonomy: The basis for true self-esteem. In M. Kernis (Ed.), *Efficacy, agency, and self-esteem* (pp. 31–49). New York: Plenum.

Delaney, J., Lupton, M. J., & Toth, E. (1988). *The curse: A cultural history of menstruation*. Urbana, IL: University of Illinois Press.

Dollard, J., Miller, N. E., Mowrer, O. H., & Sears, R. R. (1939). *Frustration and aggression*. New Haven, CT: Yale University Press.

Fausto-Sterling, A. (1992). *Myths of gender: Biological theories about women and men* (2nd ed.). New York: Basic Books.

Fiske, S. T., Bersoff, D. N., Borgida, E., Deaux, K., & Heilman, M. E. (1991). Social science research on trial: Use of sex stereotyping research in *Price Waterhouse v. Hopkins. American Psychologist, 46*, 1049–1060.

Fredrickson, B. L., & Roberts, T. (1997). Objectification theory: Toward understanding women's lived experiences and mental health risks. *Psychology of Women Quarterly, 21*, 173–206.

Fredrickson, B. L., Roberts, T., Noll, S. M., Quinn, D. M., & Twenge, J. M. (1998). That swimsuit becomes you: Sex differences in self-objectification, restrained eating and math performance. *Journal of Personality and Social Psychology, 75*, 269–284.

Freud, S. (1961). *Civilization and its discontents*. New York: Norton.

Freud, S. (1975). Medusa's head. In *Standard edition* (Vol. 18, J. Strachey, Ed.). London: Hogarth Press. (Original work published 1940)

Garner, D. M., Garfinkel, P. E., Schwartz, D., & Thompson, M. (1980). Cultural expectations of thinness in women. *Psychological Reports, 47*, 483–491.

Gilmore, D. D. (2001). *Misogyny: The male malady*. Philadelphia: University of Pennsylvania Press.

Glick, P., & Fiske, S. T. (1996). The ambivalent sexism inventory: Differentiating hostile and benevolent sexism. *Journal of Personality and Social Psychology, 70*, 491–512.

Glick, P., & Fiske, S. T. (2001). An ambivalent alliance: Hostile and benevolent sexism as complementary justifications for gender inequality. *American Psychologist, 56*, 109–118.

Goldenberg, J. L., Arndt, J., & Brown, M. (2003). *Dying to be thin: The effects of mortality salience and body-mass-index on restricted eating among women*. Manuscript under review, University of California, Davis, CA.

Goldenberg, J. L., Cox, C., Pyszczynski, T., Greenberg, J., & Solomon, S. (2002). Understanding human ambivalence about sex: The effects of stripping sex of its meaning. *Journal of Sex Research, 39*, 310–320.

Goldenberg, J. L., Hart, J., Warnica, G. M., Landau, M., Pyszczynski, T., & Thomas, L. (2004). *Terror of the body: Death, neuroticism, and the flight from physical sensation*. Manuscript under review, Boise State University, Boise, ID.

Goldenberg, J. L., McCoy, S. K., Pyszczynksi, T., Greenberg, J., & Solomon, S. (2000). The body as a source of self-esteem: The effects of mortality salience on identification with one's body, interest in sex, and appearance monitoring. *Journal of Personality and Social Psychology, 79*, 118–130.

Goldenberg, J. L., Pyszczynski, T., Greenberg, J., & Solomon, S. (2000). Fleeing the body: A terror management perspective on the problem of human corporeality. *Personality and Social Psychology Review, 4*, 200–218.

Goldenberg, J. L., Pyszczynski, T., Greenberg, J., Solomon, S., Kluck, B., & Cornwell, R. (2001). I am NOT an animal: Mortality salience, disgust, and the denial of human creatureliness. *Journal of Experimental Psychology: General, 130*, 427–435.

Goldenberg, J. L., Pyszczynski, T., McCoy, S. K., Greenberg, J., & Solomon, S. (1999). Death, sex, love, and neuroticism: Why is sex such a problem? *Journal of Personality and Social Psychology, 77*, 1173–1187.

Greenberg, J., Pyszczynski, T., & Solomon, S. (1986). The causes and consequences of a need for self-esteem: A terror management theory. In R. F. Baumeister (Ed.), *Public and private self* (pp. 189–212). New York: Springer-Verlag.

Haidt, J., Rozin, P., McCauley, C.R., & Imada, S. (1997). Body, psyche and culture: The relationship between disgust and mortality. *Psychology and Developing Societies, 9*, 107–131.

Havens, B. B., & Swenson, I. (1988). Imagery associated with menstruation in advertising targeted to adolescent women. *Adolescence, 23*, 89–97.

Hays, H. R. (1964). *The dangerous sex: The myth of feminine evil*. New York: Putnam.

Kissling, E. A. (1996). "That's Just a Basic Teen-age Rule": Girls' linguistic strategies for managing the menstrual communication taboo. *Journal of Applied Communication Research, 24*, 292–309.

Landau, M. J., Goldenberg, J. L., Greenberg, J., Gillath, O., Cox, C., Solomon, S., et al. (2003). *The siren's call: Terror management and the threat of sexual attraction*. Manuscript under review, University of Arizona, Tucson, AZ.

Lee, J. (1994). Menarche and the (hetero)sexualization of the female body. *Gender and Society, 8*, 343–362.

Margolin, L., & White, L. (1987). The continuing role of physical attractiveness in marriage. *Journal of Marriage and the Family, 49*, 21–27.

Noll, S. M., & Fredrickson, B. L. (1998). A mediational model linking self-objectification, body shame, and disordered eating. *Psychology of Women Quarterly, 22*, 623–636.

Paglia, C. (1990). *Sexual personae: Art and decadence from Nefertiti to Emily Dickinson*. New York: Random House.

Roberts, T.-A. (2004). Female trouble: The Menstrual Self-Evaluation Scale and women's self-objectification. *Psychology of Women Quarterly, 28*, 22–26.

Roberts, T.-A., Gettman, J., Konik, J., & Fredrickson, B. L. (2001, August). *"Mere exposure": Gender differences in the negative effects of priming a state of self-objectification*. Paper presented at the annual meeting of the American Psychological Association, San Francisco.

Roberts, T.-A., Goldenberg, J. L., Power, C., & Pyszczynski, T. (2002). "Feminine protection:" The effects of menstruation on attitudes toward women. *Psychology of Women Quarterly, 26*, 131–139.

Roberts, T.-A., & MacLane, C. (2002, February). *The body disgusting: How knowledge of body functions affects attitudes toward women*. Paper presented at the annual meeting of the Society for Personality and Social Psychology, Savannah, GA.

Rogers, K. M. (1966). *The troublesome helpmate*. Seattle, WA: University of Washington Press.

Routledge, C., Arndt, J., & Goldenberg, J. L. (in press). A time to tan: Proximal and distal effects of mortality salience on sun exposure intentions. *Personality and Social Psychology Bulletin*.

Rozin, P., Haidt, J., McCauley, C. R. (1993). Disgust. In M. Lewis & J. Haviland (Eds.), *Handbook of emotions* (pp. 575–594). New York: Guilford Press.

Schimel, J., Arndt, J., Pyszczynski, T., & Greenberg, J. (2001). Being accepted for who we are: Evidence that social validation of the intrinsic self reduces general defensiveness. *Journal of Personality and Social Psychology, 80*, 35–52.

Silberstein, L. R., Streigel-Moore, R., & Rodin, J. (1987). Feeling fat: A woman's shame. In H. B. Lewis (Ed.), *The role of shame in symptom formation* (pp. 89–108). Hillsdale, NJ: Erlbaum.

Snow, J. T., & Harris, M. B. (1985). Maintenance of weight loss: Demographic, behavioral and attitudinal correlates. *Journal of Obesity and Weight Regulation, 4*, 234–255.

Smith-Rosenberg, C., & Rosenberg, C. (1973). The female animal: Medical and biological views of woman and her role in 19th century America. *Journal of American History, 60*, 330–345.

Spiro, M. (1997). *Gender ideology and psychological reality: An essay on cultural reproduction*. New Yaven, CT: Yale University Press.

Sponberg, A. (1992). Attitudes toward women and the feminine in early Buddhism. In J. I. Cabezon (Ed.), *Buddhism, sexuality and gender* (pp. 3–36). Albany: State University of New York Press.

Stearns, C. A. (1999). Breastfeeeding and the good maternal body. *Gender and Society, 13*, 308–325.

Tuana, N. (1993). *The less noble sex: Scientific, religious, and philosophical conceptions of women's nature*. Indianapolis: Indiana University Press.

Thompson, S. (1956). *Motif index of folk culture*. Bloomington: Indiana University Press.

Unger, R. K. (1979). Toward a redefinition of sex and gender. *American Psychologist, 34*, 1085–1094.

Ussher, J. (1989). *The psychology of the female body*. New York: Routledge.

Weitz, R. (1998). A history of women's bodies. In R. Weitz (Ed.), *The politics of women's bodies* (pp. 3–11). New York: Oxford University Press.

Wolf, N. (1991). *The beauty myth: How images of beauty are used against women*. New York: Anchor Books.

Wooley, S. C., & Wooley, O. W. (1980). Eating disorders: Anorexia and obesity. In A.M. Brodsky & R. Hare-Mustin (Eds.), *Women and psychotherapy* (pp. 135–158). New York: Guilford Press.

Yalom, M. (1997). *A history of the breast*. New York: Knopf.

Young, I. M. (1992). Breasted experience: The look and the feeling. In D.Leder (Ed.), *The body in medical thought and practice* (pp. 215–230). Boston: Kluwer.

Chapter 6

Paradise Lost and Reclaimed

A Motivational Analysis of Human–Nature Relations

SANDER L. KOOLE
AGNES E. VAN DEN BERG

> I was snorkeling alone in the warm, sunny, clear waters of a tropical la-
> goon and experienced, as I often do in the water, a deep sense of plea-
> sure and coziness. I felt at home. The warmth of the water, the beauty of
> the coral bottom, the sparkling silver minnows, the neon-bright coral
> fish, the regal angel fish, the fleshy anemone fingers, the esthetic pleasure
> of gliding and carving through the water, all in concert created an under-
> water elysium. And then, for reasons I have never understood, I had a
> sudden radical shift in perspective. I suddenly realized that none of my
> watery companions shared my cozy experience. The regal angel fish did
> not know that it was beautiful, the minnows that they sparkled, the
> coral fish that they were brilliant. Nor for that matter did the black nee-
> dle urchins or the bottom débris (which I tried not to see) know of their
> ugliness. The at-homeness, the coziness, the smiling hour, the beauty, the
> beckoning, the comfort—none of these really existed. I had created the
> entire experience! (. . .) It was as though I peered through a rent in the
> curtain of daily reality to a more fundamental and deeply unsettling
> reality.
>
> —IRVIN YALOM, *Existential Psychotherapy* (1980, p. 219)

In his classic volume on existential psychotherapy, Yalom (1980) describes how he once had a deeply disturbing existential experience while he was on his own in a magnificent natural environment. At first glance, it seems odd that the mere circumstance of being surrounded by natural beauty could shake the very foundations of someone's existence. However, research in environmental psychology indicates that close encounters with nature quite commonly have this effect on people (Williams & Harvey, 2001). For instance, many participants of wilderness programs report that the confrontation with nature inspires feelings of awe and leads to thoughts about spiritual meanings and eternal processes (Frederickson & Anderson, 1999; Kaplan & Kaplan, 1989). Likewise, college students often report that visiting a natural setting causes them to reflect on themselves and their priorities in life (Korpela, Hartig, Kaiser, & Fuhrer, 2001). It thus appears that people's close encounters with nature are frequently accompanied by existential ruminations.

Is it by accident that so many people—like Yalom—are driven to ponder the meaning of existence when they are confronted with nature? Or, could there be something about nature itself that triggers these existential concerns? In this chapter, we argue that people's interactions with nature are indeed closely associated with some of their most basic existential struggles. Human–nature relations thus provide a window on how people cope with matters of life and death. Conversely, a consideration of people's ultimate concerns may illuminate some of the deeper grounds of modern civilization's mounting conflicts with nature. In the following paragraphs, we start by tracing some of the historical roots between existential concerns and human–nature relations. Next, we introduce an existential–motivation analysis of human–nature relations, which portrays defense and growth as two fundamental motivational systems underlying people's responses to nature. We subsequently discuss some preliminary empirical applications of this dual-motive framework. Finally, we consider some of the broader implications of the present perspective for existential psychology and contemporary human–nature relations.

A BRIEF HISTORY OF HUMAN–NATURE RELATIONS

The study of human–nature relations presumes that human beings can be contrasted with other, presumably more natural life forms. Yet from a biological point of view, the similarities between humans and other species by far outnumber any differences. Other mammals, reptiles, insects, and even plants have the same basic needs for sustenance and reproduction, self-regulate their inner functions, and interact with the environment in ways that are fundamentally comparable to members of the human species. Indeed, genetic investigations have revealed that most human genes have an ancestry that goes back to even the earliest of animals and are held in common with many other species (Freeman & Herron, 2001). Creatures as far removed from humans as the fruitfly or roundworm have genes whose DNA is recognizably similar to that of human beings. Chimpanzees, a primate species that branched off from the human species only 5 million years ago (a very short time on the evolutionary time scale), have DNA that is on average 98% identical to human DNA (Gould, 1977).

Despite the great similarities between humans and other biological species, human beings seem unique in at least one respect: their unusually large cerebral cortex, which supports a sophisticated cognitive architecture. More than any other human trait, this cognitive architecture has contributed to the way in which the human race has managed to survive natural hardships and ultimately came to dominate the rest of the planet. The cognitive sophistication of the human mind has been responsible for the invention of ever more powerful technologies, which have afforded humans with a level of control over their environment that is unsurpassed by any other species. The human mind further supports self-awareness, people's capacity to reflect on their own being. Self-awareness has many adaptive advantages, by enabling people to function as responsible and planful organisms (Pyszczynski, Greenberg, & Solomon, 1998; Silvia & Duval, 2001). However, self-awareness also forces people to confront their deepest fears about matters of life and death (Becker, 1962, 1973;

Rank, 1936/1945; Yalom, 1980). The human mind is thus responsible for both the technological achievements and the deep psychological conflicts that characterize the human species.

The driving force behind all artificiality, the human mind itself is the product of natural forces. Although the precise origins of the human mind remain shrouded in mystery, recent archeological findings have enabled researchers to reconstruct a general picture of how the human mind evolved (Sedikides & Skowronski, 1997). Between 2.5 and 3 million years ago, a general cooling of the climate and a decline in the availability of forested areas led early hominids to move from the forests toward savannahs that contained a mix of grasslands and trees. This change in habitat presumably led the hominids to adopt a different lifestyle, which included hunting for larger animals and living in larger groups. According to recent evolutionary analyses, this change in lifestyle created a new set of selection pressures that eventually led to the evolution of self-awareness (Sedikides & Skowronski, 1997). In particular, the hunting life style of the hominids favored the development of cognitive abilities to construct long-term plans, which included the sophisticated representational abilities to imagine one's current and future selves. In addition, group living favored the development of sophisticated perspective-taking abilities and symbolic communication. The change toward a savannah environment and the resulting changes in lifestyle thus gave rise to selection pressures that ultimately led to the evolution of human self-awareness.

Once the capacity for self-awareness had evolved, humans began to develop ever more sophisticated cultural practices (Leary & Cottrell, 1999). Indeed, a veritable "big bang of culture" seems to have occurred among *Homo sapiens* roughly 40,000 years ago (Mithen, 1996). Archeological excavations indicate that these late Paleolithic times were characterized not only by rapid technological developments of stone tools and weapons but also by the development of symbolic cultural practices. For instance, the Cro-Magnon people of Europe decorated their tools and sculpted small pieces of stone, bone, antler, and tusks. Necklaces, bracelets, and decorative pendants were made of bones, teeth, and shells. Moreover, the Cro-Magnons were able to make music (as indicated by findings of flutes and drums) and produced many cave paintings that contain naturalistic scenes of animals. For instance, the painting from the caves of Lascaux that is depicted in Figure 6.1 shows a man who is apparently attacked by a bison. Cave paintings of this kind suggest that the Cro-Magnon people were acutely aware of the natural dangers that surrounded them. Indeed, archeologists believe that Cro-Magnon cave paintings might have played an important function in magical or religious rituals that symbolically controlled the violent forces of nature. Cro-Magnons further had intentional burials which included grave goods, suggesting that they had a culturally shared understanding of death and perhaps even notions of an afterlife. Taken together, a wealth of archeological evidence suggests that the self-aware *Homo sapiens* had developed symbolic behavior patterns that set him apart from the natural world.

Some 10,000 years ago, people began to make the transition from hunting and gathering to settled agriculture (Diamond, 1998; Harlan, 1995; Smith, 1995). At first, this transition occurred in just a few places. Within roughly 6,000 years, however, most economies were based on settled agriculture. The reasons for this relatively rapid transition to settled agriculture are still poorly understood. Indeed, in some respects hunter–gatherer societies seemed better off than agricultural societies. For instance, relative to agricultural societies, hunter–gatherer societies spent less time and labor on food procurement and had better diets, lower rates of starvation, and fewer chronic diseases (Harlan, 1995). Possible explanations for the rise of settled agriculture include climatic changes, population growth, and cul-

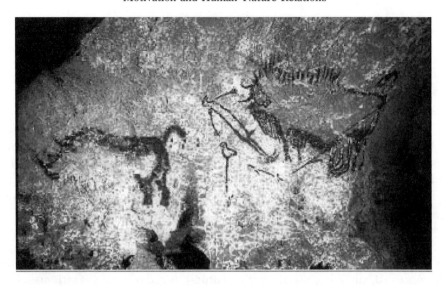

FIGURE 6.1. The shaft of the dead man, Paleolithic cave painting at Lascaux, France. The tryptich portrays the confrontation between a man (middle) and a bison (right) with a fleeing rhinoceros (left).

tural factors. Irrespective of its causes, the transition to agriculture dramatically changed people's relations with nature. The hunter–gatherer lifestyle required intimate knowledge of the locations, plant cycles, properties and uses of virtually all plants in their extended environment, as the average diet depended between 60 and 80% on plant foods (Harlan, 1995). By contrast, the agricultural lifestyle led people to settle permanently in a more limited amount of space, and to depend on a only few crops that were used for large-scale production. Agriculture also encouraged people to assume a greater amount of control over the natural world. Domestication of wild animals and plants, as well as the invention of other technologies, yielded bigger harvests.

The transition toward agriculture gradually allowed more people to depend on less land. Freed from the land, people started living together in cities. Conceivably, the formation of larger communities was also stimulated by people's mounting concerns with death, given that larger communities are better equipped to create shared meanings that endow individuals with symbolic immortality (Solomon, Greenberg, Schimel, Arndt, & Pyszczynski, 2003). City dwellers were able to pursue occupations that were removed from immediate food production, in arts, religion, sciences, or technology. Human society thus developed into a complex pattern of ordered, differentiated relationships (Baumeister, in press). Within this societal arrangement, traits such as rationality, personal responsibility, and planfulness were strongly encouraged (Martin, 1999; Woodburn, 1982). This rational emphasis further stimulated the accelerating development of science and technology. Awesome forces of nature such as electricity, atomic power, and DNA were subjugated and converted into powerful allies of human civilization. Indeed, in modern times, civilization's interference with nature has become a growing cause of concern, creating problems such as depletion of the earth's energy resources, pollution, deforestation, and accelerating rates of extinction of many species. Pure and untamed nature has become a scarce commodity, something that most people can only marvel at when it is displayed in zoos and nature documentaries. A sense of alienation from nature is increasingly felt among many members of modern society.

Indeed, large numbers are willing to expend considerable time and resources to return to nature, through activities such as growing gardens or planning a trip to the outdoors.

FEAR VERSUS GROWTH: AN EXISTENTIAL PERSPECTIVE ON HUMAN–NATURE RELATIONS

Clearly, humanity has come a long way since its prehistoric ancestors decided to move from the forests into the savannah. It seems tempting to conclude that ancient fears of nature have all but vanished from the minds of modern individuals. However, there may be more to people's relations with nature than meets the eye. As many existential thinkers recognized, nature is inherently associated with both life and death (Becker, 1973; Fromm, 1977; Jung, 1964; see also Goldenberg, Pyszczynski, Greenberg, & Solomon, 2000). Accordingly, the confrontation with nature in a deeper sense still implies a confrontation with people's ultimate existential concerns. In modern times, the most frightening aspects of nature are typically concealed, surfacing mainly during natural disasters such as earthquakes, floods, or epidemics. However, even on a more mundane level, nature remains a setting of stomach-turning cruelty and horror. Rotting corpses of animals by the road side, packs of rats in the sewers, swarms of cockroaches that plague apartment buildings—these are only a few of the natural horrors that abide even in the most urbanized environments. Despite human civilization's increased control over nature, it seems impossible to eliminate all such natural horrors completely.

The horrors of nature are enhanced by people's realization they themselves are part of the same cruel universe as all other natural phenomena. As Erich Fromm (1977, p. 320) argued, "Self-awareness, reason, and imagination have disrupted the 'harmony' that characterizes animal existence. Their emergence has made man into an anomaly, the freak of the universe. He is part of nature, subject to her physical laws and unable to change them, yet he transcends nature; he is set apart while being a part; he is homeless, yet chained to the home he shares with all creatures." The uncanny realization of being "the freak of the universe" may be too much for most people to handle. As a consequence, people's existential concerns form a powerful drive to distance themselves from the savage reality of nature. This distancing may occur quite literally, when people lock themselves away in cities. However, distancing from nature can also assume more symbolic forms. People may deny the physical, biological aspects of their being, for instance, by displaying disgust for body products or by suppressing their sexuality (Goldenberg & Roberts, Chapter 5, this volume). Alternatively, people may render the relations with nature less problematic by controlling and cultivating the forces of nature. Symbolic distancing from nature can also be achieved through cultural means. Indeed, all known cultures have presented their members with idealized images of cultivated natural environments, such as the biblical Garden of Eden and the Arcadian pastoral landscapes of the ancient Greeks (Eisenberg, 1998). Such idealized images of nature convey the reassuring notion that the savage forces of nature can be tamed and may thus alleviate the existential anxiety that is aroused by the confrontation with nature (cf. Goldenberg et al., 2000).

Despite nature's association with deep existential fears, people's interactions with nature cannot be explained by defensive motives alone. To survive in a dynamic, ever-changing environment, people had to be at least somewhat open to new experiences, to explore new grounds, and to develop new cognitive and behavioral skills. These needs for exploration and personal mastery can probably be realized to some extent in the civilized world. However, civilization is by definition preorganized and constrained by artificial boundaries. Accordingly, people's exploration needs should form a powerful drive to seek out nature, especially nature in its wild and untamed varieties. Moreover, there may be deeper reasons why people cannot afford to lose touch with wilderness altogether. According to Jung (1964), the modern mind is built on ancient, primordial psychic structures. These age-old structures contain "archetypes," collective memories and instinctual urges that refer back to the experiences of our prehuman ancestors. Although the archetypes seemed strange and mystifying to many of Jung's contemporaries, recent advances in evolutionary psychology have rendered the notion of evolved psychological structures compatible with mainstream psychology (Kenrick, Sadall, & Keefe, 1998; Öhman & Mineka, 2000). Evolved psychological structures (or archetypes) are presumably part of the deep, preconscious parts of the brain. Therefore modern humans may possess little conscious access to these structures. Yet, Jung (1964, p. 37) argued, "For the sake of mental stability and even physiological health, the unconscious and the conscious must be integrally connected and thus move on parallel lines. If they are split apart or 'dissociated', psychological disturbance follows." Thus, to function as whole persons, individuals should be prepared to overcome the artificial boundaries that civilization has placed between them and the natural world. From this perspective, the confrontation with nature may be indispensable for achieving personal growth and self-actualization.

To summarize, human–nature relations can be understood in terms of two conflicting existential motives. Close encounters with nature involve a confrontation with deeply rooted existential fears, which fuel defensive motives to distance oneself from or control the wild forces of nature. Nevertheless, nature also provides an ideal setting for exploration and personal growth. Because self-defense and growth each represents a fundamental source of human motivation (Deci & Ryan, 2000; Pyszczynski, Greenberg, & Goldenberg, 2003; Sedikides & Strube, 1997), it seems plausible that both types of motives are important determinants of people's responses to nature. Even so, self-defense may be the more basic system, in that defensive needs must be met before the growth/enrichment system may become activated. The primacy of defensive motives is based on the notion that, throughout evolutionary history, the costs of ignoring threats have outweighed the cost of ignoring opportunities for self-development (Baumeister, Bratslavski, Finkenauer, & Vohs, 2001; Taylor, 1991). Moreover, empirical investigations have shown that growth motives are short-circuited when defensive pressures are brought to bear upon the individual (Deci & Ryan, 2000; Koole, Baumann, & Kazén, 2003; Mikulincer, 1997).

EMPIRICAL EVIDENCE

Within environmental psychology, there are numerous indications that the confrontation with nature gives rise to ambivalent reactions. For instance, there are many reports of fearful reactions to wilderness environments among people who are unfamiliar with this type of environment (Kaplan & Kaplan, 1989). In a related vein, research has shown that modern urban youth commonly experience fear and discomfort when they are exposed to wilderness settings during mandatory school trips (Bixler & Floyd, 1997). At the same time, as noted earlier, many people report that the confrontation with nature inspires feelings of awe, thoughts about deep spiritual meanings, and reflections on one's priorities in life (Kaplan & Kaplan, 1989; Korpela et al., 2001). Findings within environmental psychology thus support defense and growth as important motives in people's interactions with nature.

Our existential-motives analysis assumes that the activation of self-defense and growth motives can vary substantially across situations and individuals (Koole & Van den Berg, 2003). In some situations and for some individuals, growth motives are likely to predominate. Relevant circumstances are those in which individuals feel free to explore their surroundings by themselves in an unconstrained manner, especially circumstances that trigger curiosity and exploration needs. Likewise, individuals who are chronically inclined toward autonomous self-regulation are likely to be driven by growth needs (Deci & Ryan, 2000). When growth needs are prepotent, people can be expected to respond in an open, explorative manner to the natural world, for instance, by seeking out wild and untamed nature. By contrast, self-defense needs are likely to become triggered by threatening or anxiety-arousing circumstances. Because of nature's inherent association with death, situations which trigger death concerns can be expected to be especially powerful elicitors of self-defense needs. Likewise, individuals who are chronically prone to experience high levels of threat or anxiety may be driven by self-defense needs to a greater degree than are low-anxious individuals. When self-defense needs predominate, people will respond highly defensively to nature, for instance, by psychologically distancing themselves from nature or by seeking out cultivated environments.

Defense Motivation and Distancing from Nature

The notion that defensive concerns can motivate people to distance themselves from nature is closely in line with terror management theory (TMT; Solomon, Greenberg, & Pyszczynski, Chapter 2, this volume). According to TMT, concerns with death lead people to construct and validate a set of cultural worldviews, which offer ways of achieving either literal or symbolic immortality. In support of this hypothesis, more than 100 experiments to date have shown that death reminders lead people to defend their cultural worldviews more vigorously. Insofar as culture is antithetical to nature, the worldview defense findings can be interpreted as a tendency to distance the self from nature in the face of death. In recent years, TMT research has begun to address the existential aspects of human–nature relations more directly. In particular, Goldenberg and associates showed that death reminders cause people to respond more negatively to the physical aspects of sex (Goldenberg et al., 2000; Goldenberg & Roberts, Chapter 5, this volume). Presumably, this tendency occurs because people feel a need to distance themselves from their mortal, animal nature when they have been primed with existential concerns. In line with this, death reminders caused greater aversion to the physical aspects of sex, especially after people have been primed with the similarities between humans and animals. Moreover, individuals who are reminded of death are especially likely to support beliefs that humans are distinct from animals and to report being disgusted by animals.

In parallel with the ground-breaking research by Goldenberg and associates, we have recently explored the influence of existential concerns on people's attitudes toward the natural environment. In this research, we have focused on people's responses to landscapes that varied in degree of cultivation, a well-studied landscape characteristic in environmental psychology (Van den Berg & Vlek, 1998; Van den Berg, Vlek, & Coeterier, 1998). Based on our conceptual analysis, we reasoned that wild natural environments should be more closely associated with thoughts about death than more cultivated environments. After all, cultivation imbues the natural environment with structure and order, which should affirm people's beliefs in a meaningful universe and render existential concerns less salient. In a first test of this notion, we asked a group of Dutch undergraduates to indicate in which kind of environment they thought most about various topics (Koole & Van den Berg, 2003, Study 1). For each topic, participants were asked to indicate whether they thought most about these topics when they were visiting wilderness, cultivated nature, or the city. Embedded in a list of fairly mundane topics like relation problems, politics, and studies, we included the topic of death. The results showed that around 70% of our participants reported thinking most about death when they were in a wild natural environment. Notably, wilderness did not trigger thoughts about any topic, because subjects reported thinking most about politics and studying when they were either in cultivated nature or the city. Moreover, the greater inclination to think about death in a wild natural environment did not seem to reflect a tendency to think about negative topics in general, because fewer participants reported thinking about relationship problems in the wilderness than in the city.

The aforementioned study supports the hypothesized link between thoughts of death and exposure to wilderness. However, it is unclear from this study whether wilderness inspires thoughts about death, or whether thoughts about death lead people to seek out wilderness. Moreover, according to our theoretical analysis, the link between wilderness and death should not just be apparent in people's self-reports but also should operate on more implicit levels. To clarify these issues, an additional study used the classic Stroop paradigm to document the link between wilderness and death (Koole, 2003). In this study, different types of nature were primed by exposing participants to color photographs of natural landscapes, which were rapidly flashed on a computer screen. For one half of the participants, the photos consisted of cultivated landscapes; the other half was primed with photos of wild landscapes. Following the priming task, participants were asked to name the color of red and blue words that appeared on the center of the computer screen, an adaptation of the Stroop task. Some words in the Stroop task were related to death (e.g., corpse and grave). The remaining words were unrelated to death but negatively valenced (e.g., punishment and deceit), positively valenced (e.g., reward and love), or related to positive aspects of nature (e.g., flowers and birds). In this task, heightened accessibility of death thoughts was indicated by slower color-naming latencies for death words relative to the color-naming latencies of the other word categories. Based on our theoretical analysis, then, the wilderness prime should lead to relatively slower color naming latencies of death words, whereas the cultivated prime would not elicit this effect. This pattern was indeed obtained. Thus, wilderness can prime thoughts about death, and this link is even potent on implicit levels.

Given that wilderness can trigger thoughts about death, terror management concerns seem highly relevant to understanding people's attitudes toward wilderness. In particular, salient terror management concerns may lead people to respond less favorably to wilderness, which heightens people's concerns with death. To test this prediction, we examined the influence of terror management concerns on evaluations of wild versus cultivated natural landscapes (Koole & Van den Berg, 2000). In a first study, we manipulated mortality salience by asking participants two open-ended questions about either death or television (cf. Greenberg, Solomon, & Pyszczynski, 1997). Next, participants evaluated descriptions of wild and cultivated Dutch natural landscapes, which were highly familiar to our Dutch sample. For instance, the wild landscapes included an impenetrable swamp forest and rough grasslands. The cultivated landscapes included landscapes such as green meadows and a grain field. We also included a measure of individual differences in need for structure. Past research indicates that individuals with high need for structure have a pronounced inclination to rely on simple cognitive structures and cultural worldviews (Deschesne & Kruglanski, Chapter 16, this volume; De Dreu, Koole, & Oldersma, 1999). Accordingly, we anticipated that need for structure would be negatively related to evaluations of wilderness.

As can be seen in Figure 6.2, both mortality salience and need for structure reliably predicted lower evaluations of wild natural landscapes (both p's < .05). Evaluations of cultivated natural landscapes were not reliably affected by these variables. It is further noteworthy that the effects of mortality salience and need for structure were additive. This pattern is consistent with the notion that mortality salience and need for structure relate to a single motivational system. In a follow-up study, we replicated the basic finding that mortality salience causes people to display more negative evaluations of wilderness (Koole & Van den Berg, 2003, Study 2). In this study, we also examined whether our findings were moderated by participants self-reported fear of death. Previous TMT research suggests the counterintuitive notion that individuals with low expressed fear of death may actually display stronger defensive reactions to mortality salience than individuals with high expressed fear of death (e.g., Greenberg et al., 1997). Conceivably, low expressed fear of death may reflect a tendency to deny one's existential fears, rather than a genuine absence of the fear of death. In line with this reasoning, we found that mortality salience produced stronger reductions in preference for wild over cultivated nature among participants with low expressed fear of death than among their counterparts with high expressed fear of death. Accordingly, these results suggest that defensive terror management processes indeed induce lower appreciation of wilderness.

To summarize, several lines of research have examined whether existential concerns can lead people to distance themselves from nature. First, TMT research indicates that mortality salience induces increased support of cultural worldviews (Greenberg et al., 1997) and negative reactions toward one's own biological functions and animals (Goldenberg et al., 2000). Second, there is evidence that exposure to wilderness environments can trigger thoughts about death (Koole, 2003; Koole & Van den Berg, 2003). Finally, recent experiments indicate that mortality salience and need for structure lead to less favorable evaluations of wilderness (Koole & Van den Berg, 2000, 2003). Taken together, there is preliminary support for the relevance of defensive terror management concerns to human–nature relations.

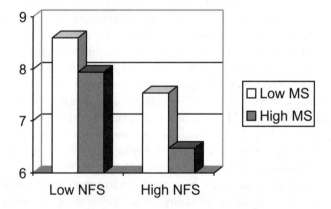

FIGURE 6.2. Effects of mortality salience (MS) and need for structure (NFS) on perceived beauty of wild natural landscapes (1 = not at all beautiful, 11 = very beautiful) (Koole & Van den Berg, 2000).

Growth Motivation and the Embracing of Nature

The idea that people may respond to nature in a nondefensive, growth-oriented manner is broadly consistent with humanistic approaches to human motivation (Deci & Ryan, 2000; Kasser & Sheldon, Chapter 29, this volume; Pyszczynski et al., 2003). In addition, environmental scientists have argued that natures provides one of the most suitable contexts in which people can explore their own potential and engage in intrinsically motivated activities (e.g., Kaplan & Kaplan, 1989; Kellert, 1997). In line with this idea, Koole and Van den Berg (2003, Study 1) found that most people think about freedom more often in wild environments than in either cultivated or urban environments. Thus, wilderness is not only strongly associated with thoughts about death but also with thoughts about freedom.

Some recent work in environmental psychology has further studied the relation between growth motivation and nature experiences. One line of research has shown that participants of wilderness programs and visitors of forests frequently report spiritual experiences (Frederickson & Anderson, 1999; Williams & Harvey, 2001). In a related vein, a recent series of interviews on nature experiences among members of a nature organization in the Netherlands found that being in the woods is associated with inner peace, the experience of connectedness, and reflections on the cycle of life and death and one's own smallness in the grand scheme of things (Van Trigt, 2002). Although suggestive, the aforementioned investigations were qualitative, limited to one kind of nature, and conducted among preselected groups of nature enthusiasts. Accordingly, we deemed it desirable further investigate the connection between growth motivation and nature experiences.

In a preliminary investigation, we focused on growth motives that are associated with recreation activities (Van den Berg & Koole, 2003). Recreation is a largely self-initiated, voluntary behavior that brings millions of modern people into close contact with nature. Accordingly, recreation seemed an ideal domain to explore the influence of growth motivation on nature evaluation. In our research, we built on Cohen's (1979) analysis of modern recreation experiences. According to Cohen, many recreation activities are primarily oriented toward the pursuit of brief, carefree pleasures (e.g., hanging in the bar with friends or exchanging jokes), the need to "recharge one's batteries," or the desire to partake in a worldwide canon of attractions (e.g., visiting the Niagara waterfalls or seeing Dutch tulip fields). Cohen argues that these recreational orientations are primarily concerned with staged representations that only provide a reflection of reality. However, Cohen (1979) also distinguishes two recreational orientations that are characterized by a deeper, more genuine search for alternative truths. First, the *experimental mode* is driven by a desire to find ultimate values that exist not within some other culture but within oneself (e.g. "When I'm on vacation I like to be alone in the natural environment for hours on end"). Second, the *existential mode* is characterized by an embracing of newly discovered truths and alternative realities (e.g., "I am not satisfied with just seeing local cultures and their habits. I want to be part of it myself as much as possible").

In our study, we assessed Cohen's recreational orientations using a validated Dutch instrument, the Modes of Experience Scale (MES; Elands & Lengkeek, 2000) among a randomly selected sample of Dutch city residents. After filling out the MES, participants were asked to rate six pairs of photographic simulations of wild and cultivated environments. Based on the notion that wild nature provides better opportunities for growth and exploration, we predicted that individuals whose recreational motives were growth-oriented (i.e., oriented toward the experimental or existential modes) would be more favorably disposed toward wild nature and less favorably disposed towards cultivated nature. Consistent with this, we found a highly reliable interaction between growth-oriented recreational modes and cultivation (see Figure 6.3).

Growth-oriented participants rated wild environments as *more* beautiful than cultivated environments. By contrast, participants low on growth-orientation rated wild environments as *less* beautiful than cultivated environments. Recreational modes that were not growth-related (e.g., amusement, recharging one's batteries) were unrelated to nature evaluations.

After this initial study, we sought to extend our analysis to a more general level of personality functioning. Accordingly, another study focused on individual differences in action orientation (Koole & Van den Berg, 2003, Study 3). Action orientation is a volitional style that is characterized by self-determined, autonomous goal striving, particularly under stressful circumstances (Kuhl, 1994; Kuhl & Koole, Chapter 26, this volume). Work on self-determination theory (Deci & Ryan, 2000) indicates that self-determination and autonomy are central elements of personal growth, so that action orientation seemed a valid indicator of the strength of the growth-motivation system. Therefore, we predicted that participants high on action orientation would provide more favorable ratings of wild nature than would participants low on action orientation. This prediction was confirmed across both participants' ratings of photographic simulations and their ratings of verbal descriptions of wild versus cultivated landscapes.

On the Dialectics between Growth and Defense

Taken together, there is preliminary evidence that both defense and growth motives exert an important influence on people's responses to nature. Accordingly, the next question that arose was how defense and growth motives might interact. As we argued earlier, there are theoretical grounds to assume that defensive motives are primary. Negative experiences are generally more urgent than positive ones, because ignoring threats can potentially be lethal to the organism (Baumeister et al., 2001; Taylor, 1991). Furthermore, experimental evidence suggests that growth motives tend to become undermined under threatening circumstances (Deci & Ryan, 2000; Kasser & Sheldon, Chapter 29, this volume; Koole et al., 2003).

We first examined the dialectics between defense and growth motives in a study that explored the effects of mortality salience on the nature evaluations of individuals with high or low action orientation (Koole & Van den Berg, 2003, Study 4). In this study, we manipulated mortality salience by means of a subliminal priming procedure (Arndt, Greenberg, Solomon, & Pyszczynski, 1997; see also Arndt, Cook, & Routledge, Chapter 3, this volume).

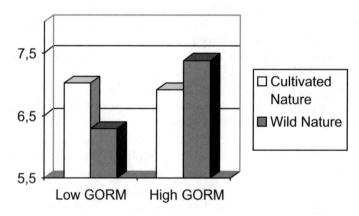

FIGURE 6.3. Effects of growth-oriented recreation motives (GORM) on perceived beauty for cultivated landscapes (Van den Berg & Koole, 2003).

In the high-mortality-salience condition, participants were subliminally primed with the word "dood" (the Dutch word for death); in the low-mortality-salience condition, participants were subliminally primed with the four x-es. To assess whether our findings were specific to death priming, we also included a third condition that subliminally primed the word "pijn" (Dutch for pain). Subsequently, participants were asked to evaluate a series of high-resolution color photos of wild versus uncultivated natural landscapes. We predicted that action-oriented participants would give higher beauty ratings to wilderness than would state-oriented participants under conditions of low mortality salience or pain salience. This prediction was based on our presumption that action-oriented individuals are more oriented toward growth and exploration. Under high mortality salience, however, we predicted that action-oriented individuals would become more similar to state-oriented individuals in giving lower ratings of wilderness. The results of the experiment supported these predictions. Moreover, the same basic pattern was replicated in two studies that used another indicator of growth/autonomy motivation, i.e., Burger's (1995) Desire for Control Scale (Van den Berg & Koole, 2002). Taken together, it appears that mortality salience eliminates the influence of growth motives on people's nature evaluations.

If defensive motives are primary, then how might growth motives come to influence people's responses to nature? Conceivably, growth motives only surface when people are fully convinced that their environment is free from any possible threat or harm. However, such idyllic circumstances seem too rare and fleeting to account for all the circumstances under people's growth motives emerge. A second possibility is that there might exist some psychological mechanisms through which people can shield their growth motivation from becoming undermined by defensive concerns (Baumann & Kuhl, 2003; Koole, 2004; Schimel, Arndt, Pyszczynski, & Greenberg, 2001). One suggestive line of research has shown that exposure to nature frequently has beneficial consequences for affective functioning and health (Ulrich, 1993). For instance, exposure to nature can provide relief from stress (Hartig, Mang, & Evans, 1991; Ulrich et al., 1991) and quicker recovery from surgery (Ulrich, 1984, 1986). These findings seem relevant to the growth motive, because various theories have argued that the growth motives orient people's functioning in a manner that is highly conducive to psychological and physical health (Deci & Ryan, 2000; Kuhl, 2001; Jung, 1964). As such, the growth motivation system might mediate some of the restorative effects of nature.

Past studies on the restorative effects of nature typically included rather mundane stressors, such as a college examination (Ulrich, 1979), everyday stress (Hartig et al., 1991), or fear of going to the dentist (Heerwagen, 1990). It thus seemed important to know whether the restorative effects of nature might be heplful in reducing the anxiety that is associated with people's ultimate concerns about death. To explore this issue, Van den Berg, Koole, and Van der Wulp (2003) examined nature's restorative effects on participants who had been exposed to gruesome reminders of death. Specifically, Van den Berg et al. (2003) first obtained baseline mood ratings from a group of participants and subsequently exposed them to scenes from "Faces of Death #1," a manipulation that has been successfully used in prior TMT research (Greenberg et al., 1992). The particular fragments included a farmer's wife decapitating a rooster and images of a slaughterhouse where sheep and bulls were killed in a very bloody fashion. After rating their moods for a second time, participants were exposed to another video fragment of a slowly paced walk through either a natural or an urban environment. Finally, participants rated their moods for a third time. Our results showed that, as might be expected, participants had more negative moods immediately after watching "Faces of Death." More important, however, participants who had subsequently watched a nature video showed significantly greater mood improvements than participants who had watched an urban video. It thus appears that the restorative effects of nature are powerful enough to extend to coping with death-related stressors.

At first glance, nature's ability to alleviate existential anxiety might seem at odds with our earlier findings that death reminders serve to reduce people's appreciation of nature. However, there are at least two ways in which these findings may be reconciled. First, our findings indicate that death reminders only lead to more negative evaluations of wild, uncultivated nature (Koole & Van den Berg, 2003). As such, our findings fit with other research showing that restorative effects of nature occur only for nonthreatening nature (Ulrich, 1993). Extrapolating from these findings, we would expect natural scenery to alleviate existential anxiety only when the scenery is not perceived as highly uncontrollable and overwhelming.

Second, our findings that death reminders can induce negative responses to wilderness have been obtained with rather subtle, cognitive death primes and on esthetic judgments of nature, which presumably involve more sophisticated cognitive processing. This paradigm is consistent with the bulk of TMT research, which has generally used subtle manipulations and dependent measures (Arndt et al., Chapter 3, this volume). By contrast, our findings that natural scenery can alleviate existential anxiety were obtained using a highly arousing death prime. There are reasons to believe that such more blatant death primes evoke qualitatively different defensive responses than more subtle death primes (Arndt et al., Chapter 3, this volume). The anxiety-buffering effects of nature were further obtained on mood ratings, which presumably are mediated primarily by affective processes that are less cognitively elaborated than beauty ratings. Taken together, it seems conceivable that anxiety-buffering effects of nature occur mainly for death reminders and responses that are highly affectively charged, whereas defensive distancing from nature may occur most strongly for death reminders and responses that are more cognitively driven. Although these speculations are intriguing, more research is required to understand how and when the confrontation with nature is anxiety-buffering versus anxiety-arousing, and how cognitive and affective defense systems are related to each other.

SUMMARY AND CONCLUSIONS

This chapter focused on some of the existential foundations of people's relations with nature. We began by arguing that people's capacity for self-awareness has been a catalyst of both people's existential concerns and people's growing alienation from nature. Thus there may exist a fundamental link between existential psychology and human–nature relations. We then analyzed the core existential motives that may underlie people's ambivalence about nature. Nature is inherently problematic for people because of its association with death and decay. Accordingly, people's defensive concerns with death provide a powerful motivation to distance themselves from the natural world. However, nature also provides an optimal setting for exploration and personal growth, both because nature is unconstrained by artificial boundaries and because the primal forces of nature are part of the deep structures of the human psyche. Although people's defensive concerns are likely to be primary, our analysis concluded that defense and growth each exert a profound influence on people's interactions with nature.

After introducing our existential motives analysis of human–nature relations, we discussed some relevant empirical research. First, people often report fearful reactions to nature, particularly wilderness settings, in line with the notion that the confrontation with nature can arouse existential concerns. Second, research within the TMT paradigm indicates that reminders of death lead people to intensify their identifications with their culture (indirectly implying a distancing from nature; Solomon et al., Chapter 2, this volume), greater support of beliefs that humans are different from animals (Goldenberg et al., 2001), and more negative reactions to animals and things that remind people of their animal nature, such as sex (Goldenberg et al., 2000; Goldenberg, Cox, Pyszczynski, Greenberg, & Solomon, 2002; Goldenberg & Roberts, Chapter 5, this volume). Third, recent studies have shown that exposure to wilderness triggers thoughts about death (Koole & Van den Berg, 2003). Finally, reminders of death lead to more negative evaluations of wilderness, especially among individuals who deny their death anxiety. Taken together, there is consistent evidence that people's responses to nature are influenced by defensive existential concerns, which induce distancing oneself from nature.

Research has similarly supported the notion that people can respond to nature in a more positive, growth-oriented manner. First, exposure to nature (as opposed to exposure to urban settings) often leads to restorative effects—that is, reductions in stress, both experienced and on psychophysiological levels, and even improved physical health (Hartig et al., 1991; Ulrich, 1993; Van den Berg et al., 2003). Second, wilderness is associated with thoughts about freedom (Koole & Van den Berg, 2003). Finally, various indicators of growth motivation, such as growth-oriented recreational motives and action orientation, are positively associated with evaluations of wilderness (Koole & Van den Berg, 2003). Given that defensive and growth motives influence people's responses to nature in opposite ways, it becomes important to ask how these motives interact. In this regard, research offers a mixed picture. Some recent studies have found that verbal reminders of death can serve to suppress the influence of autonomy-related growth motives (e.g., as indicated by individual differences in action orientation) on esthetic evaluations of wild versus cultivated nature (Koole & Van den Berg, 2003). These findings suggest that defensive motives can override the influence of growth motives on people's evaluations of nature. However, another recent study showed that exposure to nature can reduce the negative affective impact of a highly vivid, emotional charged reminder of death (Van den Berg et al., 2003). Accordingly, the interaction between growth and defense motives in human–nature relations seems complex and in need of further study.

Generally speaking, the present analysis demonstrates how basic ideas in existential and motivation psychology can have profound relevance to our understanding of human–nature relations. Although human–nature relations are traditionally considered beyond the realm of existential and motivation psychology, we believe that there is a vast potential for integration between these respective areas. The human species has lived in savage, uncultivated territories for the greater part of its evolutionary history (Appleton, 1975; Orians, 1980; Sedikides & Skowronski, 1997). It is therefore plausible that basic existential–motivational mechanisms evolved, at least originally, to cope with the risks and challenges of natural environments (Kaplan, 1987; Öhman & Mineka, 2001; Ulrich, 1993). The defense system, for instance, may have developed in conjunction with more primitive fear response systems such as the amygdalae (LeDoux, 1995), systems that originally evolved to cope with natural dangers such as insects and reptiles (Öhman & Mineka, 2000). In a related vein, some recent personality theories have proposed that the growth-motivation system in part grew out of the spatial orienting system of the hippocampus (Kuhl, 2001; LeDoux, 2002). These and other connections between existential–motivational and environmental–psychological mechanisms may be exploited in future theorizing and research.

Finally, the present analysis could have some far-ranging practical implications for people's interactions with nature. Some of the deeper roots of modern society's mounting environmental problems may lie in nature's association with ultimate concerns about death. The sharp conflict between nature and human civilization may thus be ultimately psychological, and as such seems unlikely to be solved by further scientific or technological developments. More than anything, then, humanity may need psychological wisdom to resolve its problematic relationship with nature. In the end, we humans might come to terms with the reality that we are part of nature as much as nature is part of us.

ACKNOWLEDGMENTS

Preparation of this chapter was facilitated by an Innovation Grant from the Netherlands Organization for Scientific Research (NWO) awarded to Sander Koole and by a stay of Sander Koole at the Peter Wall Institute for Interdisciplinary Studies at the University of British Columbia in Vancouver, Canada.

REFERENCES

Appleton, J. (1975). *The experience of landscape*. London: Wiley.

Arndt, J., Greenberg, J., Solomon, S., & Pyszcynski, T. (1997). Subliminal exposure to death-related stimuli increases defense of the cultural worldview. *Psychological Science, 8*, 379–385.

Becker, E. (1973). *The denial of death*. New York: Free Press.

Baumeister, R. F. (in press). *The cultural animal: Human nature, meaning, and social life*. New York: Oxford University Press.

Baumeister, R. F., Bratslavsky, E., Finkenauer, C., & Vohs, K. D. (2001). Bad is stronger than good. *Review of General Psychology, 5*, 323–370.

Baumann, N., & Kuhl, J. (2003). Self-infiltration: Confusing assigned tasks and self-selected in memory. *Personality and Social Psychology Bulletin, 29*, 487–498.

Becker, E. (1962). *The birth and death of meaning*. New York: Free Press.

Becker, E. (1973). *The denial of death*. New York: Free Press.

Bixler, R. D., & Floyd, M. F. (1997). Nature is scary, disgusting, and uncomfortable. *Environment and Behavior, 29*, 443–467.

Burger, J. M. (1995). Need for control and self-esteem: Two routes to a high desire for control. In M. Kernis (Ed.), *Efficacy, agency, and self-esteem* (pp. 217–233). London: Plenum Press.

Cohen, E. (1979). A phenomenology of tourist experiences. *Journal of the British Sociological Association, 13*, 179–201.

Deci, E. L., & Ryan, R. M. (2000). The "what" and "why" of goal pursuits: Human needs and the self-determination perspective. *Psychological Inquiry, 11*, 227–268.

De Dreu, C. K. W., Koole, S. L., & Oldersma, F. L. (1999). On the seizing and freezing of negotiator inferences: Need for closure moderates the use of heuristics in negotiation. *Personality and Social Psychology Bulletin, 25*, 348–362.

Diamond, J. (1998). *Guns, germs and steel: A short history of everybody for the last 13,000 years*. London: Vintage.

Eisenberg, E. (1998). *The ecology of Eden: An inquiry into the dream of paradise and a new vision of our role in nature*. New York: Random House.

Elands, B., & Lengkeek, J. (2000). *Typical tourists: Research into the theoretical and methodological foundations of a typology of tourism and recreation experiences*. Wageningen, The Netherlands: Mansholt Graduate School.

Frederickson, L. M., & Anderson, D. H. (1999). A qualitative exploration of the wilderness experience as a source of spiritual inspiration. *Journal of Environmental Psychology, 19*, 21–39.

Freeman, S., & Herron, J. C. (2001). *Evolutionary analysis*. Englewood Cliffs, NJ: Prentice-Hall.

Fromm, E. (1977) *The anatomy of human destructiveness*. Hardmondsworth, UK: Penguin Books.

Goldenberg, J. L., Cox, C., Pyszczynski, T., Greenberg, J., & Solomon, S. (2002). Understanding human ambivalence about sex: The effects of stripping sex of its meaning. *Journal of Sex Research, 39*, 310–320.

Goldenberg, J., Pyszczynski, T., Greenberg, J., & Solomon, S. (2000). Fleeing the body: A terror management perspective on the problem of corporeality. *Personality and Social Psychology Review, 4*, 200–218.

Goldenberg, J., Pyszczynski, T., Greenberg, J., Solomon, Kluck, B., & Cornwell, R. (2001). I am *not* an animal: Mortality salience, disgust, and the denial of human creatureliness. *Journal of Experimental Psychology: General, 130*, 427–435.

Gould, S. J. (1977). *Ontogeny and phylogeny*. Cambridge, MA: Belknap Press.

Greenberg, J., Solomon, S., & Pyszczynski, T. (1997). Terror management theory of self-esteem and cultural worldviews: Empirical assessments and conceptual refinements. In M. Zanna (Ed.), *Advances in experimental social psychology* (Vol. 29, pp. 61–139). London: Academic Press.

Greenberg, J., Solomon, S., Pyszczynski, T., Rosenblatt, A., Burling, J., Lyon, D., et al. (1992). Why do people need self-esteem? Converging evidence that self-esteem serves an anxiety-buffering function. *Journal of Personality and Social Psychology, 63*, 913–922.

Harlan, J. R. (1995). *The living fields: Our agricultural heritage*. New York: Cambridge University Press.

Hartig, T., Mang, M., & Evans, G. W. (1991). Restorative effects of natural environment experiences. *Environment and Behavior, 23*, 3–26.

Heerwagen, J. H. (1990). The psychological aspects of windows and window design. In K. H. Anthony, J. Choi, & B. Orland (Eds.), *Proceedings of the 21st annual conference of the Environmental Design Association*. Oklahoma City: EDRA.

Jung, C. G. (1964). *Man and his symbols*. New York: Dell.

Kaplan, R., & Kaplan, S. (1989). *The experience of nature: A psychological perspective*. Cambridge, UK: Cambridge University Press.

Kaplan, S. (1987). Aesthetics, affect and cognition: Environmental preference from an evolutionary perspective. *Environment and Behavior, 19*, 3–32.

Kellert, S. R. (1997). *Kinship to mastery: Biophilia in human evolution and development*. Washington, DC: Island Press.

Kenrick, D. T., Sadalla, E. K., & Keefe, R. C. (1998). Evolutionary cognitive psychology: The missing heart of modern cognitive science. In C. Crawford & D. L. Krebs (Eds.) *Handbook of evolutionary psychology* (pp. 485–514). Hillsdale, NJ: Erlbaum.

Koole, S. L. (2004). Volitional shielding of the self: Effects of action orientation and external demands on implicit self-evaluation. *Social Cognition, 22*, 117–146.

Koole, S. L. (2003). *The confrontation with wilderness triggers death-related thought*. Unpublished data, Free University Amsterdam.

Koole, S. L., Baumann, N., & Kazén, M. (2003). *When is it time to be true to your self? Effects of mortality salience and self-esteem on authenticity*. Manuscript in preparation, Free University Amsterdam.

Koole, S. L., & Van den Berg, A. E. (2000). *Effects of mortality salience and need for structure on evaluations of wild versus cultivated nature*. Unpublished data set, Free University Amsterdam.

Koole, S. L., & Van den Berg, A. E. (2003). *Lost in the wilderness: Terror management, action orientation, and evaluations of nature*. Manuscript submitted for publication, Free University Amsterdam.

Korpela, K., Hartig, T., Kaiser, F. G., & Fuhrer, U. (2001). Restorative experience and self-regulation in favorite places. *Environment and Behavior, 33*, 572–589.

Kruglanski, A. W., & Webster, D. M. (1996). Motivated closing of the mind: "Seizing" and "freezing." *Psychological Review, 103*, 263–283.

Kuhl, J. (1994). A theory of action and state orientations. In J. Kuhl & J. Beckmann (Eds.), *Volition and personality: Action versus state orientation* (pp. 9–46). Göttingen, Germany: Hogrefe & Huber.

Kuhl, J. (2001). *Motivation und Persönlichkeit: Interaktionen psychischer Systeme* [Motivation and personality: Interactions between psychic systems]. Göttingen, Germany: Hogrefe.

Leary, M. R. & Cottrell, C. A. (1999). Evolution of the self, the need to belong, and life in a delayed-return environment. *Psychological Inquiry, 10,* 229–232.

LeDoux, J. E. (1995). Emotion: Clues from the brain. *Annual Review of Psychology, 46,* 209–235.

LeDoux, J. E. (2002). *Synaptic self: How our brains become who we are.* London: MacMillan.

Martin, L. L. (1999). I-D compensation theory: Some implications of trying to satisfy immediate-return needs in a delayed culture. *Psychological Inquiry, 10,* 195–208.

Mikulincer, M. (1997). Adult attachment style and information processing: Individual differences in curiosity and cognitive closure. *Journal of Personality and Social Psychology, 72,* 1217–1230.

Mithen, S. (1996). *The prehistory of the human mind.* London: Thames & Hudson.

Öhman, A., & Mineka, S. (2000). Fears, phobias, and preparedness: Toward an evolved module of fear and learning. *Psychological Review, 108,* 483–522.

Orians, G. H. (1980). Habitat selection: General theory and applications to human behavior. In J. Nasar (Ed.), *Environmental aesthetics: Theory, research, and applications* (pp. 364–378). New York: Cambridge University Press.

Pyszczynski, T. Greenberg, J., & Goldenberg, J. L. (2003). Freedom versus fear: On the defense, growth, and expansion of the self. In M. R. Leary & J. P. Tangney (Eds.). *Handbook of self and identity* (pp. 314–343). New York: Guilford Press.

Pyszczynski, T., Greenberg, J., & Solomon, S. (1998). A terror management perspective on the psychology of control: Controlling the uncontrollable. In M. Kofta, G. Weary, and G. Sedek (Eds.), *Personal control in action* (pp. 85–107). New York: Plenum Press.

Rank, O. (1945). *Will therapy and truth and reality.* New York: Knopf. (Original work published 1936)

Schimel, J., Arndt, J., Pyszczynski, T., & Greenberg, J. (2001). Being accepted for who we are: Evidence that social validation of the intrinsic self reduces general defensiveness. *Journal of Personality and Social Psychology, 80,* 35–52.

Sedikides, C., & Skowronski, J. J. (1997). The symbolic self in evolutionary context. *Personality and Social Psychology Review, 1,* 80–102.

Sedikides, C., & Strube, M. J. (1997). Self-evaluation: To thine own self be good, to thine own self be sure, to thine own self be true, to thine own self be better. In M. P. Zanna (Ed.), *Advances in experimental social psychology* (Vol. 29, pp. 209–269). New York: Academic Press.

Silvia, P. J., & Duval, T. S. (2001). Objective self-awareness: Recent progress and enduring problems. *Personality and Social Psychology Review, 5,* 230–241.

Smith, B. D. (1995). *The emergence of agriculture.* New York: Scientific American Library.

Solomon, S., Greenberg, J., Schimel, J., Arndt, J., & Pyszczynski, T. (2003). Human awareness of mortality and the evolution of culture. In M. Schaller & C. Crandall (Eds.), *The psychological foundations of culture* (pp. 15–40). Hillsdale, NJ: Erlbaum.

Taylor, S. E. (1991). Asymmetrical effects of positive and negative events: The mobilization-minimization hypothesis. *Psychological Bulletin, 110,* 67–85.

Ulrich, R. S. (1979). Visual landscapes and psychological well-being. *Landscape Research, 4,* 17–23.

Ulrich, R. S. (1984). View through a window may influence recovery from surgery. *Science, 224,* 420–421.

Ulrich, R. S. (1986). Human responses to vegetation and landscapes. *Landscape and Urban Planning, 13,* 29–44.

Ulrich, R. S. (1993). Biophilia, biophobia and natural landscapes. In S. R. Kellert & E. O. Wilson (Eds.), *The biophilia hypothesis* (pp. 73–137). Washington, DC: Island Press.

Ulrich, R. S., Simons, R. F., Losito, B. D., Fiorito, E., Miles, M. A., & Zelson, M. (1991). Stress recovery during exposure to natural and urban environments. *Journal of Environmental Psychology, 11,* 201–230.

Van den Berg, A. E., & Koole, S. L. (2003). *Desire for control and nature evaluation.* Unpublished data, Alterra Green World Research, Wageningen, The Netherlands.

Van den Berg, A. E., Koole, S. L., & Van der Wulp, N. (2003). Environmental preference and restoration: (How) Are they related? *Journal of Environmental Psychology, 23,* 135–146.

Van den Berg, A. E., & Vlek, C. A. J. (1998). The influence of planned-change context on the evaluation of natural landscapes. *Landscape and Urban Planning*, *43*, 1–10.

Van den Berg, A. E., Vlek, C. A. J., & Coeterier, J. F. (1998). Group differences in the aesthetic evaluation of nature development plans: A multilevel approach. *Journal of Environmental Psychology*, *18*, 141–157.

Van Trigt, A. A. (2002). *Hogere sferen. Belevingsonderzoek naar de spirituele waarde van bomen en bos* [Higher grounds. An investigation into the experience of the spiritual value of trees and forests]. Unpublished master's thesis, Wageningen University, Wageningen, the Netherlands.

Williams, K. D., & Harvey, D. (2001). Transcendent experience in forest environments. *Journal of Environmental Psychology*, *96*, 18–23.

Woodburn, J. C. (1982). Egalitarian societies. *Man*, *17*, 431–451.

Yalom, I. (1980). *Existential psychotherapy*. New York: Basic Books.

Chapter 7

Risk Taking in Adolescence

"To Be or Not to Be" Is Not Really the Question

ORIT TAUBMAN - BEN-ARI

Risk-taking behaviors, such as unprotected sex, reckless driving, substance abuse, or challenging sportive activities, are the most severe threats to adolescent health and may even cause eventual death. What makes young people ready to take such major risks to their lives? Doesn't it contradict their basic self-preservation instinct? What are the basic psychological determinants of risky behaviors? To answer these questions, it is essential to understand the existential circumstances and needs of adolescence and how they affect the internal risk-taking schemas, along with the potential external influences on these behaviors.

While studying the subjective meanings of reckless driving, a 19-year-old man told me, with glowing eyes: "Driving is exactly like a bungee jump. . . . But bungee is a whole operation, you have to plan ahead, go to a particular place where you can jump. . . . Instead, I can go down, get into the car and just press the gas pedal . . . I get the same thrill out of it." I know for certain that this was the first time I truly understood what reckless driving really means to young people. It is not just an easy way to move around or a quick means to get somewhere; the danger and sensations associated with this behavior make it so attractive and enjoyable. Moreover, on a deeper level, people are frequently attracted to risky behaviors as a way to resolve their existential fear of death. It is not that they consciously decide whether they want to live or to die when they engage in a risky behavior, rather what guides the behavior is the "walking on the edge," limit testing, and a sense of aliveness. Moreover, in some cases risk-taking behavior enhances self-esteem and helps to gain a better image of one's competence and efficiency, which may even exacerbate the life-endangering behavior. Thus, the existential paradox here is that the sense of aliveness so frequently associated with risk taking might be well established in the individual's attempts to handle the ultimate anxiety—the terror of his or her own death.

Traditionally, risk taking has been explored in theoretical frameworks such as decision-making, problem behavior, and sensation-seeking patterns. Even though much can be learned from such perspectives, I would like to suggest an integrative way to organize the accumulated knowledge regarding risk taking, using an existential framework focused on the unique experiences and subjective perspective of the adolescent, to explore the motivations, emotions, and cognitions that guide risk-taking processes. This approach can benefit from all the aforementioned frameworks as well as improve our understanding of this behavior. Evidently, the distinction between the three risk-taking aspects—the cognitive, the motivational, and the affective—is not definite. Whereas decision making is a cognitive process, it may be influenced by emotions and still be explained by the motivations that guide the decision maker. Therefore, any attempt to distinguish between these aspects of risk taking is somewhat arbitrary. The purpose of this chapter is, thus, to review existing literature on adolescents' risk taking, aiming to identify and examine the set of affective, cognitive, and motivational aspects that are most likely to contribute to a decision to engage in risky behaviors. In addition, any description of risk-taking behavior will not be complete without relating to external influences. Being human means, in part, acting in a social milieu; thus family and friends constitute the basic environment for adolescents, and their role in controlling and modeling risk-taking behavior is discussed later.

Importantly, risk taking is not a unified phenomenon, it consists of a wide range of activities. Though some of the theoretical approaches attempted to comprehend a host of behaviors, many studies in this field relate to a specific behavior. In this chapter, I endeavor to integrate the knowledge in order to advance the understanding of risky behaviors as a whole, as well as to pay attention to specific behaviors. Notably, this chapter is devoted to specific risk-taking variables rather than to global personality variables.

RISK TAKING IN ADOLESCENCE

A specific behavior can lead to more than one outcome, some of which are desirable and satisfying and others undesirable and even dangerous. Risk taking involves implementation of options that could lead to negative consequences (Byrnes, Miller, & Schafer, 1999).

Risk taking can be either adaptive or maladaptive. It is maladaptive whenever the benefits of the activity are far less likely to occur than the potential hazards. It is adaptive whenever the converse is true (Byrnes et al., 1999). In other words, people cannot and should not avoid all the risks in their surroundings. Instead, they adapt successfully by systematically pursuing certain risks and avoiding others (Byrnes, 1998).

Much of the risk-taking literature is focused on adolescence. Adolescence is a fascinating phase, which entails enormous changes caused by physiological, cognitive, and psychosocial developments and changes in the nature of the social environment. Young people are going through an existential process of liberating themselves from their parents and asserting themselves as grownups and independent individuals. The young person must develop a sense of personal identity, of stable selfhood, so that experienced past and anticipated future are meaningfully connected (Erickson, 1968). This effort can be demonstrated in various lifestyles as well as in group affiliation, role expectations, and degrees of social dependence. Erickson (1968) termed the success in achieving this phase's tasks "ego identity" formation, while the failure in doing so was termed "role confusion," indicating an inability to integrate various self-images to one self-identity. The decision to engage in risk taking may stem from curiosity, thrill seeking, peer pressure and acceptance, escape from stress, and rebellion against authority, as well as from a desire for self-knowledge, self-improvement, creativity, or expansion of consciousness. When these motives are considered in terms of Erickson's theory, risk taking can be considered a normal developmental phase in adolescence, in relation to an underlying identity confusion. Thus, young people who do not know for sure who they are might find alcohol- or drug-related experiences attractive in exploring the outer boundaries of selfhood; they may think, for example, that they can find a dimension of themselves which evades them in the sober, "straight" world.

All the same, a certain degree of risk taking is considered to be essential for the development of optimal social and psychological competence, to build self-confidence, to enhance independence and self-regulation, and to provide reinforcement for taking initiatives (Baumrind, 1987; Shedler & Block, 1990). It may also fulfill the evolving needs for autonomy, mastery, and intimacy of adolescents (e.g., Deci & Ryan, 2000; Irwin & Millstein, 1986). In this respect, risk taking can be viewed as one way adolescents cope with central developmental tasks. Jessor (1982) claims that behaviors such as smoking, drinking, substance abuse, or risky sexual activity should be considered "purposeful, meaningful, goal oriented and functional rather than arbitrary or perverse." As such, problem behavior in adolescence can be regarded as instrumental in gaining peer acceptance and respect; in establishing autonomy from parents, in repudiating the norms and values of conventional authority; in coping with anxiety, frustration, and anticipation of failure; in conforming to self and significant others' certain attributes of identity, or in affirming maturity and marking a transition from childhood toward a more mature status (Jessor, 1991).

Yet, risk-taking behaviors such as driving a vehicle at high speeds or while intoxicated, having sex without contraception or with a stranger, using illegal drugs, and so on, are the most severe threats to adolescents' health and well-being. Negative potential consequences of such behaviors include unwanted pregnancy, sexually transmitted diseases, severe disability, and even death (Igra & Irwin, 1996). Still, many times, a person is willing to exchange exposure to death risks to attain other goals. Thus, health-risk choices often have an alternative, in which one choice leads to an immediate available benefit at the price of a low death risk and the other avoids risk at the cost of a postponed reward. Narcotics, high-exposure rock climbing, and reckless driving provide immediate rewards associated with low, but nonnegligible death risks, which are frequently acceptable to young individuals (Gardner, 1993). However, many scholars adopted the assumption that adolescents do not have a basic knowledge regarding health, illness, and risk (e.g., Irwin, 1993), and the way adolescents think, feel, and experience these behaviors has gained less attention.

Only a few studies offer a nonjudgmental insight into adolescents' behavior and experiences from the adolescents' own point of view (e.g., Furbey & Beyth-Marom, 1992). It is important to bear in mind that the negative connotations of "risk behavior" that dominate adult thinking are not necessarily viewed in the same manner by adolescents (Furby & Beyth-Marom, 1992; Parsons, Siegel, & Cousins, 1997). Because we are trying to figure out adolescents' thinking, it is highly important to attempt to explore their experiences, perceptions, attitudes, emotions, and motivations in order to gain a better understanding of risk taking at this life phase.

Because participating in risky behavior is not a unidimensional objective experience, it cannot be easily described as positive or negative. Risk taking is, rather, first and foremost, an internal scheme, subjective and individual, which may raise conflicts and ambivalence. Viewing the vast literature concerning adolescents' risk-taking behavior reveals three related general aspects—cognitive, motivational, and emotional. Each aspect represents another dimension of risk taking experience, but combined they reflect a full spectrum of interdependent feelings, thoughts, attitudes, values, needs, and aspirations of young persons that all focus on the most important task they have to face and cope with at the current phase in their life cycle: the need to try out experiences. The cognitive aspect relates to attitudes toward and the perceptions of risk taking, and to the decision-making process of "to be or not to be" involved in a risky behavior, including potential biases in this process. The motivational aspect relates to two facets. The first is the subjective meanings attached to risk-taking behavior and to the functions it fulfills; the second, the meanings attached to the perceptions of competence, self-esteem and self-efficacy while participating in risk-taking activities. The affective aspect relates to emotions and sensations raised by experiencing risk taking. These emotions can be positive (happiness, thrill, excitement, etc.) or negative (fear, anger, helplessness, etc.) and are probably not mutually exclusive.

INTERNAL ASPECTS OF RISK TAKING: COGNITIVE, AFFECTIVE, AND MOTIVATIONAL

Cognitive Aspects of Risk Taking

Cognitively based theories of risk-taking behavior examine ways in which individuals perceive risks and make decisions about risk taking. Often the basic premise is that adolescents are "optimistically biased" in their risk perception or that they feel "invulnerable" (Elkind, 1967), which means that they have an exaggerated sense of uniqueness and invulnerability. Yet, Furby and Beyth-Marom (1992) stress the important fact that almost every behavior is risky, because risk behavior applies to every action (or inaction) that entails some chance for loss. Smoking marijuana may be risky if it entails a chance of becoming addicted. However, not smoking is also risky if it entails a chance of being rejected by peers. In this regard, not smoking marijuana could be as risky as smoking, depending on the individual's values and tendencies.

In general, two different purposes might affect risk-related decisions (Lopes, 1983, 1987): the desire to avoid loss and the desire to maximize gain. The desire to avoid loss is motivated by fear (the more one fears loss, the more choices he or she will make that minimize the chances for loss), whereas the desire to exploit opportunity is motivated by hope (the more one hopes for gain, the more choices he or she will make that maximize the opportunity for gain). Thus, people sometimes take risks because the value of the expected gain outweighs the value of the expected loss. However, sometimes there is a tendency to focus on the potential gain and pay little attention to the potential loss. Such a choice could be made despite the awareness of the loss and the absolute value of the expected loss, which might be higher than the absolute value of the expected gain (Lopes, 1983, 1987). Moreover, findings suggest that even when youngsters are aware of the potential risks of reckless driving, they tend to disregard these negative consequences while driving, which in turn enhances their tendency to drive recklessly (Taubman - Ben-Ari, Mikulincer, & Iram, 2002). Thus, it seems that young drivers adopt a present time orientation regarding reckless driving, concentrating on the pleasure and fun and tending to ignore possible future outcomes of their behavior even though, rationally, they know it is risky and might endanger their life and the life of others. The immediate temptation seems to override the existing learned knowledge of what might be the result of reckless driving, probably due to their strong feeling of control over the situation.

Numerous studies have shown that adolescents tend to ascribe less risk to several health-risk behaviors than do adults, and adolescents estimate that the probability of a negative outcome as a result of engaging in reckless behavior is lower for themselves than for others (e.g., Arnett, 1992; Weinstein, 1987). For example, in comparison to older drivers, adolescent drivers have a higher tendency to rate themselves as less likely to be involved in accidents than their peers (e.g., Finn & Bragg, 1986), and they tend to overestimate their own driving abilities (Glendon, Dorn, Davies, Matthews, & Taylor, 1996). Younger drivers, especially men, underestimate certain traffic hazards and perceive dangerous situations as less risky than do older drivers (e.g., Finn & Bragg, 1986; DeJoy, 1992; Glendon et al., 1996; Matthews & Moran, 1986). Adolescent girls who have sex without contraception estimate the probability of getting pregnant as a result from such behavior as lower than do girls who have sex with contraception (Arnett, 1995).

Although links between perceptions and behavior are complex, there is a reasonable agreement that perceptions of risk are related to the individual's decision to engage or not to engage in reckless behaviors. Nevertheless, risk perceptions are not the only contributors to risky behavior; emotional states and reactions are certainly part of the larger picture.

Affective Aspects of Risk Taking

Risk-taking decision making has begun to incorporate affect into what used to be an almost exclusively cognitive field (Lerner & Keltner, 2001). Findings indicate that happy individuals made relatively optimistic risk-related judgments and choices, and hence they perceived less risk and made risk-seeking choices (Lerner & Keltner, 2000, 2001). In contrast, the induction of negative affect increased the tendency to choose high-risk, high-payoff options in a lottery game (Leith & Baumeister, 1996). However, a more thorough examination of the effect of negative emotions showed that whereas fearful individuals made relatively pessimistic risk-related judgments and choices, and hence tended to perceive more risk and favor risk-free options, angry individuals, in a similar way to the happy ones, made relatively optimistic risk-related judgments and choices, and thus tended to perceive less risk and made risk-seeking choices (Lerner & Keltner, 2000, 2001). It seems that a general bad mood leads people to engage in risky behaviors and to be less aware of their potential costs, as though they have nothing to lose. Anger seems to be related to risk taking, perhaps because it allows people to act out their feelings instead of coping with them in an introverted manner.

Several studies validated this assertion regarding angry persons and risky behaviors, especially in the area of reckless driving, showing that some adolescents use driving as a way of expressing aggressiveness and hostility (Arnett, 1995; Donovan, Umlaf, & Selzberg, 1988). In addition, it has been shown that more aggressive adolescents tend to drive more recklessly (Arnett, Offer, & Fine, 1997), and that adolescents drive more recklessly when they are in an angry mood (Arnett et al., 1997). Driving-related anger was associated with more frequent reckless driving (Taubman - Ben-Ari & Mikulincer, 2003b), and angry driving style was significantly associated with self-reports of more frequent involvement in car accidents and with committing driving offenses (Taubman - Ben-Ari, Mikulincer, & Gillath, 2004). Reactance theory (Brehm & Brehm, 1981) may help to explain the high levels of anger associated with risk-taking behavior. This theory attempts to explain human behavior in situations involving a threat to perceived freedom, stating that such a threat arouses a motivational state, which is directed toward the establishment of the threatened freedom. This motivation can be evidenced in behavioral efforts to reassert a threatened freedom, such as rejecting a coercive attempt at attitude change or the need to transform a restraint to one's impulses. Because the decision *not* to engage in risk-taking behaviors might be perceived as a restriction of the desire for freedom, jointed with the fact that it is possible that the attempts to shape youngsters' behavior patterns according to the adults' preferred way are perceived as coercive by the adolescents, the possible result in view of a reactance approach might be a boomerang effect, increasing the engagement in risky behaviors along with high levels of expressed aggression.

A different, yet related, frequently studied emotional aspect of risky behavior relates to sensation seeking (Arnett, 1992; Zuckerman, 1979), which implies that individual differences in risk taking reflect biological differences in optimal levels of arousal and stimulation. It assumes that the engagement in behaviors that entail a chance of loss heightens one's level of arousal. Though it is not clear whether sensation seeking leads to risk taking (Furbey & Beyth-Marom, 1992), accumulated evidence suggests a significant association between sensation seeking and a wide range of risky behaviors. In their search for novel and intense sensations and experiences, sensation seekers take physical and legal risks when they drive too fast (Zuckerman & Neeb, 1980), recklessly, or while intoxicated (e.g., Arnett et al., 1997; Jonah, 1997; Taubman - Ben-Ari et al., 2004). They tend to drink heavily, taking the social risks of disinhibited behavior (Zuckerman, 1987), they smoke, accepting the health risks (Zuckerman, Ball, & Black, 1990), and they take physical, legal, and social risks by using illegal drugs (Zuckerman, 1983).

In addition, high sensation seekers tend to perceive less risk in many activities and to anticipate more positive potential outcomes than do low sensation seekers (Igra & Irwin, 1996). Hence, risk perception may mediate the relationship between sensation seeking and risky driving. High sensation seekers may not perceive certain driving behaviors as risky and feel that they can speed, follow closely, or drive after drinking and still drive safely because of their perceived superior driving skills (Jonah, 1997). Alternatively, initially high sensation seekers may perceive their behaviors as risky but accept the risks in order to experience the thrill of engaging in them, maybe as part of their identity seeking. A lowered perception of risk level in high sensation seekers once they have experienced a risky behavior without negative consequences may cause more frequent risky driving behavior in the future (Jonah, 1997). Thus, besides the explanation of affective-related aspects of risk-taking behavior, sensation seeking provides an explanation for cognitive processes. In addition, sensation seeking, is frequently cited for being a motivator to engage in risky behaviors. It is, however, only one of many potential motivators to take risks.

Motivational Aspects of Risk Taking

Perceived Costs and Benefits of Risk Taking

According to a functional analysis, behavior is best understood in terms of the goals or needs it serves (Snyder & Cantor, 1997). Whether people engage in different behaviors to achieve the same goals or in the same behavior to achieve different goals, the key for understanding is contained within the purposes and motives that underlie and promote each behavior (Cooper, Shapiro, & Powers, 1998). Self-determination theory, for example, assumes that there are three basic psychological needs that direct individuals' behaviors: the need for autonomy, competence, and relatedness to others. It implies that people must experience the satisfaction of these needs in order to experience optimal growth and health (Deci & Ryan, 1985).

Although discussions of risky behavior often focus on its potential impairment and endangering aspects, risk taking is also a positive force in development, manifested in adventurousness, creativity, and the desire to face challenges (Moore & Parsons, 2000), and it may indeed serve as an important context that allows satisfaction of basic needs, which are theorized to promote health and well-being (Deci & Ryan, 1985). Moreover, risk taking enables youthful experimentation, which is a critical factor in a healthy development of young persons. In fact, studies have shown that experimentation with risk taking is both normative and psychologically adaptive (Baumrind, 1987). Increased self-confidence, self-esteem, stress tolerance, and initiative are all potential gains that may result from risky behaviors (Moore & Parsons, 2000).

Perceived benefits of engaging in a risky behavior, or enhancement motivators, are described most frequently. They include the motivation to show off; to achieve adult status; to undergo various experiences; to be challenged; to achieve self-esteem, personal worth, control and confidence; to gain a sense of competence and skill; to feel part of a group; and to experience thrill, adventure, and sensation. Accordingly, risky driving was found to serve as a means to increase feelings of self-determination, personal efficacy, sense of control, status, and power (Donovan et al., 1988; Taubman - Ben-Ari & Mikulincer, 2003a) and to achieve pleasure and relaxation, manage impression, show off, test limits, or compete with other drivers (Gregersen & Bjurulf, 1996; Taubman - Ben-Ari & Mikulincer, 2003a). Cars were perceived by adolescent males as "making them more powerful" (Farrow & Brissing, 1990). Young drivers tend to report more driving to "enjoy themselves and get the most out of the car," to "let off steam" (Jung & Huguenin, 1992), to "cool off after an argument" (Farrow & Brissing, 1990), or to achieve sensation-seeking thrills (Arnett et al., 1997). In addition, trying dangerous driving maneuvers may aid young men in creating gender identities (Papadakis & Moore, 1991), in a culture in which seeking risks is part of the social construction of manhood (Hopkins & Emler, 1990).

The influence of these motives on driving is governed by reinforcement, which is connected with this behavior. The relation between motives and reinforcement is quite complicated, as exceeding speed limits, for example, may most probably not result in being stopped by the police, or in involvement in an accident, but rather in arriving faster at a destination. This reinforcement helps adolescents to draw conclusions about individual safe driving that counteracts safety in statistical terms (Gregersen & Bjurulf, 1996). The same applies to other risky behaviors. When risky sexual behavior is pleasurable and does not necessarily result in contracting AIDS, or when the use of drugs results in a wonderful high feeling and group acceptance, in the absence of resenting adults around to disapprove, reinforcement for this behavior is almost a built-in mechanism.

Discussions in the literature on the costs of engaging in a risky behavior from the adolescents' point of view are fewer. They include fears of getting addicted, concerns of parents and reactions of significant others, regret for engaging in the risky behavior, helplessness, loss of control, and risk to self-esteem. More specifically, feelings of embarrassment, reduced pleasure, unnatural feeling, and inconvenience are commonly expressed in relation to the costs of condom use (Parsons, Halkitis, Bimbi, & Borkowski, 2000). Similarly, several costs of driving were found, namely, stress and loss of control, damage to self-esteem, frustration and burden, and life-endangerment (Taubman - Ben-Ari & Mikulincer, 2003a). Interestingly, Taubman - Ben-Ari and Mikulincer's (2003a) findings indicate that both costs and benefits are significantly and positively related to reckless driving behaviors, implying that complex psychological dynamics, including counterphobic mechanisms, may be involved in the decision to drive recklessly.

Most scholars refer to costs and benefits of the involvement in risky behaviors, but Furby and Beyth-Marom (1992) point out the importance of studying costs and benefits of avoiding the risky behavior (e.g., of smoking marijuana and of not smoking it): "some possible consequences of choosing to smoke marijuana are that she will feel high, she will feel part of a group, she will disappoint her parents, she will feel sick, she will get addicted, and she will enjoy trying something that is illegal. Some possible consequences of not smoking are her feeling good about not giving in to social pressure, her friends' calling her a "goody goody," and her regretting her decision later" (p. 5).

In other words, risky behaviors can serve many different goals and functions. People may engage in risky behaviors as a way to develop certain competencies or skills (e.g., by driving at high speed on a winding mountain road), to meet affiliative or intimacy needs (e.g., by having sex with a new sexual partner), or to cope with stress and dysphoric mood (e.g., by drinking to cheer up) (Cooper, Agocha, & Sheldon, 2000).

Interestingly, it has been found that adolescents' perception of positive consequences (benefits) are better predictors of involvement in risk-taking behaviors than perceived costs. Accordingly, the perceived benefits of unprotected sex are better predictors of sexual risk-taking behaviors than the perceived costs (e.g., Moore & Gullone, 1996; Parsons et al., 1997; Parsons et al., 2000; Siegel et al., 1994). In addition, in making decisions regarding sexual risk taking, adolescents tend to focus on the potential benefits of the risky, endangering activity (unprotected sex) rather than on the benefits of the safer activities (condom use), perhaps because the risky behavior is perceived as more pleasurable (Moore, Rosenthal, & Mitchell, 1996; Parsons et al., 2000). In this way, fear of costs of safer sex is more predictive of sexual behavior than fear regarding unsafe sex (Galligan & Terry, 1993), which might be explained by the fact that it is more likely that adolescents experienced the benefits of unprotected sex but did not yet experience any costs associated with this risky behavior (Moore et al., 1996).

However, one should keep in mind that, as Jessor (1991) argued, people do not typically smoke for the thrill of seeing whether they can avoid lung cancer or have unprotected sex for the thrill of beating the odds of contracting a sexually transmitted disease. Rather, they engage in these behaviors because they offer an immediate gain or benefit, which the individual judges (consciously or unconsciously) to be worth the long-term risk of negative consequences. Thus, risky behavior involves an exchange between short-term, usually affective, gains and potential long-term costs (Cooper et al., 2000). Accordingly, perceived benefits of alcohol and smoking cigarettes were found to considerably outweigh the perceived costs of these behaviors (Goldberg, Halpern-Felsher, & Millstein, 2002), presumably because adolescents adjust and base their perceptions on both their positive experiences and the failure to experience negative outcomes. Understanding the interplay between perceived risks and benefits highlights the importance of the recognition that people value different things, and that health concerns may not rank as high as social concerns for adolescents. All other things being equal, individuals are more likely to take risks if they are about to gain highly valued outcomes (benefits). Similarly, they are more likely to avoid risks when they are about to lose highly valued outcomes (Millstein & Halpern-Felsher, 2002).

Baumeister and Scher (1988) argue that self-destructive behavior patterns are characterized by a propensity to choose immediate pleasure or relief and that this propensity is exacerbated under the influence of aversive emotional states, partly because the experience of aversive emotions increases the attractiveness of immediate relief. Cooper et al. (1998) add that given that certain types of sexual behavior may provide quick and easy relief from aversive emotional states, it seems plausible that individuals who are motivated to use sex to escape aversive emotional states will weigh the immediate benefits of having sex more heavily than the possible long-term costs. Thus, individuals who are primarily motivated by needs to maintain or restore self-esteem, to regulate negative emotions, or to conform to the expectations of peers or partners tend to make suboptimal decisions about their sexual behavior. Given that, these decisions may be disproportionately influenced by the strength of their immediate psychological needs rather than by the appropriateness or advisability of engaging in a particular sexual behavior with a given partner on a given occasion. Accordingly, people who drink to cope with negative emotions experience more alcohol-related problems, even though they do not necessarily drink more (Cooper, Frone, Russell, & Mudar, 1995). Presumably, the need to escape an aversive emotional state overrides the ability to effectively regulate one's drinking behavior (Cooper et al., 1998).

Costs and benefits of risk-taking behavior constitute an important motivational base for participating in these behaviors. Nevertheless, another important part of the motivational aspect is its relation to the enhancement of self-esteem and to advancing the sense of self-efficacy.

Self-Esteem and Self-Efficacy

Besides the distinction between costs and benefits, Cooper et al. (1998) suggest the existence of another dimension, which inspires motivations in general, and with respect to risky behavior in particular: individual versus social goal-directed behaviors. Self-focused goals are primarily motivated by identity, or autonomy–competence needs such as the use of risky sex, to affirm one's sense of identity or attractiveness or to manage one's internal emotional experiences. In contrast, other-focused goals are motivated by attachment or communal needs such as having sex to achieve intimacy and communion in a relationship, or by a desire to gain or maintain social approval from significant others such as having sex to impress one's peers.

Focusing on the individual aspect of this dimension, it is important to refer to the role that self-esteem and self-efficacy play in risky behaviors. Self-esteem has often been cited as a predictor of risk-taking behavior. Lower self-esteem has been associated with sexual debut in adolescent females (Orr, Wilbrandt, Brack, Rauch, & Ingersoll, 1989), with inconsistent use of contraceptive among adolescent girls (Miller, Forehand, R., & Kotchick, 2000), and with higher rates of alcohol and substance abuse (e.g., Dielman, Campbelli, Shope, & Butchart, 1987). Possibly, low self-esteem persons, may be more inclined to highlight the benefits of risky behaviors (e.g., unprotected sex) in their decision making, which may be the way they justify their risk-taking behavior (Parsons et al., 2000). In contrast, other studies showed that high-risk-taking adolescents have better self-esteem and suffer less depression than do low adolescent risk takers (Gonzalez et al., 1994). This contradiction between the various findings may be somewhat reconciled using Deci and Ryan's (1985) self-determination theory. On one hand, high self-esteem adolescents may use risk-taking behavior as a path for the actualization of intrinsic growth needs; hence they experience a validation of their already perceived high self-esteem. On the other hand, low self-esteem adolescents may use risk-taking behaviors to satisfy extrinsic needs such as fame and positive image in the eyes of others, and hence they defend their inferior feelings by taking higher risks.

In addition, beyond any decision-making process of weighing the benefits or costs associated with a given behavior, adolescents must have the confidence, or self-efficacy, in their ability to perform the behavior (Parsons et al., 2000). Self-efficacy can be defined as the beliefs of individuals in their capability to engage successfully in a course of actions that satisfy their situational demands sufficiently (McAuley, 1992). In part, perceptions of self-efficacy are independent of the skills involved, whereas optimal functioning requires both skills and efficacy self-beliefs. People tend to undertake and perform activities with self-assurance when they judge themselves capable of handling them (Bandura, 1986). Accordingly, high perceptions of physical self-efficacy were found to be predictors of sportive risk taking (Slanger & Rudestam, 1997), high diving self-efficacy was positively related to risk taking in various recreational diving scenarios (Miller & Taubman - Ben-Ari, in press), and a belief in having suitable inner resources to handle various driving situations predicted reckless driving habits (Taubman - Ben-Ari et al., 2002). However, self-efficacy has been also identified as an important factor in the practice of safer sex behaviors and condom use (e.g., Fisher & Fisher, 1992; Goldman & Harlow, 1993; Parsons et al., 2000). This self-efficacy perception means confidence in the ability to use condoms correctly, to negotiate safer sex with a partner, and to resist situational temptations (Parsons et al., 2000).

Recognizing the guiding motivations and inner resources leading to a decision to engage in risk-taking behaviors leaves out an important question regarding another existential motivational base for taking risks, or more specifically, the associations between risk-taking and death awareness.

Risk-Taking and Death Awareness

Studies that examined the association between death anxiety and risk taking provided inconclusive results. Whereas in most of them no associations were found between death anxiety and risk taking (Alexander & Lester, 1972; Berman, 1973; Schrader & Wann, 1999; Slanger & Rudestam, 1997; Thorson & Powell, 1990; Warren, 1981–1982), one study indicated that the willingness to think about death among men was related only to lower risky sexual behavior but not to risk taking in sports and drug abuse, whereas among women it was related to higher drug abuse (Word, 1996).

However, recently, the incorporation of terror management theory (TMT) provided a better understanding of the motivational basis for risk taking (e.g., Greenberg, Pyszczynski, & Solomon, 1997; Solomon, Greenberg, & Pyszczynski, 1991; see also Solomon, Greenberg, & Pyszczynski, Chapter 2, this volume). Adopting this approach, Taubman - Ben-Ari, Florian, and Mikulincer (1999, 2000) speculated that whereas death reminders may lead people to search for potential courses of action that may validate their self-esteem, the perception that driving is relevant to self-esteem may focus this search on driving behavior. As a consequence, people may overemphasize the self-relevant gains involved in driving (e.g., validating one's sense of mastery and improving social prestige), pay little attention to potential dangers, and then take more risks while driving. In a series of five studies, we found that mortality salience led young men who perceived driving as relevant to their self-esteem to engage in more reckless driving. For them, the engagement in reckless driving probably involved the potential gain of positive self-relevant outcomes that might have increased their sense of self-esteem. On the other hand, for men who did not perceive driving as relevant to their self-esteem, this effect of mortality salience was nullified. The potential positive outcomes involved in reckless driving might have been irrelevant to their defensive efforts to increase self-esteem (Taubman - Ben-Ari et al., 1999).

Results of other studies were in line with the foregoing findings and supported the idea that death reminders may affect risk taking. Specifically, studies showed that a mortality salience manipulation increased the attraction of various risky activities (e.g., engaging in casual sex and trying heroin) for men (Hirshberger, Florian, Mikulincer, Goldenberg, & Pyszczynski, 2002), led to riskier choices in different risky contexts by individuals with external locus of control (Miller & Mulligan, 2002), and increased the willingness of divers (in a wide age range) with low self-esteem and low self-efficacy to take higher diving risks than in the control condition (Miller & Taubman - Ben-Ari, in press). However, death awareness reduced the willingness of low self-esteem - high diving-self-efficacy persons to take diving risks (Miller & Taubman - Ben-Ari, in press), caused high school students to report smoking less frequently (Kain & Nelson, 2001), and led those with internal locus of control to choose less risky options (Miller & Mulligan, 2002). Thus, the effect of death awareness on risk taking might be an inhibiting one—reducing the willingness to take risks as a consequence of the heightened awareness of the risks embedded in such a behavior, or be counterphobic, and sometimes counterintuitive, leading to decisions which may bring about a higher potential for death risk. Trying to integrate the various findings is not a simple task, as each study concentrated on another feature and examined different risk-taking behaviors. However, two potential explanation lines may lend important insights. The first relates to a person's inner resources, which may shield him or her from the fear of annihilation while confronting death awareness (see, e.g., Florian, Mikulincer, & Hirschberger, 2001). Thus, on one hand, persons with a high sense of self-efficacy or those with internal locus of control may have better mechanisms to cope with the terror of death, avoiding unnecessary risks. On the other hand, those who have external locus of control or low self-efficacy may feel helpless and therefore look for ways that can calm them down immediately, ignoring the long-term costs of such conducts. The second possible explanation relates to the joint attempts to enhance self-esteem and validate cultural worldview. Hence, men try to validate their manly worldview and self-image by taking more risks in general, and while driving in particular.

Understanding the general cognitive–motivational–emotional frame of risk-taking behavior leads the way to examine interpersonal and familial issues that may have a substantial influence on risk perceptions and practice.

EXTERNAL INFLUENCES: THE SOCIAL ENVIRONMENT

Social or environmental influences on risk-taking behavior relate to roles of peers, parents, family structure, and institutions (e.g., school and church) in providing models, opportunities, and reinforcements for adolescents' participation in risk-taking behaviors (Igra & Irwin, 1996). External sources that lend a model and encourage reckless behavior may contribute to the inner dynamics of a risk-taking behavior. Studies have shown that negative environmental determinants were related to habits of reckless driving and were associated with personal perceptions of reckless driving as challenging, and with disregarding its potential harmful consequences (Taubman - Ben-Ari et al., 2002).

Specifically, parenting behavior has been identified as an important source of influence on adolescents' risky behavior. Throughout the socialization process, parents transmit their own standards of conduct, both directly—through their parenting practices—and indirectly—through their own observable behavior. Three dimensions of parenting—parental monitoring of adolescent behavior, quality of parent–adolescent relationship, and parent–adolescent communication—have been identified as important variables in reducing adolescents' risk-taking behavior with regard to the direct transmission route (Kotchik, Shaffer, Forehand, & Miller, 2001).

First, studies have shown that parental monitoring and control are inversely associated with involvement in various risk-taking behaviors, such as substance use, sexual promiscuity, and deviant behavior of children and adolescents (Barnes & Farrell, 1992; Beck, Ko, & Scaffa, 1997; Beck, Shattuck, Haynie, Crump, & Simon-Morton, 1999; Chilcoat, Dishion, & Anthony, 1995; Dishion & Loeber, 1985; Rodgers, 1999; Smith & Krohn, 1995; Stice &

Barrera, 1995; Thombs, 1997). However, the optimal efficacy level of parental constrains has not been determined so far (excess boundaries and limitations may become less effective, cause resentment, reactance, etc.) (Rodgers, 1999).

Second, the way adolescents perceive their relationship with their parents is another important predictor of adolescents' risk-taking behavior. Research has shown that negative family relations increase adolescents' involvement in risky behavior (Bijur, Kurzon, Hamelsky, & Power, 1991; Igra & Irwin, 1996; Luster & Small, 1994; Resnick et al., 1997; Turner, Irwin, Tschann, & Millstein, 1993; White, Johnson, & Buyske, 2000; Wills, McNamara, Vaccaro, & Hirky, 1996). Emotional detachment from the family, or inability to achieve autonomy from parents while maintaining positive relationship with them, has been considered to lead adolescents to engage in risky behaviors to reduce their discomfort or stress (e.g., Turner et al., 1993). In addition, low autonomy-supportive parenting is associated with adolescents having stronger extrinsic relative to intrinsic life values, which in turn is related to higher involvement in risk behaviors (Williams, Cox, Hedberg, & Deci, 2000). Finally, poor parent–child communication was related to adolescents' risky behavior (Turner et al., 1993; Wills et al., 1996), whereas parent–child high-quality communication about sex was related to decreased sexual risk behavior among adolescents (e.g., Baumeister, Flores, & Marin, 1995; Luster & Small, 1994; Miller, Levin, Xu, & Whitaker, 1998).

Adolescents may also "learn" to engage in risk-taking behavior by observing their parents' behavior (e.g., Hardy, Astone, Brooks-Gunn, Shapiro, & Miller, 1998; Igra & Irwin, 1996). Moreover, studies support the assertion that there is a familial transmission of risky behaviors. Specifically, alcohol and drug problems tend to aggregate in families and are transmitted from parents to adolescents and adults (Ellis, Zucker, & Fitzgerald, 1997; Jacob & Johnson, 1997; Windle & Searles, 1990). In addition, an association was found between parents' and children's traffic records (Ferguson, Williams, Chapline, Reinfurt, & De Leonardis, 2001), and a significant intergenerational association was found for various driving styles, implying that a person's driving style may be shaped within his or her family of origin and may be associated with his or her father's and mother's driving styles and behaviors (Taubman - Ben-Ari, Mikulincer, & Gillath, 2003).

However, during adolescence, there is a shift from relying on parents to relying on peers, because peers become an important source of reinforcement, modeling, and support in the process of establishing value and belief systems during adolescence (Forehand & Wierson, 1993). The peak influence of peers occurs in early to middle adolescence, as reflected by the high conformity levels at this age. As a result, decisions during this period may rely more on peer than on parents' input (Igra & Irwin, 1996). Adolescent friends may "conspire" to engage in reckless behavior together (Arnett, 1992), because they desire social rewards that result from participation in risky behaviors, such as being part of the group, making friends, and having a good time (Cooper, 1994). Many risk-taking activities of young people begin with a dare from their peers, and refusing a dare is risking losing the esteem of valued friends.

Additional findings indicate that adolescents' perceptions, rather than the actual act, regarding participation of peers in risky behaviors highly predict their own behavior (Benda & DiBlasio, 1991; Benthin, Slovic, & Severson, 1993; Irwin & Millstein, 1986). Hence, adolescents' perceived role models among friends were found to be most predictive of multiple problem behavior (Jessor, Van Den Bos, Vanderryn, Costa, & Turbin, 1995); Adolescents' reports on peer alcohol and marijuana use were found to be significant predictors of adolescents' reports regarding the frequency of their own use (Kandel & Andrews, 1987); High frequency of reckless driving among family and friends were among the important predictors of reckless driving (Taubman - Ben-Ari et al., 2002), and perceptions of nonuse of safe precautions among peers have been shown to relate to increased sexual risk in adolescents (e.g., Gillmore, Lewis, Lohr, Spencer, & White, 1997; Romer et al., 1994).

CONCLUSION

Most theoretical perspectives on risk taking assume that because there is a basic desire to live, the tendency of a person to take risks is either irrational or unacceptable. Namely, it is impossible that people who know they are about to engage in life-endangering activities will consciously do it. This alleged contradiction between people's desire to live and their willingness to take risks led theoreticians to suggest that people who deny the death potential while committing the risky behavior either underestimate or are unable to calculate the prospective risks, or they may be using various defense mechanisms against the aroused anxieties. Only a few scholars have reasoned that risk taking in adolescence is part of a normal developmental process, which must be understood by virtue of its underling motivations, emotions, and cognitions, and that it enables adolescents to cope with some basic existential issues that shape the entire personal conception of him- or herself. TMT may be uniquely capable of understanding both growth motivations and the salience of death in one theoretically sound framework. It does so by relating to individuals' basic preoccupation with death as a motivating mechanism of a lifelong search for the validation and enhancement of self-esteem. By taking risks, adolescents may be satisfying a large range of existential needs, other than thrill and adventure, such as identity formation, value priorities construction, and social status placement. In other words, in many aspects, risk-taking behaviors play a major role in the process of transition to adulthood and may serve as a positive force in encouraging self-confidence and self-esteem. This understanding does not contradict in any way the overriding concern that adolescents are taking risks that are detrimental to their health and well-being. It does, however, point out that although these behaviors entail a probability of loss, certain needs are, undoubtedly, attained through the engagement in risky behavior and that, intrinsically, risk taking can be highly rewarding. Notably, in many ways this gap may reflect the discrepancy between "older" and "younger" points of view; whereas adults view risks as dangerous, adolescents perceive risks as challenging.

Because risky behaviors may serve a range of psychological functions that have little to do with health protection or promotion, and because adolescents tend to engage in risky behaviors despite their substantial knowledge regarding the dangerous consequences associated with their actions, it seems that factual knowledge concerning the health-related dangers of a risky behavior is insufficient in promoting safer behaviors. Intervention programs should, therefore, invest resources in designing multifaceted programs, which truly relate to adolescents' experiences of risk, and take into consideration emotional, cognitive, and motivational aspects of risk taking. Perception of risk, by itself, may be insufficient, as many times, avoiding risky behaviors takes its toll, and the benefits of participation outweigh the potential risks. Taken as a whole, it seems that one way to encourage behavioral change is by exchanging motivations to take risks with motivations to protect one's friends and exert responsibility over own and other's well-being and even life itself. Thus, reminding people of the worth of life, instead of the threat of death, while making use of various growth motivations to convince them of the importance of health promoting behaviors might be an effective strategy for moderating risky behaviors among adolescents.

REFERENCES

Alexander, M., & Lester, D. (1972). Fear of death in parachute jumpers. *Perceptual and Motor Skills, 34*, 338.

Arnett, J. (1992). Socialization and adolescent reckless behavior: A reply to Jessor. *Developmental Review, 12*, 391–409.

Arnett, J. (1995). The young and the reckless: Adolescent reckless behavior. *Current Directions in Psychological Science, 4*, 67–71.

Arnett, J. J., Offer, D., & Fine, M. A. (1997). Reckless driving in adolescence: "State" and "trait" factors. *Accident Analysis and Prevention, 29*, 57–63.

Bandura, A. (1986). *Social foundation of thought and action: A social cognitive theory.* Englewood Cliffs, NJ: Prentice-Hall.

Barnes, G., & Farrell, M. (1992). Parental support and control as predictors of adolescent drinking, delinquency, and related problems. *Journal of Marriage and the Family, 54*, 763–776.

Baumeister, L. M., Flores, E., & Marin, B. (1995). Sex information given to Latina adolescents by parents. *Health Education Research, 10*, 233–239.

Baumeister, R. F., & Scher, S. J. (1988). Self-defeating behavior patterns among normal individuals: Review and analysis of common self-destructive tendencies. *Psychological Bulletin, 104*, 3–22.

Baumrind, D. (1987, Fall). A developmental perspective on adolescent risk taking in contemporary America. In C. E. Irwin (Ed.), *Adolescent social behavior and health. New directions for child development* (Social and Behavioral Science Series, 37). San Francisco: Jossey-Bass.

Beck, K. H., Ko, M., & Scaffa, M. E. (1997). Parental monitoring, acceptance and perceptions of teen alcohol misuse. *American Journal of Health Behavior, 21*, 26–32.

Beck, K. H., Shattuck, T., Haynie, D., Crump, A. D., & Simon-Morton, B. G. (1999). Associations between parent awareness, monitoring, enforcement and adolescent involvement with alcohol. *Health Education Research, 14*, 765–775.

Benda, B. B., & DiBlasio, F. A. (1991). Comparison of four theories of adolescent sexual exploration. *Deviant Behavior. An Interdisciplinary Journal, 12*, 235–257.

Benthin, A., Slovic, P., & Severson, H. (1993). A psychometric study of adolescent risk perception. *Journal of Adolescence, 16*, 153–168.

Berman, A. L. (1973). Smoking behavior: How is it related to locus of control, death anxiety, and belief in afterlife? *Omega, 4*, 149–155.

Bijur, P. E., Kurzon, M., Hamelsky, V., & Power, C. (1991). Parent–adolescent conflict and adolescent injuries. *Journal of Developmental and Behavioral Pediatrics, 12*, 92–97.

Brehm, S. S., & Brehm, J. W. (1981). *Psychological reactance: A theory of freedom and control.* New York: Academic Press.

Byrnes, J. P. (1998). *The nature and development of decision-making: A self-regulatory model.* Hillsdale, NJ: Erlbaum.

Byrnes, J. P., Miller, D. C., & Schafer, W. D. (1999). Gender differences in risk taking: A meta analysis. *Psychological Bulletin, 125*, 367–383.

Chilcoat, H., Dishion, T., & Anthony, J. (1995). Parent monitoring and the incidence of drug sampling in urban elementary school children. *American Journal of Epidemiology, 141*, 25–31.

Cooper, M. L. (1994). Motivations for alcohol use among adolescents: Development and validation of a four-factor model. *Psychological Assessment, 6*, 117–128.

Cooper, M. L., Agocha, V. B., & Sheldon, M. S. (2000). A motivational perspective on risky behaviors: The role of personality and affect regulatory processes. *Journal of Personality, 68*, 1059–1088.

Cooper, M. L., Frone, M. R., Russell, M., & Mudar, P. (1995). Drinking to regulate positive and negative emotions: A motivational model of alcohol use. *Journal of Personality and Social Psychology, 69*, 990–1005.

Cooper, M. L., Shapiro, C. M., & Powers, A. M. (1998). Motivations for sex and sexual behavior among adolescents and young adults: A functional perspective. *Journal of Personality and Social Psychology, 75*, 1528–1558.

Deci, E. L., & Ryan, R. M. (1985). *Intrinsic motivation and self-determination in human behavior.* New York: Plenum Press.

Deci, E. L., & Ryan, R. M. (2000). The "what" and "why" of goal pursuits: Human needs and the self-determination of behavior. *Psychological Inquiry, 11,* 227–268.

DeJoy, D. M. (1992). An examination of gender differences in traffic accident risk perception. *Accident Analysis and Prevention, 24,* 237–246.

Dielman, T. E., Campbelli, P. C., Shope, J. T., & Butchart, A. T. (1987). Susceptibility to peer pressure, self-esteem, and health locus of control as correlates of adolescent substance abuse. *Health Education Quarterly, 14,* 207–221.

Dishion, T., & Loeber, R. (1985). Adolescent marijuana and alcohol use: The role of parents and peers revisited. *American Journal of Drug and Alcohol Abuse, 11,* 11–25.

Donovan, D. M., Umlaf, R. L., & Salzberg, P. M. (1988). Derivation of personality subtypes among high risk drivers. *Alcohol, Drugs and Driving, 4,* 233–244.

Elkind, D. (1967). Egocentrism in adolescence. *Child Development, 38,* 1025–1034.

Ellis, D. A., Zucker, R. A., & Fitzgerald, H. E. (1997). The role of family influences in development and risk. *Alcohol Health and Research World, 21,* 218–240.

Erickson, E. (1968). *Identity: Youth and crisis.* New York: Norton.

Farrow, J. A., & Brissing, P. (1990). Risk for DWI: A new look at gender differences in drinking and driving influences, experiences, and attitudes among new adolescent drivers. *Health Education Quarterly, 17,* 213–222.

Ferguson, S. A., Williams, A. F., Chapline, J. F., Reinfurt, D. W., & De Leonardis, D. M. (2001). Relationship of parent driving records to the driving records of their children. *Accident Analysis and Prevention, 33,* 229–234.

Finn, P., & Bragg, B. (1986). Perception of risk of an accident by younger and older drivers. *Accident Analysis and Prevention, 18,* 289–298.

Fisher, J. D., & Fisher, W. A. (1992). Changing AIDS-risk behavior. *Psychological Bulletin, 111,* 455–474.

Forehand, R., & Wierson, M. (1993). The role of developmental factors in planning behavioral interventions for children: Disruptive behavior as an example. *Behavior Therapy, 24,* 117–141.

Florian, V., Mikulincer, M., & Hirschberger, G. (2001). An existential view on mortality salience effects: Personal hardiness, death-thought accessibility, and cultural worldview defence. *British Journal of Social Psychology, 40,* 437–453.

Furby, L., & Beyth-Marom, R. (1992). Risk taking in adolescents: A decision-making perspective. *Developmental Review, 12,* 1–44.

Galligan, R. F., & Terry, D. J. (1993). Romantic ideals, fear of negative implications, and the practice of safe sex. *Journal of Applied Social Psychology, 23,* 1685–1711.

Gardner, W. (1993). A life-span rational-choice theory of risk taking. In N. J. Bell & R. W. Bell (Eds.), *Adolescent risk taking.* Newbury Park, CA: Sage.

Gillmore, M. R., Lewis, S. M., Lohr, M. J., Spencer, M. S., & White, R. D. (1997). Repeat pregnancies among adolescent mothers. *Journal of Marriage and the Family, 59,* 536–550.

Glendon, A. I., Dorn, L., Davis, D. R., Matthews, G., & Taylor, R. G. (1996). Age and gender differences in perceived accident likelihood and driver competences. *Risk Analysis, 16,* 755–762.

Goldberg, J. H., Halpern-Felsher, B. L., & Millstein, S. G. (2002). Beyond invulnerability: The important of benefits in adolescents' decision to drink alcohol. *Health Psychology, 21,* 477–484.

Goldman, J. A., & Harlow, L. L. (1993). Self-perception variables that mediate AIDS-preventive behavior in college students. *Health Psychology, 12,* 489–498.

Gonzalez, J., Field, T., Yando, R., Gonzalez, K., Lasko, D., & Bendell, D. (1994). Adolescent perceptions of their risk-taking behavior. *Adolescence, 29,* 701–709.

Greenberg, J., Pyszczynski, T., & Solomon, S. (1997). Terror management theory of self-esteem and cultural worldviews: Empirical assessments and conceptual refinements. In P. M. Zanna (Ed.), *Advances in experimental social psychology* (pp. 61–141). San Diego: Academic Press.

Gregersen, N. P., & Bjurulf, P. (1996). Young novice drivers: Towards a model of their accident involvement. *Accident Analysis and Prevention, 28,* 229–241.

Hardy, J. B., Astone, N. M., Brooks-Gunn, J., Shapiro, S., & Miller, T. L. (1998). Like mother like child: Intergenerational patterns of age at first birth and associations with childhood and adolescent characteristics and adult outcomes in the second generation. *Developmental Psychology, 34,* 1220–1232.

Hirschberger, G., Florian, V., Mikulincer, M., Goldenberg, J., & Pyszczynski, T. (2002). Gender differences in willingness to engage in risky behavior: A terror management perspective. *Death Studies, 26,* 117–141.

Hopkins, N., & Emler, N. (1990). Social network participation and problem behavior in adolescence. In K. Hurrelman & F. Lösel (Eds.), *Health hazards in adolescence* (pp. 385–408). Berlin, Germany: de Gruyter.

Igra, V., & Irwin, C. E. Jr. (1996). Theories of adolescent risk-taking behavior. In R. J. DiClemente, W. B. Hansen, & L. E. Ponton (Eds.), *Handbook of adolescent health risk behavior* (pp. 35–51). New York: Plenum Press.

Irwin, C. E. Jr. (1993). Adolescents and risk taking: How are they related? In N. J. Bell & R. W. Bell (Eds.), *Adolescent risk taking.* Newbury Park, CA: Sage.

Irwin, C. E. Jr., & Millstein, S. G. (1986). Biopschosocial correlates of risk taking behaviors during adolescence. *Journal of Adolescent Health Care, 7,* 82S–96S.

Jacob, J., & Johnson, S. (1997). Parenting influence on the development of alcohol abuse and dependence. *Alcohol Health and Research World, 21,* 204–209.

Jessor, R. (1982). Problem behavior and developmental transition in adolescence. *Journal of School Health, May,* 295–300.

Jessor, R. (1991). Risk behavior in adolescence: A psychosocial framework for understanding and action. *Journal of Adolescent Health Care, 12,* 597–605.

Jessor, R., Van Den Bos, J., Vanderryn, J., Costa, F. M., & Turbin, M. S. (1995). Protective factors in adolescent problem behavior: Moderator effects and development change. *Developmental Psychology, 31,* 923–933.

Jonah, B. A. (1997). Sensation seeking and risky driving: A review and synthesis of the literature. *Accident Analysis and Prevention, 29,* 651–665.

Jung, H., & Huguenin, R. D. (1992). Behaviour analysis of young drivers. *International Journal of Adolescent Medicine and Health, 5,* 267–274.

Kain, K., & Nelson, L. J. (2001). Cigarette smoking and fear of death: explaining conflicting results in death anxiety research. *Omega, 43,* 43–61.

Kandel, D. B., & Andrews, K. (1987). Processes of adolescent socialization by parents and peers. *The International Journal of the Addictions, 22,* 319–342.

Kotchick, B. A., Shaffer, A., Forehand, R., & Miller, K. S. (2001). Adolescent sexual risk behavior: A multi-system perspective. *Clinical Psychology Review, 21,* 493–519.

Leith, K. P., & Baumeister, R. F. (1996). Why do bad moods increase self-defeating behavior? Emotion, risk taking, and self-regulation. *Journal of Personality and Social Psychology, 71,* 1250–1267.

Lerner, L. S., & Keltner, D. (2000). Beyond valence: Toward a model of emotion-specific influences on judgment and choice. *Cognition and Emotion, 14,* 473–493.

Lerner, L. S., & Keltner, D. (2001). Fear, anger, and risk. *Journal of Personality and Social Psychology, 81,* 146–159.

Lopes, L. L. (1983). Some thoughts on the psychological concept of risk. *Journal of Experimental Psychology: Human Perception and Performance, 9,* 137–144.

Lopes, L. L. (1987). Between hope and fear: The psychology of risk. In L. Berkowitz (Ed.), *Advances in experimental social psychology* (pp. 255–295). San Diego: Academic Press.

Luster, T., & Small, S. A. (1994). Factors associated with sexual risk-taking behaviors among adolescents. *Journal of Marriage and the Family, 56,* 622–632.

Matthews, M. L., & Moran, A. R. (1986). Age differences in male drivers perception of accident risk: The role of perceived driving ability. *Accident Analysis and Prevention, 18,* 299–313.

McAuley, E. (1992). Understanding exercise behavior: A self efficacy perspective. In G. C. Roberts (Ed.), *Motivation in sport and exercise* (pp. 107–127). Champaign IL: Human Kinetics.

Miller, G., & Taubman - Ben-Ari, O. (in press). Scuba diving risk taking—A terror management theory perspective. *Journal of Sport and Exercise Psychology.*

Miller, K. S., Forehand, R., & Kotchick, B. A. (2000). Adolescent sexual behavior in two ethnic minority samples: A multi-system perspective. *Adolescence, 35,* 313–333.

Miller, K. S., Levin, M. L., Xu, X., & Whitaker, D. J. (1998). Patterns of condom use among adolescents: The impact of maternal–adolescent communication. *American Journal of Public Health, 88,* 1542–1544.

Miller, R. L., & Mulligan, R. D. (2002). Terror management: The effects of mortality salience and locus of control on risk-taking behaviors. *Personality and Individual Differences, 33,* 1203–1214.

Millstein, S. G., & Halpern-Felsher, B. L. (2002). Perceptions of risk and vulnerability. *Journal of Adolescent Health, 31,* 10–27.

Moore, S., & Gullone, E. (1996). Predicting adolescent risk behavior using a personalized cost-benefit analysis. *Journal of Youth and Adolescence, 25,* 343–359.

Moore, S., & Parsons, J. (2000). A research agenda for adolescent risk-taking: Where do we go from here? *Journal of Adolescence, 23,* 371–376.

Moore, S., Rosenthal, D., & Mitchell, A. (1996). *Youth, AIDS and sexually transmitted diseases.* London: Routledge.

Orr, D. P., Wilbrandt, M. L., Brack, C. J., Rauch, S. P., & Ingersoll, G. M. (1989). Reported sexual behaviors and self-esteem among young adolescents. *American Journal of Diseases of Children, 143,* 86–90.

Papadakis, E., & Moore, A. (1991). Drink-driving and adolescent lifestyles: Rethinking policy. *Australian Journal of Social Issues, 25,* 83–106.

Parsons, J. T., Halkitis, P. N., Bimbi, D., & Borkowski, T. (2000). Perceptions of the benefits and costs associated with condom use and unprotected sex among late adolescent college students. *Journal of Adolescence, 23,* 377–391.

Parsons, J. T., Siegel, A. W., & Cousins, J. H. (1997). Late adolescent risk-taking: Effects of perceived benefits and perceived risks on behavioral intentions and behavioral change. *Journal of Adolescence, 20,* 381–392.

Resnick, M. D., Bearman, P. S., Blum, R. W., Bauman, K. E., Harris, K. M., Jones, J., et al. (1997). Protecting adolescents from harm: Findings from the national longitudinal study on adolescent health. *Journal of the American Medical Association, 278,* 823–832.

Rodgers, K. B. (1999). Parenting processes related to sexual risk-taking behaviors of adolescent males and females. *Journal of Marriage and the Family, 61,* 99–109.

Romer, D., Black., M., Ricardo, L., Feigelman, S., Kaljee, L., Galbraith, J., et al. (1994). Social influences on the sexual behavior of youth at risk for HIV exposure. *American Journal of Public Health, 84,* 977–985.

Schrader, M. P., & Wann, D. L. (1999). High-risk recreation: The relationship between participant characteristics and degree of involvement. *Journal of Sport Behavior, 22,* 426–441.

Shedler, J., & Block, J. (1990). Adolescent drug use and psychological health: A longitudinal inquiry. *American Psychologist, 45,* 612–630.

Siegel, A. W., Cousins, J. H., Rubovitz, D., Parsons, J. T., Lavery, B., & Crowley, C. (1994). Adolescents' perceptions of the benefits and risks of their own risk-taking. *Journal of Emotional and Behavioral Disorders, 2,* 89–98.

Slanger, E., & Rudestam, E. (1997). Motivation and disinhibition in high risk sports: Sensation seeking and self efficacy. *Journal of Research in Personality, 31,* 355–374.

Smith, C., & Krohn, M. D. (1995). Delinquency and family life among male adolescents: The role of ethnicity. *Journal of Youth and Adolescence, 24,* 69–93.

Snyder, M., & Cantor, N. (1997). Understanding personal and social behavior: A functionalist strategy. In D. T. Gilbert, S. T. Fiske, & G. Lindzey (Eds.), *Handbook of social psychology* (pp. 635–679). New York: McGraw-Hill.

Solomon, S., Greenberg, J., & Pyszczynski, T. (1991). A terror management theory of social behavior: The psychological functions of self-esteem and cultural worldviews. In L. Berkowitz (Ed.), *Advances in experimental social psychology* (pp. 93–159). New York: Academic Press.

Stice, E., & Barrera, M. (1995). A longitudinal examination of the reciprocal effects between perceived parenting and adolescents' substance use and externalizing behaviors. *Developmental Psychology, 31,* 322–334.

Taubman - Ben-Ari, O., Florian, V., & Mikulincer, M. (1999). The impact of mortality salience on reckless driving—A test of Terror Management mechanisms. *Journal of Personality and Social Psychology, 76,* 35–45.

Taubman - Ben-Ari, O., Florian, V., & Mikulincer, M. (2000). Does a threat appeal moderate reckless driving?—A terror management theory perspective. *Accident Analysis and Prevention, 32,* 1–10.

Taubman - Ben-Ari, O., & Mikulincer, M. (2003a). Driving cognitive-emotional-motivational scheme: Part 1—Motivational aspects of driving. Manuscript in preparation.

Taubman - Ben-Ari, O., & Mikulincer, M. (2003b). Driving cognitive-emotional-motivational scheme: Part 3—Emotional aspects of driving. Manuscript in preparation.

Taubman - Ben-Ari, O., Mikulincer, M., & Gillath, O. (2004). The Multidimensional Driving Style Inventory—Scale Construct and Validation. *Accident Analysis and Prevention, 36,* 323–332.

Taubman - Ben-Ari, O., Mikulincer, M., & Gillath, O. (2003). *Intergenerational transmission of driving styles and reckless driving.* Manuscript under review.

Taubman - Ben-Ari, O., Mikulincer, M., & Iram, A. (2002). *A multifactorial framework for understanding reckless driving—Appraisal indicators and perceived environmental determinants.* Manuscript under review.

Thombs, D. L. (1997). Perception of parent behavior as correlates of teenage alcohol problems. *American Journal of Health Behavior, 21,* 279–288.

Thorson, J. A., & Powell, F. C. (1990). To laugh in the face of death: The games that lethal people play. *Omega, 21,* 225–239.

Turner, R. A., Irwin, C. E. Jr., Tschann, J. M., & Millstein, S. G. (1993). Autonomy, relatedness, and early initiation of health risk behaviors in early adolescence. *Health Psychology, 12,* 200–208.

Warren, W. G. (1981–1982). Death threats, concern, anxiety, fear and acceptance in death involved and "at risk" groups. *Omega, 12,* 359–372.

Weinstein, N. D. (1987). Unrealistic optimism about susceptibility to health problems: Conclusions from a community-wide sample. *Journal of Behavioral Medicine, 10,* 481–500.

White, H. R., Johnson, V., & Buyske, S. (2000). Parental modeling and parenting behavior effects on offspring alcohol and cigarette use—A growth curve analysis. *Journal of Substance Abuse, 12,* 287–310.

Williams, G. C., Cox, E. M., Hedberg, V. A., & Deci, E. L. (2000). Extrinsic life goals and health-risk behaviors in adolescents. *Journal of Applied Social Psychology, 30,* 1756–1771.

Wills, T. A., McNammara, G., Vaccaro, D., & Hirky, A. E. (1996). Escalated substance use: A Longitudinal grouping analysis from early to middle adolescence. *Journal of Abnormal Psychology, 105,* 166–180.

Windle, M., & Searles, J. S. (1990). (Eds.). *Children of alcoholics: Critical perspectives.* New York: Guilford Press.

Word, S. (1996). Mortality awareness and risk taking in late adolescence. *Death Studies, 20,* 133–148

Zuckerman, M. (1979). *Sensation seeking: Beyond the optimal level of arousal.* Hillsdale, NJ: Erlbaum.

Zuckerman, M. (1983). Sensation seeking: The initial motive for drug abuse. In E. Gotheil, K. A. Druley, T. E. Skoloda, & H. M. Waxman (Eds.), *Etiological aspects of alcohol and drug abuse* (pp. 202–220). Springfield, IL: Thomas.

Zuckerman, M. (1987). Is sensation seeking a predisposing trait for alcoholism? In E. Gotheil, K. A. Druley, S. Pashkey & S. P. Weinstein (Eds.), *Stress and addiction* (pp. 283–301). New York: Bruner/Mazel.

Zuckerman, M., Ball, S., & Black, J. (1990). Influences of sensation seeking, gender, risk appraisal, and situational motivation on smoking. *Addictive Behaviors, 15,* 209–220.

Zuckerman, M., & Neeb, M. (1980). Demographic influences in sensation seeking, and expression of sensation seeking in religion, smoking and driving habits. *Personality and Individual Differences, 1,* 197–206.

Chapter 8

Random Outcomes
and Valued Commitments

Existential Dilemmas and the
Paradox of Meaning

RONNIE JANOFF-BULMAN
DARREN J. YOPYK

Much has been written on people's need for meaning, but there is little clarity or consensus regarding the nature of such meaning (see, e.g., Wong & Fry, 1998, for a diversity of perspectives). A quick scan of synonyms in a thesaurus offers multiple possibilities—purport, implication, connotation, substance, intent, purpose, understanding, explanation, definition, interpretation—all of which seem to be represented, in one form or another, in the psychological literature. When psychologists discuss meaning, then, it is often unclear whether we are even talking about the same phenomenon. In the paragraphs that follow we address two primary understandings of meaning, which together comprise most of the aforementioned terms. These two interpretations of meaning derive from years of research with individuals who had experienced extreme, negative events. Their struggles and successes provide the basis for proposing that there are at least two quite distinct quests for meaning in human experience: One revolves around comprehensibility, the other around significance (Janoff-Bulman & Frantz, 1997; see also Davis, Nolen-Hoeksema, & Larson, 1998; Klinger, 1998). Survivors of traumatic life events first confront questions about how to make sense of events in their world (i.e., comprehensibility) and then address issues regarding the construction of value and worth in their life (i.e., significance). Although these two types of meaning may be quite independent, it is interesting that in the case of trauma survivors it is the recognition of meaninglessness in the first sense—incomprehensibility—that appears to serve as a catalyst for the creation of meaning in the second sense—

significance. Survivors move from a recognition of randomness in the world to the creation of value in their own lives.

MEANING AS COMPREHENSIBILITY: MAKING SENSE OF EXTREME EVENTS

In the aftermath of an extreme, negative event—debilitating accident, physical assault, natural disaster, rape, life-threatening illness, natural disaster, off-time death of a loved one—existential questions are paramount in the mind of the survivor. These questions revolve primarily around the incomprehensibility of the traumatic even. Survivors struggle to make sense of their experience: Why did this happen? Why did it happen to me? (see, e.g., Bulman & Wortman, 1977; Burgess & Holmstrom, 1979; Chodoff, Friedman, & Hamburg, 1964; Davis et al., 1998; Erikson, 1976; Kiecolt-Glaser & Williams, 1987; McIntosh, Silver, & Wortman, 1993; Parkes & Weiss, 1983; Silver, Boon, & Stones, 1983; Taylor, Lichtman, & Wood, 1984; Thompson, 1991).

The attempt to make sense of their experience does not stop with a simple causal analysis but with an understanding of the selective incidence of the event. Questions about the distribution of outcomes—"Why me?" and not simply "Why?"—occupy the mind of the survivor. Knowing he or she was seriously injured because another car jumped the highway's median strip or was assaulted because the assailant was poor and needed money is not sufficient to satisfy a survivor's need for meaning, his or her need to comprehend the event. There are loads of cars on the road and lots of people on the city's streets. The survivor asks, "Why did the wayward auto hit my car in particular?" "Why did the perpetrator specifically attack me?" These are questions about the selective incidence of extreme events.

This distinction between "Why?" and "Why me?" is also evident in the responses of parents of the Azande tribe of Sudan, as reported by anthropologist Max Gluckman (1944). When a hippo overturns a child's dugout on the river, the parent knows that the child died because water in the lungs resulted in drowning. Yet this is insufficient to satisfy the need to truly understand the event: Why did this happen to my child in particular? To fully comprehend the event, the Azande parent turns to witchcraft. People are not harmed randomly and arbitrarily; rather a sorcerer or witch, responding to past or current behaviors of the family, tragically chose to bring together the paths of the child and the hippo.

Making sense of traumatic events involves understanding the contingency between people and their outcomes. The absence of such an understanding necessitates a recognition that important events can be randomly distributed, and, by implication, that safety and security can no longer be assured. Traumatic events shatter survivors' fundamental assumptions about the world (Janoff-Bulman, 1989, 1992; see also Horowitz, 1976; Parkes, 1975). One such assumption is the meaningfulness of events, particularly events that have a marked impact on our own life. We take it for granted that what happens to us is based on who we are or what we do; we minimize the possibility of random outcomes and maximize the impact of our own control over outcomes. Specifically, we rely on our culturally constructed theories of person–outcome contingency, which in Western societies primarily reflect beliefs in justice and behavioral control.

These theories provide both explanations for past outcomes and expectancies about future events, as do accepted theories in the realm of science (Kuhn, 1962). In other words, events "make sense" if they fit our accepted theories or fundamental assumptions about the world. In science, physical laws explain outcomes; in the domain of daily human experience, "social laws," revolving around justice and behavioral control, explain human outcomes. For the nonreligious, such events are distributed in an impersonal universe; for the religious, these justice- and control-based outcomes may be meted out by a deity who is sensitive to human actions and character. The Hindu belief in karma is an interesting instance of making sense of life's outcomes via behavioral control. Previous acts determine the conditions into which a person is reborn; one's outcomes are fated, but in the sense that they are the effect of one's past deeds. Whether based on religious or nonreligious beliefs, if we are good people, we expect good things to happen to us (see, e.g., Lerner, 1980), and if we engage in appropriately careful behaviors, we similarly expect positive outcomes. In other words, by being the right kind of people who do the right kind of things, we maintain an illusion of safety and security—an illusion of relative invulnerability—because we believe we can ward off tragedy and disaster.

The psychologically powerful, painful impact of traumatic life events cannot be fully appreciated without an understanding of the extent to which we take for granted this sense of safety and security and overestimate the contingency between ourselves and our outcomes. For survivors, the force of this illusion becomes all too evident following their extreme negative experiences. They suddenly recognize the extent to which they took their immunity from misfortune for granted. Years of research with survivors reveal that the most common response in the immediate aftermath of victimization is "I never thought it could happen to me." All of a sudden the world appears malevolent and mean-ingless: The world does not make sense. Bad things can happen to anyone, not just the careless and the corrupt.

The potency of these beliefs is similarly evident in the reactions of nonvictims to victims. Years of research on victim blaming and derogation support the common nature of this response (e.g., Bennett & Dunkel-Schetter, 1992; Cann, Calhoun, & Selby, 1979; Carli & Leonard, 1989; Foley & Pigott, 2000). There is virtually a knee-jerk attempt to blame the victim by those who hear about traumatic events. It is as if we naturally assume that the victim was in some way responsible. How else could people make sense of the tragic outcome? As work on the just world theory (see, e.g., Lerner, 1980) contends, victim derogation is a powerful way to maintain beliefs in a just world, in which people get what they deserve. In a recent set of compelling studies, Hafer (2000) made use of implicit measures of victim blaming to demonstrate that innocent victims threaten people's justice beliefs. Participants performed a modified Stroop test, in which they identified word colors presented for very brief exposures. Research has show than latencies are longer (i.e., there is interference) when the stimulus words are associated with a salient threat. Hafer (2000) found that when re-spondents had been exposed to an innocent victim (via videotape), color-identification latencies were greater for justice-related words than for neutral words, indicating that the participants were threatened by the injustice of the victim's suffering. To maintain our own assumptions about the meaningfulness of the world, we strive to minimize any acceptance of randomness and uncontrollability. We therefore assume a contingency between victims and their traumatic outcomes and rely on our culturally constructed theories about justice and control in blaming the victim.

Social psychologists have demonstrated our underestimation of randomness in far more mundane domains than traumatic events. An early series of studies by Langer (1975; Langer & Roth, 1975; also see Wortman, 1975) demonstrated that people overestimated their per-sonal control when making attributions for purely chance tasks (e.g., lottery outcomes and predicting coin tosses) in the laboratory. Although the outcomes were uncontrollable, re-spondents felt inappropriately confident, for they assumed their own skills heavily influenced task results. This was particularly the case when skill-related factors, such as choice and familiarity, were present in the situation; these manipulated factors had no impact on the outcome but had a considerable impact on respondents' attributions. Subsequent research has continued to provide strong support for people's underestimation of randomness and overestimation of personal control over random, uncontrollable outcomes (e.g., Biner, Angle, Park, & Mellinger, 1995; Davis, Sundahl, & Lesbo, 2000; Friedland, Keinan, & Regev, 1992; Wohl & Enzle, 2002). Given our failure to recognize randomness and arbitrariness in such low-cost situations, we can begin to imagine how much greater our motivation would be to dismiss randomness and uncontrollability in the domain of potent life events.

Of course, countering these conclusions are people's common contrary responses when told that we take for granted our own safety and security and do not believe in randomness. "Oh," they say, "I know bad things can happen to me. Just look around. Bad things happen all the time. I could be diagnosed with cancer tomorrow, or get into an accident on the way home from work today." Yes, we know bad things happen in the world. However, we tend not to believe they happen in *our* world. As we now know from the considerable work on dual-processing models in psychology, what we maintain at the conscious, rational level may be distinctly different from what we believe at the more implicit, nonconscious level of processing (for a general overview of this work in several psychological domains, see Chaiken & Trope, 1999). As Epstein (1998) has emphasized in his cognitive–experiential theory, we have two ways of knowing—experiential and rational—and these can be quite different, as illustrated by the person who fears flying yet knows, rationally, that it is actually (statistically) quite safe. Similarly, we may rationally maintain that bad things can happen to us, even if we are good and careful, but in our guts—at the experiential level of our being—we actually maintain a belief in our relative safety and invulnerability.

It is not that we are patently pollyannish (even at the implicit, experiential level) and believe bad things simply do not happen. It is not that we do not take precautionary actions or feel they are unnecessary; rather, we believe in behavioral control and justice and overestimate the protective nature of our actions and personal character. Thus, we assume precautionary behaviors will ultimately protect us from misfortune. Walking in safe neighborhoods and sober driving will certainly minimize our risk of rape and auto accident, respectively, but they will not reduce the probability to zero. Life is inherently risky. Bad things happen to people who are careful and take precautions, yet psychologically we are ill-prepared. We maintain assumptions of a meaningful, comprehensible world, which affords us comfort and a sense of relative invulnerability.

For survivors, the breakdown of these fundamental assumptions largely defines the psychological crisis post-trauma (Janoff-Bulman, 1989, 1992; also see Horowitz, 1976; Parkes, 1975). They can no longer believe "It can't happen to me," for it has happened. Gone is the sense of safety, comfort, and security. Horrible events can happen for no reason. Disastrous random outcomes can strike even the good and worthy. Psychologically the response to these newfound realizations is terror. A meaningless world, in the sense of a random, incomprehensible world, is one that induces intense anxiety and dread, for we cannot truly protect ourselves from serious injury or death. Survivors come face to face with our own mortality and recognize the fragility of the human condition. They recognize that random, undeserved events can strike at any time and annihilate us.

The psychological state associated with meaninglessness as incomprehensibility is anxiety, and in the case of trauma, it is anxiety writ large—terror. Not only have previously accepted theories and assumptions proven to be inadequate guides in navigating the world, but survivors recognize the real possibility of future tragedy and loss. It is impossible to protect oneself against tragic outcomes that are arbitrarily distributed.

Such terror would be predicted by terror management theory (TMT) (for overviews see Greenberg, Solomon, & Pyszczynski, 1997; Pyszczynski, Greenberg, & Solomon, 1999; Solomon, Greenberg, & Pyszczynski, 1991), which asserts that people need to protect themselves from deeply rooted fears of death. Humans are programmed for self-preservation and therefore are generally able to ward off the anxiety associated with thoughts of their own mortality, most particularly through the pursuit of self-esteem and faith in cultural worldviews. From a terror management perspective, traumatic life events render mortality all too salient. There is a breakdown of our defensive systems, and the terror of our fragility is paramount.

Similarly, cultural anthropologist Ernest Becker (1973), whose work provides the basis for TMT, writes regarding our human need to deny death, "It can't be stressed, one final time, that to see the world as it really is is devastating and terrifying—it makes *routine, automatic, secure, self-confident activity impossible. . . .* It places a trembling animal at the mercy of the entire cosmos and the problem of the meaning of it" (p. 60). We guard against a recognition of our own mortality, and our fundamental assumptions about the world facilitate and validate our invulnerability; in essence they are integral components of the cultural worldviews discussed by terror management theorists (see, e.g., Greenberg et al., 1990; Greenberg, Simon, Pyszczynski, Solomon, & Chatel, 1992). Traumatic victimization forces survivors to confront the terror of their own mortality. Survivors not only dramatically realize their own vulnerability, but they also recognize that their fundamental assumptions are no longer valid, trustworthy guides to the world, which no longer makes sense; it is now a world of malevolent, arbitrary outcomes.

Perhaps not surprisingly, in the immediate aftermath of trauma, survivors' responses often include psychological attempts to minimize the perception of randomness and uncontrollability, and thus their perception of personal vulnerability. This may help account for the common occurrence of self-blame attributions following extreme, negative life events (see, e.g., Bulman & Wortman, 1977; Burgess & Holmstrom, 1974; Davis, Lehman, Silver, Wortman, & Ellard, 1996; Kiecolt & Williams, 1987; for a review, see Janoff-Bulman & Lang-Gunn, 1989). These attributions generally tend to be of two types: behavioral self-blame, which focuses on specific actions, and characterological self-blame, which focuses on a more negative view of the self (Janoff-Bulman, 1979). Survivors frequently engage in behavioral self-blame by pointing to behaviors they feel they should or should not have engaged in prior to the event. These are discrete actions—or the lack thereof—that are perceived as having contributed to the negative outcome. Such interpretations maximize survivors' beliefs in the controllability of the traumatic event; with the benefit of hindsight they overestimate the potential impact of their own behaviors. Even characterological self-blame minimizes the perception of randomness, although it does so at the risk of seeing oneself more negatively.

In the aftermath of traumatic life events, survivors struggle to rebuild a view of the world that is not wholly meaningless and threatening. Coping involves moving from a blanket perception of randomness and uncontrollability to attempts to minimize these overgeneralized views. Over time, survivors rebuild their inner worlds such that they reconstruct assumptions that can now account for the data of their traumatic experience yet enable survivors to go on with life. The world is controllable and random—but not absolutely. The world is no longer wholly threatening; rather, survivors reestablish a relative sense of safety and comfort but nevertheless continue to recognize the very real possibility of misfortune.

Thus, empirical studies of survivors' assumptions about meaning and randomness in the long-term aftermath of traumatic life events find that they are not extremely negative but are generally more negative than those of control populations. More specifically, several studies have specifically attempted to assess changes in survivors' assumptive worlds by comparing scores of survivors and nonvictims on the World Assumptions Scale (Janoff-Bulman, 1992). The meaningfulness subscale of this instrument attempts to measure meaningfulness in terms of comprehensibility and specifically taps beliefs about justice, control, and randomness in regard to the distribution of negative outcomes. Using this scale and control populations, researchers have found decreased perceptions of meaningfulness by survivors of criminal victimizations that occurred the previous year (Denkers & Winkel, 1995; also see Mitchell-Gibbs & Joseph, 1996), accident survivors 7 years after the collision (bus–train collision; Solomon, Iancu, & Tyano, 1997), survivors of torture and detention (in South Africa) 10–15 years after their traumatic experience (Magwaza, 1999; also see Dekel, Solomon, Elklit, & Ginzburg, 2002, for similar findings regarding combat veterans), and undergraduates who had experienced the untimely death of a parent during the previous 3 years (Schwartzberg & Janoff-Bulman, 1991; also see Janoff-Bulman, 1989).

A negative change in meaning-related assumptions, specifically regarding randomness and uncontrollability, is a legacy of traumatic experiences. Long after the terror and extreme anxiety subside, the assumptive world retains a psychological marker of traumatic experiences. As coping progresses, the traumatic event ceases to define the survivor's world and daily living, but it continues to serve as a touchstone, a reminder of tragedy and loss. The possibility of future tragedy is recognized but no longer dwelled on. And it is this ever-available reminder of potential loss that provides an understanding of a very different, often unexpected set of responses to traumatic life events—the perception of benefits and gains.

MEANING AS SIGNIFICANCE: CREATING LIVES OF VALUE

In the immediate aftermath of victimization, survivors' meaning-related questions largely revolve around comprehensibility and the newfound recognition that the most potent of outcomes may not make sense. With time, the existential concerns of victims begin to revolve around a second understanding of meaning—that of significance—and become evident in the positive changes that are increasingly recognized, too, as common responses to victimization.

The aftermath of victimization involves both losses and gains, changes that are both positive and negative. In considering the traumatic event in terms of comprehensibility, survivors experience losses and the negative emotions that accompany such losses; the world is more meaningless in the sense of randomness and the lack of contingency—at least at times—between actions and important outcomes. In considering the traumatic event in terms of significance, however, survivors experience gains and the positive emotions that accompany such gains. For in the long-term aftermath of victimization, survivors commonly perceive—or rather construct—benefits based on their traumatic experience. What are these reported benefits, and how can they be understood in light of the threats posed by traumatic life events and the survivors' consequent negative reactions?

In contrast to the early emphasis on the (expected) negative impact of traumatic life events, there is now a burgeoning literature on the positive impact of these events. The recent work of Calhoun and Tedeschi (1999, 2001; Tedeschi & Calhoun, 1995, 1996; Tedeschi, Park, & Calhoun, 1998) on posttraumatic growth reflects this new attention to the benefits of victimization. Empirical studies consistently find reports of benefits and positive outcomes among survivors of traumatic events, including HIV infection (Bower, Kemeny, Taylor, & Fahey, 1998; Schwartzberg, 1993), heart attacks (Affleck, Tennen, Croog, & Levine, 1987; Laerum, Johnson, Smith, & Larsen, 1987), house fires (Thompson, 1985), combat (Elder & Clipp, 1989; Sledge, Boydstun, & Rabe, 1980), rapes and sexual assaults (Burt & Katz, 1987; Frasier, Conlon, & Glaser, 2001; Veronen & Kilpatrick, 1983), bereavement (Edmonds & Hooker, 1992; Lehman et al., 1993; Nerken, 1993), cancer (Cordova, Cunningham, Carlson, & Andrykowski, 2001; Collins, Taylor, & Skokan, 1990), and accidents (Joseph, Williams, & Yule, 1993). Increasingly, research on survivors points to the benefits reported as a consequence of their victimization. It is not that some survivors experience losses and negative responses and others experience gains and positive responses; rather, these seem to be common reactions of the very same survivors.

Researchers have different ways of "cataloging" such benefits, although these typically include changes in the areas of self-perceptions, changes in relationships, and changes in life orientation (see, e.g., Davis, 2001; Lehman et al., 1993; Updegraff & Taylor, 2000). In their Posttraumatic Growth Scale, Tedeschi and Calhoun (1996) distinguish among five factors: Relating to Others, New Possibilities, Personal Strength, Spiritual Change, and Appreciation of Life. The benefits reported may reflect changes in different areas of the survivors' lives, but in general, they appear to reflect two different processes or mechanisms for positive change. One we would label "strength through suffering" and the other "appreciation through existential reevaluation." Although both are common responses to traumatic victimization, it is the second process that is related to questions of meaning, and particularly meaning in the sense of significance. We will therefore briefly address "strength through suffering" and then move on to a more complete discussion of "appreciation through existential reevaluation."

Our cultural lore includes the folk wisdom that whatever doesn't kill us makes us stronger, which is consistent with the redemptive value of suffering taught in many religions. The exercise mantra "no pain, no gain" is a popularized version of similar thinking. Underlying these messages is a belief that people get stronger through painful challenges—physically stronger when their bodies are pushed, and mentally stronger when their psychological resources are taxed. Survivors expend tremendous pain and effort in the course of their posttraumatic adjustment, and in the process they learn about their own strengths and possibilities. They know the incredible challenges posed by the victimization, and they derive a greater sense of personal strength, self-reliance, and self-respect from having been "put to the test" and coped successfully. Tedeschi and Calhoun's (1996) Personal Strength and New Possibilities factors capture the types of benefits represented by 'strength through suffering." Items in the Personal Strength factor include the following positive changes: "A feeling of self-confidence," "Knowing I can handle difficulties," "I discovered that I'm stronger than I thought I was." Items in the "New Possibilities" factor include "I'm able to do better things with my life," "I'm more likely to try to change things which need changing," and "I developed new interests." These self-perceptions, associated with a newfound sense of possibilities and personal strength, are likely to be veridical in that survivors no doubt develop new coping skills and personal resources in the process of their long-term adjustment. To date the validity of such self-assessments has rarely been addressed, although a single study that sought corroboration from close family and friends found support for these self-reported changes (Park, Cohen, & Murch, 1996).

Survivors' greater strength may also reflect the psychological advantages of a more flexible, less rigid, assumptive world; that is, in rebuilding their fundamental assumptions, sur-

vivors recognize the limits and naivete of their earlier assumptions and reconstruct fundamental schemas that can now account for their traumatic experience, without being wholly
negative. This suggests that survivors who have coped successfully by rebuilding viable, yet
comfortable inner worlds are apt to be more psychologically prepared for future tragedies. If
revictimized, they will avoid the massive expectancy disconfirmation of their earlier experience. Several studies have found support for this type of "inoculation effect" (see
Meichenbaum, 1985) of a first trauma in adulthood (see, e.g. Aldwin, Sutton, & Lachman,
1996; Burgess & Holmstrom, 1978; Elder & Cripp, 1989; Shanan & Shahar, 1983), although empirical tests are limited to date. Further, research studies have generally not
focused on the terror/anxiety component of trauma, which is what is most apt to be minimized in subsequent traumas, given that the randomness and meaninglessness of the world
have already been confronted. Survivors' assumptions have been severely challenged and
shattered and consequently are rebuilt to be more resistant to future onslaughts.

A second set of benefits more directly reveals the existential struggle of survivors, and
this is the development of appreciation-related evaluations in the process of coping with
traumatic life events. Survivors commonly report greater appreciation of life, and of particular life domains, including, especially, their close relationships (close family and friends) as
well as nature and spirituality. It is not at all uncommon to hear victims talk about life as a
gift, of their newfound enjoyment of simple pleasures, and of the preciousness of living.
Three of Tedeschi and Calhoun's (1996) posttraumatic growth factors—Appreciation of
Life, Relating to Others, and Spiritual Change—reflect this second set of benefits based on
existential reevaluations. The first factor includes positive changes related to life in general:
"My priorities about what is important in life," "An appreciation for the value of my own
life," and "Appreciating each day." The second and third factors relate to increased sensitivity to and appreciation of specific life domains: close relationships and spirituality (which is
often related to nature).

The term "appreciation" refers to an appraisal of increased value or worth. From the
perspective of economics, when goods appreciate they increase in value; from the perspective of psychology, when we appreciate something, we increase its perceived value in our
eyes (Janoff-Bulman, 2000; Singer, 1996). Appreciation involves evaluation processes, or
more typically reevaluation processes, which accord significance and worth. To appreciate
something is to construe it as special; we typically do not value the ordinary but rather the
extraordinary.

There is a sense of joy in survivors' expressions of life as precious, of living as a valued
gift, which surely seems to belie their negative postvictimization responses. One might expect that their confrontation with incomprehensibilty and human fragility would fuel dis-
heartening appraisals of human insignificance, the inconsequentiality of life, and the futility
of daily living. And in the immediate aftermath of victimization, such responses are surely
common, reflecting survivors' sense of being overwhelmed by the meaninglessness and ma-
levolence of the world. Yet over time they come to recognize the other side of their experience, its implications for their own life and their own choices. Reviews of empirical studies
suggest that between 75 and 90% of survivors report benefits (see, e.g., Davis, 2001;
Tedeschi et al., 1998; Updegraff & Taylor, 2000), and although intense anxiety and
posttraumatic stress are extremely common in the immediate aftermath of extreme events,
the incidence of debilitating chronic posttraumatic stress disorder (PTSD) is relatively low,
affecting approximately 5–15% of victimized populations (see, e.g., Keane, Litz, & Blake,
19990; Kilpatrick, Saunders, Veronon, Best, & Vron, 1987; also see Kulka et al., 1988, a
particularly comprehensive evaluation of PTSD in Vietnam veterans).

Over time, most survivors report heartening appraisals of existential consequence and significance. Yet these new assessments may be fundamentally tied to the recognition of human mortality, random outcomes, and the very real knowledge of possible future loss. In a world that is not wholly comprehensible, outcomes are no longer assumed to be completely controllable or predictable, and thus survivors realize that living can no longer be taken for granted. In the face of possible loss and annihilation, life takes on new value. As philosopher Irving Singer (1996) writes in discussing ontological anxiety, "Fortunately, this type of anxiety can have a positive side. Once our hopeless questioning has reverberated in us, we may also intuit the mystery and wonder in everything being what it is. The source of our anxiety will not have changed but our attention will now be focused on the mere fact of existence rather than the obscure possibility of non-existence" (p. 80).

From a less philosophical and more psychological perspective, survivors' appraisals of life's newfound significance derive from a recognition of "potential unavailability"; we come to value that which we know we may lose. Such reevaluations are no doubt related to a "scarcity principle" of sorts, by which we accord greater value to opportunities and objects that are less available. Lay notions of economic value include beliefs that objects and experiences are valued to the extent that they are unavailable (Brock, 1968), and scarce commodities do and should cost more (Lynn, 1992). Cialdini (1993) persuasively points out that retailers use this scarcity principle through a "limited number" tactic to increase the value, and thus sales, of their products.

Of relevance as well is research indicating that value-related appraisals are particularly affected by perceptions of possible future loss, or potential unavailability. As demonstrated by Kahneman and Tversky (1979, 2000) in their important work on prospect theory, there are distinct value functions for gains versus losses; the function is concave for gains and convex for losses and is also steeper for losses than gains. Thus, in making decisions under uncertainty, we are more motivated by the possibility of losing something than gaining something of equal value; we are essentially risk-averse. That which we might lose we appear to value all the more.

For survivors, existence is taken off automatic. They are shaken from the complacency that often defines people's daily routines and instead become exquisitely sensitive to living. It is as if they begin to live life more deeply. Survivors reprioritize what is important; they make conscious choices about how to live their newly valued lives. In a fundamental way, they have shifted from a concern with the meaning *of* life to a focus on meaning *in* life.

The value now perceived as inherent in living becomes the basis for choices about how to spend one's life—about the activities and domains that will translate this sense of significance and worth into daily existence. Survivors know they do not have complete control over major life outcomes such as traumatic life events, but they *do* have control over the choices they make about how to live their lives. In a sort of "top-down" process, survivors' realization of life's value provides the basis for creating newfound significance through their choices, goals, and activities. They become *committed* to living.

Survivors demonstrate this commitment by consciously considering how to live their lives and by choosing to engage in those activities they deem worthy of their time and effort. Research on "personal projects" in the general population has found that the types of activities people regard as most meaningful are interpersonal and spiritual projects involving a goal of intimacy or connection, and "altruistic" activities engaged in for the sake of others, such as community projects; such tasks as household maintenance are consistently regarded as least meaningful (Little, 1998). In the aftermath of traumatic life events, survivors make active choices about their commitments and, not surprisingly, most often appear to place special emphasis on these particularly worthy domains—family and friends, spiritual activities, and altruistic endeavors. Personality psychologists who have studied people's self-articulated tasks—their personal concerns, projects, and strivings—maintain that such activities not only provide structure and sources of identity but a sense of purpose and meaning (Canter, 1990; Emmons, 1989; Klinger, 1977; Little, 1983; Pervin, 1989). In essence, by formulating and completing goals, we create value, for our activities function as carriers of personal meaning. For survivors, the meaning derived from passionately engaging in significant life tasks and projects is also a reflection of the survivor's greater commitment to living in general.

The survivor's confrontation with meaninglessness, in the sense of incomprehensibility, essentially serves as a catalyst for the construction of meaningfulness, in the sense of significance. It is through a terrifying realization of fragility, mortality, and loss as ever-present possibilities that survivors recognize their own power to create lives of value and commitment. Though seemingly paradoxical, the survivor's existential struggle and resolution have interesting parallels in the historical unfolding of existential philosophy itself.

Existentialism emerged largely in response to the trauma of World War II. With roots in 19th-century romanticism, with its revolt again science and reason, existentialists recognize no rational basis for our lives and maintain that feelings of apprehension and dread are a part of our human experience. In characterizing existentialism, Barrett (1962) argues, "This philosophy embodies the self-questioning of the time. . . . Alienation and estrangement; a sense of the basic fragility and contingency of human life; the impotence of reason confronted with the depths of existence; the threat of Nothingness, and the solitary and unsheltered condition of the individual before this threat . . . A single atmosphere pervades them all like a chilly wind: the radical feeling of human finitude" (p. 36). One could be describing the terror of the survivor in the immediate aftermath of a traumatic experience.

Yet, in the face of this dread existentialism does not advocate a withdrawal from life or an acceptance of passive existence. It simultaneously recognizes human weakness as one side of the coin, human power the other (Barrett, 1962), and strongly advocates human choice and self-determination. We are to embrace a passionate involvement in life. Through freedom and choice we create our own existence, for in the absence of any ultimate justification for our choices, we are what we make of ourselves (e.g., Sartre, 1957, 1966). Here are strong echoes of the shift in meaning-making experienced by survivors; in an incomprehensible world, we create our own meaning and lives of significance through our choices and commitments.

SOME THOUGHTS ON MEANING AND EMOTION

In the aftermath of victimization, survivors experience both positive and negative changes. They now know there is no necessary contingency between people and their outcomes, for humans lead an uncertain existence in which events are neither wholly predictable nor controllable. Survivors know that they cannot fully comprehend why tragedy strikes particular people, and they know it can strike at any time. This acknowledgment of loss and future vulnerability is encoded in the survivors' reconstructed assumptive worlds, but it is also the basis for a process of existential reevaluation that generates considerable benefits and gains. These new appraisals create an appreciation for life and living and consequent commitments of personal value and significance.

The coexistence of losses and gains may in part account for a somewhat unexpected set of findings in the literature on posttraumatic growth. Research has failed to find a consistent positive relationship between the benefits reported by survivors posttrauma and indices of well-being and decreased psychological stress. The evidence is mixed; although most studies have found the expected positive relationship, some find no relationship (for a review of this research, see Park, 1998). A closer look at these studies reveals that there was no uniformity of measures in assessing well-being or psychological distress; measures included assessments of depression, general symptomatology, anxiety, daily mood, self-esteem scores, and global satisfaction. And in considering the positive and negative changes associated with traumatic life events, it seems quite conceivable that the nature of the outcome measure may strongly influence the association found between reported benefits and well-being. To understand why, we turn to a brief consideration of meaning and emotion.

The two types of meaning or meaninglessness—cognitions related to comprehensibility or significance—are apt to be associated with distinct clusters of emotions and psychological symptomatologies. More specifically, comprehension-based meaninglessness is likely to be manifested in anxiety and anxiety disorders. A world in which tragic outcomes can be uncontrollable and random is a threatening world. It is a world in which an acknowledgment of threat and personal vulnerability is ever-present, sometimes beneath the surface, waiting to be activated, sometimes above the surface and powerfully in one's consciousness. In contrast, significance-based meaninglessness is likely to be manifested in depression rather than anxiety. A life without value or significance is one without commitment, direction, purpose, or fulfillment, which is emotionally experienced as hopelessness and despair.

Although clinically anxiety and depression are often comorbid disorders (e.g., Dobson, 1985; Kendall, Kortlander, Chansky, & Brady, 1992; Kendall & Watson, 1989), research on the structure of these emotions makes a strong case for the largely independent nature of these psychological responses. In their tripartite model of anxiety and depression, Clark and Watson (1991; Watson et al., 1995) theorized and empirically supported distinct structural dimensions for each; in particular, although both depression and anxiety are characterized by negative affect (NA), depression is characterized by low positive affect (PA), and anxiety is characterized by physiological hyperarousal. NA reflects displeasurable engagement with the environment and a sense of subjective distress, whereas PA reflects pleasurable engagement with the environment and the sense that one is enthusiastic, active, and alert. These dimensions are believed to be orthogonal (Tellegen, 1985; Watson & Tellegen, 1985), separate dimensions in the affective domain.

This approach has proved useful for distinguishing between anxiety and depression; research has found that individuals with anxiety and depressive disorders report high levels of NA, but only individuals with a depressive disorder report low levels of PA, and only individuals with anxiety disorders have high physiological hyperarousal (e.g., Brown, Chorpita, & Barlow, 1998; Jolly, Dyck, Kramer, & Wherry, 1994; Watson, Clark, & Carey, 1988). Thus, although anxiety and depression are both subjectively unpleasant, only anxiety is related to hyperarousal, and only depression is related to low levels of positive emotions.

These patterns may help us better understand the complex emotional responses of most trauma survivors, who simultaneously experience greater meaninglessness, in the sense of incomprehensibility, and greater meaningfulness, in the sense of significance. In the long-term aftermath of victimization, survivors are thus apt to be more anxious and less depressed than they were before the traumatic event. They are likely to feel the NA and arousal associated with anxiety; yet they are also likely to feel the more PA associated with the deceased depression that follows their newfound assessment of value and commitment in their lives. The inconsistent results (see earlier) found in studies that assessed the association between survivors' reports of benefits and their psychological well-being or distress could thus be attributable to the choice of outcome measures. Well-being or distress measures that assessed depression or self-esteem would presumably find greater "well-being" among survivors, whereas those that assessed general negative symptomatology or anxiety would more likely find evidence of decreased "well-being." Although this distinction has not previously been applied to the inconsistent findings regarding survivors' reported benefits and psychological well-being, when we examined the studies reviewed by Park (1998) we found considerable support for these hypotheses.

For survivors, the negative and positive emotions they experience posttrauma should comfortably coexist, given the largely independent structure of the emotions involved. Just as survivors' rebuilt assumptive worlds are richer and more complex than their more rigid, absolutist preexisting assumptions, their affective lives appear to be richer and more complex as well. The juxtaposition of positive and negative affect, evident in greater anxiety as well as greater engagement and enthusiasm, seems to reflect a kind of "emotional creativity" (Averill & Thomas-Knowles, 1991) involving innovation and change. In this case, although seemingly contradictory or at best unrelated, these affective responses are instead closely associated, with anxiety fueling the survivor's more positive emotions.

Traumatic life events confront survivors with challenges that are initially terrifying, yet ultimately life affirming. From a recognition of human mortality and fragility in the face of an uncontrollable, arbitrary universe, survivors reevaluate life and enthusiastically embrace living. By realizing the real and ever-present possibility of loss, survivors create value in their lives. Surely, some are more readily able to accomplish this creative reconstruction than others, based on either the nature of the traumatic event or pretrauma resources. Unfortunately, to date we know little about the role of the trauma itself—its nature and extent—in the process of constructing meaning. Although there have been suggestions that it is easier to find benefits in the aftermath of impersonal events (e.g., illnesses and natural disasters) than those involving the malevolent actions of others (e.g., rape and other criminal assaults), this remains a research hypothesis that has yet to be adequately tested and supported. Similarly, the severity of the extreme event has been linked to both greater coping difficulties and greater possibility of benefits (see Updegraff & Taylor, 2000, for review), leaving unresolved the nature of this relationship as well. Researchers have discussed pretrauma psychological resources believed to be associated with posttrauma well-being, with some typical coping candidates selected for review (e.g., optimism, ego strength, perceptions of control, social support, explanatory style, and coping style). Unfortunately, these factors are associated with positive coping and adjustment in general (and not specifically in the case of traumatic events) and provide few additional clues as to the nature of the process involved in creating perceptions of meaningfulness from meaninglessness. For our purposes, it seems most important to emphasize that the process of reevaluation and value creation is extremely common in the aftermath of extreme life events, as is the terror of victimization. Together these seem to define two interdependent sides of the traumatic experience.

Interestingly, the work of terror management theorists has sensitized us to our strong defensive reactions in the face of reminders of our mortality and vulnerability. Such threats lead us to cling to cultural ideologies and practices, to old, comfortable patterns rather than to any creative development of new approaches to living. Traumatic life events do not simply threaten our assumptive worlds, particularly our assumptions about controllability and meaning, but shatter them. Survivors are forced to confront their own mortality in an intensely emotional, deeply experienced way; ordinary defenses are powerless in the face of such an overwhelming onslaught. Yet it is the dramatic undermining of the survivor's worldview that generates not only an acceptance of human fragility and vulnerability but a sense of human significance as well. Over time these newfound perceptions no doubt take a back seat to the daily routines of living, yet they remain beneath the surface, ready to be tapped. As painful as it is, trauma is a route to value creation. Surely it is not the only route, but, paradoxically, it is one very effective path. A future task for psychologists is to discover alternative routes, so that we may learn to live lives of greater depth and commitment in the absence of traumatic life experiences.

REFERENCES

Affleck, G., Tennen, H., Croog, S., & Levine, S. (1987). Causal attribution, perceived benefits, and morbidity following a heart attack: An eight year study. *Journal of Consulting and Clinical Psychology*, *55*, 29–35.

Aldwin, C. M., Sutton, K. J., & Lachman, M. (1996). The development of coping resources in adulthood. *Journal of Personality*, *64*, 837–871.

Averill, J. A., & Thomas-Knowles, C. (1991). Emotional creativity. In K. T. Strongman (Ed.), *International review of studies of emotion* (Vol. 1, pp. 269–299). London: Wiley.

Barrett, W. (1962). *Irrational man: A study in existential philosophy*. Garden City. New York: Doubleday.

Becker, E, (1973). *The denial of death*. New York: Free Press.

Bennett, H. Y., & Dunkel-Schetter, C. (1992). Negative social reactions to victims: An overview of responses and their determinants. In L. Montada, S. Fillip, & M. J. Lerner (Eds.), *Life crises and experiences of loss in adulthood* (pp. 497–518). Hillsdale, NJ: Erlbaum.

Biner, P., Angle, S. T., Park, J. H., & Mellinger, A. E. (1995). Need state and the illusion of control. *Personality and Social Psychology Bulletin*, *21*, 899–907.

Bower, J. E., Kemeny, M. E., Taylor, S. E., & Fahey, J. L. (1998). Cognitive processing, discovery of meaning, CD 4 decline, and AIDS-related mortality among bereaved HIV-seropositive men. *Journal of Consulting and Clinical Psychology*, *66*, 979–986.

Brock, T. C. (1968). Implications of commodity theory for value change. In A. G. Greenwald, T. C. Brock, & T. M. Ostrom (Eds.), *Psychological foundations of attitudes* (pp. 243–275). New York: Academic Press.

Brown, T. A., Chorpita, B. F., & Barlow, D. H. (1998). Structural relations among dimensions of the DSM-IV anxiety and mood disorders and dimensions of negative affect, positive affect, and autonomic arousal. *Journal of Abnormal Psychology*, *107*, 179–192.

Bulman, R., & Wortman, C. B. (1977). Attributions of blame and coping in the "real world": Severe accident victims react to their lot. *Journal of Personality and Social Psychology*, *35*, 351–363.

Burgess, A. W., & Holmstrom, L. L. (1974). *Rape: Victims of crisis*. Bowie, MD: Robert J. Brady.

Burgess, A. W., & Holmstrom, L. L. (1978). Recovery from rape and prior life stress. *Research in Nursing and Health*, *1*, 165–74.

Burgess, A. W., & Holmstrom, L. L. (1979). Adaptive strategies and recovery from rape. *American Journal of Psychiatry*, *136*, 1278–1282.

Burt, M. R., & Katz, B. L. (1987). Dimensions of recovery from rape: Focus on growth outcomes. *Journal of Interpersonal Violence*, *2*, 57–81.

Calhoun, L. G., & Tedeschi, R. G. (1999). *Facilitating posttraumatic growth:A clinicians'guide*. Mahwah, NJ: Erlbaum.

Calhoun, L. G., & Tedeschi, R. G. (2001). Posttraumatic growth: The positive lessons of loss. In R. A. Neimeyer (Ed.), *Meaning reconstruction and the experience of loss* (pp. 157–172). Washington, DC: American Psychological Association.

Cann, A., Calhoun, L., & Selby, L. (1979). Attributing responsibility to the victim of rape: Influence of information regarding past sexual experiences. *Human Relations*, *32*, 57–67.

Cantor, N. (1990). From thought to behavior: "Having" and "doing" in the study of personality and cognition. *American Psychologist*, *45*, 735–750.

Carli, L. L., & Leonard, J. B. (1989). The effect of hindsight on victims derogation. *Journal of Social and Clinical Psychology*, 8, 331–343.

Chaiken, S., & Trope, Y. (Eds.). (1999). *Dual-process models in social psychology*. New York: Guilford Press.

Chodoff, P. S., Friedman, S. B., & Hamburg, D. A. (1964). Stress, defense, and coping behavior: Observations in parents of children with malignant disease. *American Journal of Psychiatry*, 120, 743–749.

Cialdini, R. B. (1993). *Influence: Science and practice*. New York: HarperCollins.

Clark, L. A., & Watson, D. (1991). Tripartite model of anxiety and depression: Psychometric evidence and taxonomic implications. *Journal of Abnormal Psychology*, 100, 316–336.

Collins, R. L., Taylor, S. E., & Skokan, L. A. (1990). A better world or a shattered vision: Changes in life perspective following victimization. *Social Cognition*, 8, 263–285.

Cordova, M. J., Cunningham, L. L. C., Carlson, C. R., & Andrykowski, M. A. (2001). Posttraumatic growth following breast cancer: A controlled comparison study. *Health Psychology*, 20, 176–185.

Davis, C. G. (2001). The tormented and the transformed: Understanding responses to loss and trauma. In R. A. Neimeyer (Ed.), *Meaning reconstruction and the experience of loss* (pp. 137–155). Washington, DC; American Psychological Association.

Davis, C. G., Lehman, D. R., Silver, R. C., Wortman, C. B., & Ellard, J. H. (1996). Self-blame following a traumatic event: The role of perceived avoidability. *Personality and Social Psychology Bulletin*, 22, 557–567.

Davis, C. G., Nolen-Hoeksema, S., & Larson, J. (1998). Making sense of loss and benefiting from the experience: Two construals of meaning. *Journal of Personality and Social Psychology*, 75, 561–574.

Davis, D., Sundahl, I., & Lesbo, M. (2000). Illusory personal control as a determinant of bet size and type in casino crap games. *Journal of Applied Social Psychology*, 30, 1224–1242.

Dekel, R., Solomon, Z., Elklit, A., & Ginzburg, K. (2002). World assumptions and combat-related PTSD.

Denkers, A. J. M., & Winkel, F. W. (1995). Reactions of criminal victimization: A field study of the cognitive effects on victims and members of their social network. In D. Graham, S. Bostock, M. McMurran, & C. Wilson (Eds.), *Psychology, law and criminal justice: International developments in research and practice* (pp. 374–383). Oxford, UK: Walter de Gruyter.

Dobson, K. S. (1985). An analysis of anxiety and depression scales. *Journal of Personality Assessment*, 49, 522–527.

Edmonds, S., & Hooker, K. (1992). Perceived changes in life meaning following bereavement. *Omega*, 25, 307–318.

Elder, G. H., & Clipp, E. C. (1989). Combat experience and emotional health: Impairment and resilience in later life. *Journal of Personality*, 57, 311–322.

Emmons, R. A. (1989). The personal striving approach to personality. In L. Pervin (Ed.), *Goal concepts in personality and social psychology* (pp. 87–126). Hillsdale, NJ: Erlbaum.

Epstein, S. (1998). Cognitive-experiential self-theory. In D. F. Barone, M. Hersen, & V. B. Van Hasselt (Eds.), *Advanced personality* (pp. 35–47). New York: Plenum Press.

Erikson, K. T. (1976). *Everything in its path: Destruction of community in the Buffalo Creek flood*. New York: Simon & Schuster.

Foley, L. A., & Pigott, M. A. (2000). Belief in a just world and jury decisions in a civil rape trial. *Journal of Applied Social Psychology*, 30, 935–951.

Frazier, P., Conlon, A., & Glaser, T. (2001). Positive and negative life changes following sexual assault. *Journal of Consulting and Clinical Psychology*, 69, 1048–1055.

Friedland, N., Keinan, G., & Regev, Y. (1992). Controlling the uncontrollable: Effects of stress on illusory perceptions of controllability. *Journal of Personality and Social Psychology*, 63, 923–931.

Gluckman, M. (1944, June). The logic of African science and witchcraft: An appreciation of Evans-Pritchard's "Witchcraft Oracles and Magic among the Azande" of the Sudan. *The Rhodes-Livingstone Institute Journal*, pp. 61–71.

Greenberg, J., Pyszczynski, T., Solomon, S., Rosenblatt, A., Veeder, M., Kirkland, S., et al. (1990). Evidence for terror management theory II: The effects of mortality salience on reactions to those who threaten or bolster the cultural worldview. *Journal of Personality and Social Psychology, 58,* 308–318.

Greenberg, J., Simon, L., Pyszczynski, T., Solomon, S., & Chatel, D. (1992). Terror management and tolerance: Does mortality salience always intensify negative reactions to others who threaten one's worldview? *Journal of Personality and Social Psychology, 63,* 212–220.

Greenberg, J., Solomon, S., & Pyszczynski, T. (1997). Terror management theory of self-esteem and cultural worldviews: Empirical assessments and conceptual refinements. In M. Zanna (Ed.), *Advances in experimental social psychology* (Vol. 29, pp. 61–139). San Diego: Academic Press.

Hafer, C. (2000). Do innocent victims threaten the belief in a just world? Evidence from a modified Stroop task. *Journal of Personality and Social Psychology, 79,* 165–173.

Horowitz, M. J. (1976). *Stress response syndromes.* New York: Jason Aronson.

Janoff-Bulman, R. (1979). Characterological versus behavioral self-blame: Inquiries into depression and rape. *Journal of Personality and Social Psychology, 37,* 1798–1809.

Janoff-Bulman, R. (1989). Assumptive worlds and the stress of traumatic events: Applications of the schema construct. *Social Cognition, 7,* 113–136.

Janoff-Bulman, R. (1992). *Shattered assumptions: Towards a new psychology of trauma.* New York: Free Press.

Janoff-Bulman, R. (2000). The other side of trauma: Towards a psychology of appreciation. In J. H. Harvey & E. D. Miller (Eds.), *Loss and trauma: General and close relationship perspectives* (pp. 29– 44). Philadelphia: Brunner-Routledge.

Janoff-Bulman, R., & Frantz, C. M. (1997). The impact of trauma on meaning: From meaningless world to meaningful life. In M. Power & C. Brewin (Eds.), *The transformation of meaning in psychological therapies* (pp. 91–106). London: Wiley.

Janoff-Bulman, R., & Lang-Gunn, L. (1989). Coping with disease and accidents: The role of self-blame attributions. In L. Y. Abramson (Ed.), *Social–personal inference in clinical psychology.* New York: Guilford Press.

Jolly, J. B., Dyck, M. J., Kramer, T. A., & Wherry, J. N. (1994). Integration of positive and negative affectivity and cognitive content-specificity: Improved discrimination of anxious and depressed symptoms. *Journal of Abnormal Psychology, 103,* 544–552.

Joseph, S., Williams, R., & Yule, W. (1993). Changes in outlook following disaster: The preliminary development of a measure to assess positive and negative change. *Journal of Traumatic Stress, 6,* 271–279.

Kahneman, D., & Tversky, A. (1979). Prospect theory: An analysis of decision under risk. *Econometrica, 47,* 263–291.

Kahneman, D., & Tversky, A. (Eds.). (2000). *Choices, values, and frames.* New York. New York: Cambridge University Press.

Keane, T. M., Litz, B. T., & Blake, D. D. (1990). Post-traumatic stress disorder in adulthood. In M. Hersen & C. G. Last (Eds.), *Handbook of child and adult psychopathology: A longitudinal perspective.* New York: Pergamon.

Kendall, P. C., Kortlander, E., Chansky, T. E., & Brady, E. U. (1992). Comorbidity of anxiety and depression in youth: Treatment implications. *Journal of Consulting and Clinical Psychology, 60,* 869–880.

Kendall, P. C., & Watson, D. (Eds.). (1989). *Anxiety and depression: Distinctive and overlapping features.* San Diego: Academic Press.

Kiecolt-Glaser, J. K., & Williams, D. A. (1987). Self-blame, compliance, and distress among burn patients. *Journal of Personality and Social Psychology, 53,* 187–193.

Kilpatrick, D. G., Saunders, L. J., Veronen, L. J., Best, C. L., & Vron, J. M. (1987). Criminal victimization: Lifetime prevalence, reporting to police, and psychological impact. *Crime and Delinquency, 33,* 479–489.

Klinger, E. (1977). *Meaning and void: Inner experience and the incentives in people's lives.* Minneapolis: University of Minnesota Press.

Klinger, E. (1998). The search for meaning in evolutionary perspective and its clinical implications. In P. T. P. Wong & P. S. Fry (Eds.), *The human quest for meaning: A handbook of psychological research and clinical applications.* Mahwah, NJ: Erlbaum.

Kuhn, T. S. (1962). *The structure of scientific revolutions*. Chicago: University of Chicago Press.

Kulka, R. A., Schlenger, W. E., Fairbank, J. A., Hough, R. L., Jordan, C. R., Marmar, et al. (1988). *NationalVietnam veterans readjustment study (NVVRS): Description, current status, and initial PTSD prevalence rates*. Washington, DC: Veterans Administration.

Laerum, E., Johnson, N., Smith, P., & Larsen, S. (1987). Can myocardial infarction induce positive changes in family relationships? *Family Practice, 4*, 302–305.

Langer, E. J. (1975). The illusion of control. *Journal of Personality and Social Psychology, 32*, 311–328.

Langer, E. J., & Roth, J. (1975). Heads I win, tails it's chance: the illusion of control as a function of sequence of outcomes in a purely chance task. *Journal of Personality and Social Psychology, 32*, 951–955.

Lehman, D. R., Davis, C. G., Delongis, A., Wortman, C., Bluck, S., Mandel, D. R., et al. (1993). Positive and negative life changes following bereavement and their relations to adjustment. *Journal of Social and Clinical Psychology, 12*, 90–112.

Lerner, M. J. (1980). *The belief in a just world*. New York: Plenum Press.

Little, B. R. (1983). Personal projects: A rationale and method for investigation. *Environment and Behavior, 15*, 273–309.

Lynn, M. (1992). Scarcity's enhancement of desirability: The role of naive economic theories. *Basic and Applied Social Psychology, 13*, 67–78.

Magwaza, A. S. (1999). Assumptive world of traumatized South African adults. *Journal of Social Psychology, 139*, 622–630.

Meichenbaum, D. (1985). *Stress inoculation training*. New York: Pergamon.

McIntosh, D. N., Silver, R. C., & Wortman, C. B. (1993). Religion's role in adjustment to a negative life event: Coping with the loss of a child. *Journal of Personality and Social Psychology, 65*, 812–821.

Mitchell-Gibbs, J., & Joseph, S. (1996). Occupational trauma in the British police: Preliminary analyses. *Issues in Criminology and legal Psychology, 19*, 54–58.

Nerken, I. R. (1993). Grief and the reflective self: Toward a clearer model of loss and growth. *Death Studies, 17*, 1–26.

Park, C. L. (1998). Implications of posttraumatic growth for individuals. In R. G. Tedeschi, C. L. Park, & L. G. Calhoun (Eds.), *Posttraumatic growth: Positive change in the aftermath of crisis* (pp. 153–177). Mahwah, NJ: Erlbaum.

Park, C. L., Cohen, L. H., & Murch, R. (1996). Assessment and prediction of stress-related growth. *Journal of Personality, 64*, 71–105.

Parkes, C. M. (1975). What becomes of redundant world models? A contribution to the study of adaptation to change. *British Journal of Medical Psychology, 48*, 131–137.

Parkes, C. M., & Weiss, R. S. (1983). *Recovery from bereavement*. New York: Basic Books.

Pervin, L. A. (1989). *Goal concepts in personality and social psychology*. Hillsdale, NJ: Erlbaum.

Pyszczynski, T., Greenberg, J., & Solomon, S. (1999). A dual-process model of defense against conscious and unconscious death-related thoughts: An extension of terror management theory. *Psychological Review, 106*, 835–845.

Sartre, J. P. (1957). *Existentialism and human emotions*. New York: Philosophical Library.

Sartre, J. P. (1966). *Being and nothingness: A phenomenological study of ontology*. New York: Washington Square Press.

Schwartzberg, S. S. (1993). Struggling for meaning: How HIV-positive gay men make sense of AIDS. *Professional Psychology: Research and Practice, 24*, 483–490.

Schwartzberg, S. S., & Janoff-Bulman, R. (1991). Grief and the search for meaning: Exploring the assumptive worlds of bereaved college students. *Journal of Social and Clinical Psychology, 10*, 270–288.

Shanan, J., & Shahar, O. (1983). Cognitive and personality functioning of Jewish Holocaust survivors during the midlife transition (46–65) in Israel. *Archiv fur die Gesamte Psychologie, 135*, 275–294.

Silver, R. C., Boon, C., & Stones, M. H. (1983). Searching for meaning in misfortune: making sense of incest. *Journal of Social Issues, 39*, 81–102.

Singer, I. (1996). *The creation of value*. Baltimore: Johns Hopkins University Press.

Sledge, W. H., Boydstun, J. A., & Rabe, A. J. (1980). Self-concept changes related to war captivity. Archives of General Psychiatry, *37*, 430–443.

Solomon, S., Greenberg, J., & Pyszczynski, T. (1991). A terror management theory of social behavior: The psychological functions of self-esteem and cultural worldviews. In M. P. Zanna (Ed.), *Advances in experimental social psychology* (Vol. 24, pp. 91–159). San Diego: Academic Press.

Solomon, Z., Iancu, I., & Tyano, S. (1997). World assumptions following disaster. *Journal of Applied Social Psychology, 27*, 1765–1798.

Taylor, S. E., Lichtman, R. R., & Wood, J. V. (1984). Attributions, beliefs about control, and adjustment to breast cancer. *Journal of Personality and Social Psychology, 46*, 489–502.

Tedeschi, R. G., & Calhoun, L. G. (1995). *Trauma and transformation: growing in the aftermath of suffering*. Thousand Oaks, CA; Sage.

Tedeschi. R. G., & Calhoun, L. G. (1996). The posttraumatic growth inventory: measuring the positive legacy of trauma. *Journal of Traumatic Stress, 9*, 455–471.

Tedeschi, R. G., Park, C., L., & Calhoun, L. G. (1998). *Posttraumatic growth: Changes in the aftermath of crisis*. Mahwah, NJ: Erlbaum.

Tellegen, A. (1985). Structures of mood and personality and their relevance to assessing anxiety with an emphasis on self-report. In A. H. Tuma & J. D. Maiser (Eds.), *Anxiety and the anxiety disorders* (pp. 681–706). Hillsdale, NJ: Erlbaum.

Thompson, S. C. (1985). Finding positive meaning in a stressful event and coping. *Basic and Applied Social Psychology, 6*, 279–295.

Thompson, S. C. (1991). The search for meaning following a stroke. *Basic and Applied Social Psychology, 12*, 81–96.

Updegraff, J. A., & Taylor, S. E. (2000). From vulnerability to growth: Positive and negative effects of stressful events. In J. H. Harvey & E. D. Miller (Eds.), *Loss and trauma: general and close relationship perspectives* (pp. 3–28). Philadelphia: Brunner-Routledge.

Veronen, L. J., & Kilpatrick, D. G. (1983). Rape: A precursor of change. In E. J. Callahan & K. A. McCluskey (Eds.), *Life span developmental psychology: Non-normative events* (pp. 167–191). San Diego: Academic Press.

Watson, D., Clark, L. A., & Carey, G. (1988). Positive and negative affectivity and their relation to anxiety and depressive disorders. *Journal of Abnormal Psychology, 97*, 346–353.

Watson, D., Clark, L. A., Weber, K., Assenheimer, J. S., Strauss, M. E., & McCormick, R. A. (1995). Testing a tripartite model: II. Exploring the symptom structure of anxiety and depression in student, adult, and patient samples. *Journal of Abnormal Psychology, 104*, 15–25.

Watson, D., & Tellegen, A. (1985). Toward a consensual structure of mood. *Psychological Bulletin, 98*, 219–235.

Wohl, M., & Enzle, M. (2002). The deployment of personal luck: Sympathetic magic and illusory control in games of pure chance. *Personality and Social Psychology Bulletin, 28*, 1388–1397.

Wong, P. T. P., & Fry, P. S. (Eds.). (1998). *The human quest for meaning: A handbook of psychological research and clinical applications*. Mahwah, NJ: Erlbaum.

Wortman, C. B. (1975). Some determinants of perceived control. *Journal of Personality and Social Psychology, 31*, 282–294.

Part III

Systems of Meaning and Value

Chapter 9

Religion

Its Core Psychological Functions

C. DANIEL BATSON
E. L. STOCKS

> Here is the real core of the religious problem: Help! Help!
> —WILLIAM JAMES, *The Varieties of Religious Experience* (1902, p. 137)

Religion may be broadly defined as whatever a person does to deal with existential questions. Existential questions are those that arise from our awareness that we and others like us are alive and that we will die. They are questions that arise from our awareness of what is sometimes called the human predicament. Examples of existential questions include the following: What is the meaning and purpose of my life? What is my responsibility to others? How do I deal with the fact that I am going to die? What should I do about my shortcomings? These questions refer to matters we care about deeply but cannot fully control. Often, but certainly not always, answers to these questions invoke some higher power (e.g., God) or spiritual force. They come in the form of religious myth, ritual, and practice. They appeal to a dimension of reality beyond the everyday.

Existential questions rise out of a person–situation interaction. On the one hand, we humans have certain basic needs and desires; on the other, we live in a situation that is less than totally accommodating. Our physical and social environment poses problems as well as opportunities—hence, the human predicament. Existential questions take many different forms and reflect the range of different problems and opportunities provided by our environment. The core psychological functions of religion may, in turn, be characterized in terms of response to the existential questions raised by this range of human problems and opportunities.

Abraham Maslow (1954, 1970) provided one of the most comprehensive descriptions of human problems and opportunities. He proposed a hierarchy of basic conative (motivational) needs, including physiological, safety, belongingness, esteem, and self-actualization needs. He also described basic cognitive needs to know and to understand. Maslow believed that as lower-level needs are met, higher-level needs emerge, although he did not consider this pattern invariant. Maslow's analysis went well beyond the existing empirical evidence; it still does. We invoke his analysis not as an accurate and exhaustive description of human needs but as a broad heuristic frame on which to stretch our thinking about the psychological functions of religion.

We propose that religion in its various forms can function to address each of Maslow's needs because each of these needs can raise existential questions. Table 9.1 presents examples of the existential questions raised. We also propose that religion can function to challenge the individual to transcend all of these needs through subjugation of oneself and one's personal needs to a higher purpose or cause.

RELIGIOUS RESPONSES TO QUESTIONS RAISED BY HUMAN NEEDS

Physiological Needs

At the base of Maslow's hierarchy of human needs are physiological needs, including needs for food, drink, warmth, sex, and so on, as well as the need to avoid pain. These needs are a product of the interaction between our biological nature and an environment that may provide insufficient food and shelter, the chance for injury, and the possibility of disease.

TABLE 9.1. Basic Psychological Needs and Resulting Existential Questions, Which Religion Can Function to Address

Psychological needs arising from person–situation interaction[a]	Existential questions raised by these needs
Conative needs	
Physiological needs—Needs for food, drink, warmth, sex, etc.	How do I satisfy my hunger and thirst? What if the crop fails? How do I stay warm and dry? How do I deal with this injury or disease?
Safety needs—Needs to keep oneself and one's possessions safe.	What can and should I do to protect myself? Are there powerful forces that I can and should appeal to for safety? How can I control the future?
Belongingness and love needs—Needs to have a place in the social world, to be loved, and to love.	Where do I belong? Who are my people? Who loves me? Whom do I love? What is my responsibility to others?
Esteem needs—Needs for a sense of strength and competence, as well as for reputation, status, and appreciation.	Am I a person of worth? Am I valued by others? How am I to live with my shortcomings, mistakes, and inabilities?
Need for self-actualization—Need to become everything one is capable of becoming, to express one's true nature.	What is my true nature? What will make me truly happy? How can I be fulfilled?
Cognitive needs	
Need to know and understand—Need to have a sense of meaning and purpose in one's life.	What is the meaning and purpose of my life? What will happen to me when I die? What should I do, given my inevitable death?

[a]Adapted from Maslow (1954, 1970).

Maslow (1970) considered these needs to be "the most prepotent of all needs" (p. 36). That is, "a person who is lacking food, safety, love, and esteem would most probably hunger for food more strongly than for anything else. . . . All other needs may become simply nonexistent or be pushed into the background" (Maslow, 1970, p. 37).

As Maslow noted, for the chronically hungry person, his or her vision of Utopia becomes a place where there is plenty of food. In this observation, one catches a glimpse of the nature of existential questions raised by physiological needs and of the religious response. Existential questions raised by such needs are typically concrete and pointed: How do I satisfy my hunger and thirst? What do we do if the rains do not come and the crop fails? How do I stay warm and dry? How do I deal with this injury or disease?

If a person is confident that the environment is so benign that such problems can never arise, or that when they arise resources are at hand to meet them, then such questions are not existential; they are only practical. If, however, one believes that satisfaction of these needs is not fully under one's control, these questions can become existential.

The religious response to such questions is often as concrete and pointed as the questions themselves. Consider the prayer of a Native American chief:

> Great Sun Power! I am praying for my people, that they may be happy in the summer and that they may live through the cold of winter. Many are sick and in want. Pity them, and let them survive. Grant that they live long and have abundance. May we go through these ceremonies correctly, as you taught our forefathers to do in the days that are past. If we make mistakes, pity us!
>
> Help us, Mother Earth! For we depend upon your goodness. Let there be rain to water the prairies, that the grass may grow long and the berries be abundant.
>
> O Morning Star! When you look down upon us, give us peace and refreshing sleep.
>
> Great Spirit! Bless our children, friends, and visitors through a happy life. May our trails lie straight and level before us. Let us live to be old. We are all your children, and we ask these things with good hearts. (Burtt, 1957, p. 42)

In early civilizations, when the food supply was far from certain, planting was a time for religious rituals, a time to ask God or the gods for a successful crop. Harvest was a time for religious celebration and prayers of thanksgiving. If during the growing season rains did not come, people turned to priests and shamans to appeal for divine intervention. (In many farm communities, prayers for rain continue today, perhaps because the efficacy of such prayers is quite difficult to confirm or disconfirm—if one prays long enough, rain will fall.)

For nomadic herders and early farmers living in arid stretches of the Middle East, the Promised Land was often described as "a land flowing with milk and honey." And who had promised this land? It was promised by Yahweh (God), the One who could provide manna in the Wilderness. The initial petition in the famous prayer Jesus taught his disciples, the Lord's Prayer, is "give us this day our daily bread" (Matthew 6: 11). Offering a prayer of thanks to God before meals is less common today than a century ago, but the practice often reappears when disasters strike and food becomes scarce. Thanks to God for meeting our need for food was the basis for Abraham Lincoln's proclamation that established Thanksgiving Day as a holiday in the United States.

Religious responses to sexual needs have been far less simple and direct. They run the gamut from (1) praying for God to provide a sexual partner to (2) asking God to help one resist sexual urges to (3) renouncing sex as a sign of religious devotion to (4) fulfilling one's sexual desires either literally or symbolically in a religious context. In early religions it was not unusual to incorporate sexual activity into sacred ceremonies or to offer virgins to the gods. In the Middle Ages, nuns were consecrated as "brides of Christ." Nor have seemingly incompatible responses to sexual desires been mutually exclusive, as is highlighted by recent revelations of the sexual activities of some celibate Catholic priests.

Psychologists studying religion have given some but not extensive attention to the role of religion in enabling individuals to address existential questions raised by physiological needs. Freud (1927/1964, 1930/1961) recognized this function of religion, even though he focused his attention more on religion as a response to safety needs. More recently, Pargament (1990, 1997; Pargament & Park, 1995), McIntosh and Spilka (1990), Koenig (Koenig & Cohen, 2002), and others have provided correlational evidence that at least some forms of religious activity and belief can help people cope with illness, disease, and disaster, and may promote physical health. Even when some of the more obvious confounds are controlled (e.g., demographic factors, socioeconomic status, social stress, and health status), modest positive correlations have been found (for a thoughtful review, see George, Ellison, & Larson, 2002).

What about those of us who are fortunate enough not to have to worry about where our next meal will come from, about where we will sleep, about staying warm, or about our health—at least for now? To the extent that we find our physiological needs satisfied, a major psychological function of religion becomes moot. This does not, however, mean that religion ceases to serve important psychological functions. Rather, new needs arise that raise new existential questions. In Maslow's (1970) words:

> It is quite true that man lives by bread alone—when there is no bread. But what happens to man's desires when there *is* plenty of bread and when his belly is chronically filled? *At once other (and higher) needs emerge* and these, rather than physiological hungers, dominate the organism. And when these in turn are satisfied, again new (and still higher) needs emerge, and so on. (p. 38, emphasis in original)

Safety Needs

As soon as our stomachs are full and we have enough for the days to come, as soon as we have something to lose, concerns may arise about keeping our something and ourselves safe. Unless we are confident that we can forestall all threats—and who is, if we stop and think—we may find ourselves asking existential questions such as: What can and should I do to protect myself? Are there powerful forces that I can and should appeal to for safety? How can I control the future?

Threats, whether from nature, from our peers, or from signs of illness in our own bodies, lead us to fear the future and to wish for a world that is safe, reliable, and predictable. As children, we may have assumed that our parents could and would protect us. Once we begin to recognize their limitations, we may long to know that someone or something even more powerful is in control and has our welfare at heart. We may look to God or gods.

Many psychologists have recognized that religion can function to meet safety needs. Freud (1927/1964), in *The Future of an Illusion*, focused on religion as a source of safety. He suggested that the first task of the gods is to "exorcize the terrors of nature" (p. 24). Similarly, Maslow (1954) suggested that religion often speaks to the desire to see the universe as organized, coherent, and meaningful. He believed that this desire was motivated in part by basic safety needs. Allport (1966) made an important distinction between extrinsic and intrinsic approaches to religion. According to Allport, when approached extrinsically, religion functions as an instrumental means to self-serving ends. When approached intrinsically, it functions as an end in itself and "strives to transcend all self-centered needs" (Allport, 1966, p. 455). We shall have more to say about Allport's concept of intrinsic religion shortly. For now, we can note that, according to Allport, a sense of safety is one of the most important of the self-serving ends promoted by extrinsic religion. Kirkpatrick (1994, 1999), in his applications of attachment theory to religion, noted that God often functions as a "safe haven," much as the primary caregiver does for the secure child. Kirkpatrick provided empirical evidence consistent with this suggestion. In two longitudinal studies, he found that adults with insecure attachment styles due to negative models of self were especially likely to turn to God as a substitute attachment figure (Kirkpatrick, 1997, 1998).

Once again, both as individuals and as a society we work hard to keep threats to our safety at bay. To the degree that we succeed in creating an environment in which we do not fear wild animals, severe weather or extremes of temperature, robbery or assault, or terrorist attacks or war, we may find less relevance in reassurance that "God's in His heaven; All's right with the world." We may feel that we do not need religion—at least not religion that functions to provide a sense of security in the face of the perils of life. Of course, when the perils break through our defenses, we may change our mind. As is said: "There are no atheists in foxholes."

Belongingness and Love Needs

A full belly and a sense of safety provide the basis for a new hunger, which Maslow (1970) described graphically:

> If both the physiological and the safety needs are fairly well gratified, there will emerge the love and affection and belongingness needs, and the whole cycle already described will repeat itself with this new center. Now the person will feel keenly, as never before, the absence of friends, or a sweetheart, or a wife, or children. He will hunger for affectionate relations with people in general, namely, for a place in his group, and he will strive with great intensity to achieve this goal. He will want to attain such a place more than anything else in the world and may even forget that once, when he was hungry, he sneered at love as unreal or unnecessary or unimportant. (p. 43)

The existential questions evoked by this need include not only "Who loves me?" but also "Whom do I love?" And at a more general level: "Where do I belong?" "Who are my people?" "What is my responsibility to others?"

For millenia, a core function of all the major world religions has been to respond to this need. Judaism early on focused on the special relationship between the Israelites and their God. Theirs was "a jealous god," whom they should love with all their heart and before whom they should have no other; they, in turn, were God's "Chosen People." And how should they relate to other people? In the Holiness Code found in the second half of the book of Leviticus, the faithful are instructed: "You shall love your neighbor as yourself" (Leviticus 19: 18). Even at this early date (about 550 B.C.), the concept of neighbor was broad: "The stranger who sojourns with you shall be to you as the native among you, and you shall love him as yourself: for you were strangers in the land of Egypt" (Leviticus 19: 34).

Six centuries later Jesus repeated, elaborated, and extended the command to love neighbor as self. He asserted that it applied not only to strangers but even to enemies: "Love your enemies, and do good to those who hate you" (Luke 6: 27). Christian theologians have

made much of the New Testament reference to God using the Aramaic word *abba*, a familiar form of father, more akin to daddy or poppa. As Christianity spread into the Greek
world, one hears that "God is love, and he who abides in love abides in God, and God
abides in him" (I John 4: 16). The Greek word used is not *eros* or *philia* but *agape*, selfless
attention to the welfare of the other. Islam also offers the faithful an ever-present, compassionate, and merciful God, as well as a sense of brotherhood of believers and a special place
in the social order of this world and the world to come. Religions of the East such as Buddhism place less emphasis on a loving relationship with God, and more emphasis on a loving, compassionate relationship with all living things. James (1902) recounts a legend:

> Where the future Buddha, incarnated as a hare, jumps into the fire to cook himself for a meal for
> a beggar—having previously shaken himself three times, so that none of the insects in his fur
> should perish with him. (p. 224n)

As a key defining aspect of who one is, religious identity is less important today than a
century ago for people in most developed countries (the United States is a conspicuous exception), but religion remains a highly important aspect of identity for people in many parts
of the world. In the United States, the various New Age trends in contemporary Christianity
seem especially oriented toward addressing needs for belongingness and love. As Maslow
(1970) observed, "We still underplay the deep importance of the neighborhood, of one's territory, of one's clan, of one's own 'kind,' one's class, one's gang, one's familiar working
colleagues" (pp. 43–44).

Given the centrality of belongingness and love in most religious traditions, it is surprising that this function has not received more attention from psychologists of religion. (In
contrast, sociologists of religion have long emphasized the role of religion in promoting social stability and a sense of belonging; see de Tocqueville, 1835/1969; Durkheim, 1915).
James (1902) did recognize this function; Freud (1930/1961, pp. 56–61) offered a provocative, skeptical analysis of the religious call to universal, other-oriented love; and Allport
(1966) identified satisfaction of the need to belong as a second key extrinsic benefit of religion. As attachment theory has been extended beyond its initial focus on the infant's attachment to a primary caregiver (Ainsworth, Blehar, Waters, & Wall, 1978; Bowlby, 1969) to
include adult relationships, there has been increasing emphasis not only on the enduring
need for an attachment figure to provide a safe haven but also on the reciprocal nature of
adult relationships, which include caregiving as well as attachment (Mikulincer & Shaver,
2003). Thus far, however, consideration of the other-oriented side of love reflected in
care-giving has not figured prominently in attachment theory analyses of religion (e.g.,
Granqvist, 1998, 2002; Kirkpatrick, 1994, 1999). Application of social identity theory
(Tajfel, 1982; Tajfel & Turner, 1986) and self-categorization theory (Turner, 1987) may
prove fruitful in analysis of religious response to the need to belong (see DeConchy, 1984,
and Burris & Jackson, 2000, for initial attempts), although these theories have little to say
about love.

Esteem Needs

With belongingness and love needs met, esteem needs come to the fore. According to
Maslow (1970), esteem needs take two forms. First, there is a need for strength, achievement, mastery, and competence. Second, there is a need for reputation, prestige, status, recognition, and appreciation. Satisfaction of these needs leads to a sense of self-confidence,

worth, capability, and value to the world. To fully satisfy our esteem needs, both forms of esteem must be achieved. Positive reputation not accompanied by a perception of true ability is too fragile and lacking in stability to provide a healthy sense of self-esteem. Esteem needs can raise a number of existential questions, such as: Am I a person of worth? Am I valued by others? How am I to live with my shortcomings, mistakes, and inabilities?

At least in the United States, feeling good about oneself and seeing oneself as a person of worth and value play a major role in much contemporary religion. Historically, however, the religious response to the desire for self-esteem has been mixed at best. On the one hand, religion has offered assurance of personal worth simply because one is a person—not because of anything in particular one has done—and has questioned the value of reputation. On the other hand, religion has provided an alternative set of standards of worth, capability, and value—standards based not on dominance and power but on devotion, piety, and service—and it has issued a call to excellence in this new domain. Thus, one may be assured that he or she was created by and is valued by God: "Look at the birds of the air; they neither sow nor reap nor gather into barns, and yet your heavenly Father feeds them. Are you not of more value than they?" (Matthew 6: 26). At the same time, one is challenged: "For if you love those who love you, what reward do you have? Do not even the tax collectors do the same? . . . Be perfect, therefore, as your heavenly Father is perfect" (Matthew 5: 46, 48).

Further indicating a suspicion of the need for self-esteem, most religious traditions are harsh in their judgment of those who see themselves as especially worthy in God's eyes or who make a public show of their devotion.

> Beware of practicing your piety before others in order to be seen by them; for then you have no reward from your Father in heaven.
>
> So whenever you give alms, do not sound a trumpet before you, as the hypocrites do in the synagogues and in the streets, so that they may be praised by others. Truly I tell you, they have received their reward. But when you give alms, do not let your left hand know what your right hand is doing, so that your alms may be done in secret; and your Father who sees in secret will reward you.
>
> And whenever you pray, do not be like the hypocrites; for they love to stand and pray in the synagogues and at the street corners, so that they may be seen by others. Truly I tell you, they have received their reward. But whenever you pray, go into your room and shut the door and pray to your Father who is in secret; and your Father who sees in secret will reward you. (Matthew 6: 1–6)

False piety is castigated; authentic humility is extolled. To seek to excel in devotion, piety, and service is a sign that one has failed. Fortunately, one of the hallmarks of all major religious traditions is that means are provided through which personal failures and shortcomings are forgiven—sacrifice, confession, and penance.

Among psychologists, James (1902) and Allport (1950, 1966) have been the most sensitive to the perverse use of religion to meet esteem needs. Allport considered the need for reputation and social standing to be one of the most important self-serving ends motivating an extrinsic orientation to religion. Consistent with the idea that active pursuit of esteem through religion is doomed to failure, subsequent research has indicated that measures of extrinsic religion tend to correlate negatively with measures of self-esteem. Measures of intrinsic religion tend to correlate positively (see Batson, Schoenrade, & Ventis, 1993, for a review). Does this mean that the measures of intrinsic religion tap authentic humility that bestows esteem as an unintended byproduct ("your Father who sees in secret will reward you")? This was Allport's (1966) belief, but there is some reason for doubt. It may be that, contrary to Allport's intent, measures of intrinsic religion actually reflect an instrumental use of religion to enhance self-esteem—one's sense of oneself as a good, righteous person—even more than do measures of extrinsic religion (Batson et al., 1993; also see Crocker, 2002).

Need for Self-Actualization

At the top of Maslow's (1970) hierarchy of basic conative needs is the need for self-actualization. Even if all four of the preceding needs are met, an individual may feel restless and unsatisfied unless doing what he or she is fitted for. To be at peace, "a musician must make music, an artist must paint, a poet must write" (Maslow, 1970, p. 46). One needs to "become everything one is capable of becoming" (p. 46). This may be expressed in the desire to be an ideal parent; it may be expressed athletically, in the arts, or in science. Maslow's criterion for who had met this need was basically circular: People who are not only highly productive but also satisfied and at peace with themselves are self-actualized. Existential questions raised by this need include: What is my true nature? What will make me truly happy? How can I be fulfilled?

Historically, the promotion of self-actualization or expression of one's unique, individual nature has not been a function of religion. It is too self-centered. Promotion of self-actualization has, however, been a major function of the New Age mixture of Jungian and humanistic psychology that became popular in the last quarter of the 20th century among some liberal Protestants in the United States. Jung (1935) emphasized individuality and individuation:

> In so far as "individuality" embraces our innermost, last, and incomparable uniqueness, it also implies becoming one's own self. We could therefore translate individuation as "coming to selfhood" or "self-realization." (p. 173)

For Jung (1938), religion was perhaps the most effective means of achieving individuality. We find a similar sentiment expressed by humanistic psychologists such as Rollo May (1953) and Erich Fromm (1950, 1960). For example, Fromm (1960) believed that humanistic religion (in contrast to authoritarian religion) holds the key to "overcoming the limitations of an egotistical self, achieving love, objectivity, and humility and respecting life so that the aim of life is living itself, and man becomes what he potentially is" (p. 80). Maslow's discussion of self-actualization was also an important precursor of New Age religion. It is not clear that Maslow would have been happy about this because he was quite suspicious of organized religion.

One of the reasons that Maslow doubted the value of organized religion was that he felt it provided little support for the pursuit of self-actualization. Still, he was convinced that there was often a religious dimension to the life of self-actualized individuals. They were likely to have what Maslow (1964) called peak experiences—nontraditional "core-religious" experiences of a somewhat mystical nature in which one has a sense of wholeness and integration both within oneself and with one's world, a sense of effortless and creative involvement in the here and now. The mystical aspects of such experiences seem to have much in common with the experiences of wholeness and integration in the meditative traditions of Buddhism, although Buddhism puts much less emphasis on the self. The effortless and creative involvement in the here and now has much in common with what Csikszentmihalyi (1990) has called flow.

Cognitive Needs: The Desire to Know and Understand

At one level, Maslow (1970) viewed cognitive capacities as a set of tools used in the service of satisfying the basic conative needs. "Acquiring knowledge and systematizing the universe" serves to provide a sense of basic safety in the world, and in the intelligent, serves the expression of self-actualization (p. 48). At a second level, however, the desire to know and understand forms a hierarchy of needs in its own right. "Even after we know, we are impelled to know more and more minutely and microscopically on the one hand, and on the other, more and more extensively in the direction of a world philosophy, theology, etc. . . . This process has been phrased by some as the search for meaning" (p. 50). Maslow (1970) cautioned against creating a sharp dichotomy between cognitive and conative needs, for two reasons. First, the desire to know and understand has a strong motivational character; it is often experienced as a passionate drive, a desperate longing for meaning and purpose, not simply as a philosophical puzzle. Second, the two types of needs are intertwined.

For many, the most salient core psychological function of religion is to provide a sense of meaning and purpose in life. Sharp and pressing existential questions arise from the clash between the desire to know and understand and two key characteristics of the human predicament—awareness of our individual existence and awareness of our mortality. Who does not at some point face questions such as the following: What is the meaning and purpose of my life? Is my life no more than "a tale told by an idiot, full of sound and fury, signifying nothing"? What will happen to me when I die? What should I do, given my inevitable death?

These questions can shake the foundation of even the most secure, successful, and seemingly self-actualized life. Tolstoy (1904) was at the height of his career as a novelist—productive, wealthy, and acclaimed—when it all collapsed in terror and despair:

> I felt that something had broken within me on which my life had always rested, that I had nothing left to hold on to, and that morally my life had stopped. . . .
>
> One can live only so long as one is intoxicated, drunk with life; but when one grows sober one cannot fail to see that it is all a stupid cheat. What is truest about it is that there is nothing even funny or silly in it; it is cruel and stupid, purely and simply. . . .
>
> What will be the outcome of what I do today? Of what I shall do tomorrow? What will be the outcome of my life? Why should I live? Why should I do anything? Is there in life any purpose which the inevitable death which awaits me does not undo and destroy? (pp. 20–22)

These questions pushed Tolstoy to the brink of suicide:

> It cannot be said exactly that I *wished* to kill myself, for the force which drew me away from life was fuller, more powerful, more general than any mere desire. It was a force like my old aspiration to live, only it impelled me in the opposite direction. It was an aspiration of my whole being to get out of life. (Tolstoy, 1904, p. 20)

Religion provided the answers that eventually led Tolstoy away from the abyss.

Malinowski (1954) described the role of religion in providing meaning and purpose in more general terms:

> Into this supreme dilemma of life and final death, religion steps in, selecting the positive creed, the comforting view, the culturally valuable belief in immortality, in the spirit independent of the body, and in the continuance of life after death. In the various ceremonies at death, in commemo-

ration and communion with the departed, and the worship of ancestral ghosts, religion gives body and form to the saving beliefs. (p. 51)

Among psychologists studying religion, James (1902), Freud (1927/1964, 1930/1961), and Jung (1964) all recognized the importance of religion as a source of meaning and purpose in life. Allport (1950), in his classic discussion of mature religion, made this function of religion central. In contrast to immature religion, Allport believed that mature religion provides an overarching sense of meaning and purpose that integrates and orders the personality, allows the individual honestly to face the human predicament, and provides a master-motive for living. However, when Allport (1966) translated his concepts of immature and mature religion into his later concepts of extrinsic and intrinsic religion, and especially when he and his students developed questionnaire items to provide objective measures of these later concepts, subtle but important omissions occurred. The role of religion in providing meaning in life was clearly reflected in the Intrinsic scale, but the open-ended, tentative, heuristic nature of the search for meaning was not. This led Batson (1976) to propose a third dimension of personal religion to complement the extrinsic and intrinsic dimensions, religion as a quest. As a quest, religion is experienced not as a solution but as a search. Gandhi (1948) described the role of religion in his life in these words:

> I worship God as Truth only. I have not yet found Him, but I am seeking after Him. I am prepared to sacrifice the things dearest to me in pursuit of this quest. . . . But as long as I have not realized this Absolute Truth, so long must I hold to the relative truth as I have conceived it. That relative truth must, meanwhile, be my beacon, my shield and buckler. (pp. 5–6)

Subsequent research has revealed that many of the social benefits that Allport (1966) thought would be associated with an intrinsic orientation to religion are associated with the quest dimension instead. Scores on the quest dimension seem to be associated with reduced prejudice and with increased responsiveness to the needy—not only on self-report measures but also in behavior (Batson, Eidelman, Higley, & Russell, 2001; Batson, Flink, Schoenrade, Fultz, & Pych, 1986; Batson et al., 1989). On the other hand, personal benefits in the form of satisfaction in life and reduced anxiety are more likely to be associated with the clear sense of meaning and purpose reflected in an intrinsic orientation than with a quest orientation. Perhaps because it is associated with these personal benefits, an intrinsic orientation to religion is also more likely to be associated with rigid adherence to the religious meaning system. Religious freedom from anxiety, fear, and anomie may come at the price of bondage to one's religious beliefs themselves (see Batson et al., 1993, for a discussion of this possibility and review of the relevant research).

Over the past two decades, the psychological perspective that has focused most directly on the human response to awareness that one is destined to die is terror management theory (TMT; Solomon, Greenberg, & Pyszczynski, 1991; see also Chapter 2, this volume). TMT suggests that self-esteem and culture work together to form an anxiety buffer against the reality of mortality. The cultural worldview provides a system of meaning that accords value and significance to events, activities, attributes, and objects. As a result, the worldview provides a framework in which one can achieve a sense of self-worth and value by participation in specified events and activities and by possession of prescribed attributes and objects. Within this framework, one can quiet those terrifying whispers that haunted Tolstoy: Why should I live? Why should I do anything? Is there in life any purpose which the inevitable death which awaits me does not undo and destroy?

TMT accords a major role to religion both as a cultural institution and as a personal belief system. But, although there is much research consistent with various predictions of TMT, research designed to test the role of religion as an anxiety buffer remains limited and inconclusive (see Burling, 1993). The best relevant research is, we believe, an experiment done over 30 years ago by Osarchuk and Tatz (1973; also see Schoenrade, 1989; Atran, 2002, pp. 177–181).

We should, perhaps, comment briefly on our placement of TMT in our discussion of cognitive needs rather than basic conative physiological and safety needs. Solomon et al. (1991) suggested that the motive underlying terror management is a primitive and basic one, an inclination toward self-preservation. Moreover, they suggested that this inclination is common to all life forms. In making this suggestion, we believe that Solomon et al. have run afoul of a misinterpretation of natural selection common among psychologists. They have assumed that when some life form acts in a manner that promotes its survival, this life form is seeking self-preservation.

Natural selection often leads animals to act as if they were motivated to achieve some goal when, in fact, they are not. Their actions may be reflexive or in the service of another, more concrete motive. Self-preservation is a prime example. As recent work on the theory of mind underscores, it is not clear that any species other than our own has a concept of self or individual existence or an ability to imagine unexperienced states such as one's own death (the only serious contenders seem to be some of our nearest primate relatives—see Tomasello, 1999). Without a concept of self or individuality, and of one's own death, it makes no sense to speak of an inclination toward self-preservation, or fear of death, or fear of annihilation. There may be relatively hard-wired fears that are likely midbrain (amygdala) based and shared with other species (LeDoux, 1996). These include fear of heights, dark places, loud noises, or certain animals (e.g., snakes). But a fear of death or annihilation requires more than an amygdala; it also requires concepts that rely on the (prefrontal) cortex and are likely uniquely human. Even in humans, these concepts only develop after several years of life.

Animals (ourselves included) often act to escape or avoid pain or discomfort; these actions can produce the result of self-preservation without that result being their goal. Rather than being a primitive and ancient motive shared with other species, our concern for self-preservation is almost certainly a recent evolutionary development. It is dependent on the cognitive capacities to (1) understand oneself as an existing person and (2) imagine the radically altered reality in which this person no longer exists. These capacities can, in turn, produce truly terrifying doubts such as Tolstoy's about the meaning and purpose of life. For this reason, we have discussed terror management under the desire to know and understand.

RELIGION AS A CALL TO SELF-TRANSCENDENCE

Thus far, we have been following James's diagnosis, that the core of the religious problem lies in the piteous cry, "Help! Help!" We have reviewed the way religion functions to address basic needs, ranging from deficiency needs (physiological, safety, belongingness and love, esteem) to the higher growth needs (self-actualization), from conative needs to cognitive. This review has enabled us to at least touch on the core functions of religion highlighted by most major psychological studies of religion. Still, there is an extremely important psychological function of religion that we have not yet addressed, one that has received relatively little attention from psychologists. Religion may also function to promote self-transcendence. All the needs we have considered are needs of the person or individual. There is little doubt that religion has functioned to address personal needs that arise from the human predicament. But religion can do more. It can function to call the individual to reorient priorities away from meeting one or another—or even all—of these needs. It can call the individual to place value outside oneself, to pursue some higher purpose or cause.

Sometimes this call takes the form of a paradoxical suggestion that the way to effectively satisfy your needs is to quit trying to do so, to focus instead on meeting others' needs, and to trust God. For example, concerning physiological needs, Jesus taught, "Do not worry, saying, 'What will we eat?' or 'What will we drink?' or 'What will we wear?' . . . Your heavenly Father knows that you need all these things. But strive first for the kingdom of God and his righteousness, and all these things will be given to you as well" (Matthew 6: 31–33). Similarly, concerning safety needs, "So do not worry about tomorrow, for tomorrow will bring worries of its own. Today's trouble is enough for today" (Matthew 6: 34). Or in the words of a Taoist poem:

> . . . The sage puts himself last,
>   And finds himself in the foremost place;
> Regards his body as accidental,
>   And his body is thereby preserved.
> Is it not because he does not live for Self
>   That his Self achieves perfection? (Burtt, 1957, p. 191)

At other times the call to self-transcendence takes the form of a recommendation that one shift to a new set of values. "Do not store up for yourselves treasures on earth, where moth and rust consume and where thieves break in and steal; but store up for yourselves treasures in heaven, where neither moth nor rust consumes and where thieves do not break in and steal. For where your treasure is, there your heart will be also" (Matthew 6: 19–21). A similar value reorientation is central to Islam, a word that means "submission to God." Muhammed's last command to his followers was clear:

> My last command to you is that you remain united, that you love, honor, and uphold one another, that you exhort one another to faith, and constancy in belief, and to the performance of pious deeds. By these alone, men prosper. All else leads to destruction. (Burtt, 1957, p. 425)

At still other times this call takes the form of an appeal to discipline oneself to eliminate personal needs and desires. This path to self-transcendence is found in Taoism, and it is especially prominent in various forms of Buddhism, where the goal of the eightfold path is Nirvana, a state of nothingness and oneness with the Universe without personal desire. Here, religion functions not to save oneself but to free oneself from oneself.

Finally, at still other times this call can take the form of an invitation to lose oneself in participation in and service to a religious community, institution, or ideal. Subjugation of self to a religious community or ideal can go far beyond a mere sense of belongingness, affiliation, and identity. It can lead to unhesitating devotion even to the point of martyrdom, as in the Jonestown and Heaven's Gate communities. Joan of Arc (Jeanne d'Arc, 1412–1431) heard voices that led her out of herself—and into battle and, ultimately, to the stake.

Psychologists interested in religion, especially empirically oriented psychologists, have paid little attention to the role of religion in promoting self-transcendence. James (1902) presented a long list of examples of saints and others in whom religious devotion seemed to change the value-structure away from personal needs and even from personal growth and self-preservation. But this saints' gallery has been visited by later psychologists more as a one might stop by a wax museum, simply to marvel and pass on. James (1902) also considered mystical self-transcendence. Maslow (1964) hinted at the possibility of transcendence, but consistent with his emphasis on personal needs, he conceived it as a "need for transcendence" (p. xiv). The self-transcendence to which we refer is a more radical process, one in which personal needs and the self itself are transcended. It comes through active involvement and subjugation to something outside oneself, not through Maslow's passive acceptance of being. Allport (1950, pp. 63–64) included some consideration of self-transcendence in his reflections on mature religion. But self-transcendence is not clearly represented in his later empirical work on intrinsic religion. Eric Hoffer (1951) presented an insightful analysis of the dark side of self-subjugation to a religious cause or community in *The True Believer* (also see Fromm's, 1941, 1950, discussions of escape from freedom and of authoritarian religion). Beyond these and similar reflections, psychologists have given little attention to religion as a source of self-transcendence.

Perhaps it is because the life of the individual is the stock and trade of psychology that psychologists have paid so little attention to the self-transcendent function of religion. This seems regrettable because it may be the self-transcendent function that holds the most promise for shedding new light on the nature of the human psyche. The other functions, important as they are, fit relatively comfortably within existing psychological conceptions of human nature; they point to religion as one way of meeting our various needs. Self-transcendence, however, seems qualitatively different. If self-transcendence is possible, then we must face the prospect that meeting needs, even so-called growth needs, is but one way of approaching life—and at least for some, perhaps not the best way.

CONCLUSION

We have offered an untidy melange of core psychological functions of religion. Is one of these functions the true one, or at least truer than the others? We think not. Rather, depending on who one is and what needs are prepotent at the time, only one of a few functions of religion may seem deeply relevant and profoundly true. Others may seem infantile; still others, irrelevant or obscure. Which functions seem relevant and true, and which seem infantile, irrelevant, or obscure, are, however, likely to vary over time, person, situation, and culture. The matters we care about deeply but cannot fully control are not always the same. Different needs and interests raise different existential questions, which, in turn, bring different functions of religion to the fore. If the human predicament does not pose a single problem but many, then we should not expect a single religious response, but many. Nor is religion content to respond to our calls for help; it also calls us to lift our eyes from our own needs and to set our sights on higher matters, beyond ourselves.

REFERENCES

Ainsworth, M. D. S., Blehar, M. C., Waters, E., & Wall, S. (1978). *Patterns of attachment: A psychological study of the strange situation.* Hillsdale, NJ: Erlbaum.

Allport, G. W. (1950). *The individual and his religion.* New York: Macmillan.

Allport, G. W. (1966). Religious context of prejudice. *Journal for the Scientific Study of Religion, 5,* 447–457.

Atran, S. (2002). *In gods we trust: The evolutionary landscape of religion.* New York: Oxford University Press.

Batson, C. D. (1976). Religion as prosocial: Agent or double agent? *Journal for the Scientific Study of Religion, 15*, 29–45.

Batson, C. D., Eidelman, S. H., Higley, S. L., & Russell, S. A. (2001). "And who is my neighbor?" II: Quest religion as a source of universal compassion. *Journal for the Scientific Study of Religion, 40*, 39–50.

Batson, C. D., Flink, C. H., Schoenrade, P. A., Fultz, J., & Pych, V. (1986). Religious orientation and overt versus covert racial prejudice. *Journal of Personality and Social Psychology, 50*, 175–181.

Batson, C. D., Oleson, K. C., Weeks, J. L., Healy, S. P., Reeves, P. J., Jennings, P., et al. (1989). Religious prosocial motivation: Is it altruistic or egoistic? *Journal of Personality and Social Psychology, 57*, 873–884.

Batson, C. D., Schoenrade, P. A., & Ventis, W. L. (1993). *Religion and the individual: A social-psychological perspective.* New York: Oxford University Press.

Bowlby, J. (1969). *Attachment and loss: Vol 1. Attachment.* New York: Basic Books.

Burling, J. W. (1993). Death concerns and symbolic aspects of the self: The effects of mortality salience on status concern and religiosity. *Personality and Social Psychology Bulletin, 19*, 100–105.

Burris, C. T., & Jackson, L. M. (2000). Social identity and the true believer: Responses to threatened self-stereotypes among the intrinsically religious. *British Journal of Social Psychology, 39*, 257–278.

Burtt, E. A. (1957). *Man seeks the divine: A study in the history and comparison of religions.* New York: Harper.

Crocker, J. (2002). The costs of seeking self-esteem. *Journal of Social Issues, 58*, 597–615.

Csikszentmihalyi, M. (1990). *Flow: The psychology of optimal experience.* New York: Harper & Row.

DeConchy, J.-P. (1984). Rationality and social control in orthodox systems. In H. Tajfel (Ed.), *The social dimension* (Vol. 2, pp. 425–445). New York: Cambridge University Press.

de Tocqueville, A. (1969). *Democracy in America.* New York: Doubleday. (Original work published 1835)

Durkheim, E. (1915). *The elementary forms of religious life.* London: George Allen & Unwin.

Freud, S. (1961). *Civilization and its discontents.* New York: Norton. (Original work published 1930)

Freud, S. (1964). *The future of an illusion.* Garden City, NY: Doubleday. (Original work published 1927)

Fromm, E. (1941). *Escape from freedom.* New York: Rinehart.

Fromm, E. (1950). *Psychoanalysis and religion.* New Haven: Yale University Press.

Fromm, E. (1960). Psychoanalysis and Zen Buddhism. In D. T. Suzuki, E. Fromm, & R. De Martino (Eds.), *Zen Buddhism and psychoanalysis* (pp. 77–141). London: George Allen & Unwin.

Gandhi, M. K. (1948). *Gandhi's autobiography: The story of my experiments with truth* (M. Desai, Trans.). Washington, DC: Public Affairs Press.

George, L. K., Ellison, C. G., & Larson, D. B. (2002). Explaining the relationships between religious involvement and health. *Psychological Inquiry, 13*, 190–200.

Granqvist, P. (1998). Religiousness and perceived childhood attachment: On the question of compensation or correspondence. *Journal for the Scientific Study of Religion, 37*, 350–367.

Granqvist, P. (2002). Attachment and religiosity in adolescence: Cross-sectional and longitudinal evaluations. *Personality and Social Psychology Bulletin, 28*, 260–270.

Hoffer, E. (1951). *The true believer.* New York: Harper.

James, W. (1902). *The varieties of religious experience.* New York: Longmans.

Jung, C. G. (1935). The relations between the ego and the unconscious. In *Collected works* (Vol. 7, pp. 121–241). Princeton, NJ: Princeton University Press.

Jung, C. G. (1938). Psychology and religion. In *Collected works* (Vol. 11, pp. 558–575). Princeton, NJ: Princeton University Press.

Jung, C. G. (Ed.). (1964). *Man and his symbols.* London: Aldus Books.

Kirkpatrick, L. A. (1994). The role of attachment in religious belief and behavior. In K. Bartholomew & D. Perlman (Eds.), *Attachment processes in adulthood* (Vol. 5, pp. 239–265. Bristol, PA: Kingsley.

Kirkpatrick, L. A. (1997). A longitudinal study of changes in religious belief and behavior as a func-
    tion of individual differences in adult attachment style. *Journal for the Scientific Study of Reli-
    gion, 36*, 207–217.

Kirkpatrick, L. A. (1998). God as a substitute attachment figure: A longitudinal study of adult attach-
    ment style and religious change in college students. *Personality and Social Psychology Bulletin,
    24*, 961–973.

Kirkpatrick, L. A. (1999). Attachment and religious representations and behavior. In J. Cassidy & P.
    R. Shaver (Eds.), *Handbook of attachment: Theory, research, and clinical applications* (pp. 803–
    822). New York: Guilford Press.

Koenig, H. G., & Cohen, H. J. (Eds.). (2002). *The link between religion and health:
    Psychoneuroimmuniology and the faith factor.* London: Oxford University Press.

LeDoux, J. E. (1996). *The emotional brain.* New York: Simon & Schuster.

McIntosh, D., & Spilka, B. (1990). Religion and physical health: The role of personal faith and con-
    trol beliefs. In M. L. Lynn & D. O. Moberg (Eds.), *Research in the social scientific study of reli-
    gion: A research annual* (Vol. 2, pp. 167–194). Greenwich, CT: JAI Press.

Malinowski, B. (1954). *Magic, science, and religion.* New York: Doubleday.

Maslow, A. H. (1954). *Motivation and personality.* New York: Harper.

Maslow, A. H. (1964). *Religions, values, and peak-experiences.* Columbus: Ohio State University
    Press.

Maslow, A. H. (1970). *Motivation and personality* (2nd ed.). New York: Harper & Row.

May, R. (1953). *Man's search for himself.* New York: Norton.

Mikulincer, M., & Shaver, P. R. (2003). The attachment behavioral system in adulthood: Activation,
    psychodynamics, and interpersonal processes. In M. P. Zanna (Ed.), *Advances in experimental
    social psychology* (Vol. 35, pp. 53–152). San Diego: Academic Press.

Osarchuk, M., & Tatz, S. J. (1973). Effect of induced fear of death on belief in afterlife. *Journal of
    Personality and Social Psychology, 27*, 256–260.

Pargament, K. I. (1990). God help me: Toward a theoretical framework of coping for the psychology
    of religion. In M. L. Lynn & D. O. Moberg (Eds.), *Research in the social scientific study of reli-
    gion: A research annual* (Vol. 2, pp. 195–224). Greenwich, CT: JAI Press.

Pargament, K. I. (1997). *The psychology of religion and coping: Theory, research, practice.* New York:
    Guilford Press.

Pargament, K. I., & Park, C. L. (1995). Merely a defense? The variety of religious means and ends.
    Journal of Social Issues, 51(2), 13–32.

Schoenrade, P. A. (1989). When I die . . . : Belief in afterlife as a response to mortality. *Personality and
    Social Psychology Bulletin, 15*, 91–100.

Solomon, S., Greenberg, J., & Pyszczynski, T. (1991). A terror-management theory of social behavior:
    The psychological functions of self-esteem and cultural worldviews. In M. P. Zanna (Ed.), *Ad-
    vances in experimental social psychology* (Vol. 24, pp. 95–159). San Diego: Academic Press.

Tajfel, H. (1982). Social psychology of intergroup relations. *Annual Review of Psychology, 33*, 1–39.

Tajfel, H., & Turner, J. C. (1986). The social identity theory of intergroup behavior. In S. Worchel &
    W. Austin (Eds.), *Psychology of intergroup relations* (p. 7–24). Chicago: Nelson Hall.

Tolstoy, L. N. (1904). *My confessions.* Boston: Dana Estes.

Tomasello, M. (1999). *The cultural origins of human cognition.* Cambridge, MA: Harvard University
    Press.

Turner, J. C. (1987). *Rediscovering the social group: A self-categorization theory.* London: Blackwell.

Chapter 10

In Search of the Moral Person

Do You Have to Feel Really Bad to Be Good?

JUNE PRICE TANGNEY
DEBRA J. MASHEK

Pride ruined the angels,
Their shame them restores.
—RALPH WALDO EMERSON, *The Sphinx*

A fundamental existential question facing humanity concerns the nature of morality. What does it mean to be a good, "moral" person? For many, the paragon of morality is embodied by the Saints. However, as is apparent throughout human history, saints are few and far between—statistical anomalies, as it were. The vast majority of us fall far short of sainthood, and are therefore, by definition, "sinners." To err is human. In the course of day-to-day life, we all occasionally choose the wrong path. Intentionally or not, we periodically do things that are wrong, destructive, or harmful to others.

Still, all sinners are not equally rotten. Among mere mortals, there clearly is a continuum of goodness. How does one evaluate a person's relative position on this continuum of moral worth? Some would argue that the primary focus should be on the severity of one's sins. From this perspective, a person who sins occasionally and confines him or herself to relatively minor transgressions (e.g., the lust in Jimmy Carter's heart) would rank higher than a person whose sins are more morally weighty (e.g., the lust in Bill Clinton's oval office). At the extreme lower end of the moral continuum, one would find perpetrators of the most egregious acts (violent rape, genocide, premeditated murder, etc.).

Another metric for measuring moral worth is the degree to which one feels moral angst. Many religions emphasize the importance of feeling bad for one's transgressions. According to some views, the strength of a person's moral fiber can be measured by the depth of their moral distress. Having sinned, "good" people feel intense remorse and regret, a grinding sense of shame, and denouncement of the self. "Bad" people just brush it off. Some might feel a twinge of remorse, but "good" people don the hair shirt—and *suffer*. In short, suffering is good. It wipes away sins and cleanses to soul.

This is not an idiosyncratic view. The value of suffering is highlighted in quotes from across the centuries:

> They merit more praise who know how to suffer misery than those who temper themselves in contentment. (Pietro Aretino, letter to the King of France, 1525)

> God will not look you over for medals, degrees or diplomas, but for scars. (Elbert Hubbard, *The Note Book*, 1927)

> Whilst shame keeps its watch, virtue is not wholly extinguished in the heart. (Edmund Burke, *Reflections on the Revolution in France*, 1790)

> Only good people feel guilt. (Dr. Laura Schlesinger, 2003)

Without question, it is often appropriate—even useful—to feel bad about our wrongdoings. In fact, we worry about people who *don't* seem to experience moral emotions such as shame and guilt in the wake of blatant sins and transgressions. Nonetheless, recent empirical research argues strongly against this notion that the better person one is, the worse one will feel. In fact, if anything, the data suggest the contrary. In the realm of moral emotions, more is not necessarily better. Suffering is not all it is cracked up to be. The most direct evidence of this kinder, gentler view of morality comes from our research on shame and guilt.

SHAME AND GUILT: MORE ANGST IS NOT NECESSARILY BETTER

Shame and guilt are members of a family of self-conscious emotions that are evoked by self-reflection and self-evaluation (Tangney & Fischer, 1995). In the face of transgression or error, the self turns toward the self, evaluating and rendering judgment in reference to standards, rules, and goals. As a result, shame and guilt are often cited as two key moral emotions because of the presumed role they play in fostering moral behavior and in inhibiting antisocial behavior and aggression. Although both shame and guilt are negative, self-relevant emotions precipitated by failures and transgressions, the two emotions are not synonymous.

Shame is qualitatively different from guilt in that shame focuses on the self, whereas guilt focuses on behavior (Lewis, 1971). Over the past decade, a plethora of empirical research has supported the notion that how people *frame* their failures and transgressions influences profoundly the subsequent emotional experience (Ferguson, Stegge, & Damhuis, 1990; Lindsay-Hartz, 1984; Lindsay-Hartz, deRivera, & Mascolo, 1995; Tangney, 1992; Tangney, Marschall, Rosenberg, Barlow, & Wagner, 1994; Tangney, 1993; Tangney, Miller, Flicker, & Barlow, 1996; Wallbott & Scherer, 1988, 1995; Wicker, Payne, & Morgan, 1983). In particular, shame ensues when people negatively evaluate the *global self*, whereas guilt arises when people negatively evaluate a *specific behavior* (Lewis, 1971).

This differential emphasis on self ("*I* did that horrible thing") versus behavior ("I *did* that horrible *thing*") leads to distinct phenomenological experiences, different patterns of motivations, and ultimately different behaviors. Shame is the more painful and distressing emotion because, in the face of failure and transgression, the entire self is viewed as deficient and imperfect. The shame experience is typified by a sense of shrinking or of "becoming small," and by feelings of worthlessness, powerlessness, and the desire to disappear. In addition, shamed people often report ruminating on how defective they must appear to other people.

In contrast to shame, guilt does not affect one's core identity. Rather, guilt is primarily concerned with a specific behavior. Because of this differential emphasis on the behavior, guilt is typically less crushing than shame. The guilt experience is colored by a sense of tension, remorse, and regret over the "bad thing done." People in the midst of a guilt experience are often preoccupied with the transgression—mentally replaying the transgression time and again, wishing they had behaved differently. Importantly, rather than encouraging escape and avoidance, guilt motivates reparative behavior—confessions, apologies, and attempts to fix the situation and undo the harm that was done.

Clearly, shame and guilt are two distinct emotions experienced by most people in the course of daily life. A multitude of factors may determine whether a person experiences shame, guilt, or both in the face of a particular transgression or error. These factors may represent aspects of the situation (e.g., the enormity of the behavior's consequences, social feedback, the victim of the transgression) as well as aspects of the person (e.g., preexisting levels of self-esteem or other genetic or socialization-influenced predispositions). Regarding dispositions, it is clear that individuals differ in their degree of proneness to these different emotions. Different people react very differently in the face of similar failures or transgressions. For example, Shame-Prone Samantha might feel intense shame on learning that her scathing e-mail about office politics was mistakenly sent to her boss. In response to such a transgression, Samantha might brand herself a worthless person and avoid her boss at all costs, possibly even missing work as a means of escaping. Guilt-Prone Guilda, on the other hand, might respond to the same transgression with profound guilt. Guilda would be inclined to reflect on the specific behavior, thinking about it over and over with a sense of remorse and regret. In turn, this focus on the behavior is likely to prompt her to make amends with her boss, possibly by writing an apology or addressing her concerns about office politics in a more open forum.

Importantly, empirical research on shame and guilt suggests strongly that these are not equally "moral" emotions. As summarized in Table 10.1, guilt seems to be the more adaptive emotion in that it benefits individuals (and their relationships) in diverse ways (Baumeister, Stillwell, & Heatherton, 1994, 1995a, 1995b; Tangney, 1991, 1995). In contrast, the shame experience appears to carry with it a number of hidden costs (Tangney, 1995; Tangney & Dearing, 2002; Tangney, Wagner, & Gramzow, 1992; Tangney, Wagner, Fletcher, & Gramzow, 1992).

The motivational, behavioral, and psychological constellations of people who are shame-prone and guilt-prone differ in at least four ways. First, as discussed earlier, guilt prompts apologies and reparation, whereas shame prompts denial and escape. Second, guilt-prone people tend to be empathic individuals, whereas shame-prone people seem to be oblivious to the emotional experiences of others. This link between guilt proneness and empathy (and the inverse association between shame proneness and empathy) has been replicated across studies of children, college students, and adults (Leith & Baumeister, 1998; Tangney, 1991, 1994, 1995; Tangney, Wagner, Burggraf, Gramzow, & Fletcher, 1991; Tangney, Wagner, & Barlow, 2004). Third, shame-prone and guilt-prone people experience and respond differently to feelings of anger and hostility. Compared to guilt-prone individuals, shame-prone people are both more inclined to experience feelings of anger and hostility *and* more apt to manage their anger in a destructive fashion (Tangney et al., 1992; Tangney, 1994, 1995; Tangney et al., 1991; Tangney, Wagner, Barlow, Marschall, & Gramzow, 1996). In particular, shame-prone individuals are inclined to blame others and engage in a

TABLE 10.1. Comparison of Correlates with Shame versus Guilt

Attribute	Shame	Guilt
Behavioral and motivational responses	Deny, hide, and escape from the situation Defensive responses Distancing and separation	Repair the damage done Constructive responses
Empathy	Inversely associated with empathy	Positively associated with empathy
Anger	Prone to anger and hostility Maladaptive and nonconstructive responses to anger Engage in aggressive behavior in romantic relationships	Constructive approaches to handling anger Better able to elicit conciliatory behavior from romantic partners
Psychological distress	Depression Anxiety Obsessive patterns of thought Paranoid ideation Disordered eating Low self-esteem	Unrelated Unrelated Unrelated Unrelated Unrelated Unrelated

broad range of aggressive behaviors. Fourth, and finally, the empirical data clearly indicate that whereas shame is positively associated with distressing psychological symptoms (e.g., depression, anxiety, eating disorder symptoms, subclinical psychopathy, narcissism, and low self-esteem), guilt is simply not related to these same symptoms (Allan, Gilbert, & Goss, 1994; Brodie, 1995; Gramzow & Tangney, 1992; Harder, 1995; Harder, Cutler, & Rockart, 1992; Harder & Lewis, 1987; Hoblitzelle, 1987; Sanftner, Barlow, Marschall, & Tangney, 1995; Tangney, 1993; Tangney, Burggraf, & Wagner, 1995; Tangney & Dearing, 2002; Tangney et al., 1991; Tangney, Wagner, & Gramzow, 1992).

DO FEELINGS OF SHAME AND GUILT KEEP US "ON THE STRAIGHT AND NARROW"?

At the heart of this chapter is a fundamental question: Do you have to feel bad to be a good person? A common belief is that because they are painful emotions, feelings of shame and guilt keep people "on the straight and narrow," decreasing the likelihood of transgression and impropriety (Barrett, 1995; Ferguson & Stegge, 1995; Zahn-Waxler & Robinson, 1995). Surprisingly little research has directly evaluated this assumption.

Compared to their less guilt-prone peers, guilt-prone individuals were more likely to endorse such items from the Conventional Morality Scale (Tooke & Ickes, 1988) as "I would not steal something I needed, even if I were sure I could get away with it," "I will not take advantage of other people, even when it's clear that they are trying to take advantage of me," and "Morality and ethics don't really concern me" (reversed) (Tangney, 1994). In other words, guilt emerged as the "good" moral emotion. In contrast, there was no evidence for the "moral," self-regulatory functions of shame.

Research on aggression, delinquency, and substance abuse further supports the idea that shame and guilt are distinctively related to moral behavior. Across the lifespan, aggression and delinquency are positively related to shame proneness (Ferguson, Stegge, Miller, & Olsen, 1999; Tangney, Wagner, et al., 1996; Tibbetts, 1997). Prospectively, Stuewig and McCloskey (2002) found that shame-prone teen delinquents were more likely than non–shame-prone teen delinquents to be subsequently arrested for a violent act according to juvenile court records. Similarly, shame proneness is also linked to substance use and abuse (Tangney & Dearing, 2002; Meehan et al., 1996; O'Connor, Berry, Inaba, Weiss, & Morrison, 1994). In contrast, guilt proneness has been negatively related to alcohol and drug problems (Tangney & Dearing, 2002) and negatively related (Merisca & Bybee, 1994; Stuewig & McCloskey, 2002; Tangney, Wagner, et al., 1996), or inconsistently related (Ferguson et al., 1999), to aggression and delinquency.

The most direct evidence linking moral emotions with moral behavior comes from our large-scale, ongoing longitudinal family study of moral emotions. In this prospective study of 380 children, moral emotional style in the fifth grade predicted critical "bottom-line" behaviors in young adulthood, including substance use, risky sexual behavior, involvement with the criminal justice system, and suicide attempts. Specifically, shame proneness in the 5th grade predicted risky behaviors later in life such as dangerous driving, trying alcohol earlier in life, using drugs, attempting suicide, and practicing not-so-safe sex. In contrast, the guilt-prone 5th-graders tried alcohol later in life, were less likely to attempt suicide, less likely to use marijuana as well as "hard core" drugs such as heroin and hallucinogens, and were less likely to drive under the influence. Moreover, guilt-prone children were, in adolescence, less likely to be arrested and convicted; they had fewer sexual partners and were more likely to practice "safe sex."

In sum, there is virtually no direct evidence supporting the presumed adaptive function of shame, the more painful of the self-conscious moral emotions. Rather, recent research has linked shame with a range of illegal, risky, or otherwise problematic behaviors. In contrast, the capacity for guilt about specific behaviors seems to foster a lifelong pattern of generally following a moral path, motivating individuals to accept responsibility and take reparative action in the wake of the inevitable if only occasional failure or transgression. Moreover, there does not appear to be a substantial personal cost for the interpersonally beneficial effects of guilt. Guilt is the moral emotion of choice at multiple levels—when considering the individual, relationships, and society at large.

In other words, in the realm of moral emotions, an ounce of angst seems sufficient. In many instances, global, overwhelming feelings of shame represent a case of overkill—the equivalent of using a sledgehammer where a tack hammer would do. The result is not a job done well but a self with a gaping hole.

MORE EVIDENCE THAT YOU DON'T HAVE TO FEEL REALLY BAD TO BE GOOD

Several other lines of research similarly hint at the notion that feeling bad—especially feeling *very* bad—is not necessarily good for one's character, for one's behavior, nor for the welfare of society. In the areas of empathy and humility, more pain does not necessarily a better person make.

Empathy is generally regarded as a positive, relationship-enhancing process—a critical element, for example, in happy marriages, successful parenting, and effective therapy. Researchers interested in empathy have found it useful to distinguish between true other-oriented empathy versus "self-oriented" personal distress (Batson, 1990; Batson & Coke, 1981; Davis, 1983; Fultz, Batson, Fortenbach, McCarthy, & Varney, 1986). In the case of true "other-oriented" empathic responses, the observer takes another person's perspective, vicariously experiencing feelings similar to those of the other (e.g., sympathy and concern). All told, the focus of truly empathic individuals remains on the experiences and needs of the other person. In contrast, self-oriented personal distress involves an initial intense empathic reaction to another person's distress, which is then followed by "egoistic drift" to the feelings, needs, and experiences of the *empathizer* (Hoffman, 1984). Several empirical studies have shown that other-oriented empathic concern prompts altruistic helping behavior, whereas "self-oriented" personal distress is unrelated to altruism (Batson et al., 1988). Personal distress appears to interfere with prosocial behaviors in both children (Eisenberg et al., 1993; Eisenberg et al., 1990) and adolescents (Estrada, 1995). Similarly, among romantic couples, personal distress has been associated with negative interpersonal behaviors (Davis & Oathout, 1987). In short, one can be too "empathic"—one can feel too much of another person's pain, ultimately to the detriment of all involved.

Current conceptions of humility further underscore that one does not necessarily have to feel bad to be good (Tangney, 2002). Although humility is often equated with low self-regard, philosophers, theologians, sociologists, and psychologists have a different—and much richer—notion of this construct. Specifically, the key elements of true humility seem to include an accurate assessment of one's abilities and achievements, an ability to acknowledge one's mistakes and limitations, a corresponding openness to new ideas and advice, and a relatively low self-focus, a "forgetting of the self." Emmons (1998) clearly articulated this alternative view of humility by stating:

> Although humility is often equated in people's minds with low self-regard and tends to activate images of a stooped-shouldered, self-deprecating, weak-willed soul only too willing to yield to the wishes of others, in reality humility is the antithesis of this caricature. To be humble is not to have a low opinion of oneself, it is to have an accurate opinion of oneself. It is the ability to keep one's talents and accomplishments in perspective (Richards, 1992), to have a sense of self-acceptance, an understanding of one's imperfections, and to be free from arrogance and low self-esteem (Clark, 1992). (p. 33).

Paradoxically, the excessively self-deprecating person actually lacks humility. This lack of humility is especially apparent when one considers the degree of self-focus typically involved in self-denouncements—the person remains at the center of attention, with the self as the focus of consideration and evaluation. For example, consider the person who protests, "These cookies? Oh, I just whipped up a batch last night. *I'm* really no good at baking; *I* simply can't get the proportions correct. *I* actually failed my home-ec class! *I* hope they don't make anyone sick!" These apparently humble protests divulge a marked self-focus, a decidedly uncharacteristic feature of true humility.

Feeling bad—in this case, self-debasement—does not bring us closer to God *or* Good. Rather, true humility shifts our attention outward, opening our eyes to the beauty and potential in those around us.

WHY DOESN'T SUFFERING RESULT IN MORAL SUPERIORITY?

Although a good deal of social lore emphasizes the value of moral suffering, several psychological theories and associated findings illuminate *why* feeling bad does not necessarily lead people to act in a more moral direction. Perhaps most relevant is Berkowitz's (1989) reformulated frustration–aggression hypothesis. Early theories of aggression (Dollard, Doob,

Miller, Mowrer, & Sears, 1939) emphasized the importance of frustration of goals as a critical precursor of anger and aggressive behavior. In his landmark theoretical reformulation, Berkowitz (1989) argued persuasively that it is negative affect, more generally, that leads to aggression. Frustration of goals is just one example of such negative affect. Research has shown that noxious noise, environmental heat, and physical pain, for example, similarly precipitate aggressive acts, even though no goal appears to be frustrated. Taken together, a substantial body of evidence supports Berkowitz's reformulation. Clearly, negative affect is more likely to promote hostility and harm to others, rather than the more moral path of altruistic care and concern.

Moreover, a recent review of the literature, following up on work by Peeters and Czapinski (1990), indicates that when it comes to pain, a little can go a long way. Citing evidence from diverse areas of psychological research including interpersonal relationships, child development, learning, information processing, memory, stereotyping, impression formation, and health, Baumeister, Bratslavsky, Finkenauer, and Vohs (2001) conclude that bad is stronger than good. "In everyday life, bad events have stronger and more lasting consequences than comparable good events" (p. 355). Baumeister et al. argue that this principle is universal, evident in both human and non-human animals, and observed across a wide range of cognitive, emotional, and social domains. In the realm of moral emotion, a little "bad" may be sufficient to keep us on the straight and narrow, whereas too much "bad" may be counterproductive. Across numerous studies, people report that experiences of shame (about the self) are much more painful than experiences of guilt (about a specific behavior) (Lewis, 1971; Tangney, 1992; Tangney, Miller, et al., 1996; Wicker et al., 1983). Given that bad is stronger than good, it follows that the relatively less painful nature of guilt is sufficient in most instances to steer us in a moral direction. By the same token, it is not surprising that the much more painful, overwhelming experience of shame often backfires in the moral sense, leading to denial, distancing, and sometimes downright aggressive behavior.

In the context of child discipline, more is not necessarily better. Good parents intuitively know this, and developmental psychologists have empirically demonstrated that moderately negative feedback and consequences are more effective than severe punishment. When children transgress, some degree of induced negative emotion may be necessary to cause them to sit up and take notice that they have transgressed, to reflect on their behavior and its consequences, and to make positive changes for the future. In contrast, punishment that is too much or too severe often becomes counterproductive, leaving the child angry and disregulated—too overwhelmed to process the event and take reparative action (Grusec & Goodnow, 1994). The paradoxical result can be a less moral child.

BEYOND INTENSITY OF AFFECT

Thus far, we have been focusing on intensity of negative affect as a problematic feature of shame. But shame is not simply a more negative version of guilt. A key difference is the focus on self versus behavior, which we believe is at the root of many of the costs of shame, including intense negative affect. Compared to negative evaluation of one's behavior, negative evaluation of the self is (1) more painful, (2) more difficult to resolve (repair of the self is much more difficult than repair of a behavior), and therefore (3) more difficult to regulate. Moreover, feelings of shame are apt to impair or inhibit the self (Lewis, 1971; Lindsay-Hartz, 1984; Tangney & Dearing, 2002), further compounding the difficulties inherent in "down-regulating" shame (Kuhl, 2000; Kuhl & Koole, Chapter 26, this volume).

In fact, research has shown that adults rate personal shame experiences as less controllable than personal guilt experiences (Tangney, 1993). In short, some of the documented "effects" of shame may be due more specifically to frustrated efforts to down regulate such painful emotion (e.g., denial, externalization of blame, drug and alcohol abuse, and suicide).

SUMMARY AND CONCLUSIONS

In sum, in the realm of moral emotions—more is not necessarily better. Moderately painful feelings of guilt about specific behaviors motivate people to behave in a moral, caring, socially responsible manner. In contrast, intensely painful feelings of shame do *not* appear to steer people in a constructive, moral direction. Painful feelings of shame about the self cut to our core, exacting a heavy "penance" perhaps. But rather than motivating reparative action, shame often motivates denial, defensiveness, anger, and aggression. Neither is intense pain useful in the context of moral emotions or virtues, such as empathy and humility. These findings are consistent with current social psychological theory emphasizing the power of bad versus good, and the link between negative affect and aggression. Taken together, theory and research seriously challenge the notion that suffering is a useful barometer of moral worth. Instead, the psychological literature underscores that feeling good is not incompatible with being good. Some guilt now and then is appropriate and useful to help keep us on the moral path and, more important, to motivate us to correct and repair. But, ultimately, people need to be able to get on with the business of life, taking care of one another rather than condemning the self.

REFERENCES

Allan, S., Gilbert, P., & Goss, K. (1994). An exploration of shame measures II: Psychopathology. *Personality and Individual Differences, 17*, 719–722.

Barrett, K. C. (1995). A functionalist approach to shame and guilt. In J. P. Tangney & K. W. Fischer (Eds.), *Self-conscious emotions: The psychology of shame, guilt, embarrassment, and pride* (pp. 25–63). New York: Guilford Press.

Batson, C. D. (1990). How social an animal? The human capacity for caring. *American Psychologist, 45*, 336–346.

Batson, C. D., & Coke, J. S. (1981). Empathy: A source of altruistic motivation for helping? In J. P. Rushton & R. M. Sorrentino (Eds.), *Altruism and helping behavior: Social, personality, and developmental perspectives* (pp. 167–187). Hillsdale, NJ: Erlbaum.

Batson, C. D., Dyck, J. L., Brandt, J. R., Batson, J. G., Powell, A. L., McMaster, M. R., et al. (1988). Five studies testing two new egoistic alternatives to the empathy-altruism hypothesis. *Journal of Personality and Social Psychology, 55*, 52–77.

Baumeister, R. F., Bratslavsky, E., Finkenauer, C., & Vohs, K. D. (2001) Bad is stronger than good. *Review of General Psychology, 5*, 323–370.

Baumeister, R. F., Stillwell, A. M., & Heatherton, T. F. (1994). Guilt: An interpersonal approach. *Psychological Bulletin, 115*, 243–267.

Baumeister, R. F., Stillwell, A. M., & Heatherton, T. F. (1995a). Interpersonal aspects of guilt: Evidence from narrative studies. In J. P. Tangney & K. W. Fischer (Eds.), *Self-conscious emotions: The psychology of shame, guilt, embarrassment, and pride* (pp. 255–273). New York: Guilford Press.

Baumeister, R. F., Stillwell, A. M., & Heatherton, T. F. (1995b). Personal narratives about guilt: Role in action control and interpersonal relationships. *Basic and Applied Social Psychology, 17*, 173–198.

Berkowitz, L. (1989). Frustration-aggression hypothesis: Examination and reformulation. *Psychological Bulletin, 106,* 59–73.

Brodie, P. (1995). *How sociopaths love: Sociopathy and interpersonal relationships.* Unpublished doctoral dissertation, George Mason University, Fairfax VA.

Clark, A. T. (1992). Humility. In D. H. Ludlow (Ed.), *Encyclopedia of Mormonism* (pp. 663–664). New York: Macmillan.

Davis, M. H. (1983). Measuring individual differences in empathy: Evidence for a multidimensional approach. *Journal of Personality and Social Psychology, 44,* 113–126.

Davis, M. H., & Oathout, H. A. (1987). Maintenance of satisfaction in romantic relationships: Empathy and relational competence. *Journal of Personality and Social Psychology, 53,* 397–410.

Dollard, J., Doob, L. W., Miller, N. E., Mowrer, O. H., & Sears, R. R. (1939). *Frustration and aggression.* New Haven: Yale University Press.

Eisenberg, N., Fabes, R. A., Carlo, G., Speer, A. L., Switzer, G., Karbon, M., et al. (1993). The relations of empathy-related emotions and maternal practices to children's comforting behavior. *Journal of Experimental Child Psychology, 55,* 131–150.

Eisenberg, N., Fabes, R. A., Miller, P. A., Shell, R., Shea, C., & Mayplumlee, T. (1990). Pre-schoolers' vicarious emotional responding and their situational and dispositional prosocial behavior. *Merrill–Palmer Quarterly, 36,* 507–529.

Emerson, R. W. (1841). *The sphinx.* Retrieved January 23, 2004, from: *http://www.americanpoems.com/poets/emerson/thesphinx.html.*

Emmons, R. A. (1998). *The psychology of ultimate concern: Personality, spirituality, and intelligence.* Unpublished manuscript, University of California at Davis.

Estrada, P. (1995). Adolescents' self-reports of prosocial responses to friends and acquaintances: The role of sympathy-related cognitive, affective, and motivational processes. *Journal of Research on Adolescence, 5,* 173–200.

Ferguson, T. J., & Stegge, H. (1995). Emotional states and traits in children: The case of guilt and shame. In J. P. Tangney & K. W. Fischer (Eds.), *Self-conscious emotions: The psychology of shame, guilt, embarrassment, and pride* (pp. 174–197). New York: Guilford Press.

Ferguson, T. J., Stegge, H., & Damhuis, I. (1990). Guilt and shame experiences in elementary school-age children. In R. J. Takens (Ed.), *European perspectives in psychology* (Vol. 1, pp. 195–218). New York: Wiley.

Ferguson, T. J., Stegge, H., Miller, E. R., & Olsen, M. E. (1999). Guilt, shame, and symptoms in children. *Developmental Psychology, 35,* 347–357.

Fultz, J., Batson, C. D., Fortenbach, V. A., McCarthy, P. M., & Varney, L. L. (1986). Social evaluation and the empathy altruism hypothesis. *Journal of Personality and Social Psychology, 50,* 761–769.

Gramzow, R., & Tangney, J. P. (1992). Proneness to shame and the narcissistic personality. *Personality and Social Psychology Bulletin, 18,* 369–376.

Grusec, J. E., & Goodnow, J. (1994). Impact of parental discipline methods on the child's internalization of values: A reconceptualization of current points of view. *Developmental Psychology, 30,* 4–19.

Harder, D. W. (1995). Shame and guilt assessment, and relationships of shame- and guilt-proneness to psychopathology. In J. P. Tangney & K. W. Fischer (Eds.), *Self-conscious emotions: The psychology of shame, guilt, embarrassment, and pride* (pp. 368–392). New York: Guilford Press.

Harder, D. W., Cutler, L., & Rockart, L. (1992). Assessment of shame and guilt and their relationship to psychopathology. *Journal of Personality Assessment, 59,* 584–604.

Harder, D. W., & Lewis, S. J. (1987). The assessment of shame and guilt. In J. N. Butcher & C. D. Spielberger (Eds.), *Advances in personality assessment* (Vol. 6, pp. 89–114). Hillsdale, NJ: Erlbaum.

Hoblitzelle, W. (1987). Attempts to measure and differentiate shame and guilt: The relation between shame and depression. In H. B. Lewis (Ed.), *The role of shame in symptom formation* (pp. 207–235). Hillsdale, NJ: Erlbaum.

Hoffman, M. L. (1984). Interaction of affect and cognition in empathy. In C. E. Izard, J. Kagan, & R. Zajonc (Eds.), *Emotion, cognition, and behavior* (pp. 103–131). Cambridge, UK: Cambridge University Press.

Hubbard, E. (1927). *The note book of Elbert Hubbard: Mottoes, epigrams, short essays, passages, orphic sayings and preachments.* New York: Wm. H. Wise.

Kuhl, J. (2000). A functional-design approach to motivation and volition: The dynamics of personality systems interactions. In M. Boekaerts, P. R. Pintrich & M. Zeidner (Eds.), *Self-regulation: Directions and challenges for future research* (pp. 111–169). New York: Academic Press.

Leith, K. P., & Baumeister, R. F. (1998). Empathy, shame, guilt, and narratives of interpersonal conflicts: Guilt-prone people are better at perspective taking. *Journal of Personality, 66,* 1–37.

Lewis, H. B. (1971). *Shame and guilt in neurosis.* New York: International Universities Press.

Lindsay-Hartz, J. (1984). Contrasting experiences of shame and guilt. *American Behavioral Scientist, 27,* 689–704.

Lindsay-Hartz, J., deRivera, J., & Mascolo, M. (1995). Differentiating shame and guilt and their effects on motivation. In J. P. Tangney & K. W. Fischer (Eds.), *Self-conscious emotions: Shame, guilt, embarrassment, and pride* (pp. 274–300). New York: Guilford Press.

Meehan, M. A., O'Connor, L. E., Berry, J. W., Weiss, J., Morrison, A., & Acampora, A. (1996). Guilt, shame, and depression in clients in recovery from addiction. *Journal of Psychoactive Drugs, 28,* 125–134.

Merisca, R., & Bybee, J. S., (1994, April). *Guilt, not moral reasoning, relates to volunteerism, prosocial behavior, lowered aggressiveness, and eschewal of racism.* Poster presented at the annual meeting of the Eastern Psychological Association, Providence, RI.

O'Connor, L. E., Berry, J. W., Inaba, D., Weiss, J., & Morrison, A. (1994). Shame, guilt, and depression in men and women in recovery from addiction. *Journal of Substance Abuse Treatment, 11,* 503–510.

Peeters, G., & Czapinski, J. (1990). Positive-negative asymmetry in evaluations: The distinction between affective and informational negativity effects. In W. Stroebe & M. Hewstone (Eds.), *European review of social psychology* (Vol. 1, pp. 33–60). Chichester: Wiley.

Richards, N. (1992). *Humility.* Philadelphia: Temple University Press.

Sanftner, J. L., Barlow, D. H., Marschall, D. E., & Tangney, J. P. (1995). The relation of shame and guilt to eating disorders symptomotology. *Journal of Social and Clinical Psychology, 14,* 315–324.

Schlesinger, L. (2003). *Moral and inspirational quotes, sayings, and observations.* Retrieved January 23, 2004, from: *http://www.geocities.com/Hollywood/Set/8534/quotes.html.*

Stuewig, J., & McCloskey, L. (2002). *Do shame and guilt predict antisocial behavior in late adolescence? Findings from a prospective study.* Paper presented at the meeting of the American Society of Criminology, Chicago.

Tangney, J. P. (1991). Moral affect: The good, the bad, and the ugly. *Journal of Personality and Social Psychology, 61,* 598–607.

Tangney, J. P. (1992). Situational determinants of shame and guilt in young adulthood. *Personality and Social Psychology Bulletin, 18,* 199–206.

Tangney, J. P. (1993). Shame and guilt. In C. G. Costello (Ed.), *Symptoms of depression* (pp. 161–180). New York: Wiley.

Tangney, J. P. (1994). The mixed legacy of the super-ego: Adaptive and maladaptive aspects of shame and guilt. In J. M. Masling, & R. F. Bornstein, (Eds.), *Empirical perspectives on object relations theory* (pp. 1–28). Washington, DC: American Psychological Association.

Tangney, J. P. (1995). Shame and guilt in interpersonal relationships. In J. P. Tangney & K. W. Fischer (Eds.), *Self-conscious emotions: The psychology of shame, guilt, embarrassment, and pride* (pp. 114–139). New York: Guilford Press.

Tangney, J. P. (2002). Humility. In C. R. Snyder & S. J. Lopez (Eds), *The handbook of positive psychology* (pp. 411–419). New York: Oxford University Press.

Tangney, J. P., Burggraf, S. A., & Wagner, P. E. (1995). Shame-proneness, guilt-proneness, and psychological symptoms. In J. P. Tangney & K. W. Fischer (Eds.), *Self-conscious emotions: The psychology of shame, guilt, embarrassment, and pride* (pp. 343–367). New York: Guilford Press.

Tangney, J. P., & Dearing, R. (2002). *Shame and guilt.* New York: Guilford Press.

Tangney, J. P., & Fischer, K. W. (Eds.). (1995). *Self-conscious emotions: The psychology of shame, guilt, embarrassment, and pride.* New York: Guilford Press.

Tangney, J. P., Marschall, D. E., Rosenberg, K., Barlow, D. H., & Wagner, P. E. (1994). *Children's and adults' autobiographical accounts of shame, guilt and pride experiences: An analysis of situational determinants and interpersonal concerns*. Manuscript under review.

Tangney, J. P., Miller, R. S., Flicker, L., & Barlow, D. H. (1996). Are shame, guilt and embarrassment distinct emotions? *Journal of Personality and Social Psychology, 70*, 1256–1269.

Tangney, J. P., Wagner, P. E., & Barlow, D. H. (2004). *The relation of shame and guilt to empathy: An intergenerational study*. Unpublished data.

Tangney, J. P., Wagner, P. E., Barlow, D. H., Marschall, D. E., & Gramzow, R. (1996). The relation of shame and guilt to constructive vs. destructive responses to anger across the lifespan. *Journal of Personality and Social Psychology, 70*, 797–809.

Tangney, J. P., Wagner, P. E., Burggraf, S. A., Gramzow, R., & Fletcher, C. (1991, June). *Children's shame-proneness, but not guilt-proneness, is related to emotional and behavioral maladjustment*. Poster presented at the meetings of the American Psychological Society, Washington DC.

Tangney, J. P., Wagner, P. E., Fletcher, C., & Gramzow, R. (1992). Shamed into anger? The relation of shame and guilt to anger and self-reported aggression. *Journal of Personality and Social Psychology, 62*, 669–675.

Tangney, J. P., Wagner, P. E., & Gramzow, R. (1992). Proneness to shame, proneness to guilt, and psychopathology. *Journal of Abnormal Psychology, 103*, 469–478.

Tibbetts, S. G. (1997). Shame and rational choice in offending decisions. *Criminal Justice and Behavior, 24*, 234–255.

Tooke, W. S., & Ickes, W. (1988). A measure of adherence to conventional morality. *Journal of Social and Clinical Psychology, 6*, 310–334.

Wallbott, H. G., & Scherer, K. R. (1988). How universal and specific is emotional experience? Evidence from 27 countries and five continents. In K. R. Scherer (Ed.), *Facets of emotion: Recent research* (pp. 31–56). Hillsdale, NJ: Erlbaum.

Wallbott, H. G., & Scherer, K. R. (1995). Cultural determinants in experiencing shame and guilt. In J. P. Tangney & K. W. Fischer (Eds.), *Self-conscious emotions: The psychology of shame, guilt, embarrassment, and pride* (pp. 465–487). New York: Guilford Press.

Wicker, F. W., Payne, G. C., & Morgan, R. D. (1983). Participant descriptions of guilt and shame. *Motivation and Emotion, 7*, 25–39.

Zahn-Waxler, C., & Robinson, J. (1995). Empathy and guilt: Early origins of feelings of responsibility. In J. P. Tangney & K. W. Fischer (Eds.), *Self-conscious emotions: The psychology of shame, guilt, embarrassment, and pride* (pp. 143–173). New York: Guilford Press.

Chapter 11

An Existentialist Approach to the Social Psychology of Fairness

The Influence of Mortality and Uncertainty Salience on Reactions to Fair and Unfair Events

KEES VAN DEN BOS

Sex, Drank, en Dood, deze drie, maar de meeste van deze is de dood. [Sex, Booze, and Death, this three, but of this three, death is the greatest.]
—GERARD REVE, *In Gesprek: Interviews* (1983, pp. 124–125)

This quote (inspired by the Bible's 1st Corinthians, Chapter 13) highlights the key role that death plays in the work by Gerard Reve, my favorite Dutch novelist (a Dutch mixture, one could say, of Arthur Miller, Charles Bukowski, and Ernest Hemingway). The work by this author has not only given me huge literary enjoyment but also taught me a lesson or two about mankind, the most important being the fascinating role that death plays in human life and the intriguing albeit sometimes strange way with which people may deal with this issue. Other literary work that I read as an adolescent and as a student, such as the novels by Louis-Ferdinand Céline, as well as some important experiences in my private life, also convinced me of the importance of the darker side of humankind in general and death in particular. As a student I was excited about social psychology but sometimes dissatisfied with the fact that social psychology seemed to neglect these important topics. It was as if there was a discrepancy between issues that social psychologists studied and concepts that were very important in the arts and—even more important of course—in real life.

I was thrilled, therefore, when I read about the pioneering work in social psychology by Jeff Greenberg, Tom Pyszczynski, and Sheldon Solomon and their colleagues on terror management theory (e.g., Greenberg, Solomon, & Pyszczynski, 1997; Pyszczynski, Greenberg, & Solomon, 1999; Solomon, Greenberg, & Pyszczynski, 1991). Here there was this theoretical framework that explicitly focused on these important issues in human existence, and, what is more, here there were several ingenious experiments that thoroughly tested several of the predictions derived from the framework's theorizing. All this I thought was very exciting. Furthermore, I could see interesting parallels with my own work on the social psychology of fairness and justice judgments. For all these reasons, I started talking about terror management with my colleagues at my department, defended the terror management framework against skeptics, and began conducting terror management studies myself. In this chapter I would like to discuss these experiments and the studies and insights that followed from it. The issues I focus on in this research program are all nicely illustrated in the following quote by Erich Fromm:

> The state of anxiety, the feeling of powerlessness and insignificance, and especially the doubt concerning one's future after *death*, represent a state of mind which is practically unbearable for anybody. Almost no one stricken with this fear would be able to relax, enjoy life, and be indifferent as to what happened afterwards. One possible way to escape this unbearable state of *uncertainty* and the paralyzing feeling of one's own insignificance is the very trait which became so prominent in Calvinism: the development of a frantic activity and a striving to do something. . . . In Calvinism this meaning of effort was part of the religious doctrine. Originally it referred essentially to *moral* effort. (1942/2002, pp. 78–80, emphasis added)

This quotation illustrates the core of what I concentrate on in this chapter: death, uncertainty, and fairness concerns (and related concepts such as justice, morality, and ethics). As it turned out, combining the insights from the first terror management experiments I conducted with insights from my earlier work (e.g., Van den Bos, Lind, Vermunt, & Wilke, 1997; Van den Bos, Wilke, & Lind, 1998) and other articles (esp. Martin, 1999; McGregor, Zanna, Holmes, & Spencer, 2001) led me to propose that important (albeit perhaps not all) elements of terror management theory and at least some mortality salience effects seemed to fit into a broader framework of uncertainty management.

I would like to repeat here that I was and still am very enthusiastic about terror management theory and that I do think that the predictions that follow from the theory are accurate, insightful, and among the best in modern social psychology. Therefore, the purpose of the research program I discuss here is certainly not to falsify or attack terror management theory. Rather the idea is to take the framework very seriously and see how and to what extent we can build on and extend the theory to understand other issues previously not explored by the theory, and how we can use the experimental paradigms developed within the terror management domain to study these new issues.

The research program I review here is clearly work in progress. I think it is important, therefore, to prevent jumping to theoretical conclusions and that first the studies my colleagues and I conducted should be thoroughly discussed. After this overview, I would like to draw conclusions from the research findings that were reviewed and discuss the implications for the social psychology of terror and uncertainty management. Before I do this it is important to briefly introduce the social psychology of fairness judgments.

FAIRNESS

For a long time scientists from various disciplines have been intrigued by fairness and related concepts, such as justice, morality, and ethics. Social psychologists have shown convincingly that when people feel they have experienced fair or unfair events this may strongly affect their subsequent reactions (see, e.g., Brockner & Wiesenfeld, 1996; Folger & Cropanzano, 1998; Lind & Tyler, 1988; Tyler & Lind, 1992; Van den Bos & Lind, 2002). For instance, it has been reported that the belief that one has been fairly treated by judges, the police, organizational managers, or other social authorities enhances acceptance of legal decisions, obedience to laws, and evaluations of public policies, whereas the belief that one has been treated in an unfair way has been found to prompt antisocial behavior, recidivism among spouse abuse defendants, and the initiation of lawsuits (Lind & Van den Bos, 2002). These empirical investigations have been very important because, as a result, social psychologists know quite a lot about what the effects of fair and unfair treatment are. However, these advances may have been achieved at the expense of deeper insights into what may be thought of as one of the most fundamental topics in the psychology of social justice: why fairness matters so much to people (Van den Bos & Lind, 2002). Because fairness judgments influence so many important attitudes and behaviors, studying why fairness matters is a crucial issue for understanding how humans think, feel, and behave in their social environments. In the research program I discuss here, the psychology of why fairness is important is the primary focus of attention. Specifically, findings of experiments are presented in which it is manipulated whether people experience fair or unfair events and in which the antecedents of people's reactions to these fair and unfair events are assessed. The first set of studies that I discuss here explored whether insights and manipulations from terror management theory could successfully be used to study the social psychology of why fairness matters to people.

MORTALITY SALIENCE AND FAIRNESS

According to terror management theory (e.g., Greenberg et al., 1997; Pyszczynski et al., 1999; Solomon et al., 1991), the fear of death is rooted in an instinct for self-preservation that humans share with other species. Although human beings share this instinct with other species, only humans are aware that death is inevitable. This combination of an instinctive drive for self-preservation with an awareness of the inevitability of death creates the potential for paralyzing terror. Terror management theory posits that this potential for terror is managed by a cultural anxiety buffer, a social psychological structure consisting of things like one's worldview and self-esteem. To the extent that this buffer provides protection against death concerns, reminding individuals of their death should increase their need for that buffer. Thus, reminders of death should increase the need for the protection provided by the buffer and therefore lead to strong negative evaluations of people whose behaviors and beliefs threaten on that worldview and lead to strong positive evaluations of those whose behaviors and beliefs uphold or provide an opportunity to reconstruct the worldview. (For more extensive introductions to terror management theory, see, e.g., Greenberg et al., 1997; Pyszczynski et al., 1999; Solomon et al., 1991.)

On the basis of terror management theory, Van den Bos and Miedema (2000) argued that participants who are asked to think about their mortality would react more negatively toward violation of norms and more positively toward things that uphold or bolster cultural norms and values. It is reasonable to assume that most people judge unfair events to be in violation with cultural norms and values and think of fair events as being in correspondence with norms and values of good behavior and conduct (Lind & Tyler, 1988). Van den Bos and Miedema, therefore, predicted that participants would show stronger reactions toward fairness manipulations in mortality salient conditions than in mortality nonsalient conditions.

Van den Bos and Miedema (2000) describe three experiments, but here I discuss only the first. In this experiment, we used an experimental paradigm that was similar to previous fairness experiments (e.g., Van den Bos et al., 1997, 1998). In the first part of the instructions, participants were informed that they would participate in the study with another person. The participants were told that after the work round the experimenter would divide some lottery tickets between them and the other participant. After the work round, participants were told how many tasks they had completed in the work round, and—to ensure that participants compared themselves to the other participant—the participants were told that the other participant had completed an equivalent number of tasks.

After this, the participants were told that before the experimenter divided the lottery tickets between them and the other participant, they would be asked to answer some questions supposedly unrelated to the experiment, and that after they had completed these questions, the experiment would continue. Mortality salience was then manipulated. As in most previous terror management studies, the mortality salient condition was induced by having participants respond to two open-ended questions concerning their thoughts and feelings about their death: (1) "Please briefly describe the emotions that the thought of your death arouses in you" and (2) "Please write down, as specifically as you can, what you think physically will happen to you as you die." Participants in the mortality nonsalient condition were not asked to write something down; a manipulation which is in correspondence with previous terror management studies (e.g., Greenberg et al., 1990, Study 1; Rosenblatt, Greenberg, Solomon, Pyszczynski, & Lyon, 1989, Studies 1–5).

After all participants had completed the Positive and Negative Affect Schedule (PANAS; Watson, Clark, & Tellegen, 1988), on which they reported on 20 items how they felt at the moment, participants were told that by pushing the return button on the keyboard the study would continue. Following previous terror management studies (see Greenberg et al., 1997; Solomon et al., 1991), the PANAS was included in all the studies discussed in this chapter as a filler task and to determine whether the salience manipulations engendered positive and negative affect (which they generally did not). This indicates that affective states as a result of the salience manipulations cannot explain the research findings discussed here.

The fairness manipulation was then induced. In the fair condition, the experimenter asked participants to type in their opinions about the percentage of tickets that they should receive relative to the other participant. Participants in the unfair condition were informed that they would not be asked to type such an opinion. Dependent variables and manipulation checks were then assessed. The main dependent variables were participants' positive affective reactions toward the way they were treated (i.e., how happy, content, and satisfied participants felt about the way they were treated).

As expected, a significant interaction between mortality salience and the fairness manipulation was found. In the mortality nonsalient condition, participants' affective reactions were significantly more positive following an opportunity to voice their opinion than following no such opportunity, but this fair process effect was stronger in the mortality salient condition. Findings of Experiments 2 and 3 of Van den Bos and Miedema (2000) replicated and extended these results (using other fairness manipulations and other ratings of affect). Thus, as predicted, when people have been thinking about their own mortality they react more strongly to fairness of treatment than when they have not been thinking about this subject.

Thus, in line with predictions derived from terror management theory, these research findings show that mortality salience leads people to react more negatively toward violation and more positively toward things that uphold or bolster their cultural norms and values. Moreover, this work extends previous work on terror management theory, in that it used that theoretical framework to explicitly investigate why fairness—one of the most important social norms and values (Folger, 1984; Folger & Cropanzano, 1998; Tyler & Smith, 1998)—matters to people. By showing effects of mortality salience on people's reactions to perceived procedural fairness in ways that were predicted on the basis of terror management theory, the findings provided important new insights into the antecedents of reactions to fair and unfair events: Fairness matters more when mortality has been made salient.

UNCERTAINTY SALIENCE AND FAIRNESS

In subsequent research articles, I argued that the Van den Bos and Miedema (2000) findings fit into a line of research that shows that people pay more attention to fairness when they are uncertain about things such as authority's trustworthiness (Van den Bos et al., 1998), distributive issues (Van den Bos et al., 1997), or procedural issues (Van den Bos, 1999). For example, Van den Bos et al. (1998) argued that, because ceding authority to another person raises the possibility of exploitation and exclusion, people frequently feel uneasy about their relationship with authorities. Furthermore, these authors proposed that this implies that people want to have information about whether they can trust the authority. As a consequence, when information about whether an authority can be trusted is not available, people will rely heavily on perceived procedural fairness, yielding strong fair process effects. However, when people receive information that the authority either can or cannot be trusted, they are less in need of procedural fairness information, yielding less strong fair process effects. This suggests that when people move from uncertainty to certainty, people end up needing fairness less.

Being reminded about one's mortality will lead one to be more uncertain, of course, than not being reminded about this fundamental vulnerable aspect of one's life. In fact, results collected by Martin (1999) show that asking people to think about their mortality—in the same way as we did in—leads them to be more uncertain than not asking them to think about this subject. McGregor et al. (2001) also found that mortality salience caused uncertainty-related feelings. These are important data because they suggest that an important psychological mechanism underlying mortality salience effects may be perceived uncertainty.

This position is strengthened by the results of research (Van den Bos 2001a) showing that reminding people about their own mortality does indeed make them feel uncertain about themselves and that these feelings of uncertainty explain how people react toward subsequent events. One of the Van den Bos (2001a) experiments was based on the fact that there is good evidence that state self-esteem is an indicator of the extent to which people are uncertain about themselves (see, e.g., Heatherton & Polivy, 1991; see also Baumgardner, 1990; cf. Sedikides & Strube, 1997). Therefore, state self-esteem measures were taken as indicators of perceived uncertainty in the experiment, and it was predicted that these measures would reveal that participants' state self-esteem was lower in mortality salient, as opposed to nonsalient, conditions. Furthermore, it was hypothesized that state self-esteem would mediate the relationship between manipulations of mortality salience and fairness. The results indeed showed that reminding participants about their death lowered their levels of state self-esteem, and that state self-esteem mediated participants' reactions to subsequent varia-

tions in distributive fairness (participants received an outcome that was equal to the outcome of a comparable other participant or that was worse than the outcome of the comparison other). These findings lend further support to the hypothesis that mortality salience may
lead people to become more uncertain about themselves (as indicated by lower levels of state
self-esteem; see also McGregor et al., 2001) and hence react more strongly to variations in
fairness.

In additional research that supports and extends this line of thought, Miedema, Van
den Bos, and Vermunt (2003) recently collected data that show that people react more
strongly toward variations in fairness when their self-image has been threatened (by having them think of situations in which important aspects of their selves were questioned by
other people who are very important for them). The findings of these studies show that
reminding people of things that threaten their ego (e.g., being judged as not intelligent)
leads to stronger procedural fairness effects than does reminding people of events that do
not threaten their ego (e.g., being judged as intelligent). These results are in accordance
with our suggestion that fairness is more important for people when they are uncertain
about important aspects of their lives. It is now time, however, to move to a review of
studies that provide very direct evidence that uncertainty is a key antecedent of why
fairness matters.

Van den Bos (2001b) extended the aforementioned studies by focusing explicitly on uncertainty as a factor in people's reactions to perceived fairness. The findings by Van den Bos
and Miedema (2000; Van den Bos, 2001a; Miedema et al., 2003) suggest that when people
are reminded of aspects of their lives that lead them to feel uncertain they will react more
strongly to variations in fairness. An interesting and potentially important implication of
this is that fairness matters especially to people when their uncertainties have been made
salient. However, in the Van den Bos and Miedema studies the implication is just that: an
implication. The studies showed that mortality salience, which was *presumed* to increase
feelings of uncertainty, is a moderator of fair process effects, but the Van den Bos and
Miedema research did not present direct evidence of the importance of uncertainty salience
for people's reactions to perceived fairness.

Van den Bos (2001b) conducted three experiments. Each experiment provides evidence
that uncertainty salience itself is an important determinant of people's reactions to perceived
fairness. In this chapter I discuss only the first experiment in the series. In this experiment,
the same setup was used as in Van den Bos and Miedema (2000, Experiment 1). Instead of a
mortality salience manipulation, however, uncertainty salience was manipulated directly.
Participants in the uncertainty salient condition were asked two questions that solicited participants' thoughts and feelings of their being uncertain: (1) "Please briefly describe the emotions that the thought of your being uncertain arouses in you," and (2) "Please write down,
as specifically as you can, what you think physically will happen to you as you feel uncertain." Participants in the uncertainty nonsalient condition were asked two questions that
were similar in format but did not remind participants about their uncertainties (see Van den
Bos, 2001b): (1) "Please briefly describe the emotions that the thought of your watching TV
arouses in you," and (2) "Please write down, as specifically as you can, what you think
physically will happen to you as you watch TV." As in Van den Bos and Miedema (2000,
Experiment 1), the fairness manipulation varied whether participants received or did not receive an opportunity to voice their opinions about the percentage of tickets that they should
receive relative to the other participant. The main dependent variables were participants'
negative affective reactions toward their treatment in the experiment (i.e., how disappointed
and sad participants felt about the way they were treated).

Following the line of reasoning I reviewed earlier, participants' reactions should be influenced more strongly by perceived fairness in the uncertainty salient conditions than in the nonsalient conditions. In fact, this prediction was supported by a significant interaction between uncertainty salience (salient vs. nonsalient) and procedure (voice vs. no voice). As expected, the effect of the procedural fairness manipulation was stronger in the uncertainty salient condition than in the nonsalient condition.

Two judges coded whether the answers that participants wrote down had anything to do with death. As in the experiments by Miedema et al. (2003) and in the other uncertainty salience experiments presented in this chapter, the judges agreed that answers had nothing to do with death. Thus, as expected, death-related thoughts cannot explain the findings reported in the uncertainty salience experiments.

Findings of Experiments 2 and 3 of Van den Bos (2001b) replicated and extended these results (using other operationalizations of uncertainty salience, procedural fairness, and ratings of affect). Thus, data from three experiments show that uncertainty salience influences reactions to perceived fairness: Asking people to think about their uncertainties leads to stronger effects of perceived fairness on affective reactions to treatment. These findings reveal that fairness matters more to people when they have been focused on uncertain aspects of their lives. Thus, these findings tell us something that is very fundamental to the point I am making in this section: Fairness has particularly strong effects for people when they have been thinking about issues that are related to their uncertainties. This in turn suggests a novel answer to the question posed earlier about why fairness matters so much to people: It may well be the case that fairness is attended to and fair situations are sought out because fairness may provide protection against things people are uncertain about and/or because it makes uncertainty more tolerable. In other words, fairness is important for people because they use fairness judgments in processes of managing uncertainty (Van den Bos & Lind, 2002).

MORTALITY AND UNCERTAINTY SALIENCE

We have seen that two theoretical frameworks focus on different antecedents of people's reactions to upholding and transgressions of cultural norms and values in general and fair and unfair treatment in particular: Terror management theory highlights the impact of mortality salience (e.g., Greenberg et al., 1997; Rosenblatt et al., 1989; Van den Bos & Miedema, 2000) whereas the uncertainty management model pays special attention to the influence of uncertainty salience (Van den Bos, 2001b; Van den Bos & Lind, 2002).

The uncertainty management model provides a novel social psychological explanation of why fairness matters to people and has been constructed especially to explain people's reactions toward variations in perceived fairness. However, the model has never been tested against good other accounts. A recent paper by Van den Bos and Miedema (2003) provides an attempt to do this. Specifically, although the uncertainty management model never has claimed uncertainty to be the sole cause of people's reactions toward fair and unfair treatment, the model does suggest that it is one of the key determinants of these reactions. It would be interesting, therefore, to investigate within one experimental setup the impact of both uncertainty and mortality salience, the latter being another, perhaps even more influential, antecedent of people's reactions toward fair and unfair experiences (cf. Van den Bos & Miedema, 2000). Related to this, on the basis of terror management theory (cf. Greenberg et al., 1997; Pyszczynski et al., 1999; Solomon et al., 1991) one

would expect especially mortality salience to cause the kinds of reactions to fair and unfair treatment reviewed earlier, and this is another reason why it is important to study
within one setup the influence of mortality and uncertainty salience on people's reactions
to variations in procedural fairness.

Others have speculated about the importance of uncertainty management processes to
account for people's reactions to culture-related events (e.g., Martin, 1999; McGregor et al.,
2001) but never explored people's reactions toward fair and unfair events and, more important, never studied the impact of both mortality and uncertainty salience within one study
(Martin, 1999) or did so by operationalizing the latter by using temporal discontinuity as a
self-integrity-threat induction (McGregor et al., 2001). This latter manipulation asked participants to compare events or persons from their childhood or adolescence with how these
events or people would be in the year 2035 and hence was very different from the mortality
salience manipulation commonly used in terror management studies (cf. Van den Bos &
Miedema, 2000) and thus, methodologically speaking, did not yield a very clean
comparison with the usual mortality salience manipulations.

In the paper by Van den Bos and Miedema (2003), these authors constructed a clear uncertainty salience manipulation that closely paralleled the mortality salience manipulations
most often used in terror management studies. That is, following most previous terror management studies, the mortality salient condition was induced by having participants respond
to the usual two open-ended questions concerning their thoughts and feelings about their
death (cf. Van den Bos & Miedema, 2000): (1) "Please briefly describe the emotions that the
thought of your death arouses in you," and (2) "Please write down, as specifically as you
can, what you think physically will happen to you as you die." Participants in the uncertainty salient condition were asked two questions that were highly similar in format but
asked participants about their thoughts and feelings of their being uncertain (cf. Van den
Bos, 2001b): (1) "Please briefly describe the emotions that the thought of your being uncertain arouses in you," and (2) "Please write down, as specifically as you can, what you think
physically will happen to you as you feel uncertain." By thus replacing "death" with "uncertain" in the most commonly used manipulations of mortality salience, while leaving everything else the same, the uncertainty salience manipulation was constructed such that it very
closely resembled the mortality salience manipulation and that, as a result, the impact of
these two manipulations on people's reactions toward fair and unfair treatment could be
investigated in a way that scientifically made sense.

In Experiment 1, participants ostensibly participated in two unrelated studies. In the
first study, either mortality or uncertainty was made salient (cf. Van den Bos, 2001b; Van
den Bos & Miedema, 2000). After this, the second study started in which participants were
asked to imagine that they applied for a job and that the selection process for this job consisted of nine parts. Participants then learned that the procedures used to make the decision
entailed the use of information that was either highly accurate (all parts were graded) or not
so accurate (only one part was graded). Because it is important to measure people's affective
reactions to perceived fairness (Tyler & Smith, 1998; Weiss, Suckow, & Cropanzano, 1999),
and following previous justice research (e.g., Folger, Rosenfield, Grove, & Corkran, 1979;
Van den Bos & Spruijt, 2002; Van den Bos & Van Prooijen, 2001), main dependent variables in both experiments reported here were participants' affective reactions toward the
way they were treated (cf. Van den Bos, 2001b; Van den Bos & Miedema, 2000). Specifically, because careful pilot testing revealed that mortality salience yielded the strongest
effects of procedural fairness on participants' anger toward the way they were treated, and
because it is important to assess anger following perceived fairness (e.g., Folger &

Cropanzano, 1998; Folger et al., 1979), main dependent variables assessed participants' anger toward treatment (cf. Van den Bos, 2001b, Experiments 2 and 3).

The reported findings show that when people have been thinking about their being uncertain *and* when they have been thinking about their own death, their ratings of anger toward treatment are significantly affected by variations in procedural fairness (viz., accurate vs. inaccurate procedures). This indicates supportive evidence for the impact of both mortality and uncertainty salience on people's reactions toward fairness of treatment, thus supporting both terror management theory and the uncertainty management model. Interestingly, the findings of the experiment further reveal a significant interaction effect between the salience manipulation (mortality vs. uncertainty) and the procedure manipulation (accurate vs. inaccurate) showing that even stronger fair process effects are to be found following uncertainty salience than following mortality salience. The results thus provide supportive evidence for uncertainty management model's reasoning that uncertainty-related thought is a key cause of people's reactions toward variations in procedural fairness and even suggest that uncertainty salience is a more important cause of people's reactions to experiences of procedural fairness than a strong other account (viz. mortality salience). Findings of the second experiment reported in Van den Bos and Miedema (2003) replicated the results of the first experiment. The second experiment used a different fairness manipulation and again showed a significant interaction effect between the salience and procedure manipulations, revealing that people reacted stronger to variations in procedural fairness under conditions of uncertainty salience as opposed to mortality salience. These findings contribute to the robustness of the results reported in the first experiment.

Thus, the findings of both experiments show that asking people to think about issues that are related to their own uncertainties or their own mortality leads their anger toward treatment ratings to be strongly affected by variations in procedural fairness. Thus, in support of both terror management theory and the uncertainty management model, evidence has been obtained that both mortality and uncertainty salience lead to strong fair process effects on people's reactions. Furthermore, in both experiments it was found that uncertainty salience has an even bigger impact on people's reactions than does mortality salience. This supports the uncertainty management model's reasoning that reminders of uncertainty are a key determinant of people's reactions toward fair and unfair experiences and even suggests that uncertainty salience is a more important cause of people's reactions to fairness of treatment than mortality salience.

It can be noted here that manipulation-check findings revealed that what participants wrote down during the salience manipulations showed that although all participants in the mortality salient condition had been thinking about death, some of the participants in the mortality salient condition had also been thinking of the same uncertainty-related issues as all participants in the uncertainty salient condition had. Uncertainty was clearly more salient in the uncertainty salient condition than in the mortality salient condition, but the fact that some uncertainty-related thought could be detected in the mortality salient condition is in line with arguments that have been put forward that an effect (but not the only effect) of manipulations of mortality salience may be the activation of uncertainty-related thought (e.g., Martin, 1999; McGregor et al., 2001; Van den Bos & Lind, 2002).

Interestingly, recently collected data (Van den Bos & Poortvliet, 2003) show that it is also when experimental paradigms (other than fairness paradigms) are used that are the same as those typically used in terror management studies that uncertainty salience can have a bigger impact on people's reactions than does mortality salience. Van den Bos and Poortvliet measured participants' reactions toward essays that either violated or bolstered their cultural worldviews and found similar effects of the uncertainty and mortality salience manipulations as Van den Bos and Miedema (2003) did: Students from Utrecht University who were reminded about their mortality reacted more negatively toward an essay that stated very negative things about Utrecht University and the students at that university and reacted very positively toward an essay that was very positive about this university and the students. More important for the current purposes, a significant interaction effect between the salience manipulation (mortality vs. uncertainty) and the essay manipulation (positive vs. negative) was found, showing that participants in the uncertainty salient condition reacted even more strongly toward these essays. The findings of these studies indicate that the impact of uncertainty salience is not restricted to reactions toward fair and unfair events and can be found also on cultural worldview issues that have served a more prominent role in previous terror management studies and theorizing (e.g., Dechesne, Janssen, & Van Knippenberg, 2000).

It should be noted that, of course, it is always difficult to compare the impact of different manipulations (such as mortality and uncertainty salience) with each other. This said, however, in the experiments by Van den Bos and Miedema (2003) and Van den Bos and Poortvliet (2003), the uncertainty salience manipulation was constructed in such a way that it very closely paralleled the mortality salience manipulation most commonly used in terror management studies (the only thing that we did was to replace the word "death" with "uncertain"), thus making it possible to simultaneously investigate the impact of these two salience manipulations in a way that scientifically made sense. Furthermore, dependent variables were used that extensive pilot testing had shown to yield the strongest effects of mortality salience among the population of participants used. Future research—with other dependent variables, other populations of research participants, and other cultural norms and values and other concepts related to terror and uncertainty management (for suggestions, see, e.g., Greenberg et al., 1997; McGregor et al., 2001; Pyszczynski et al., 1999; Solomon et al., 1991; Van den Bos & Lind, 2002)—is needed, of course, but the findings of *the studies reviewed here* converge on the same point: The uncertainty management model highlights the role of uncertainty in people's reactions toward events that violate or bolster their cultural norms and values. Terror management theory focuses strongly on the importance of death to account for social psychological effects and states, among other things, that mortality salience is a very important antecedent of people's reactions toward transgressions and upholding of cultural norms and values (e.g., Greenberg et al., 1997; Pyszczynski et al., 1999; Solomon et al., 1991). On the basis of terror management theory one would therefore be inclined to expect mortality salience to be a prime, perhaps even the main, cause of people's reactions to things that violate or bolster their cultural worldview. After reviewing the consistent findings of the experiments reviewed in this section the conclusion seems warranted that mortality salience is important in predicting cultural worldview reactions but that uncertainty salience can be even more important, and in fact was more important in the studies reviewed here.

This does not rule out, of course, the possibility that mortality salience may well have unique effects that cannot be subsumed under the heading of an uncertainty framework, and this does not imply that there will not be circumstances in which mortality salience (as opposed to uncertainty salience) may exert stronger effects on reactions to other violations and bolstering of cultural worldviews than the issues and variables studied in the experiments reviewed here. This said, however, what I think matters most for our current insights regarding terror and uncertainty management is that the experiments reviewed here have shown that particular effects may occur. Other studies will be needed to investigate the full implications of these studies. It is my true hope, therefore, that more studies will be conducted to explore the exciting issues of mortality and uncertainty salience.

CONCLUSIONS AND DISCUSSION

I think that there are good conceptual reasons why uncertainty has a big impact on people's reactions toward persons and events that violate or bolster their cultural worldviews. That is, various social psychological theories have pointed at the crucial role that uncertainty plays in diverse important social psychological processes and have noted that uncertainty is an aversive state that people feel needs to be managed, at least to some extent (see, e.g., Festinger, 1954; Fiske & Taylor, 1991; Hogg & Mullin, 1999; Lopes, 1987; Sorrentino & Roney, 1986). The uncertainty management model notes that fairness judgments are particularly well suited to help in processes of uncertainty management (for details, see Lind & Van den Bos, 2002; Van den Bos & Lind, 2002), and the research findings reviewed here corroborate this prediction.

Furthermore, recently collected data (Van den Bos & Poortvliet, 2003) suggest that salience of uncertainty considerations may also have a big impact on other reactions toward violations and bolstering of cultural worldviews; reactions more commonly studied in terror management experiments than reactions toward fair and unfair events. It is noteworthy that these research findings fit into lines of thought of other, nonfairness papers that recently have explored the relationship between terror and uncertainty management processes and that have argued for the important role of uncertainty in social psychology. Martin (1999), for example, discussed research findings that indicated that individuals who had been reminded about their mortality experienced more uncertainty than did those who had not been thinking about mortality. Related to this, McGregor et al. (2001) found that mortality salience caused uncertainty-related feelings and reported that in pilot studies they found that responses in mortality salient conditions were more strongly related to uncertainty than to "fear, pain, or anything resembling annihilation terror" (p. 480). In their uncertainty management chapter, Van den Bos and Lind (2002) argued that these findings suggest that an important (albeit not the only) consequence of mortality salience manipulations may be the activation of uncertainty-related thought. In other words, an important aspect (but not the sole story) of mortality salience may be that it may be conceived of as an indirect manipulation of uncertainty salience. When developing the Van den Bos and Miedema (2003) and Van den Bos and Poortvliet (2003) experiments, my colleagues and I reasoned that if this line of logic would be true, it should imply that directly reminding people about their uncertainties would constitute a more direct manipulation of uncertainty salience and hence should have a bigger impact on reactions to fair and unfair treatment. The findings of all experiments reviewed here suggest that asking people to think about their uncertainties is indeed a more direct manipulation of uncertainty salience, and the findings of the experiments discussed here show that this manipulation indeed yielded stronger effects on people's reactions toward events that violated or bolstered their cultural worldview.

Related to this, in two out of three experiments of the Van den Bos and Miedema (2003) and Van den Bos and Poortvliet (2003) papers it was found that among participants where mortality salience triggered uncertainty-related thought, anger reactions were stronger influenced by the procedure or article manipulations, whereas for participants where mortality salience did not activate uncertainty-related thought weaker or nonsignificant differences between the procedure or article conditions were obtained. This suggests that, at least sometimes, it may be the uncertainty component of mortality salience manipulations that may be driving people's reactions to violations and bolstering of cultural worldviews.

I hasten to note here that, in my opinion, all this should not necessarily be taken as a refutation of terror management theory, but, rather, as an attempt to incorporate at least some elements of it into a broader framework. Notable in this respect, I think, are research findings that, in correspondence with the theory's predictions, show that reminders of mortality lead to a decrease in situational self-esteem (e.g., Koole, Dechesne, & Van Knippenberg, 2002; Van den Bos, 2001a). If people with low self-esteem are more uncertain about themselves than those with high self-esteem (see, e.g., Heatherton & Polivy, 1991; see also Baumgardner, 1990; cf. Sedikides & Strube, 1997), then self-esteem measures can be taken as indicators of perceived uncertainty, which would imply that the terror and uncertainty management perspectives converge on the important role of self-related uncertainty in social psychological processes. Paradoxically, the fact that we will die some day is almost the only thing we humans can be absolutely certain about. However, this does not imply that being reminded about one's own mortality may not make people uncertain about themselves (cf. Martin, 1999; McGregor et al., 2001). I would therefore like to make a plea for broadening the scope of terror management theory to explicitly encompass the role of self-related uncertainty and would urge researchers to explore this implication of the findings reviewed here. Again, I would like to emphasize that, in my opinion, this may not imply an alternative to terror management theory but rather the incorporation of pivotal aspects of the model (such as important elements of mortality salience manipulations) in a broader framework.

It is important to emphasize here that it would not really be accurate to say that terror management theory predicts that only thoughts of death would produce increased striving to maintain aspects of the cultural anxiety buffer. What the theory does claim is that the problem of death lies at the root of the need for self-esteem and faith in one's worldview, which does not imply that no other class of aversive events would increase striving for these psychological entities. This chapter (see also Martin, 1999; McGregor et al., 2001) reveals that uncertainty may well be one of these entities and may sometimes even yield bigger effects on human reactions than reminders of mortality do.

Related to this, I would like to stress that I am not saying here that the research findings that were reviewed in this chapter imply that uncertainty concerns underlie all terror management effects. In all likelihood, I would predict that future research will show that nonexistence does have a motivational force, over and beyond the uncertainty aspects that may be related to reminders of mortality, and I am therefore not arguing that fear of the termination of life, nonexistence, and decay are just side effects of uncertainty with no motivational properties. There are no data that speak to this latter position, and personally I think that it would be unreasonable to expect that in the future there will be data that will show this.

Furthermore, I am not implying here that uncertainty accounts for all of findings that have come out of the terror management literature. The mortality salience paradigm is probably the most widely used paradigm in the terror management field (for overviews, see, e.g., Greenberg et al., 1997; Pyszczynski et al., 1999; Solomon et al., 1991), but there are definitely other approaches to testing the theory as well. For example, Mikulincer, Florian, Birnbaum, and Malishkevich (2002) showed that imagining to be separated from a relationship partner enhanced subsequent death-thought accessibility, and it may be difficult to explain these findings from an uncertainty management account. This suggests that some elements of theory and research on terror management are unrelated to uncertainty and are specific to death-related thought. However, I do argue that there is also the possibility that sometimes and/or some aspects of mortality salience effects may be caused by uncertainty concerns, and I do think the research findings reviewed here may help us in our progress toward understanding the subtle and intriguing relationship between uncertainty and terror management effects. This may yield the conclusion that some elements of terror management theory (cf. Van den Bos & Miedema, 2003; Van den Bos & Poortvliet, 2003) may be part of a broader conceptual framework related to uncertainty management, whereas other core elements of the theory (cf. Mikulincer et al., 2002) clearly are not related to uncertainty and may be uniquely associated with the psychology of death.

I hope that these implications of this chapter will further future theorizing and new empirical work. This may yield more thorough insights into the psychology of uncertainty. For example, one could argue that we are always faced with uncertainties but that they may vary greatly in importance and level of uncertainty, and that this may affect people's reactions considerably. Furthermore, the uncertainty of whether one will enjoy the next Pokemon game is not the same as uncertainty about layoffs or death. Thus, all uncertainties are not the same and cannot be expected to have the same effects. However, the research findings reviewed here have revealed that just asking participants two questions about their being uncertain leads to very strong reactions toward events that are good or bad for one's cultural worldview.

Related to this, one may argue that uncertainty management seems like a more "proximal" motive for justice striving than terror management, in that justice bears more of a logical and semantic connection to the problem of uncertainty than it does to the problem of death. Most of the aspects of the cultural worldview and self-esteem that terror management theory views as functioning to provide protection from the fear of death have little or no logical connection to the problem of death (see Pyszczynski et al., 1999). Thus one difference between death and uncertainty, when it comes to justice and perhaps other important cultural norms and values (cf. Van den Bos & Poortvliet, 2003), might be in the extent to which justice helps solve the problem in a logical as opposed to symbolic way.

Future research is needed to further investigate the boundaries of the uncertainty management model (see, e.g., Van den Bos & Lind, 2001; Van Prooijen, Van den Bos, & Wilke, 2003), but for now the model seems to work pretty well in the fairness domain and in other domains as well (Van den Bos & Poortvliet, 2003). I hope that future researchers will be stimulated by this chapter to further explore the uncertainty and terror management implications of the findings reviewed here. As research accumulates concerning the psychology of cultural worldview reactions, as it has in this chapter and in other articles (e.g., Greenberg et al., 1997; Pyszczynski et al., 1999; Solomon et al., 1991), we begin to understand the conditions when the effects to cultural worldview violations are strong and when they are very strong, why these effects occur at all, and why they are so potent when they do occur. This knowledge in turn promises to advance our understanding of fundamental issues in the social psychology of cultural norms and values in basic social relations.

At the end of the day, though, there is at least one finding of the studies reviewed here that promises to have enduring importance: Across multiple studies, it was revealed that both mortality and uncertainty salience have strong effects on reactions to fairness of treatment, with uncertainty salience consistently having a bigger impact. I hope, therefore, that the existentialist approach to the social psychology of fairness reviewed here may stimulate social psychologists to better understand the principles of cultural norms and values.

REFERENCES

Baumgardner, A. H. (1990). To know oneself is to like oneself: Self-certainty and self-affect. *Journal of Personality and Social Psychology, 58,* 1062–1072.

Brockner, J., & Wiesenfeld, B. M. (1996). An integrative framework for explaining reactions to decisions: Interactive effects of outcomes and procedures. *Psychological Bulletin, 120,* 189–208.

Dechesne, M., Janssen, J., & Van Knippenberg, A. (2000). Derogation and distancing as terror management strategies: The moderating role of need for closure and permeability of group boundaries. *Journal of Personality and Social Psychology, 79,* 923–932.

Festinger, L. (1954). A theory of social comparison processes. *Human Relations, 7,* 117–140.

Fiske, S. T., & Taylor, S. E. (1991). *Social cognition* (2nd ed.). New York: McGraw-Hill.

Folger, R. (1984). Preface. In R. Folger (Ed.), *The sense of injustice: Social psychological perspectives* (pp. ix–x). New York: Plenum Press.

Folger, R., & Cropanzano, R. (1998). *Organizational justice and human resource management.* Thousand Oaks, CA: Sage.

Folger, R., Rosenfield, D., Grove, J., & Corkran, L. (1979). Effects of "voice" and peer opinions on responses to inequity. *Journal of Personality and Social Psychology, 37,* 2253–2261.

Fromm, E. (2002). *The fear of freedom.* London: Routledge. (Original work published 1942)

Greenberg, J., Pyszczynski, T., Solomon, S., Rosenblatt, A., Veeder, M., Kirkland, S., et al. (1990). Evidence for terror management theory II: The effects of mortality salience on reactions to those who threaten or bolster the cultural worldview. *Journal of Personality and Social Psychology, 58,* 308–318.

Greenberg, J., Solomon, S., & Pyszczynski, T. (1997). Terror management theory of self-esteem and cultural worldviews: Empirical assessments and conceptual refinements. In M. P. Zanna (Ed.), *Advances in experimental social psychology* (Vol. 29, pp. 61–139). New York: Academic Press.

Heatherton, T. F., & Polivy, J. (1991). Development and validation of a scale for measuring state self-esteem. *Journal of Personality and Social Psychology, 60,* 895–910.

Hogg, M. A., & Mullin, B.-A. (1999). Joining groups to reduce uncertainty: Subjective uncertainty reduction and group identification. In D. Abrams & M. A. Hogg (Eds.), *Social identity and social cognition* (pp. 249–279). Oxford, UK: Blackwell.

Koole, S. L., Dechesne, M., & Van Knippenberg, A. (2002). *The sting of death: Evidence that reminders of mortality undermine implicit self-esteem.* Manuscript submitted for publication.

Lind, E. A., & Tyler, T. R. (1988). *The social psychology of procedural justice.* New York: Plenum Press.

Lind, E. A., & Van den Bos, K. (2002). When fairness works: Toward a general theory of uncertainty management. In B. M. Staw & R. M. Kramer (Eds.), *Research in organizational behavior* (Vol. 24, pp. 181–223). Greenwich, CT: JAI Press.

Lopes, L. L. (1987). Between hope and fear: The psychology of risk. *Advances in Experimental Psychology, 20,* 255–295.

Martin, L. L. (1999). I-D compensation theory: Some implications of trying to satisfy immediate-return needs in a delayed-return culture. *Psychological Inquiry, 10,* 195–208.

McGregor, I., Zanna, M. P., Holmes, J. G., & Spencer, S. J. (2001). Compensatory conviction in the face of personal uncertainty: Going to extremes and being oneself. *Journal of Personality and Social Psychology, 80,* 472–488.

Miedema, J., Van den Bos, K., & Vermunt, R. (2003). *The influence of ego threat on reactions to perceived fairness.* Manuscript submitted for publication.

Mikulincer, M., Florian, V., Birnbaum, G., & Malishkevich, S. (2002). The death-anxiety buffering function of close relationships: Exploring the effects of separation reminders on death-thought accessibility. *Personality and Social Psychology Bulletin, 28,* 287–299.

Pyszczynski, T. A., Greenberg, J., & Solomon, S. (1999). A dual-process model of defense against conscious and unconscious death-related thoughts: An extension of terror management theory. *Psychological Review, 106,* 835–845.

Reve, G. (1983). *In gesprek: Interviews* [In conversation: Interviews]. Baarn, the Netherlands: De Prom.

Rosenblatt, A., Greenberg, J., Solomon, S., Pyszczynski, T., & Lyon, D. (1989). Evidence for terror management theory I: The effects of mortality salience on reactions to those who violate or uphold cultural values. *Journal of Personality and Social Psychology, 57,* 681–690.

Sedikides, C., & Strube, M. J. (1997). Self-evaluation: To thine own self be good, to thine own self be sure, to thine own self be true, and to thine own self be better. In M. P. Zanna (Ed.), *Advances in experimental social psychology* (Vol. 29, pp. 209–269). San Diego: Academic Press.

Solomon, S., Greenberg, J., & Pyszczynski, T. (1991). A terror management theory of social behavior: The psychological functions of self-esteem and cultural worldviews. In L. Berkowitz (Ed.), *Advances in experimental social psychology* (Vol. 24, pp. 93–159). New York: Academic Press.

Sorrentino, R. M., & Roney, C. J. R. (1986). Uncertainty orientation, achievement-related motivation and task diagnosticity as determinants of task performance. *Social Cognition, 4,* 420–436.

Tyler, T. R., & Lind, E. A. (1992). A relational model of authority in groups. In M. P. Zanna (Ed.), *Advances in experimental social psychology* (Vol. 25, pp. 115–191). San Diego: Academic Press.

Tyler, T. R., & Smith, H. J. (1998). Social justice and social movements. In D. Gilbert, S. T. Fiske, & G. Lindzey (Eds.), *Handbook of social psychology* (4th ed., Vol. 2, pp. 595–629). Boston: McGraw-Hill.

Van den Bos, K. (1999). What are we talking about when we talk about no-voice procedures? On the psychology of the fair outcome effect. *Journal of Experimental Social Psychology, 35,* 560–577.

Van den Bos, K. (2001a). Reactions to perceived fairness: The impact of mortality salience and self-esteem on ratings of negative affect. *Social Justice Research, 14,* 1–23.

Van den Bos, K. (2001b). Uncertainty management: The influence of uncertainty salience on reactions to perceived procedural fairness. *Journal of Personality and Social Psychology, 80,* 931–941.

Van den Bos, K., & Lind, E. A. (2002). Uncertainty management by means of fairness judgments. In M. P. Zanna (Ed.), *Advances in experimental social psychology* (Vol. 34, pp. 1–60). San Diego: Academic Press.

Van den Bos, K., Lind, E. A., Vermunt, R., & Wilke, H. A. M. (1997). How do I judge my outcome when I do not know the outcome of others? The psychology of the fair process effect. *Journal of Personality and Social Psychology, 72,* 1034–1046.

Van den Bos, K., & Miedema, J. (2000). Toward understanding why fairness matters: The influence of mortality salience on reactions to procedural fairness. *Journal of Personality and Social Psychology, 79,* 355–366.

Van den Bos, K., & Miedema, K. (2003). *An enquiry concerning the principles of cultural norms and values: The impact of uncertainty and mortality salience on reactions to fair and unfair treatment.* Manuscript submitted for publication.

Van den Bos, K., & Poortvliet, M. (2003). Unpublished raw data.

Van den Bos, K., & Spruijt, N. (2002). Appropriateness of decisions as a moderator of the psychology of voice. *European Journal of Social Psychology, 32,* 57–72.

Van den Bos, K., & Van Prooijen, J.-W. (2001). Referent cognitions theory: The role of closeness of reference points in the psychology of voice. *Journal of Personality and Social Psychology, 81,* 616–626.

Van den Bos, K., Wilke, H. A. M., & Lind, E. A. (1998). When do we need procedural fairness? The role of trust in authority. *Journal of Personality and Social Psychology, 75,* 1449–1458.

Van Prooijen, J.-W., Van den Bos, K., & Wilke, H. A. M. (2003). *Knowing where we stand in a group enhances reactions to procedures: On the psychology of procedural justice and intragroup status.* Manuscript submitted for publication.

Watson, D., Clark, L. A., & Tellegen, A. (1988). Development and validation of brief measures of positive and negative affect: The PANAS scales. *Journal of Personality and Social Psychology, 54,* 1063–1070.

Weiss, H. M., Suckow, K., & Cropanzano, R. (1999). Effects of justice conditions on discrete emotions. *Journal of Applied Psychology, 84,* 786–794.

Chapter 12

Zeal, Identity, and Meaning

Going to Extremes to Be One Self

IAN MCGREGOR

The starting premise of the research described in this chapter is that humans need an authoritative guide for navigating uncertainty about what to do in life. Drawing on identity consolidation (IC) theory (McGregor, 1998) I propose that people in individualist cultures turn to their identities for this purpose, and they rely on four IC strategies to maintain them. IC strategies are personally rewarding because they take people's minds off of identity threats and promote self-regulatory efficiency, but they may also feed a pernicious dark side, of narcissism, intergroup bias, and zealous extremism. This chapter begins with an outline of IC theory assumptions, then presents theoretical and empirical support for the existence and effectiveness of each IC strategy. It concludes with a comparison of IC and other theories of self-threat and defensiveness and a discussion of the multifaceted IC value of romantic relationships and monotheistic religions.

IC theory begins with the defining premise of existential philosophy, that human existence precedes human essence. This means that we humans find ourselves existing in a universe that does not provide a priori guidance about what kind of person to be. Put another way, from a more anthropological perspective, attenuated instincts and enlarged neocortexes have left us with the highly adaptive capacity to simulate alternative goals and possible selves without having to allocate concrete resources to each. A nagging side effect, however, is the potential for overwhelming personal uncertainty (PU) about what to prioritize. Accordingly, existentialists highlight the predicament of anguished freedom in a world that seems absurd.

It is important to emphasize the difference between PU and focal uncertainty about specific issues or goals. Focal uncertainty (e.g., about how to dress or behave at work) can be engaging and enjoyable because it brings opportunity for novelty and exploration (Sorrentino & Roney, 2000) and the self-determined exercise of choice and autonomy

(Kasser & Sheldon, Chapter 29, this volume). It can also be resolved by appealing to higher-level self-elements (i.e., values, priorities, and identifications). Indeed, doing so is associated with a meaningful sense that one has chosen one's direction and is "being oneself" (McGregor & Little, 1998). In contrast, PU is a kind of identity crisis that arises from awareness of conflict or lack of clarity about self-elements—about what kind of person to be (Baumeister, 1985). Without a clear identity to serve as an authoritative guide for setting priorities, humans face the potential for chronic, multiple approach–avoidance conflicts among imagined alternatives and possible selves, and the associated negative affect and immobilization (see McGregor, 2003).[1]

Anxiety and immobilization are part of an adaptive response mediated by the Behavioral Inhibition System (BIS) in all vertebrates, which prompts disengagement from goals that are impeded by failure or uncertainty, and vigilant scanning for viable alternatives (Gray, 1982). For humans, BIS integration with the neocortex has vastly expanded the capacity to generate alternatives when a focal goal is disrupted. The human BIS response provides adaptive flexibility when applied to relatively low-level, focal goals that can be easily abandoned and replaced. Anxiety and immobilization associated with existential PU, however, is potentially more problematic. PU about abstract, super-ordinate goals (e.g., "be myself") raises the specter of self-regulatory collapse because it can disrupt the entire chain of subordinate, nested, priorities, goals, and behaviors (Scheier & Carver, 1988). Thus, for optimal functioning, humans in individualistic cultures need ways of consolidating clear identities so that the adaptive capacity for focal goal flexibility can be reliably guided by identity stability.

This chapter focuses on four IC strategies—integration, self-worth, group identification, and conviction—that people use to cope with PU about how to be. Each consolidates a clear sense of identity via unique mechanisms that are discussed in turn, but they also share three common mechanisms. First, and most directly, each reduces PU by focusing awareness on a referent for action. When navigating PU about what to prioritize, one might turn to thoughts related to integration (e.g., "What fits with my story of who I am?"), self-worth (e.g., "What am I likely to succeed and be good at?"), group identification (e.g., "What are the norms and values of my group?"), or conviction (e.g., "What are my strongest values and priorities?"). Authoritative answers to these questions quell uncertainty by providing unambiguous guides for prioritizing alternatives. After repeated association and reinforcement, answers to these questions become automatic, habitual responses to PU and self-threats that expose PU.

Second, IC strategies provide an opportunity to distract oneself from PU by focusing attention on a clear subset of self-elements. Focusing on alternative thoughts is a mental control strategy that, in contrast to unfocused thought suppression efforts, does not cause rebound hyperaccessibility of unwanted thoughts (Wenzlaff & Bates, 2000). Moreover, thoughts related to the IC strategies are subjectively appealing because of repeated association with relief from PU. Thinking about appealing thoughts when confronted with troubling ones can be a spontaneous and effective way to repair mood (Dodgson & Wood, 1998; Smith & Petty, 1995), presumably because the pleasant thoughts inhibit or at least distract attention from the unpleasant ones.

The third shared mechanism is that each IC strategy highlights important, self-relevant thoughts that provide a trivializing frame for reducing importance of PUs and self-threats (cf. Simon, Greenberg, & Brehm, 1995). Lower importance translates into lower accessibility to awareness (Bizer & Krosnick, 2001). Thus, in addition to directly ameliorating PU, the identity-consolidation strategies serve as *hyperdistracters* because they (1) effectively draw the focus attention away from uncertainty without risk of rebound hyperaccessibility, (2) are subjectively appealing, and (3) are subjectively important. In the sections that follow, a brief theoretical precedent for each IC strategy is reviewed. Each section then describes research showing that people adopt the strategy when confronted with PU and that doing so reduces the subjective salience (importance and accessibility) of PUs. Past research has shown that accessibility of cognitive conflicts determines how uncomfortable they feel (Newby-Clark, McGregor, & Zanna, 2002).

IC STRATEGY 1: PERSONAL INTEGRATION

Building on ancient Greek injunctions to know and be oneself but mindful of the self's often disparate agendas, clinical–developmental theorists have long promoted the benefits of personal integration. Freud proposed *sublimation* as an integrative solution to conflicting agendas of the id and super ego, and Jung promoted *individuation*—harmonization of contradictory personality aspects and strivings. Gordon Allport claimed that the mature personality acts in accordance with a "unifying philosophy of life" (1949/1937, pp. 225–231), and Murray proposed that "time-binding," acting in accord with one's remembered past and anticipated future, provides life with continuity and purpose (1938, p. 49). Seminal humanistic theories of Fromm, Rogers, Maslow, and Erickson's similarly posited that optimal functioning required commitment to discovering and being one's true self through critical self-reflection and exploration (cf. McGregor & Little, 1998).

Following this historical emphasis on personal integration, contemporary personologists propose that identity is a life story that helps integrate disparate aspects of the self into a meaningful whole that suffuses life with purpose and direction (e.g., McAdams, 1993). Coherent stories tend to make story-consistent information more memorable and psychologically consequential (e.g., McGregor & Holmes, 1999). Thus, in addition to the shared mechanisms for ameliorating PU described in the introduction, narrative integration of self-elements allows individuals to focus on a coherent life story and to let loose ends and inconsistencies fade from awareness. As coherent life-story identities gain epistemic momentum, they can serve as authoritative guides to help individuals navigate focal uncertainties with aplomb.

In Study 1a, McGregor and Little (1998) investigated whether integration among self-elements would be associated with self-regulatory clarity (i.e., the experience of purpose and meaning in life). Participants first listed 10 personal projects—midlevel goals that they were engaged in or planning for—and then rated each project on "integrity" dimensions referring to the extent to which the project was consistent with other aspects of the self (e.g., values and identifications). They then completed a variety of well-being scales. A principal-components analysis of the scale scores revealed two orthogonal factors corresponding to purpose/meaning in life and to happiness (positive affect, negative affect, and life satisfaction). Mean personal project integrity was specifically correlated with purpose/meaning but not with happiness. (For discussion of the independence of happiness and meaning, see Baumeister, 1991; McGregor & Little, 1998.)

In Study 1b (McGregor, Zanna, Holmes, & Spencer, 2001, Study 2), PU was manipulated by having participants in the PU condition deliberate about one of their current, difficult personal dilemmas and the conflicting values and possible selves associated with it. In other research, this manipulation significantly elevated feelings of uncertainty[2] but did not affect general negative affect or state self-esteem (McGregor et al., 2001, Study 1). Participants in the control condition deliberated about a friend's dilemma instead of their own. For one of the dependent variables, participants then listed 10 personal projects and rated them on the integrity dimensions described in Study 1a. Results indicated that participants faced with the uncertainty of their own dilemmas reacted by planning to engage in projects that were significantly higher in integrity than did control participants. On another dependent variable, participants rated the importance of various values as guiding priorities in their lives. Mirroring the results for personal project integrity, participants in the PU condition described their values as more thematically consistent than did control participants (see Tesser, Crepaz, Collins, Cornell, & Beach, 2000, Study 2, for similar value-clarification results after PU was induced in a classic cognitive dissonance experiment).

Study 1c investigated whether focusing on personal integrity would reduce subjective salience of PUs (McGregor, 2002). All participants first briefly described an important dilemma in their life. They were then randomly assigned either to a PU condition (as in Study 1b) or to a no-PU condition in which they completed materials that were not related to the dilemma. Participants in the PU condition were then randomly assigned to either an integrity condition or a control condition. In the integrity condition, they wrote a paragraph about how past actions and future plans were consistent with their most important personal values (most participants wrote about communal values). In the control condition they instead wrote about how values that were important, but not their most important, could be most important for other people. All participants in the no-PU condition also completed the control materials. For the dependent variable, participants then rated the subjective salience of their personal dilemmas. Six subjective salience items referred to the extent to which the dilemmas felt preoccupying, hard to ignore, urgent, significant, big, and important "right now, at this very moment." The scale was unifactorial, with Cronbach alpha reliability = .89. Results indicated a significant difference in subjective salience across the three conditions. There was significantly higher subjective salience in the PU/control condition than in either the PU/integrity, or no-PU/control conditions. This finding demonstrates that focusing on personal integrity can take people's minds off of their troubling PUs.

Together, Studies 1a–c demonstrate that identity integration is associated with a sense of purpose and direction in life, that PU causes a quest for integration, and that integration decreases the subjective salience of PUs. One challenge associated with sole reliance on integration as an IC strategy, however, may be that it requires unwavering clarity about how one's priorities and values fit together. Such decisions rest on subjective assessments of human nature and one's relation to other people and the world that may be difficult to make on one's own (Festinger, 1954). Attempting to form a static, independent, and integrated self-identity may be difficult because self-elements are collected over time and diverse contexts. Indeed, several theorists have proposed that it is virtually impossible to independently arrive at authoritative answers to the "who am I?" question based on introspection and self-analysis, and that attempting to do so requires self-focus, deliberation, and immersion in potentially overwhelming PU (Baumeister, 1987; Cushman, 1990; Durkheim, 1951). Furthermore, even if authoritative conclusions could be independently reached, individuals in a social group, with their differing dispositions and experiences, would likely arrive at differing priorities (cf. Roberts & Robins, 2000). Thus, the competing identity commitments of others could introduce a symbolic threat by highlighting the arbitrary subjectivity of one's own commitments; a predicament reflected in the existentialist lament (Sartre, 1989) that hell is other people. The three following IC strategies can function independently but may also be used to bolster personal integrity by making it seem authoritative.

IC STRATEGY 2: SELF-WORTH

Sartre (1956) proposed that people try to escape from the nauseating uncertainty associated with radical freedom and subjective self-construction by objectifying the self and trying to be God. Seeing oneself as superior belittles others' competing claims on how to be and adds authority to an identity. Successes and positive self-evaluations may also contribute to a kind of *self-worth myopia* because they are associated with relatively low levels of vigilant and ruminative self-focus (Gray, 1982; Greenberg & Pyszczynski, 1986). This may be a reason for the robust association between self-esteem and self-concept clarity (e.g., Campbell, 1990). Self-worth myopia may shrink the subset of salient self-elements, making it less likely that PUs and inconsistencies are noticed. The appeal of this mechanism may contribute to the positive illusions and exaggerated self-esteem that characterize individualist cultures (Heine, Lehman, Markus, & Kitayama, 1999). Repeatedly reminding oneself of one's strengths to keep threats out of awareness may cause a cumulative bias toward conceit (Smith & Petty, 1995, p. 1104).

Recent research has found that people defensively enhance their self-image when confronted with PU-related threats (cf. cognitive dissonance; Festinger, 1957), and that self-worth salience eliminates subsequent defensiveness. Tesser et al. (2000) found that dissonance caused participants to exaggerate their self-worth via self-enhancing social comparisons. Steele, Spencer, and Lynch (1993) found that reminding participants of their self-worth decreased their defensiveness after a dissonance threat. Study 2 (McGregor, 2002) tested the hypothesis that self-worth affirmations decrease subjective salience of PUs. Participants completed a self-esteem scale and then deliberated about PUs (as in Study 1b and 1c). They were then randomly assigned either to write a paragraph about an important personal success (success salience), or to write about an important success of a public figure (control). They then rated the subjective salience of their PUs (as in Study 1c). Results revealed a significant interaction such that subjective salience of dilemmas was significantly lower among participants with high self-esteem (HSEs) in the success condition than among HSEs in the control condition or those with low self-esteem (LSEs) in either condition.

The finding that the success affirmation reduced salience of PUs for HSEs but not for LSEs is consistent with the finding that HSEs are particularly likely to self-promote after self-threats. LSEs are just as troubled by self-threats but may be less willing to risk the drop in likability that can be associated with defensive self-promotion (Vohs & Heatherton, 2001; Wood, Giordano-Beech, Taylor, Michela, & Gaus, 1994). This unwillingness to mask PU with self-promotion may be one reason for LSEs' particularly high PU (i.e., low self-concept clarity; Campbell, 1990). It is important to note that the defensive integration effects in Studies 1b and 1c were *not* moderated by self-esteem. This may be because the integration in those studies tended to revolve around consensual, communal themes (like helping and loving others), which LSEs *are* willing to invoke when threatened (Vohs & Heatherton). Finally, relying on exaggerated self-worth may feel personally rewarding for HSEs insofar as it helps take their minds off of threats and PUs, but given its social costs (Vohs & Heatherton), and link with defensive narcissism (Jordan, Spencer, Zanna, Hoshino-Brown, & Correl, 2003), self-worth as an IC strategy may be most effective when tempered with integration or an IC strategy that facilitates social inclusion, such as group identification.

IC STRATEGY 3: GROUP IDENTIFICATION

Using group identification as a template for self-construction reduces the need for self-analysis and deliberation and also increases the chances of intragroup consensus about meanings and ends to pursue. Instead of having to forge coherence and derive self-worth from the vagaries of personal idiosyncrasies, one can adopt the norms, values, ideals, and narratives of a group (Abrams & Hogg, 1999) and use them as internalized guides for behavior (Terry & Hogg, 2000). Indeed, Fromm (1941) proposed that the desire to escape from the painful PU of existential freedom was the impetus behind fascism, and Sartre (1956) asserted that people attempt to escape from the nausea of radical freedom and choice by living in bad faith as pillars of society. Cleaving to dominant, positive, societal norms provides a sense of purpose and direction, without having to confront the existential predicament of self-construction in an absurd world. Knowing others share those norms helps "bolster" them and makes discrepant cognitions less consequential (Festinger, 1957, p. 177). Imagined agreement of ingroup others also directly fortifies opinion certainty (Holtz & Miller, 1985; Kruglanski, Shah, Pierro, & Mannetti, 2002). If after being bolstered and fortified one's personal views are still shaky, groups also often have authoritative figureheads that one can submit to (e.g., President, Pope, Guru, or God), thereby relinquishing responsibility for choice. Finally, group identification may also help people disidentify from idiosyncratic aspects of the self that are threatened or uncertain (Mussweiller, Gabriel, & Bodenhausen, 2000; cf. Shah, Kruglanski, & Thompson, 1998).

In Study 3a (McGregor et al., 2001, Study 2), participants in a PU condition (as in Studies 1b and 1c) described their self-elements as being more communal in theme than did control-condition participants. Study 3b (Haji & McGregor, 2002) investigated whether thinking about PU and failure would cause intergroup bias (about Canada and Islam), especially among high "personal need for structure" (PNS) individuals who are particularly drawn to cognitive clarity (Neuberg & Newsom, 1993). After filling out the PNS scale, participants were randomly assigned to either a PU or a control condition (as in Studies 1b, 1c, and 3a) and then to either a failure or success condition. In the failure condition they wrote about a recent vocational failure, and in the success condition they wrote about a recent vocational success. They then evaluated the outgroup and ingroup institutions, Islam and Canada.

Results for evaluations of Islam indicated two significant main effects (with no PNS effects). Evaluations of Islam were most negative in the PU and failure conditions. Results for evaluations of Canada revealed a significant three-way interaction. Evaluations of Canada were most positive among high PNS individuals in the PU and failure conditions. These results indicate that people respond to PU and failure (which presumably exposes uncertainty) by leaning on group identifications. Future research is needed to determine why defensive derogation of Islam was not moderated by PNS. Perhaps the post-911 media coverage rendered Islam a clear outgroup institution for North Americans, regardless of PNS level.

If group identification is an effective IC strategy, then focusing on important group identifications should decrease the subjective salience of problematic aspects of one's individual identity, and should also reduce subsequent defensiveness. So-Jin Kang and I conducted two studies to investigate these ideas. In both studies, after having participants think about their PUs, we assessed the extent to which making important group identifications salient would decrease participants' bias in a different intergroup context. In Study 3c (Kang & McGregor, 2003, Study 1), after writing about their difficult personal dilemmas, Canadian participants were randomly assigned to either describe a meaningful (i.e., personally important) or a nonmeaningful group to which they belonged. Participants in the meaningful-group condition subsequently showed less derogation of anti-Canadian targets than those in the non–meaningful-group condition. As in Studies 3a and b, this effect was not moderated by self-esteem.

In Study 3d (aspects reported in Kang & McGregor, 2003 Study 2; McGregor, Kang, & Marigold, 2004, Study 3), all participants completed a self-esteem scale, then wrote about a personal dilemma, and then described the positive qualities of a group to which they belonged. They were then randomly assigned to either describe their similarities to or differences from the group as a means of manipulating group identification. The manipulation check indicated that participants in the similarities condition indeed rated themselves as being more similar to the group than participants in the differences condition (i.e., more similar in attitudes, beliefs, values, priorities, and core qualities). Most important, on the main dependent variable there was more intergroup bias in the differences condition than the similarities condition, i.e., more superior ratings of ingroup over outgroup targets. (The targets were not related to the group described in the initial group-identification manipulation.)

Study 3d also assessed whether ingroup-similarity salience would reduce subjective salience of PUs (as assessed in Study 1c and Study 2). Results indicated a significant ingroup-similarity salience x HSE interaction. Subjective salience of PUs was significantly lower in the ingroup similarities condition than the differences condition among HSEs, but not among LSEs. This result suggests that HSEs are not only able to mask PUs with successes (as in Study 2) but that they are also able to mask them with positive group identifications (cf. Crocker, Thompson, McGraw, & Ingerman, 1987; Mussweiler et al., 2000).

Together the results of Studies 3a–d are consistent with the view that group identification is an IC strategy that can, at least among HSEs, help reduce the subjective salience of PUs. Future research is needed to determine why, in Study 3d, group identification decreased defensiveness for all participants but decreased salience of PUs only for HSEs. One possibility is that whereas HSEs use group identification to take their mind off PUs, LSEs use it to feel safe, close, and connected with others. Another possibility is that whereas the group identification in Studies 3a, 3b, and 3c was a non-self-aggrandizing form that even LSEs could have been comfortable with, in 3d the instructions explicitly required participants to discuss positive qualities of their ingroup, which may have made LSEs self-conscious and thus unable to hide from their PUs (cf. Vohs & Heatherton, 2001). Other research also suggests that LSEs may engage in defenses yet not reap the cognitive benefits of them. Mikulincer and Florian (2000) found that participants with an anxious attachment style responded to threatening death thoughts by becoming more judgmental of social deviants, but that this kind of worldview defense did not decrease death-thought accessibility for them. It did decrease death-thought accessibility for participants with an avoidant attachment style, however. Anxious and avoidant attachment styles have been linked to LSE and HSE, respectively (Brennan, Clark, & Shaver, 1998)

In any case, one challenge associated with group identification may be that there are many groups one could identify that promote mutually exclusive norms for guiding behavior. Thus, group identification may help to alleviate PU when a dominant ingroup is salient but may leave individuals vulnerable to conflict and PU when competing groups vie for relative legitimacy. The intergroup bias response to PU found in the foregoing research may represent people's attempts to bolster the relative legitimacy of their groups.

IC STRATEGY 4: CONVICTION AND EXTREMISM

The finding that PU and self-threats can cause zealous group identification raises the question of whether individuals might also react to PU with other kinds of zeal. Indeed, a theme of exaggerated conviction seems to run through the three previously mentioned IC strategies. There is a rich theoretical precedent for the hypothesis that people defend against PU and self-threats with defensive zeal and conviction (see McGregor, 2003, for review). Indeed, in Freud's earliest theorizing, he proposed that repression is most often accomplished by filling one's conscious mind with an "excessively intense train of thought . . . contrary to the one which is to be repressed" and that the "reactive thought keeps the objectionable one under repression by means of a certain surplus of intensity" (translated by Gay, 1989, p. 200). Later, he more specifically referred to such reactive thoughts as "reaction formations" that form "mental dams" to block awareness of unwanted thoughts (translated by Gay, 1989, pp. 261–262). Rokeach (1960, pp. 690–70) similarly concluded "the closed system is . . . the total network of psychoanalytic defense mechanisms organized together to . . . shield a vulnerable mind." The following experiments investigated whether participants would respond to PU with defensive conviction and false consensus about their opinions and self-definitions, and whether doing so would decrease subjective salience of PUs. Exaggerated perceptions of social consensus can be a means of bolstering conviction (Holtz & Miller, 1985).

In Study 4a (McGregor & Marigold, 2003, Study 2), after filling out a self-esteem scale, participants were randomly assigned to a PU or control condition (as in Studies 1b, 1c, 3a, and 3b). For the main dependent variables, they rated their conviction (certainty and absence of ambivalence) about their capital punishment and abortion opinions and perceived consensus (percent of social agreement) for the same opinions. Results indicated a significant interaction, with significantly higher conviction among HSEs in the PU than in the control condition, but no difference between conditions among LSEs. There were no significant effects for consensus.

Study 4b (McGregor & Marigold, 2003, Study 1) assessed whether HSEs would respond to the same PU threat with implicit conviction about self-definition as assessed by a reaction time measure of self-concept clarity. For the dependent variable, participants responded as quickly and accurately as possible to trait adjectives that appeared on a computer screen, by pressing "me" or "not me" buttons. Faster responses were taken as evidence of self-concept clarity, a kind of conviction about the self (Campbell, 1990). A significant interaction mirrored the result found in Study 4a. Highest self-concept clarity was at HSE in the PU condition.

Studies 4a and b demonstrate that HSEs respond to PU with heightened conviction about their opinions and self-definitions but not with heightened consensus. Study 4c (McGregor & Grippen, 2003) and 4d (McGregor et al., 2004, Studies 1) investigated a "matching hypothesis" that whereas reminding participants of their inner-ongoing PUs in Studies 4a and 4b caused exaggerated inner convictions, other-imposed (i.e., by the researcher) PUs should cause participants to turn outward and exaggerate social consensus. This hypothesis was based on the idea that the domain of the defense should match the general domain of the threat because threats are poignant primes that orient people to the originating domain.

In Study 4c, other-imposed PU was induced in a classic dissonance experiment. After completing self-esteem measures, undergraduates wrote essays in favor of mandatory comprehensive exams at their university (a very unpopular idea among undergraduates). Those in the dissonance condition were told that it was their choice as to whether they agreed to write the essay, but that the experimenter would appreciate their help. Once participants agreed to write the essay (39/40 complied), the experimenter again reminded them that it was their own free choice. Participants in the control condition were simply instructed to write the essay, and were not given any choice. The logic of this classic procedure is that dissonance condition participants notice themselves "freely" writing their essays, which implies that they must have a favorable attitude toward comprehensive exams. The cognitive conflict between this implied positive attitude and their original negative one makes them feel like they do not know what they stand for, which causes a kind of PU. Consistent with the matching hypothesis, results revealed that compensatory consensus was significantly higher in the dissonance than control condition among HSEs, but not among LSEs. There were no significant conviction effects.

Study 4d (McGregor et al., 2003, Study 2) further assessed the matching hypothesis with a different manipulation of other- imposed PU, and also explored whether HSEs with low implicit self-esteem would be most defensive in the face of PU. Jordan et al. (2003) found HSEs with low implicit self-esteem to be particularly narcissistic and defensive. Following Jordan et al., we used the implicit associations test (IAT; Greenwald & Farnham, 2000) to measure implicit self-esteem. Implicit self-esteem scores are typically not correlated with explicit, self-reported self-esteem scores. They are derived from response latencies to stimuli that involve pairings of self-words with positive and negative words. After completing explicit and implicit self-esteem measures, participants were randomly assigned to either an academic-PU condition or a control condition. In the academic-PU condition they summarized a highly confusing passage about LISREL from a graduate stats textbook that was designed to shake their student identities. In the control condition they summarized a very easy passage from an undergraduate stats textbook. Dependent variables were the same as in Study 4a and 4c, conviction and consensus for opinions about capital punishment and abortion. Regression analysis results for consensus indicated a significant two-way interaction between explicit self-esteem and PU condition that was qualified by a significant three-way interaction with implicit self-esteem. The highest predicted value (PV) of consensus was at low implicit self-esteem and high explicit self-esteem in the academic-PU condition (PV = 76%). PVs ranged between 43 and 59% at the other seven combinations of implicit and explicit self-esteem and condition. There were no significant effects for conviction. Thus, consistent with the matching hypothesis, inner-ongoing uncertainties in Studies 4a and 4b caused defensive conviction and other-imposed uncertainties in Studies 4c and 4d caused defensive consensus.

Following the procedure used in Studies 1c, 2, and 3c, Study 4e investigated whether manipulated conviction salience would reduce the subjective salience of PUs (McGregor & Marigold, 2003, Study 4). All participants completed a self-esteem scale and then described a difficult personal dilemma that they were currently facing. They were then randomly assigned to either a conviction condition or a control condition. In both conditions, participants viewed a list of social issues. In the conviction condition, they wrote a paragraph about the one they had strongest convictions for. In the control condition, they wrote a paragraph about the one for which they thought politicians would have strongest conviction. In both conditions, participants were instructed to elaborate on why they (or politicians) held the opinion so strongly. Results indicated a significant self-esteem by conviction interaction on subjective salience of PUs (as assessed in Studies 1c, 2, and 3d). Subjective salience was significantly lower at HSE in the conviction condition than at any other combination of self-esteem and condition.

These results indicate that as with the self-worth and positive group-identification IC strategies, opinion conviction and consensus only reduce subjective salience for HSEs (cf. Vohs & Heatherton, 2001), and especially defensive HSEs with low implicit self-esteem. Overall, the results of Studies 4a–4e are consistent with the view that conviction and perceived consensus (which presumably bolsters conviction; cf. Holtz & Miller, 1985) can be an IC strategy that helps people cope with PU. As with the other three IC strategies, however, conviction may be difficult to maintain on its own because of awareness that other people's convictions can vary so dramatically from one's own. Thus, convictions may be more easily held if (1) they are part of one's integrated identity, (2) one esteems oneself highly, and (3) they are bolstered by group identifications. The following section describes research on a phenomenon that incorporates aspects of all four IC strategies—close personal relationships.

CLOSE PERSONAL RELATIONSHIPS: A COMPOSITE IC STRATEGY

Echoing classic themes from early symbolic interactionist perspectives on the self, Backman (1988, p. 253) argued that the "relationships persons have with kin, friends, and lovers are their strongest identity props." Indeed, self-verification research indicates that satisfied relationship partners scaffold each others' self views (Swann & Predmore, 1985). Hermans (1996) further proposed that identity is situated in interpersonal dialogue, and that identities are "polyphonic narratives" that emerge from the perspectives of both partners. Relationships may also afford some of the IC benefits of group identification. Like groups, relationship dyads often entail normative and idiosyncratic values and prescriptions for behavior and allow partners to escape from threatened personal identities (Gardner, Gabriel, & Hoschild, 2002). Further, by making each other "number one" and reflecting positive illusions to one another, partners may effectively leverage each others' feelings of self-worth (Murray, Holmes, & Griffin, 1996). Finally, relationships in individualist cultures seem to provide a socially acceptable outlet for extreme conviction. Western media abounds with maxims such as "love is the answer" and "all you need is love," and images of passionate lovers acting as purveyors of ultimate meaning for one another. In sum, the multifaceted IC value of relationships may account for Durkheim's (1951, p. 12) contention that "the more the family and community become foreign to the individual, so much the more does he become a mystery to himself, unable to escape the exasperating and agonizing question: to what purpose?"

If relationships do have IC value, then relationship threats should increase reliance on other IC strategies. In Study 5a (McGregor et al, 2004, Study 2), we categorized participants as either securely attached or nonsecurely attached, based on their attachment-style questionnaire responses (Brennan, Clark, & Shaver, 1998). They were then randomly assigned to one of two visualization conditions. In the separation condition they visualized a novel, hypothetical scenario that involved being isolated from loved ones and surrounded by strangers (an other-imposed threat). In the togetherness condition, they visualized an interaction with a loved one. For the main dependent variables, participants rated their consensus and conviction for unrelated opinions, as in Studies 4a, c, and d. Results indicated a significant interaction between attachment security and condition. Among insecure but not secure participants there was higher consensus in the separation condition than in the togetherness condition.[3] Consistent with the matching hypothesis, there were no significant conviction effects.

Study 5b (McGregor & Marigold, 2003, Study 3) investigated whether reminding participants of an inner-ongoing, relationship-related PU would cause compensatory conviction, but not consensus. The effect was expected to be highest among individuals with defensive HSE (i.e., high explicit and low implicit, as in Study 4c). After completing measures of explicit and implicit self-esteem participants were randomly assigned to a relationship-PU condition or a control condition. In the relationship-PU condition they described thoughts and feelings associated with a close relationship that they felt uncertain about. In the control condition they instead described thoughts and feelings about a friend's relationship that was uncertain. Regression results revealed a significant three-way interaction between implicit self-esteem, explicit self-esteem, and PU-condition on conviction, mirroring the pattern in Study 4c. At *high implicit self-esteem* there were no differences in conviction between the four possible combinations of condition and explicit self-esteem (all PVs were between 7.5 and 7.6 on a 10-point scale). At *low implicit self-esteem*, however, there was significantly higher conviction in the relationship-PU condition at HSE (PV = 8.4) than in either the relationship-PU condition at LSE (PV = 6.7) or the control condition at HSE (PV = 6.7). This result indicates that people with defensive HSE react to inner-ongoing relationship-related PU with heightened conviction. Consistent with the matching hypothesis there were no significant consensus effects.

To more directly assess the hypothesis that relationships serve an IC function, Study 5c (Haji & McGregor, 2003) investigated whether salience of validating relationships would decrease subjective salience of academic-PUs. Romantic partners first completed a measure of the extent to which they felt validated by their partners. They were then randomly assigned to either an academic PU or control condition (as in Study 4c). Then, to make their love relationships salient, they all wrote a paragraph about a time they felt in love with their partner. For the main dependent variable, participants then rated the subjective salience (adapted from Studies 1c, 2, 3c, and 4e) of the academic-PU threat. Regression results revealed a significant interaction such that in the academic-PU condition, subjective salience of the academic-PU threat was significantly lower for high validation partners (PV = 1.8) than low validation partners (PV = 2.4), almost as low as for low (PV = 1.5) and high (PV = 1.7) validation partners in the control condition. This result indicates that salience of validating relationships helps take people's minds off PUs.

SUMMARY AND DISCUSSION

The main results of the 16 studies described in this chapter are as follows:

1a. Integration of goals and values was associated with purpose and meaning in life.
1b. PU heightened integration of goals, values, and identifications.
1c. Integration reduced PU salience.
2. Self-worth-salience reduced PU salience.
3a. PU caused more communal goals, values, and identifications.
3b. PU and failure caused intergroup bias (especially among high PNS participants).

3c. Group identification eliminated unrelated intergroup biases after a PU threat.

3d. Group identification eliminated intergroup bias and reduced PU-salience among HSEs.

4a. PU caused compensatory conviction among HSEs.

4b. PU caused compensatory, implicit self-concept clarity among HSEs.

4c. Dissonance caused compensatory consensus among HSEs.

4d. Academic PU caused compensatory consensus among low implicit self-esteem HSEs.

4e. Conviction salience decreased PU salience.

5a. Relationship threat caused compensatory consensus among defensively attached participants.

5b. Relationship PU caused compensatory conviction among low implicit self-esteem HSEs.

5c. Love salience reduced academic-PU-salience for participants with validating relationships.

These results are consistent with the IC theory view that integration, self-worth, group identification, conviction, and romantic relationships are IC strategies that can help decrease subjective salience of PUs and self-threats. All the strategies but integration appear to be most effective for HSEs, who are most willing to risk the interpersonal censure that can be associated with self-promotion (Vohs & Heatherton, 2001). The finding that IC responses take peoples' minds off their PUs suggests an integrative perspective on theories of self-threat and defensiveness.

Self-affirmation theory (SAT) research (e.g., Steele & Liu, 1983; Steele, Spencer, & Lynch, 1993) has shown that affirmations of personal values and self-worth decrease defensiveness after topically unrelated dissonance threats. This *fluid compensation* finding has been interpreted as evidence that multifarious self-threats and affirmations trade on a common intrapsychic currency of *global self-integrity*—the superordinate image of oneself as adaptive and good. Self-evaluation maintenance (SEM) model theorists similarly interpret their fluid compensation findings as evidence that self-threats and defenses serve a superordinate need to feel good about oneself (e.g., Tesser et al., 2000). From the present perspective, however, fluid compensation arises from the ability of value and worth affirmations to take people's minds off self-threats. The parsimony of IC theory is that it does not need to posit an intrapsychic currency exchange that translates all self-relevant motives into a vague concept such as global self-integrity. According to IC theory, specific affirmations of integration, self-worth, group identification, and values reduce defensiveness because they distract attention from threats. Indeed, Studies 1c, 2, 3d, 4e, and 5c resurrect the distraction hypothesis that Steele and Liu (1983) disposed of and confirm that self-affirmations take people's minds off dissonant self-thoughts. These findings are not necessarily incompatible with SAT and SEM; rather, they illuminate the underlying mechanism.[4]

The personality systems interactions (PSI) theory concept of *extension memory* (Kuhl & Koole, Chapter 26, this volume) also has considerable theoretical overlap with the functional view of identity proposed by IC theory. According to PSI theory, the *implicit self-representation* aspect of extension memory is a collection of self-central needs, motives, values, and autobiographical experiences, and focusing on it provides a means of shaking off negative implicit affect and maintaining an *action orientation*. The IC research presented in this chapter could be seen as testing whether components of the implicit self-representation construct (integration, self-worth, group identifications, and convictions) are capable of decreasing subjective salience of PUs and threats. Although PSI theory puts more emphasis on implicit processes, both theories highlight the ability of adaptive people to use aspects of the self to redirect attention and restore self-regulatory efficiency.

Finally, from the IC perspective, the mortality salience threats used in terror management theory (TMT; Greenberg, Solomon, & Pyszczynski, 1997; Solomon, Greenberg, & Pyszczynski, Chapter 2, this volume) research may be such poignant causes of defensiveness because mortality salience is a composite threat that highlights PU and simultaneously undercuts several ambient IC strategies. Mortality salience highlights PU about what happens after death and about the meaning of one's goals and life. It conflicts with *all* personal goals, thereby likely activating the BIS. It humiliates grandiose pretensions. And it presents the final separation from one's valued groups and relationships. Worldview-defense responses to mortality salience, such as derogating outgroup members who do not share one's values, are viewed as composite IC reactions that bolster self-worth, group identification, and conviction. Indeed, TMT research has found that worldview defenses serve the same function as IC strategies—they take people's minds off threatening thoughts (Greenberg, Arndt, Schimel, Pyszczynski, & Solomon, 2001). Further, worldview defenses may be viable for LSEs as well as HSEs because zeal for culturally consensual values brings less risk for social censure (which LSEs fear; Vohs & Heatherton, 2001) than does idiosyncratic zeal.[5]

In sum, morality salience may be a powerful composite threat that fans the flames of PU and simultaneously strips away the varied strands of defensive insulation that people use to defend against it. Worldview defense may be appealing because it is a powerful composite defense that helps restore the various IC strands that have been stripped way. TMT theorists propose that that death has special status as a psychological threat, because in past research other threats such as thinking about pain, failure, social exclusion, or future worries have failed to cause the same kinds of defensiveness. One of the insights afforded by the research described in this chapter is that specific self-threats related to uncertainty, failure, and separation *can* cause defensive reactions that resemble worldview defenses. Moreover, it isolates what I propose are specific active ingredients in worldview defense—integration, self-worth, group identification, and conviction—and shows how each serves the same psychological function as worldview defense. As such, it could be viewed as empirically unpacking both the mortality salience and worldview defense constructs and rendering them compatible with other research on self-threat and defensiveness. In doing so, it holds promise for integrating self-related theories in social psychology that, in my view, have remained unnecessarily distinct.

IC, CULTURE, ROMANTIC LOVE, AND RELIGION

The starting assumption of IC theory is that people need to feel clear about who they are so that they can use their identities as reliable guides for action. In the foregoing experiments Canadian undergraduates responded to PU with IC strategies that mask uncertainties and sharpen the clarity and authority of the independent self. Recent cross-cultural research provides additional, indirect support for the self-regulatory assumptions of IC theory. Whereas defensive self-worth and intergroup bias are ubiquitous in individualist cultures such as Canada and the United States, they are less apparent in interdependent cultures such as Japan (Heine et al., 1999). Indeed, in Japan, effect sizes of worldview defenses after morality salience (Heine, Harihara, & Niiya, 2002) are about a third as big as they typically are in the United States. From the present perspective, this is because people in collectivist cultures rely less on personal identity as a guide for action. Indeed, it has been suggested that in collectivist cultures "behavior is . . . organized by what the actor perceives to be the thoughts, feelings, and actions of *others*" (Markus & Kitayama, 1991, p. 226). The Western reliance on personal identity for guiding action, and the attendant need to defensively consolidate personal identity when it is threatened, may arise from the influence of analytic, Greek philosophical emphases on separation of parts (i.e., self from others), abstract essence, and personal agency. Eastern reliance on social and contextual cues for guiding action, and absence of self-defensiveness, may arise from the influence of holistic, Confucian philosophical emphases on the individual as an inseparable part of a complex social system, and the idea that "the behavior of the individual should be guided by the expectations of the group" (Nisbett, Peng, Choi, & Norenzeyan, 2001, p. 292).

The differential use of the personal identity as a guide for action in individualist and collectivist cultures may explain why romantic love and monotheistic religions are more prominent in contemporary individualist cultures that have been influenced by Greek philosophy than in collectivist Eastern ones that have not (Armstrong, 1993; Dion & Dion, 1993; Durant, 1954). From the IC perspective, romantic love and monotheism are composite IC strategies that decrease subjective salience of PUs. They are particularly appealing to independent individuals living in individualist cultures that emphasize personal autonomy and control because for them, IC and absence of PU are critical for making decisions about what to do.

Romantic love facilitates personal integration as lovers co-construct life stories together (Hermans, 1996). It facilitates self-worth as lovers reflect positive illusions to one another (Murray et al., 1996). Romantic lovers also "fall" and become "lost" in love, notions that imply a surrender of the self to identification with the dyad. Moreover, romantic lovers often indulge in extremes of passionate devotion.

Monotheistic religions similarly provide multifaceted IC support. They facilitate personal integration by advocating truth, prayer, humility, and confession—practices to help the individual integrate self-awareness with revealed scriptural truth. They scaffold self-worth by reminding individuals that they are worthy of love from the ultimate source of goodness, and that this worthiness is not contingent upon personal status or success. They encourage brotherhood and identification with the community of believers and participation in group rituals and worship. Finally, monotheistic religions have historically encouraged faith, self-sacrifice, martyrdom, and zealous conviction. Indeed, the first three commandments shared by Judaism, Christianity, and Islam highlight the importance of single-minded devotion to God. Future research should investigate whether PU and self-threats lead religious individuals to heighten their religious identification and conviction, and whether salience of religious convictions can decrease subjective salience of PUs and self-threats.

CONCLUDING COMMENTS

The IC theory presented in this chapter proposes that defensiveness is rooted in the need to maintain an authoritative guide for navigating PU about what to do and be. The results presented are consistent with this view but do not conclusively rule out alternative explanations that posit self-esteem threat, separation, or fear of death as master motivators of defensiveness. The search for a foundational motive is complicated by the theoretical interrelatedness of all of the candidate threats, and by the fact that priming of one likely activates the others due to shared negative valence and self-relevance. Nevertheless, if there is a master motive, aversion to uncertainty and goal conflict seems most evolutionarily primal. Even relatively nonsocial pigeons and fish show evidence of distress when their goals are blocked or uncertain, a response that seems to be rooted in the hippocampus (Gray, 1982). Needs for the kinds of status and belongingness that characterize human culture, however, seem likely to have evolved later, in the context of primate social groups (Sedikides & Skowronski, 1997). Furthermore, if fear of death is innate, it must have evolved even later, because death is an abstract concept that one must have a neocortex to comprehend. Animals that do not have a neocortex can fear pain but not death. Finally, even if an annihilation-anxiety module had recently evolved, it would have to have served an adaptive (nonparalyzing) function significant enough for those who had it to outlive and outmate their more sanguine fellows. It is not clear then, why worldview defenses that serve to block awareness of mortality and the related anxiety should also be adaptive.

In any case, evolutionary primacy does not guarantee motivational primacy, and the possibility remains that threats related to uncertainty, self-evaluation, separation, and death are aversive for unique reasons. Future research will determine whether the IC account of self-defensiveness is parsimonious and generative or overly reductionistic. In the meantime, at very least, the research reviewed in this chapter indicates that PU is a poignant self-threat that people spontaneously mask with integration, self-worth, intergroup bias, and conviction. It further suggests the possibility that social phenomena such as zealous nationalism and religious fundamentalism may be animated by their ability to provide relief from PU and self-threats.

NOTES

1. This may be most true for people in individualist cultures who have independent self-construals. People with interdependent self-construals may be more inclined to rely on external guides for deciding, such as situational cues or traditional norms.
2. The 19-item felt-uncertainty scale (*mixed, uneasy, torn, bothered, preoccupied, confused, unsure of self or goals, contradictory, distractible, unclear, of two minds, muddled, restless, confused about identity, jumbled, uncomfortable, conflicted, indecisive, and chaotic*) was unifactorial and highly reliable (Cronbach alpha = .91).
3. As in Mikulincer and Florian (2000), anxious and avoidant participants were equally defensive.
4. One apparent inconsistency is that Steele et al. (1993) found HSEs to be *least* defensive, but in the present research they were *most* defensive. It may be that the Steele et al. findings were unique to their unusual measure of HSE, which specifically assessed secure and stable HSE. Secure and stable HSE has been associated with low defensiveness in other research (Jordan et al., 2003; Kernis, Cornell, Sun, Berry, & Harlow, 1993).
5. Harmon-Jones et al. (1997) found HSEs to be *least* defensive after mortality salience, but their procedure also ensured temporally stable subset of HSE, which has been found to be particularly nondefensive (Kernis et al., 1993).

REFERENCES

Abrams, D., & Hogg, M. A. (1999). *Social identity and social cognition*. Oxford, UK: Blackwell.

Allport, G. W. (1949/1937). *Personality: A psychological interpretation*. London: Constable.

Armstrong, K. (1993). *A history of God: The 4,000–year quest of Judaism, Christianity, and Islam*. New York: Ballantine Books.

Backman, C. W. (1988). The self: A dialectical approach. In L. Berkowitz (Ed.), *Advances in experimental social psychology* (pp. 229–257). San Diego: Academic Press.

Baumeister, R. F. (1987). How the self became a problem: A psychological review of historical research. *Journal of Personality and Social Psychology, 52,* 163–176.

Baumeister, R. F. (1991). *Meanings of life.* New York: Guilford Press.

Bizer, G. Y., & Krosnick, J. A. (2001). Exploring the structure of strength-related attitude features: The relation between attitude importance and attitude accessibility. *Journal of Personality and Social Psychology, 81,* 566–586.

Brennan, K. A., Clark, C. L., & Shaver, P. R. (1998). Self-report measurement of adult attachment: An integrative overview. In J. A. Simpson & W. S. Rholes (Eds.), *Attachment theory and close relationships* (pp. 46–76). New York: Guilford Press.

Campbell, J. D. (1990). Self-esteem and clarity of the self-concept. *Journal of Personality and Social Psychology, 59,* 538–549.

Crocker, J., Thompson, L. L., McGraw, K. M., & Ingerman, C. (1987). Downward comparison, prejudice, and evaluations of others: Effects of self-esteem and threat. *Journal of Personality and Social Psychology, 52,* 907–917.

Cushman, P. (1990). Why the self is empty. *American Psychologist, 45,* 599–611.

Dion, K. K., & Dion, K. L. (1993). Individualistic and collectivistic perspectives on gender and the cultural context of love and intimacy. *Journal of Social Issues, 49,* 53–69.

Dodgson, P. G., & Wood, J. V. (1998). Self-Esteem and the cognitive accessibility of strengths and weaknesses after failure. *Journal of Personality and Social Psychology, 75,* 178–197.

Durant, W. (1954). *Our oriental heritage.* New York: Simon & Schuster.

Durkheim, E. (1951). *Suicide: A study in sociology.* Glencoe, IL: Free Press. (Original work published 1897)

Festinger, L. (1954). A theory of social comparison processes. *Human Relations, 7,* 117–140.

Festinger, L. (1957). *A theory of cognitive dissonance.* Evanston, IL: Row, Peterson & Co.

Fromm, E. (1941). *Escape from freedom.* New York: Holt, Rinehart, & Winston.

Gardner, W. L., Gabriel, S., & Hochschild, L. (2002). When you and I are "we," you are not threatening: The role of self-expansion in social comparisons. *Journal of Personality and Social Psychology, 82,* 239–251.

Gay, P. (1989). *The Freud reader.* New York: Norton.

Gray, J. A. (1982). *The neuropsychology of anxiety: An enquiry into the functions of the septo-hippocampal system.* New York: Oxford University Press.

Greenberg, J., Arndt, J., Schimel, J., Pyszczynski, T., & Solomon, S. (2001). Clarifying the function of mortality salience-induced worldview defense: Renewed suppression or reduced accessibility of death-related thoughts? *Journal of Experimental Social Psychology, 37,* 70–76.

Greenberg, J., & Pyszczynski, T. (1986). Persistent high self-focus after failure and low self-focus after success: The depressive self-focusing style. *Journal of Personality and Social Psychology, 50,* 1039–1044.

Greenberg, J., Solomon, S., & Pyszczynski, T. (1997). Terror management theory of self-esteem and cultural worldviews: Empirical assessments and conceptual refinements. In M. P. Zanna (Ed.), *Advances in experimental social psychology* (pp. 61–139). Hillsdale, NJ: Academic Press.

Greenwald, A. G., & Farnham, S. D. (2000). Using the implicit association test to measure self-esteem and self-concept. *Journal of Personality and Social Psychology, 79,* 102–1038.

Haji, R., & McGregor, I. (2002). *Compensatory conviction and extremism about Canada and Islam: Responses to uncertainty and self-worth threat.* Poster presented at the annual meeting of the Society for the Psychological Study of Social Issues, Toronto.

Haji R., & McGregor, I. (2003). Raw data, York University, Toronto.

Harmon-Jones, E., Simon, L., Greenberg, J., Pyszczynski, T., Solomon, S., & McGregor, H. (1997). Terror management theory and self-esteem: Evidence that increased self-esteem reduces mortality salience effects. *Journal of Personality and Social Psychology, 72,* 24–36.

Heine, S. J., Harihara, M., & Niiya, Y. (2002). Terror management in Japan. *Asian Journal of Social Psychology, 5,* 187–196.

Heine, S. J., Lehman, D. R., Markus, H. R., & Kitayama, S. (1999). Is there a universal need for positive self-regard? *Psychological Review, 106,* 766–794.

Hermans, H. J. M. (1996). Voicing the self: From information processing to dialogical interchange. *Psychological Bulletin, 119,* 31–50.

Holtz, R., & Miller, N. (1985). Assumed similarity and opinion certainty. *Journal of Personality and Social Psychology, 48,* 890–898.

Jordan, C. H., Spencer, S. J., Zanna, M. P., Hoshino-Browne, E., & Correll, J. (2003). Secure and defensive self-esteem. *Journal of Personality and Social Psychology, 85,* 969–978.

Kang, S., & McGregor, I. (2003). *Belonging and tolerance: Group-identification can decrease intergroup bias.* Unpublished manuscript, York University, Toronto, Canada.

Kernis, M. H., Cornell, D. P., Sun, C. R., Berry, A., & Harlow, T. (1993). There's more to self-esteem than whether it is high or low: The importance of stability of self-esteem. *Journal of Personality and Social Psychology, 65,* 2290–1204.

Kruglanski, A. W., Shah, J. Y., Pierro, A., & Mannetti, L. (2002). When similarity breeds content: Need for closure and the allure of homogeneous and self-resembling groups. *Journal of Personality and Social Psychology, 83,* 648–662.

Markus, H. R., & Kitayama, S. (1991). Culture and the self: Implications for cognition, emotion, and motivation. *Journal of Personality and Social Psychology, 98,* 224–253.

McAdams, D. P. (1993). *The stories we live by: Personal myths and the making of the self.* New York: Morrow.

McGregor, I. (1998). *An identity consolidation view of social phenomena: Theory and research.* Unpublished doctoral dissertation, University of Waterloo, Waterloo, ON Canada.

McGregor, I. (2002, October). *Compensatory conviction as repression: Masking personal uncertainties with defensive zeal.* Paper presented at the annual meeting of the Society for Experimental Social Psychology, Columbus, OH.

McGregor, I. (2003). Defensive zeal: Compensatory conviction about attitudes, values, goals, groups, and self-definition in the face of personal uncertainty. In S. J. Spencer, S. Fein, M. P. Zanna, & J. M. Olson (Eds.), *Motivated social perception: The Ontario Symposium* (Vol. 9, pp. 73–92). Mahwah, NJ: Erlbaum.

McGregor, I., & Crippen, M. (2003). Raw data, York University, Toronto, Canada.

McGregor, I., & Holmes, J. G. (1999). How storytelling shapes memory and impressions of relationship events over time. *Journal of Personality and Social Psychology, 76,* 403–419.

McGregor, I., Kang, S., & Marigold, D. C. (2004). Exaggerated consensus after self-threats: Strength in imaginary numbers. Unpublished manuscript, York University, Toronto, Canada.

McGregor, I., & Little, B. R. (1998). Personal projects, happiness, and meaning: On doing well and being yourself. *Journal of Personality and Social Psychology, 74,* 494–512.

McGregor, I., & Marigold, D. C. (2003). Defensive zeal and the uncertain self: What makes you so sure? *Journal of Personality and Social Psychology, 85,* 838–852.

McGregor, I., Zanna, M. P., Holmes, J. G., & Spencer, S. J. (2001). Compensatory conviction in the face of personal uncertainty: Going to extremes and being oneself. *Journal of Personality and Social Psychology, 80,* 472–488.

Mikulincer, M., & Florian, V. (2000). Exploring individual differences in reactions to mortality salience: Does attachment style regulate terror management mechanisms? *Journal of Personality and Social Psychology, 79,* 260–273.

Murray, H. A. (1938). *Explorations in personality.* New York: Oxford University Press.

Murray, S. L., Holmes, J. G., & Griffin, D. W. (1996). The self-fulfilling nature of positive illusions in romantic relationships: Love is not blind, but prescient. *Journal of Personality and Social Psychology, 71,* 1155–1180.

Mussweiler, T., Gabriel, S., & Bodenhausen, G. V. (2000). Shifting social identities as a strategy for deflecting threatening social comparisons. *Journal of Personality and Social Psychology, 79,* 398–409.

Neuberg, S. L., & Newsom, J. T. (1993). Personal need for structure: Individual differences in the desire for simple structure. *Journal of Personality and Social Psychology, 65,* 113–131.

Newby-Clark, I. R., McGregor, I., & Zanna, M. P. (2002). Thinking and caring about cognitive inconsistency: When and for whom does attitudinal ambivalence feel uncomfortable? *Journal of Personality and Social Psychology, 82,* 157–166.

Nisbett, R. E., Peng, K., Choi, I., & Norenzayan, A. (2001). Culture and systems of thought: Holistic versus analytic cognition. *Psychological Review, 108,* 291–310.

Roberts, B. W., & Robins, R. W. (2000). Broad dispositions, broad aspirations: The intersection of personality traits and major life goals. *Personality and Social Psychology Bulletin, 26*, 1284–1296.

Rokeach, M. (1960). *The open and close mind: Investigations into the nature of belief systems and personality systems.* New York: Basic Books.

Sartre, J. P. (1989). *No exit and three other plays* (Stuart Gilbert, Trans.). New York: Vintage.

Sartre, J. P. (1956). *Being and nothingness* (Hazel Barnes, Trans.). New York: Pocket Books.

Scheier, M. F., & Carver, C. S. (1988). A model of behavioral self regulation: Translating intention into action. In L. Berkowitz (Ed.), *Advances in experimental social psychology* (pp. 303–339). New York: Academic Press.

Sedikides, C., & Skowronski, J. J. (1997). The symbolic self in evolutionary context. *Personality and Social Psychology Review, 1*, 80–102.

Shah, J. Y., Kruglanski, A. W., & Thompson, E. (1998). Membership has its (epistemic) rewards: Need for closure effects on in-group bias. *Journal of Personality and Social Psychology, 75*, 383–393.

Simon, L., Greenberg, J., & Brehm, J. (1995). Trivialization: The forgotten mode of dissonance reduction. *Journal of Personality and Social Psychology, 68*, 247–260.

Smith, S. M., & Petty, R. E. (1995). Personality moderators of mood congruency effects on cognition: The role of self-esteem and negative mood regulation. *Journal of Personality and Social Psychology, 68*, 1092–1107.

Sorrentino, R. M., & Roney, C. J. R. (2000). *The uncertain mind: Individual differences in facing the unknown.* Philadelphia: Psychology Press.

Steele, C. M., & Liu, T. J. (1983). Dissonance processes as self-affirmation. *Journal of Personality and Social Psychology, 45*, 5–19.

Steele, C. M., Spencer, S. J., & Lynch, M. (1993). Self-image resilience and dissonance: The role of affirmational resources. *Journal of Personality and Social Psychology, 64*, 885–896.

Swann Jr., W. B., & Predmore, S. C. (1985). Intimates as agents of social support: Sources of consolation or despair. *Journal of Personality and Social Psychology, 49*, 1609–1617.

Terry, D. J., & Hogg, M. A. (2000). *Attitudes, behavior, and social context: The role of norms and group membership.* Mahwah, NJ: Erlbaum.

Tesser, A., Crepaz, N., Collins, J. C., Cornell, D., & Beach, S. R. H. (2000). Confluence of self-esteem regulation mechanisms: On integrating the self-zoo. *Personality and Social Psychology Bulletin, 26*, 1476–1489.

Vohs, K. D., & Heatherton, T. F. (2001). Self-esteem and threats to self: Implications for self-construals and interpersonal perceptions. *Journal of Personality and Social Psychology, 81*, 1103–1118.

Wenzlaff, R. M., & Bates, D. E. (2000). The relative efficacy of concentration and suppression strategies of mental control. *Personality and Social Psychology Bulletin, 26*, 1200–1212.

Wood, J. V., Giordano-Beech, M., Taylor, K. L., Michela, J. L., & Gaus, V. (1994). Strategies of social comparison among people with low self-esteem: Self-protection and self-enhancement. *Journal of Personality and Social Psychology, 67*, 713–731.

Chapter 13

Nostalgia

Conceptual Issues and Existential Functions

CONSTANTINE SEDIKIDES
TIM WILDSCHUT
DENISE BADEN

> SAMMLER: I see you have these recollections.
> WALLACE: Well, I need them. Everybody needs his memories. They keep
> the wolf of insignificance from the door.
> —SAUL BELLOW, *Mr. Sammler's Planet* (1970, p. 190)

Approximately 2,800 years ago, a blind poet wandered from city to city in Greece telling a tall tale—that of a nobleman, war hero, and daring adventurer who did not catch sight of his homeland for 20 long years. The poet was Homer and the larger-than-life character was Odysseus. Homer sang the epic adventures of cunning Odysseus who fought the Trojan War for 10 years and labored for another 10 on a die-hard mission to return to his homeland, the island of Ithaca, and reunite with his loyal wife, Penelope, and their son, Telemachus. Three of the 10 return years were spent on sea, facing the wrath of Gods, monsters, and assorted evil-doers. The other 7 were spent on the island of Ogygia, in the seducing arms of a nymph, the beautiful and possessive Calypso. Yet, despite this *dolce vita*, Odysseus never took his mind off Ithaca, refusing Calypso's offer to make him immortal. On the edge of ungratefulness, he confided to his mistress, "Full well I acknowledge Prudent Penelope cannot compare with your stature or beauty, for she is only a mortal, and you are immortal and ageless. Nevertheless it is she whom I daily desire and pine for. Therefore I long for my home and to see the day of returning" (Homer, *The Odyssey*, trans. 1921, Book V, pp. 78–79). [1]

Return was continually on Odysseus' mind, and the Greek word for it is *nostos*. His burning wish for *nostos* afflicted unbearable suffering on Odysseus, and the Greek word for it is *algos*. Nostalgia, then, is the psychological suffering caused by unrelenting yearning to return to one's homeland. The term "nostalgia" was actually coined by the Swiss physician Johannes Hofer (1688/1934), although references to its meaning can be found in Hippocrates, Caesar, and the Bible.

HISTORICAL AND CONTEMPORARY CONCEPTUALIZATIONS OF NOSTALGIA

In its 300 years of scholarly treatment, nostalgia has journeyed from the conceptual lows of brain disease and despair to the conceptual highs of positive emotionality and happiness. We briefly review these perspectives next.

Historical Conceptions

Nostalgia as Medical Disease

Initially, nostalgia was conceptualized as a *medical or neurological disease*. Hofer (1688/1934) studied the behavioral symptoms of Swiss mercenaries fighting on behalf of various European rulers in far-away lands. Characteristic symptoms included emotional lability ranging from despondency to bouts of weeping, anorexia, and suicide attempts. Searching for physiological and neuroanatomical explanations, Hofer (1688/1934) suggested that the mercenaries suffered from nostalgia (or homesickness), "a cerebral disease of essentially demonic cause" (p. 387). The cause of the disease was "the quite continuous vibration of animal spirits through those fibers of the middle brain in which impressed traces of ideas of the Fatherland still cling" (p. 384). It did not get much better for a while. In 1732, the German–Swiss physician J. J. Scheuchzer argued that nostalgia was due to "a sharp differential in atmospheric pressure causing excessive body pressurization, which in turn drove blood from the heart to the brain, thereby producing the observed affliction of sentiment" (cited in Davis, 1979, p. 2; see also Zwingmann, 1959). It was widely believed at that time that nostalgia was a disease confined to the Swiss. In a race to offer the most bizarre explanation of them all (and our personal favorite), military physicians speculated that the cause of the disease was the unremitting clanging of cowbells in the Alps, which inflicted damage to the eardrum and brain cells (Davis, 1979).

The definition of nostalgia as a medical disease persisted in the 18th and 19th centuries, although the condition was no longer considered specific to the Swiss. Other populations, most notably soldiers fighting in the French armies and the American Civil War, were loosely studied and occasionally treated by physicians (Rosen, 1975).

Nostalgia as Psychiatric Disorder

By the end of the 19th century and the beginning of the 20th century, the definition of nostalgia had shifted from brain to *psychiatric or psychosomatic disorder* (Batcho, 1998). The symptoms now included anxiety and sadness, weakness and loss of appetite, insomnia and fever (Havlena & Holak, 1991). Nostalgia was regarded as a form of melancholia (McCann, 1941).

This latter conception of nostalgia was carried into the mid-20th century by the psychodynamic tradition (Sohn, 1983). Nostalgia was branded an "immigrant psychosis" (Frost, 1938, p. 801), a "monomaniacal obsessive mental state causing intense unhappiness" (Fodor, 1950, p. 25), arising from a subconscious yearning to return to one's fetal state, and a "mentally repressive compulsive disorder" (Fodor, 1950, p. 25). These perceptions drifted into the late part of the century. Kaplan (1987) considered nostalgia a variant of depression, and Castelnuovo-Tedesco (1980) labeled it "a regressive manifestation closely related to the issue of loss, grief, incomplete mourning, and, finally, depression" (p. 110). It is worth noting that this perspective equated nostalgia with homesickness and bounded it to four populations: soldiers, seamen, immigrants, and first-year boarding or university students (Cox, 1988; Jackson, 1986).

Contemporary Conceptions

Nostalgia as Distinct from Homesickness

In the latter part of the 20th century, nostalgia acquired a distinct conceptual status among both laypeople and researchers. The majority of college students regard nostalgia as different from homesickness. For example, they associate the words "warm, old times, childhood, and yearning" more frequently with the term "nostalgia" than with the term "homesickness" (Davis, 1979). Likewise, researchers make a clear distinction between the two terms. Along with Davis, Werman (1977) argued in favor of separate empirical traditions. Indeed, the two literatures have now diverged, with homesickness focusing mostly on the psychological difficulties accompanying the transition to boarding school or university, at home or abroad (Brewin, Furhnam, & Howes, 1989; Fisher, 1989; Van Tilburg, Vingerhoets, & van Heck, 1996). This divergeness would perhaps disappoint Odysseus, as, for him, nostalgia and homesickness were one and the same.

With all due respect to history's most famous émigré, we also conceptualize nostalgia as distinct from homesickness. Nostalgia is yearning for aspects of one's past, a yearning that may include but is not limited to one's homeland. This yearning may pertain, for example, to events, persons, or sights. Furthermore, we maintain that nostalgia is an experience that transcends a rather small, if not marginalized, set of groups (e.g., soldiers, seamen, immigrants, and students on the move). In addition, we maintain that nostalgia transcends age, as findings contradict the notion that nostalgia is limited to well-functioning adults or a specific age group such as elderly (Batcho, 1995, 1998; Mills & Coleman, 1994). Nostalgia is a universal experience, present and prevalent across the lifespan.

Nostalgia as a Positive Emotion

The New Oxford Dictionary of English defines nostalgia as "a sentimental longing or wistful affection for the past, typically for a period or place with happy personal associations" (1998, p. 1266). The nostalgic experience, then, involves positivity and even happiness. Researchers' definitions of nostalgia follow suit, although they are substantially more differentiated (Batcho, 1998; Davis, 1979; Jackson, 1986).

We are also inclined to regard nostalgia a positive experience. Specifically, we consider nostalgia an emotion—a predominantly positive, self-relevant emotion. As such, nostalgia has an affective structure and fulfills crucial functions.

The Existential Function of Nostalgia

We propose that nostalgia serves existential functions. Nostalgia is an existential exercise in search for identity and meaning, a weapon in internal confrontations with existential dilemmas, and a mechanism for reconnecting with important others. Nostalgia keeps "the wolf of insignificance from the door" (Bellow, 1970, p. 190).

THE EMOTION OF NOSTALGIA: STRUCTURE AND FUNCTIONS

We proceed by considering the affective structure and psychological functions of nostalgia.

Affective Structure of Nostalgia

Is Nostalgia an Emotion?

Emotion theorists are unanimous in labeling nostalgia an emotion, and we concur. When it comes, however, to more nuanced classifications, there is disagreement.

Authors who endorse the distinction between basic and nonbasic emotions argue that nostalgia belongs to the latter category. For example, Kemper (1987) regarded nostalgia as a secondary, culturally influenced, emotion, whereas Frijda (1986) argued that nostalgia lacks specificity of modes of physiological activation, action readiness, and expression. Theorists, however, who reject or are skeptical of the basic–nonbasic emotion dichotomy provide a more textured script, in our opinion. Ortony, Clore, and Collins (1988) cast nostalgia in the group of well-being emotions. They argue that these emotions represent valenced reactions to outcomes rather than guiding goals or action. In particular, nostalgia is part of the negative subgroup of well-being emotions, and more specifically it belongs either to the distress emotions or loss emotions. In either case, nostalgia involves sadness or mourning about the past. Along similar lines, Johnson-Laird and Oatley (1989) highlight the dual nature of nostalgia, a positive experience with tones of loss. They cast nostalgia in the complex emotion category. Such emotions differ from basic emotions in that they reflect high-level cognitive appraisal and have propositional content. Nostalgia, they argue, is a happiness-related emotion. However, induction of nostalgia brings about mild discontent and sadness, due to the contrast between a desirable past and an undesirable present.

Our own view resonates partially with that of Johnson-Laird and Oatley (1989). Like them, we think that nostalgia involves a high degree of cognitive appraisal. Also like them, we regard nostalgia as a positive emotion, and we suggest that nostalgia involves a contrast between the present and the past. Unlike them, however, we do not think that this contrast is always direct or explicit, nor do we think that nostalgia always, or even typically, induces sadness. Instead, we suggest that nostalgia is often triggered by intrapersonal, social, or environmental stimuli and that it may sometimes involve minimal or implicit comparison of the past with the present. In addition, we think that nostalgia spawns more positive than negative intrapsychic (e.g., affective) outcomes. Finally, in disagreement with Ortony et al. (1988), we believe that nostalgia can have a bearing on goals and action.

Who Is the Referent of Nostalgia?

The referent of the nostalgic experience can range from the specific to the general. At the most specific level, nostalgia refers to a direct, individual experience. We call this case personal nostalgia. The experience can also pertain to an organization with which one is affiliated, and seemingly organizational nostalgia is quite prevalent (Gabriel, 1993). Furthermore, the referent may be a generational cohort, the culture independently of cohorts, or a historical period within a culture (Batcho, 1995; Holbrook, 1993; Lears, 1998; Stern, 1992).

Our focus here is on *personal nostalgia*, the emotion whose "brooding" ground is an important experience that involves directly the self. This experience may include a specific episode, a person, a place, moods, sights, or smells.

Is Nostalgia a Self-Relevant Emotion?

We regard nostalgia as a prima-facie self-relevant emotion. The central and defining character of the nostalgic experience is the self. At the same time, however, we acknowledge and emphasize the social dimension of nostalgia. In the nostalgic experience, the self is surrounded by people, typically close others such as family members, friends, and romantic partners (Holak & Havlena, 1998).

There is another way in which nostalgia is self-relevant while being social. We suggest that nostalgia serves crucial existential functions that range from individual (e.g., clarity and continuity of identity) to social (e.g., connectedness and meaning) ones.

Is Nostalgia a Positive, Negative, or Bittersweet Emotion?

"Nostalgia is memory with the pain removed," exclaimed the columnist Herb Caen (1975). Similarly, Davis (1979) termed nostalgia "a positively toned evocation of a lived past" (p. 18) and stated that "the nostalgic . . . experience . . . is infused with imputations of past beauty, pleasure, joy, satisfaction, goodness, happiness, love. . . . Nostalgic feeling is almost never infused with those sentiments we commonly think of as negative—for example, unhappiness, frustration, despair, hate, shame, abuse" (p. 14). Paralleling this view, Kaplan (1987) considered nostalgia a "warm feeling about the past, a past that is imbued with happy memories, pleasures, and joy" and maintained that the feeling is "basically one of joyousness, producing an air of infatuation and a feeling of elation" (p. 465). Several other theorists have highlighted the positive side of nostalgia, such as Gabriel (1993) and Holak and Havlena (1998). Chaplin (2000), in particular, argued that nostalgia reflects appreciation, if not reenjoyment, of past experiences.

Other theorists, however, posit that nostalgia is a negative emotion. Along with Johnson-Laird and Oatley (1989), authors such as Best and Nelson (1985), Hertz (1990), and Holbrook (1993, 1994) argued that the experience of nostalgia is immersed in sadness, as the nostalgic individual realizes that the past is irredeemably lost. Peters (1985) gave a more vivid description of the attributed negative content of the nostalgic experience, stating that it varies from "a fleeting sadness and yearning to an overwhelming craving that persists and profoundly interferes with the individual's attempts to cope with his present circumstances" (p. 135).

Still a third group of theorists emphasize the bittersweet flavor of the nostalgic experience. Despite labeling nostalgia a positive emotion, Davis (1979) acknowledged the ambivalence involved in yearning for an experience while full well recognizing that it is bygone. Nostalgia involves a "wistful pleasure, a joy tinged with sadness," Werman (1977, p. 393) asserted. Socarides (1977) added that nostalgia involves psychological pain, a view shared by Fodor (1950).

Our take on nostalgia is a hybrid of the positive and bittersweet views: We regard nostalgia as a disproportionately positive emotion, with bittersweet elements. There is some preliminary support for our conceptualization. In a study by Holak and Havlena (1998), participants detailed the circumstances and feelings that they experienced during each of three nostalgic episodes, pertaining to persons, events, and objects. Two judges rated the participants' accounts on the basis of several emotions. The accounts were described mostly by positive emotions (e.g., warmth, joy, elation, tenderness, and gratitude), although a link with a few negative emotions (e.g., sadness, irritation, and fear) also emerged.

Does Nostalgia Reflect Redemption or Contamination?

McAdams and colleagues (McAdams, Diamond, de St. Aubin, & Mansfield, 1997; McAdams, Reynolds, Lewis, Patten, & Bowman, 2001) distinguished between two strategies that people use to imbue their life stories with meaning and coherence. These strategies are redemption and contamination. In redemption, the story progresses from a bad or difficult life scene to a good or triumphant one. "The bad is redeemed, salvaged, mitigated, or made better in light of the ensuing good" (McAdams et al., 2001, p. 474). In contamination, the story progresses from a good or uncomplicated life situation to a problematic or bad one. "The good is spoiled, ruined, contaminated, or undermined by what follows it" (McAdams et al., 2001, p. 474).

These strategies have notable emotional implications. In a redemption sequence, the resulting emotion is positive, as the individual feels content, happy, or ecstatic. In a contamination sequence, the resulting emotion is negative, as the individual feels sad, dejected, or depressed. In light of our conceptualization of nostalgia as a predominantly positive emotion, we predict that nostalgic episodes are characterized mostly by redemption rather than by contamination sequences. We are in the process of testing this hypothesis.

Is Nostalgia Different from Reminiscence and Autobiographical Memory?

We think that there is a distinction to be drawn between reminiscence (Havighurst & Glasser, 1972; Reis-Bergan, Gibbons, Gerrard, & Ybema, 2000) and autobiographical memory (Brown & Schopflocher, 1998; Skowronski, Walker, & Betz, 2003), on one hand, and nostalgia, on the other. The former two involve "cold" processing (i.e., cognition), whereas the last involves "hot" processing (i.e., affect) (Castelnuovo-Tedesco, 1980; Cavanaugh, 1989).

Reminiscence and autobiographical memory are acts of remembering specific events in one's life, including the order of their occurrence. These events do not have to be, and typically are not, important or affect-laden. Nostalgia, however, goes well beyond memory veracity or temporal ordering of past events. It is centered around personally relevant events, is dipped in affect, and serves vital existential functions which we specify below.

What Triggers Nostalgia?

Nostalgia can be fortuitous, that is, triggered passively by external stimuli associated with one's recent or distant past. These stimuli can be social (e.g., friends, family members, picnics, birthday parties, reunions, and lost loved ones) or nonsocial (e.g., objects, music, scents, products, and possessions) (Havlena & Holak, 1991; Holak & Havlena, 1998; Holbrook, 1993, 1994). Alternatively, nostalgia may be deliberate, or initiated actively through reflection.

In either case, a direct (i.e., explicit) or indirect (i.e., implicit) comparison is made between past and current experiences (e.g., events, psychological states, and lifestyles) (Davis,

1979). This juxtaposition is a defining feature of the nostalgic experience. We elaborate on this feature when discussing functions of nostalgia, a topic to which we now turn.

Psychological Functions of Nostalgia

We propose that nostalgia fulfills existential functions. We think of nostalgia as a positive emotional and experiential reservoir that people delve into to deal with existential threat. We briefly review relevant literature and link it to our suggested functions of nostalgia.

Rank (1941) and Becker (1973) articulated the intrapersonal struggles that humans face when confronting their own mortality. Their ideas formed the foundation for an influential theory, terror management theory (TMT; Solomon, Greenberg, & Pyszczynski, 1991; Chapter 2, this volume). According to TMT, the knowledge, inevitability and imminence of death, if pondered consciously and deliberately, can induce paralyzing feelings of terror. In self-preservation, humans deflect death-related thoughts and existential terror by engaging in two symbolic strategies (Greenberg, Pyszczynski, & Solomon, 1997; Pyszczynski, Greenberg, & Solomon, 1999). First, they suppress thoughts of their death or relegate such thoughts to the non-foreseeable future (*proximal strategy*). Second, they implement self-esteem maintenance and elevation tactics or adhere to cultural norms and values (*distal strategy*). Mikulincer, Florian, and Hirschberger (2003, Chapter 18, this volume) added a third symbolic and distal strategy: close relationships. They reported that relationship dissolution induces, whereas relationship involvement shields off, existential terror. Further, death awareness increases one's motivation to affiliate and initiate or strengthen close relationships.

The central thesis of our chapter is that nostalgia is a process that facilitates the implementation of the above-mentioned distal strategies, namely, enhancement of the self, support of the cultural worldview, and bolstering of relational bonds. Nostalgia soothes the self from existential pangs by solidifying and augmenting identity, regenerating and sustaining a sense of meaning, and buttressing and invigorating desired connectedness with the social world. We review theoretical notions next and offer our own as well.

Existential Function 1: Nostalgia Solidifies and Augments Identity

An important way in which nostalgia "quiet[s] our fears of the abyss" (Davis, 1979, p. 41) is through the solidification of identity. To begin with, nostalgia is a source of identity uncertainty–reduction or identity attainment (Cavanaugh, 1989; Mills & Coleman, 1994). One can derive a stronger sense of selfhood, an increasingly unified self, by putting together pieces of past lives through nostalgia.

Moreover, nostalgia serves to protect identity. Kaplan (1987) thought of nostalgia as a mechanism for coping with loss of self-esteem. He speculated that nostalgia increases one's ability to deal with the present and restores self-worth perhaps by resorting, at least momentarily, to an idealized past (Kleiner, 1977) and "bestowing an endearing luster on past selves that may not have seemed all that lustrous at the time" (Davis, 1979, p. 41). Relatedly and importantly, nostalgia is thought to augment self-worth and identity (Gabriel, 1993). Kaplan, for example, labeled nostalgia "an ego ideal" (p. 471). Indeed, nostalgia likely is an effective self-affirmation tool (Steele, 1988; Tesser & Cornell, 1991).

The redeeming value of nostalgia is also worth emphasizing. Nostalgia enables a person to escape present mediocrity by resorting to a splendid past. Through reflected glory or vicarious fulfilment, the present identity acquires value and veneer and becomes more tolerable (Gabriel, 1993). A has-been becomes somebody again. Schwartz (1987) termed this "ontological function" (p. 328), and Becker (1962) illustrated it with commendable clarity:

> Anthony Quinn in his great role in *Requiem for a Heavyweight* earned his inner sense of self-value by constantly reminding himself and others that he was "*fifth*-ranking contender for the heavyweight crown." (p. 84)

This assertion gave the character some substance, some personal and social standing: It lifted him from nobody to somebody. It infused him with a wave of self-worth (Greenberg et al., 1997; Pyszczynski et al., 1999).

Existential Function 2: Nostalgia Regenerates and Sustains a Sense of Meaning

Another existential function of nostalgia is to regenerate and sustain a sense of meaning, in part through identification with the cultural worldview (Greenberg et al., 1997; Pyszczynski et al., 1999). In instances of felt loneliness, separateness, and alienation, resorting to nostalgic engagement can be therapeutic. Nostalgia alleviates these existential fears by reinforcing the value of cultural traditions and rituals of which one was once a part. This can be achieved by revelling in past Thanksgiving dinners, school fares, parades, and disco nights, or by collecting old baseball cards and movie or war memorabilia. Through such practices, one increases his or her sense of cultural belongingness (Baumeister & Leary, 1995), while restoring direction and the belief that one is living a purposeful life in a meaningful cultural context.

In the process, identity continuity will be facilitated (Chaplin, 2000; Davis, 1979). Continuity of identity across time is fostered through both a more appreciative attitude toward past selves and an improved understanding of how one fits into the cultural jigsaw puzzle, of how culture has shaped one's personality and value system. An increased sense of mastery and control over one's life may ensue.

Existential Function 3: Nostalgia Buttresses and Invigorates Social Connectedness

The third major existential function of nostalgia is the bolstering of relational bonds. In nostalgic reverie, "the mind is 'peopled' " (Hertz, 1990, p. 195). One reestablishes a symbolic connection with significant others (Batcho, 1998; Castano, Yzerbyt, & Paladino, Chapter 19, this volume; Cavanaugh, 1989; Kaplan, 1987; Mills & Coleman, 1994). Figures of the past are brought to life and become part of one's present.

This reignition of meaningful relational bonds satisfies one's need for interpersonal belongingness, thus benefiting self-esteem and identity (Leary & Baumeister, 2000). It also affords the individual a sense of safety and secure attachment (Mikulincer et al., 2003, Chapter 18, this volume). Finally, it allows for a symbolic celebration of life—both past and present.

Summary

We suggested that the core existential functions of nostalgia are (1) enhancement of the self, through identity solidification and augmentation; (2) support of the cultural worldview, through meaning regeneration and sustenance; and (3) bolstering of relational bonds though invigoration of interpersonal connectedness. Although no direct, systematic program of research has scrutinized these notions so far, there is indeed a relevant, albeit scant, literature to which we now turn.

The Discontinuity Hypothesis

Davis's (1979) discontinuity hypothesis is consistent with our argument that nostalgia is an effective resource for coping with existential threat. The hypothesis states that nostalgia is an emotional reaction to discontinuity in people's lives. Stated alternatively, people who experience disruption in their lives will rate the past more favorably than those who experience continuity.

What are the sources of discontinuity? We would speculate that they include death of a loved one, health deterioration, relationship breakup or divorce, occupational crises (e.g., layoffs), and drops in standards of living. What are the emotional or existential consequences of discontinuity? Davis (1979) named "fears, discontents, anxieties, or uncertainties" (p. 34). We would add loneliness, alienation, and fear of death to the list. Nostalgia, then, is a coping mechanism for dealing with these highly uncomfortable psychological states.

Three studies have tested the discontinuity hypothesis. Best and Nelson (1985) analyzed data from four national sample surveys. Each survey contained one or two statements that the authors operationalized as indicators of nostalgia. In the National Senior Citizens Survey (conducted in 1968; $N = 4,000$ adults ages 64 or over), participants responded with a *yes* or *no* to two statements: "You are as happy now as you were when you were younger" and "People had it better in the old days." In the National Council on Aging study (conducted in 1974; $N = 1,500$ adults ages 18 or over), participants expressed their agreement or disagreement with each of two statements: "I am as happy as when I was younger" and "These are the best years of my life." In the Americans View Their Mental Health survey (conducted in 1976; $N = 2,000$ adults ages 21 or over), participants responded to a single question: "What do you think of as the happiest time in your life?" Participants were classified as nostalgic if they selected a period in their past rather than the present. Finally, in the General Social Survey (conducted in 1980; $N = 1,500$ adults ages 18 or over), participants responded with *agree* or *disagree* to the statement: "In spite of what some people say, the lot of the average man is getting worse, not better."

The results offered weak support for the discontinuity hypothesis. Consistent with the hypothesis, deteriorating circumstances (e.g., death of a child or sibling, personal health problems, divorce) were associated with increased nostalgia. Also, African Americans (who were deemed to have experienced more discontinuity in the changing times of the Civil Rights movement) were more nostalgic than whites. Other predictions, however, were not supported. One such prediction was that men would be more nostalgic than women. As Davis (1979) put it, "traditionally, women's status passages occur in the familiar and re-assuring context of home, family, and kin, whereas those of men are more likely to involve abrupt shifts of locale, reference group, life style, and interpersonal atmospheres" (p. 56). Although this prediction is rather controversial, given that the Feminist Movement was well under way at the time the surveys were carried out, the results did not support the prediction anyway: Women were more nostalgic than men on four statements, whereas women and men did not differ on the remaining two statements. More pointedly, working women were equally or more nostalgic than women who stayed at home. The discontinuity hypothesis was not supported on three more grounds: Neither occupational nor geographic mobility predicted nostalgia, and no relation was found between work interruption and nostalgia.

Another test of the discontinuity hypothesis was reported by Batcho (1995). She assessed nostalgia in a two-part survey which included 684 participants ages 4–80 (median age = 20 years). In the first part of the survey, evaluated the world as it is now (1 = pretty bad, 5 = pretty great), as it will be 20 years from now (1 = a lot worse, 5 = a lot better), and as it was when they were younger (1 = a lot worse, 5 = a lot better). In the second part of the survey, participants completed the Nostalgia Inventory. They indicated (1 = not at all, 5 = very much) how much they missed each of 20 items from when they were younger. Items ranged from concrete (toys, your house, friends) to abstract (the way society was, not knowing sad or evil things, not having to worry).

The first part of the survey yielded no significant results: Evaluations of the world across the three periods did not differ by age or gender. However, when the upper and lower quartiles of the Nostalgia Inventory were examined, high nostalgics rated the world when they were younger as better than did low nostalgics. Also, 87% of the high nostalgics rated the future as less favorable than the past, whereas 63% of the low nostalgics rated the future as more favorable than the past. Furthermore, the overall nostalgia score, although uncorrelated with judgments of the present or the future, was correlated with judgments of the past. In general, nostalgia was associated with the view that the past was better and not necessarily with substantial dissatisfaction with the present or anxieties concerning the future. Regardless, support for the discontinuity hypothesis was weak.

The second part of the survey did not yield gender differences either. Age main effects, however, were significant for 14 of the 20 items of the Nostalgia Inventory: friends, family, school, house, music, heroes/heroines, feelings, having someone to depend on, not knowing sad or evil things, holidays, toys, pets, not having to worry, and the way people were. Rather surprisingly, on all but two (family, music) of these items, younger adults were more nostalgic than older ones. The age main effect was not significant for the following six items: places, someone you loved, things you did, church/religion, the way society was, and TV shows/movies. The results were inconsistent with the discontinuity hypothesis.

In a follow-up investigation, Batcho (1998) ventured another two-study test of the discontinuity hypothesis. The first study used the same procedure as that of Batcho (1995). In addition, participants completed self-descriptiveness ratings of the items: happy, risk or thrill seeking, emotional, good memory, and preferring activities with people rather than alone. High and low nostalgics did not differ on happiness, leading Batcho (1998) to infer that unhappiness does not qualify as an etiology of nostalgia. Also, high and low nostalgics did not differ on risk or thrill seeking, leading Batcho to disqualify dread for the future as an etiology of nostalgia. However, high (compared to low) nostalgics described themselves as more emotional, having stronger memory, and more likely to prefer activities with people rather than alone. Based on these findings, Batcho speculated that susceptibility to nostalgia is related to greater capacity for emotionality, to proneness to continuity with the past, and to greater need for involving others in one's activities.

In the second study, Batcho (1998) tested recall of high and low nostalgics based on a list of eight negative, eight neutral, and eight positive nouns. Participants also completed scales of optimism, hopelessness, emotionality, and affect intensity. The two groups did not differ in memory for words. However, the memories of high nostalgics were more people-directed than those of low nostalgics. The individual-difference scales yielded null results.

Although we acknowledge the pioneering character and usefulness of the above-mentioned studies, we cannot conceal a few points of criticism. Best and Nelson's (1985) six statements were not ideal indicators of nostalgia, and their data were underanalyzed. Furthermore, Batcho's (1995, 1998) findings were preliminary. These researchers were not concerned exclusively with personal nostalgia, and their approach was survey-based rather than experimental.

As matters stand, then, support for the discontinuity hypothesis is weak. We hope that future empirical tests will evaluate the hypothesis in a controlled, laboratory setting. For example, existential threat (e.g., a mortality salience manipulation; Solomon et al., 1991, Chapter 2, this volume) would need to be introduced, and corresponding changes in the level of nostalgia would need to be observed. The prediction is that awareness of one's own death will induce nostalgic engagement, which in turn will augment self-esteem, reaffirm the meaningfulness of the cultural worldview, and reestablish connection with close others. We are in the process of preparing such experimental procedures.

NOSTALGIA IN CONTEXT: FURTHER CONSIDERATIONS

Our view of nostalgia can be summarized as follows. Nostalgia is a universal experience: It concerns all persons, regardless of age, gender, social class, ethnicity, or other social groupings. Nostalgia is a self-relevant emotion that involves reliving one's past, and in particular events involving one's important but bygone relationships. Its bittersweet content notwithstanding, nostalgia is predominantly positive. Furthermore, nostalgia is typically triggered by a threatening stimulus (e.g., death of a loved one, health problems, relationship dissolution, and income loss) or is a deliberate response to an uncomfortable psychological state (e.g., sadness, loneliness, anxiety, and alienation), although it can also be triggered by fortuitous stimuli (e.g., old photographs, letters, or CDs). Most important, nostalgia, by being a stock of positive feelings, can ward off external threat or distressing thoughts. Nostalgia serves three core existential functions: self-enhancement, alignment with the cultural worldview, and fostering of close relationships. Successful fulfillment of one or more of these functions contributes to positive affectivity and a state of reassurance, warmth, and security.

We do not wish to argue that nostalgia has uniquely beneficial effects on psychological functioning. As stated earlier, nostalgia is somewhat associated with ambivalence and confusion. Also, nostalgia may, if excessive and uncontrollable, interfere with enjoyment of the present. It may also make one feel closed to new opportunities, experiences, and relationships.

These rather extreme cases aside, however, we do expect for nostalgia to be associated with psychological well-being. As a predominantly positive emotion, nostalgia may contribute to a broader thought–action repertoire (Fredrickson, 2001; Fredrickson, Tugade, Waugh, & Larkin, 2003), fostering creative and productive thinking. Indeed, if nostalgia clarifies and enhances the positivity of identity, while cementing close relationships, we would expect it to be linked with several markers of psychological well-being, such as feeling content or happy, being able to grow, and being able to plan and achieve (Taylor, Lerner, Sherman, Sage, & McDowell, 2003). Contrary, then, to Ortony et al.'s (1988) argument, we believe that nostalgia can have a bearing on goals and action. It can have motivational implications.

We also expect nostalgia to be associated with physical well-being. Although there is no direct evidence addressing this question, we can speculate based on the results of a study by Danner, Snowdon, and Friesen (2001). These researchers coded for emotional content the handwritten diaries of Catholic nuns (ages 75–95) which were composed at an early age (Mean age = 22 years). Early positive emotionality predicted survival rates 60 years later. In a similar vein, Emmons and McCullough (2003) demonstrated that positive emotions (e.g., gratitude, counting one's blessings) predicted psychological and physical well-being. Assuming that nostalgia is a typically positive emotion, it is likely to have long term implications for physical health.

Finally, who are the persons most likely to wax nostalgic? Although extant research has not succeeded in relating individual differences in nostalgia proneness to other personality variables (e.g., Batcho, 1998), we think that the issue deserves additional consideration. For example, are anxious–ambivalent persons more likely to engage in nostalgia than their securely attached counterparts? Are low self-esteem individuals more nostalgic than high self-esteem ones? Are individuals with interdependent self-construals more likely to be nostalgic than those with independent self-construals? We hope that future research addresses these and other questions pertaining to the emotion of nostalgia and its relevance to daily life.

ACKNOWLEDGMENT

Preparation of this chapter was supported by British Academy Grant No. LRG-33566 to Constantine Sedikides and Tim Wildschut.

NOTE

1. We are pleased to be able to offer some narrative relief for the hooked-up reader. The story has more steam, culminating in a Hollywood-type happy-ever-after finale. Calypso is ordered by Zeus to release Odysseus. She helps him build a raft, and Odysseus sails away toward Ithaca, but his raft is wrecked by Poseidon near the island of Scheria (current Corfu), home of the Phaeacians and princess Nausicaa. Despite her unrequited infatuation with Odysseus, Nausicaa graciously orders the Phaeacian seamen to take him to his homeland. They lay Odysseus near an olive tree on Ithaca's shore and depart without waking him. In plotting and sinister mood, Odysseus traps into death the brazen fellows who dallied with Penelope, is reunited with his wife and son, and is reinstated as the ruler of Ithaca. (For the latest scholarship on Homer and *The Odyssey*, see *http:// www.perseus.tufts.edu/*.)

REFERENCES

Batcho, K. I. (1995). Nostalgia: A psychological perspective. *Perceptual and Motor Skills, 80,* 131–143.

Batcho, K. I. (1998). Personal nostalgia, world view, memory, and emotionality. *Perceptual and Motor Skills, 87,* 411–432.

Baumeister, R. F., & Leary, M. R. (1995). The need to belong: Desire for interpersonal attachments as a fundamental human motivation. *Psychological Bulletin, 117,* 497–529.

Becker, E. (1962). *The birth and death of meaning.* Harmondsworth, UK: Penguin.

Becker, E. (1973). *The denial of death.* New York: Free Press.

Bellow, S. (1970). *Mr. Sammler's planet*. New York: Viking Press.

Best, J., & Nelson, E. E. (1985). Nostalgia and discontinuity: A test of the Davis hypothesis. *Sociology and Social Research, 69,* 221–233.

Brewin, C. R., Furhnam, A., & Howes, M. (1989). Demographic and psychological determinants of homesickness. *British Journal of Psychology, 80,* 467–477.

Brown, N. R., & Schopflocher, D. (1998). Event clusters: An organization of personal events in autobiographical memory. *Psychological Science, 9,* 470–475.

Caen, H. (1975, April 15). [Editorial]. *San Francisco Chronicle.*

Castelnuovo-Tedesco, P. (1980). Reminiscence and nostalgia: The pleasure and pain of remembering. In S. I. Greenspan & G. H. Pollack (Eds.), *The course of life: Psychoanalytic contributions toward understanding personality development: Vol. III: Adulthood and the aging process* (pp. 104–118). Washington, DC: U.S. Government Printing Office.

Cavanaugh, J. C. (1989). I have this feeling about everyday memory aging . . . *Educational Gerontology, 15,* 597–605.

Chaplin, S. (2000). *The psychology of time and death*. Ashland, OH: Sonnet Press.

Cox, J. L. (1988). The overseas student: Expatriate, sojourner or settler? *Acta Psychiatrica Scandinavica, 78,* 179–184.

Danner, D. D., Snowdon, D. A., & Friesen, W. V. (2001). Positive emotions in early life and longevity: Finding from the nun study. *Journal of Personality and Social Psychology, 80,* 804–813.

Davis, F. (1979). *Yearning for yesterday: A sociology of nostalgia*. New York: Free Press.

Emmons, R. A., & McCullough, M. E. (2003). Counting blessings versus burdens: An experimental investigation of gratitude and subjective well-being in daily life. *Journal of Personality and Social Psychology, 84,* 377–389.

Fisher, S. (1989). *Homesickness, cognition, and health*. London: Erlbaum.

Fodor, N. (1950). Varieties of nostalgia. *Psychoanalytic Review, 37,* 25–38.

Fredrickson, B. L. (2001). The role of positive emotions in positive psychology: The broaden-and-build theory of positive emotions. *American Psychologist, 56,* 218–226.

Fredrickson, B. L., Tugade, M. M., Waugh, C. E., & Larkin, G. R. (2003). What good are positive emotions in crises?: A prospective study of resilience and emotions following the terrorist attacks on the United States on September 11th, 2001. *Journal of Personality and Social Psychology, 84,* 365–376.

Frijda, N. H. (1986). *The emotions*. New York: Cambridge University Press.

Frost, I. (1938). Homesickness and immigrant psychoses. *Journal of Mental Science, 84,* 801–847.

Gabriel, Y. (1993). Organizational nostalgia: Reflections on "The Golden Age." In S. Fineman (Ed.), *Emotion in organizations* (pp. 118–141). London: Sage.

Greenberg, J., Pyszczynski, T., & Solomon, S. (1997). Terror management theory of self-esteem and cultural worldviews. Empirical assessments and conceptual refinements. In P. M. Zanna (Ed.), *Advances in experimental social psychology* (Vol. 29, pp. 61–141). San Diego: Academic Press.

Havighurst, R. J., & Glasser, R. (1972). An exploratory study of reminiscence. *Journal of Gerontology, 27,* 245–253.

Lewis, C. N. (1971). Reminiscing and self-concept in old age. *Journal of Gerontology, 26,* 240–243.

Havlena, W. J., & Holak, S. L. (1991). "The good old days": Observations on nostalgia and its role in consumer behavior. *Advances in Consumer Research, 18,* 323–329.

Hertz, D. G. (1990). Trauma and nostalgia: New aspects of the coping of aging holocaust survivors. *Israeli Journal of Psychiatry and Related Sciences, 27,* 189–198.

Hofer, J. (1934). Medical dissertation on nostalgia. (C. K. Anspach, Trans.). *Bulletin of the History of Medicine, 2,* 376–391. (Original work published 1688)

Holak, S. L., & Havlena, W. J. (1998). Feelings, fantasies, and memories: An examination of the emotional components of nostalgia. *Journal of Business Research, 42,* 217–226.

Holbrook, M. B. (1993). Nostalgia and consumption preferences: Some emerging patterns of consumer tastes. *Journal of Consumer Research, 20,* 245–256.

Holbrook, M. B. (1994). Nostalgia proneness and consumer tastes. In J. A. Howard (Ed.), *Buyer behavior in marketing strategy* (2nd ed., pp. 348–364). Englewood Cliffs, NJ: Prentice-Hall.

Homer. (1921). *The Odyssey*. (F. Caulfield, Trans.). London: G. Bell and Sons.

Jackson, S. W. (1986). *Melancholia and depression: from Hippocratic times to modern times*. New Haven, CT: Yale University Press.

Johnson-Laird, P. N., & Oatley, K. (1989). The language of emotions: An analysis of semantic field. *Cognition and Emotion, 3*, 81–123.

Kaplan, H. A. (1987). The psychopathology of nostalgia. *Psychoanalytic Review, 74*, 465–486.

Kemper, T. (1987). How many emotions are there? Wedding the social and autonomic components. *American Journal of Sociology, 93*, 263–289.

Kleiner, J. (1977). On nostalgia. In C. W. Socarides (Ed.), *The world of emotions* (pp. 471–498). New York: International University Press.

Lears, J. (1998). Looking backward: In defense of nostalgia. *Lingua Franca, 7*, 59–66.

Leary, M. R., & Baumeister, R. F. (2000). The nature and function of self-esteem: sociometer theory. In M. Zanna (Ed.), *Advances in experimental social psychology* (Vol. 32, pp. 1–62). San Diego: Academic Press.

McAdams, D. P., Diamond, A., de St. Aubin, E., & Mansfield, E. (1997). Stories of commitment: The psychosocial construction of generative lives. *Journal of Personality and Social Psychology, 72*, 678–694.

McAdams, D. P., Reynolds, J., Lewis, M., Patten, A. H., & Bowman, P. J. (2001). When bad things turn good and good things turn bad: Sequences of redemption and contamination in life narratives and their relation to psychosocial adaptation in midlife adults and in students. *Personality and Social Psychology Bulletin, 27*, 474–485.

McCann, W. H. (1941). Nostalgia: A review of the literature. *Psychological Bulletin, 38*, 165–182.

Mikulincer, M., Florian, V., & Hirschberger, G. (2003). The existential function of close relationships: Introducing death into the science of love. *Personality and Social Psychology Review, 7*, 20–40.

Mills, M. A., & Coleman, P. G. (1994). Nostalgic memories in dementia: A case study. *International Journal of Aging and Human Development, 38*, 203–219.

Ortony, A., Clore, G. L., & Collins, A. (1988). *The cognitive structure of emotions*. Cambridge, UK: Cambridge University Press.

Peters, R. (1985). Reflections on the origin and aim of nostalgia. *Journal of Analytical Psychology, 30*, 135–148.

Pyszczynski, T., Greenberg, J., & Solomon, S. (1999). A dual process model of defense against conscious and unconscious death-related thoughts: An extension of terror management theory. *Psychological Review, 106*, 835–845.

Rank, O. (1941). *Beyond psychology*. New York: Dover.

Reis-Bergan, M., Gibbons, F. X., Gerrard, M., & Ybema, J. F. (2000). The impact of reminiscence on socially active elderly women's reactions to social comparisons. *Basic and Applied Social Psychology, 22*, 225–236.

Rosen, G. (1975). Nostalgia: A "forgotten" psychological disorder. *Psychological Medicine, 5*, 340–354.

Schwartz, H. S. (1987). Anti-social actions of committed organizational participants: An existential psychoanalytic perspective. *Organization Studies, 8*, 327–340.

Skowronski, J. J., Walker, W. R., & Betz, A. L. (2003). Ordering our world: An examination of time in autobiographical memory. *Memory, 11*, 247–260.

Socarides, C. W. (1977). (Ed.). *The world of emotions: Clinical studies of affects and their expression*. New York: International University Press.

Sohn, L. (1983). Nostalgia. *International Journal of Psychoanalysis, 64*, 203–211.

Solomon, S., Greenberg, J., & Pyszczynski, T. (1991). A terror management theory of social behavior: The psychological functions of self-esteem and cultural worldviews. In L. Berkowitz (Ed.), *Advances in experimental social psychology* (Vol. 24, pp. 93–159). New York: Academic Press.

Steele, C. M. (1988). The psychology of self-affirmation: Sustaining the integrity of the self. In L. Berkowitz (Ed.), *Advances in experimental social psychology* (pp. 261–302). Hillsdale, NJ: Erlbaum.

Stern, B. B. (1992). Historical and personal nostalgia in advertising text: The *fin de siecle* effect. *Journal of Advertising, 21*, 11–22.

Taylor, S. E., Lerner, J. S., Sherman, D. K., Sage, R. M., & McDowell, N. K. (2003). Portrait of the self-enhancer: Well adjusted and well liked or maladjusted and friendless? *Journal of Personality and Social Psychology, 84,* 165–176.

Tesser, A., & Cornell, D. P. (1991). On the confluence of self processes. *Journal of Experimental Social Psychology, 27,* 501–526.

The New Oxford Dictionary of English. (1998). (J. Pearsall, Ed.). Oxford, UK: Oxford University Press.

Werman, D. S. (1977). Normal and pathological nostalgia. *Journal of the American Psychoanalytic Association, 25,* 387–398.

Van Tilburg, M. A. L., Vingerhoets, J. J. M., & van Heck, G. L. (1996). Homesickness: A review of the literature. *Psychological Medicine, 26,* 899–912.

Zwingmann, C. A. A. (1959). *"Heimweh" or "Nostalgic reaction": A conceptual analysis and interpretation of a medico-psychological phenomenon.* Unpublished Ph.D. dissertation, School of Education, Stanford University.

Chapter 14

Existential Meanings
and Cultural Models

The Interplay of Personal and Supernatural Agency in American and Hindu Ways of Responding to Uncertainty

MAIA J YOUNG
MICHAEL W. MORRIS

> The race is not to the swift
> or the battle to the strong,
> nor does food come to the wise
> or wealth to the brilliant
> or favor to the learned;
> but time and chance happen to them all.
> —ECCLESIASTES 9: 11

Ecclesiastes presents a discomforting view of the human condition. It challenges our cherished presumptions of existential meaning and moral order, evoking feelings of injustice, weariness, and despair. The observations of Ecclesiastes are chilling, because we recognize they are empirically true. Who can deny that chance and timing account for considerable variance in life outcomes. Evidence for the absurdity of the human condition is everywhere. That said, people who hold this worldview are a small minority; the majority of people strive and take risks even when there appears to be scant justification for optimism. How does this occur? How do so many individuals avoid the conclusions their experience warrants? We argue that it does not happen independently for each person; rather, it happens through collective-level processes involving culture. Through culture, people collude to forget some aspects of reality and to remember others.

This chapter takes the approach of cultural psychology in distinguishing patterns of beliefs, judgments, and decisions that reflect the shared mental models of cultural groups. Like water to the fish, cultural models are largely invisible to us. They surround and support our acts of cognition and communications so ubiquitously that we never notice them. In this chapter, we argue that cultural models are essential to understanding the ways in which people construct and sustain a view of existence as orderly and meaningful. We describe research that tested hypotheses about cultural differences in meaning-making patterns. For instance, as we shall see, although the temptation to judge others' misfortunes as deserved is felt everywhere, Judeo-Christian Americans and Hindu Indians perceivers do so under different circumstances, following different cultural models of "just deserts" or "karma."

At the same time, we argue that existential problems are crucial to understanding why cultures have much in common. A cultural universal that plays a central role in the current argument is religion. Virtually all human groups studied by anthropologists have religions—traditions concerning supernatural forces that influence human ends (Boyer, 2001). This ubiquity may indicate that religion serves a necessary function—that trust and cooperation in social organization requires a group to have a shared interpretive system for masking the inequity of fortunes and the uncontrollability of risks (Geertz, 1966). Regardless of its societal function, religion certainly operates at the level of individual psychology to buffer against existential threats. Demographic surveys reveal that religiosity increases with age and thoughts of death (Roth, 1978). Experiments find that even brief reminders of their mortality make people more likely to adopt habits of social judgment and ritual practices associated with their religion/culture (Greenberg, Arndt, Simon, Pyszczynski, & Solomon, 2000, Solomon, Greenberg, & Pyszczynski, Chapter 2, this volume). In sum, the notion that religious understandings play a role in adaptive sense making and coping is supported by a variety of evidence from past social science research, although those insights are not well integrated with the way that social psychologists have primarily understood sense making and coping.

Social psychology and existential psychology grew out of the same mid-20th-century Western milieu in which religion, that traditional wellspring of existential meaning, seemed increasingly obsolete to social thinkers. Perhaps for this reason, psychologists have focused on perceiving personal control as the central way people seek order (rather than absurdity) and hope (rather than despair). Many influential models hold the perception of personal control to be the linchpin of psychological adjustment, a necessary and sufficient condition for adaptive coping. We review this research and raise questions about what may be left out of the picture. As we shall see, research in other cultures, primarily East Asian settings, finds that personal control plays a lesser role in people's construal of the environment and coping with uncertainty.

This chapter takes the argument one step further by suggesting that past psychological models miss important pieces of the processes at work in American settings as well. In other words, the same cultural tendencies that magnify the role of personal control in people's lives may have affected the science of psychology, limiting researchers' attention to personal agency rather than supernatural agency. We draw on Dennett's notions of basic interpretive stances to distinguish two types of supernatural agency—influence by a person-like deity and influence by preordained destiny. We then describe American and Hindu cultural models of the interplay between personal and supernatural control. A key difference lies in which type of supernatural agency is most salient, and many differences in judgment and practice follow from this. In sum, we contend that the valorization of personal control in social psychology presents an incomplete and distorted picture of people's interpretive theories and habits.

PERCEIVING PERSONAL CONTROL

Farewell to the monsters, farewell
to the saints. Farewell to pride. All
that is left is men.
—Jean-Paul Sartre, *The Devil and the Good Lord* (1951;
Act 10, Sc. 4)

The way in which a man accepts his fate and all the suffering it entails
. . . gives him ample opportunity . . . to add a deeper meaning to his life.
—Viktor Frankl, *Man's Search for Meaning* (1963, p.
88)

For many mid-20th-century social thinkers, such as the Existentialists, the entire metaphysical foundation of the Western Judeo-Christian tradition seemed to have fallen away. Bidding adieu to Gods, devils, and other supernatural agents, and any cosmic designs beyond the human realm, they suggested that the only faith left is in human freedom and human intentions. The existentialists' view was not a naive faith in untrammeled free will; they were well aware of the exigencies of poverty, class, health, and war that cut short human ambitions. However, they maintained that individuals make choices at the margin that color their experience, such as choices about how to see themselves. In this way, perceiving oneself as having control is a step toward actually being free. Yet, the consequences of perceiving personal control are not entirely salutary; recognition of one's freedom brings a weighty responsibility. Recognizing the self, rather than God or Fate, as the author of one's life can lead to anxiety about making the right choices.

Another product of mid-20th-century Western *Zeitgeist*, social psychology has similarly emphasized the importance of perceiving personal control. Perceiving control has been held to be the key to motivation and engagement with the environment (Rotter, 1966), to avoiding a response of helplessness and depression (Seligman, 1975; Peterson & Seligman, 1983, 1984), and psychological adjustment (Taylor & Brown, 1999; Taylor 2000). In this way, personal control beliefs manifest in a variety of constructs such as self-efficacy, illusory optimism, and self-esteem.

It is worth distinguishing two levels at which researchers have approached the problem of measuring people's self-perceptions. One tradition initiated by Rotter (1966) focuses on the level of explicit verbal understandings. It has measured people's agreement or disagreement with general statements about control. Another tradition associated with Langer (1975) focuses on the level of implicit expectancies that guide action. It has measured people's tendency to take actions or make judgments that reflect an implicit belief that a particular outcome can be influenced by personal will. In recent years, social psychologists have become increasingly aware that explicitly espoused generalities often differ from implicit, contextual beliefs that drive individuals' behavior (see Wilson, 2002). In both traditions, as we shall see, recent research increasingly suggests that cultures differ in tendencies to perceive personal control.

Explicit General Beliefs

Studies of explicit beliefs about control begin with the work of Rotter (1966). He argued that the most fundamental dimension separating well-functioning and poorly functioning individuals lies in basic beliefs about the locus of control over the life outcomes. He developed a survey instrument to measure the extent to which respondents endorse general statements concerning the possibility of personal control, such as "What happens to me is my own doing" and "In the long run people get the respect that they deserve in this world" (markers of an internal orientation) as opposed to "Most people don't realize the extent to which their lives are controlled by accidental happenings" and "There will always be wars no matter how hard people try to prevent them" (markers of an external orientation). Rotter (1966) found that internal orientations were associated with higher levels of educational achievement and political engagement. However, the validity of the evidence was critiqued on a number of grounds—for example, that the measure tapped variation in respondents' objective opportunities, not just their subjective perceptions of control (Gurin, Gurin, & Morrison, 1978).

Although Rotter (1966) maintained that beliefs in many external factors—accidents, political forces, supernatural forces—all fell on the opposite pole from internal personal control, subsequent research suggested that people's control beliefs had to be understood within a more complex framework. Levenson (1981) introduced a revised instrument that separated external control into two factors tapping political forces and chance respectively; however, this chance construct still encompassed a broad range of qualitatively different statements, some referring more to the chance of accidents and some referring to supernatural forces such as fate or luck. Another tack was developing scales for specific domains, such as academic performance (Lefcourt, 1982). Despite these moves, researchers in the locus of control tradition retained the premise an individual must "perceive himself as the determiner of his fate if he is to live comfortably with himself" (Lefcourt, 1982, p. 3).

Numerous cross-cultural studies have been conducted with Rotter's locus of control instrument in Europe, East Asia, and Latin America. Factor analyses have not generally supported a unidimensional scale, and myriad country differences have been reported. A general finding, however, is that Asians tend to score lower than North Americans on internality or personal control items (for a review, see Dyal, 1984). Seeking to understand the country differences, Smith, Trompenaars, and Dugan (1995) regressed country-level means from a worldwide sample on a number of variables for each country tapping its economic, social, and religions features. Interestingly, personal control belief was more strongly predicted by an indicator of exposure to Christian theology (percentage of population Christian) than by indicators of economic and social conditions (income level, system of government, literacy rate, etc.). It may be that exposure to theological teachings and texts shapes people's agreements with explicit statements about control (like Rotter's items), because religion is one of the few discourses that deals in such abstract general propositions. Let us turn now to a different kind of knowledge encoding belief about one's control that has been widely studied, that is the context-specific expectancies that guide action.

Implicit Contextual Expectancies

A different tradition of research has focused on people's expectancies of efficacy or control in particular contexts (Bandura, 1977). This knowledge is less an abstract, reflective belief about one's general level of control and more a feeling of confidence in being able to affect a particular outcome in a given context. Consider the case of illusions of control, in which a person behaves as though one's actions can affect outcomes, due to motivations to control them. Ethnographic studies of people dealing with continual risk—whether tribal fisherman, aviation test pilots, or gamblers—typically find superstitious behaviors. Psychological experiments investigated how such illusions of personal control depend on features of a behavioral context. Rothbart and Snyder (1970) found that participants in a gambling experiment bet more money on the outcome of a dice roll when the dice had not yet been tossed (the "open fate" condition) than when the dice had already been rolled but not yet revealed (the "sealed fate" condition). Interestingly, a more explicit measure—their judged probabilities of particular dice outcomes—did not reveal the control illusion. In a series of studies, Langer (1975) found that participants' illusions of personal control can be increased by introducing various features that suggest the relevance of skill, such as rolling the dice rather than merely observing them rolled, or playing alongside an inept fellow participant (actually a confederate).

Whereas gambling studies highlighted that illusory control expectancies may lead to regrettable behavior in the context of casinos, research in other contexts pointed to positive consequences. Langer and Rodin (1976) found that an intervention elevating the control expectancies of residents in a nursing home increased their longevity. Studies of breast cancer patients by Taylor, Lichtman, and Wood (1984) found that positive adjustment comes from perceiving personal control over one's cancer as well as perceiving that others (e.g., physicians) have control. In other studies, Taylor and Brown (1999) found that American students are prone to unrealistic optimism about their personal chances of attaining positive outcomes and avoiding negative ones and that this tendency is correlated with self-esteem. From a broader lens, self-efficacy, illusory optimism, and self-esteem are all manifestations of a belief in personal control, and they are useful in buffering individuals from lapsing into helplessness and depression (Seligman, 1975; Peterson & Seligman, 1983, 1984).

In the last decade a great deal of research has examined whether personal control and these related control expectancies—such as self-efficacy and self-esteem—differ across cultures, most of it focusing on the contrast between American and East Asian settings. Numerous studies by Heine and colleagues (Heine & Lehman, 1995; Heine, Lehman, Markus, & Kitayama, 1999) have found that Japanese, compared to Americans, have lower levels of unrealistic optimism about their personal outcomes and lower levels of self-esteem. Yet evidence from a number of research programs suggests that East Asians, compared to Americans, have higher levels of perceived efficacy and illusory optimism in groups as well as more positive feelings about their relationships to groups (Earley, 1993; Morris, Menon, & Ames, 2001; Yamaguchi, 2001).

Recent research has sought to go beyond country-level explanations in order to understand East Asian's lesser expectancies of personal agency and greater expectancies of group agency expectancies. Is it childhood socialization into the sociocentric, Confucian belief systems or is it the daily experience of participation in social institutions that prioritize the group (such as norms, the roles, and scripts) that guide interactions in schools and workplaces? Striking evidence has recently emerged from studies by Heine (1999) of respondents who have recently moved to another cultural setting. Heine observed higher self-esteem scores among Japanese exchange students in Canada than the same Japanese students in Japan, whereas Canadians after half a year in Japan had lower self-esteem scores than before leaving home. Insight about the mechanism for these effects comes from studies by Kitayama and colleagues (Kitayama, Markus, Matsumoto, & Norasakkunkit, 1997; Morling, Kitayama, & Miyamoto, 2002) of the social situations that constitute American and Japanese social environments. In the first stage, Americans and Japanese were asked to describe successes and failures; in the second stage, new groups of Americans and Japanese were presented with a sample of situations that originated from both cultures and imagined how the situation would make them feel. Among the findings were that American-origin situations evoked greater feelings of self-esteem for both American and Japanese participants, suggesting that there are more intensely self-esteem bolstering situations in the American cultural ecology. Overall, these results suggest that participation in everyday practices and institutions is the key determinant of implicit expectancies of control. Given that implicit expectancies guide behavior, it fits that they would be tuned by behavioral experiences.

Conclusion from Research on Culture and Personal Control

There is abundant evidence that the role of perceived personal control in psychological adaptation differs across cultures. Moreover the evidence suggests a tentative conclusion about respective aspects of culture that proximally shape explicit control beliefs versus implicit control expectancies, which is illustrated in Figure 14.1.

This tentative conclusion yields predictions about the association of the two kinds of measures that have been used to study perceived control. Measures of perceived control in espoused general beliefs and in implicit expectancies about particular contexts should hang together in comparisons at the country level of analysis. Homeostatic cultural processes ensure that in general the theologies and belief systems in a country match its social institutions and practices. However, the measures need not hang together in individual-level analyses. The individuals who are most steeped in theologies and other formalized belief systems are not necessarily those most engaged in the social institutions and situations that shape control expectancies. For sake of illustration, let us consider the teenagers in an Amish community in rural Ohio and an artists' colony in coastal California. Our bet is that the Amish, inculcated into theological axioms stressing individual responsibility, would score higher than the hippies in a measure of explicit beliefs in personal control like that of Rotter (1966). Yet we wager that the hippies would hold their own in a contest of illusory overcon-

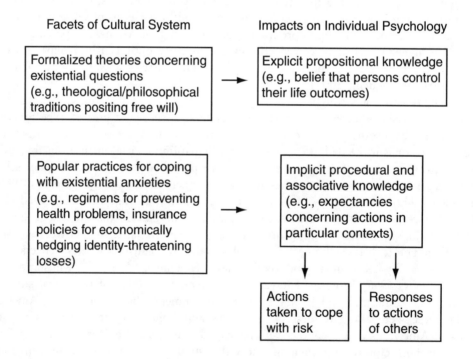

FIGURE 14.1. Different aspects of one's psychology may be shaped by different facets of a religious tradition. That is, exposure to formal theology may inculcate one's explicit beliefs about control, whereas participation in popular practices may instill the expectancies about context-appropriate action paths that proximally shape one's coping behaviors and one's responses to others.

fidence and self-esteem, the reason being that their social institutions and practices are richer in situations that prop up the individual's sense of freedom, efficacy, and esteem.

We have argued that the obsession with perceived personal control in social psychology reflects the place and moment of the field's origin—the place being Western Europe and the United States and moment being the mid-20th-century modernism. Cultural and historical ideologies bias what social scientists notice and what they overlook (Sampson, 1988). In seeking to compare the psychology of control in the American setting to that in Indian Hindu settings, we first reflected on what is missing.

A first need was greater clarity in conceptualizing external orientations. Although control research has come to distinguish external human forces (e.g., groups and powerful others) from external nonhuman factors, this latter category still encompassed too much. Factors such as fate, God, destiny, and chance seem psychologically very different; some are control perceptions in that they refer to factors having agency, yet some (e.g., chance) are not really references to control. We turned to theories about cognition to build a model of two basic conceptions of supernatural agency.

A second need was considering that people might have theories encompassing both personal control and external supernatural forces. For example, the Christian ethos that had been discussed as personal control may really consist of a belief that individuals directly influence their outcomes through a direct interaction with a higher power. This is overt in the petitionary prayer that occurs within the direct relationship to God that individuals have in the Judeo-Christian tradition. Yet it may be present at other moments. For example, a gambler's "illusions of control" might not reflect a belief that the dice can be directly controlled by one's wishes; it might reflect a sense that they can be altered by the combination of one's personal wish and the magical powers of some supernatural wish granter. Similarly, it seemed important to make progress in understanding the ways personal control and supernatural control beliefs combine in Hindu Indian culture. Several social scientists had advanced neo-Weberian arguments that Indian economic underdevelopment reflects an ethos of fatalistic passivity that arises from Hindu understandings of destiny (e.g., Kapp, 1963; Myrdal, 1968). Based on secondhand interpretations of Hindu beliefs, rather than direct research, these books were roundly critiqued by anthropologists. However, perhaps because of the lingering controversy, no one had followed up by actually studying Hindu folk theories about control and their links to economic judgments and decisions.

PERCEIVING SUPERNATURAL CONTROL

Our theorizing about cultural variation in notions of supernatural influence began with the assumption that there are limited ways that cultural groups forge understandings of a domain (Wellman & Gelman, 1992). Commonalities across different cultures or religions do not have to be explained in terms of one tradition influencing the other, although of course this happens frequently; commonalities can be explained in terms of the variation and selection stages of cultural evolution. Variation does not occur through random mutation as in biological evolution but through an individual innovating and getting the innovation established as routine. These cognitive and communicative stages are fostered when preestablished (perhaps hardwired) understandings of a core domain serve as a template or analogy (Sperber, 1994; Boyer, 2001). Further constraint comes from the selection stage; some ways of thinking about a domain may be weeded out.[1] As a result, for many domains, the differences among cultures consist largely of several basic possibilities that became established.

In a useful distinction, Dennett (1987) proposed that understandings of many domains either involve an intentional stance or a design stance. Using the intentional stance is to treat something like a person—to read its intentions and interact with it as though it has perceptions, emotions, and goals. Using the design stance is to treat something as if it is a device, apparatus, or system that was has been put together to serve a particular function. In approaching a novel domain, one could take either of these stances. For example, when trying to understand our personal computer we might impute intentions and desires to predict its behavior ("It wants me to click OK before it will let me close the file"), and sometimes we analyze how the system was designed ("It's designed so that the default is always to save something").

The distinction between these two basic interpretive stances was our point of departure in theorizing about the elements that constitute theories of control in religious traditions. The design stance leads to seeing outcomes as caused by preordained destinies and other complicated systems of forces—destiny control. The intentional stance leads to seeing outcomes as caused by a person-like entity—deity control. We suggest that there are traditions of both stances in all religious-cultural traditions, but traditions inevitably emphasize one over the other.

In the Judeo-Christian tradition that saturates American culture, the locus of supernatural agency is the person-like deity. God is seen as watchful and easily provoked or moved to mercy. Although there are some prophecies that have been determined, God is assumed to be fairly free to alter the course of events at his discretion. In the Hindu tradition, there are many deities or at least many avatars of a deity. The deities themselves are constrained by a higher power, which is the law of karma that they are obliged to enact (see Young, Morris, Krishnan, & Regmi, 2003).

Importantly, however, neither stance toward supernatural agency is inconsistent with perceiving one's own personal control; neither should be opposite to internal personal control. One can navigate a system or a bureaucracy based on an understanding of the functions for which it was designed. Or one can negotiate with intentional beings based on an understanding of their perceptions, goals, emotions, and actions.

STUDIES OF EXPLICIT BELIEFS

The first studies in our research tested our hypotheses about American and Hindu conceptions by measuring explicit beliefs about control. The strongest beliefs were in personal control for both groups, belying any notion that Hindu beliefs lack personal control. Americans, however, were higher than Hindus in their belief in personal control.

The two proposed forms of belief in supernatural agency revealed themselves as psychologically separate and yet not opposite to personal control. Americans endorsed deity control more than destiny control. Hindu participants equally endorsed the notions of deity control and destiny control.

The higher American levels of personal control enabled us to examine a slight tangent to the argument. A key idea in existentialist philosophy and psychology is that freedom carries responsibility that is weighty enough that people seek to escape from freedom (Fromm, 1942). A heightened sense of personal control, then, may be associated with decision anxiety, because choices are thought to have momentous consequences in the future. If an individual endorses the notion of destiny control and events are seen as predetermined, however, he or she may see choices as inconsequential in steering toward destined outcomes. Our findings (Young et al., 2003) also suggest that personal control can be associated with more angst over life choices; American participants in our studies report having more anxiety about lifestyle choices than do Hindu participants. In a related finding, American participants in our studies also reported more anxieties about past choices and regrets about foregone alternative paths in academics and life.

STUDIES OF IMPLICIT EXPECTANCIES

Ways of Coping with Risk

As we have argued, individuals may find opportunities to exercise personal control within the rubric of their external control beliefs. Many kinds of practices for coping with risks exist in both the American and Hindu contexts, such as the following:

1. Petitioning for divine intervention in one's future outcomes,
2. Consulting seers who divine one's fate and suggest mitigating steps,
3. Buying insurance to hedge against devastating losses, and
4. Engaging in ritual superstition to align the self with desired ends.

Based on our notion that theories guiding control attempts combine a sense of personal agency with notions of supernatural forces that are conceived from intentional or design stances, we studied the kinds of practices that are regarded as normal or appropriate in the two contexts. We predicted that individuals' normative beliefs would mediate cultural differences in their willingness to use the practices and to associate with others who use the practices.

The intentional stance engenders a view that coping with risks should be like negotiating with an intentional being—making promises in order to influence the other's emotions, perceptions, and actions. The prototypical risk coping strategy within the intentional stance framework is petitioning divine intervention through prayer; it often involves making promises to a deity about changing one's own behaviors for more immediate favorable outcomes. Petitionary prayer makes reference to two intentional beings—the deity who is addressed and the future self that is promised.

Another practice that involves an intentional stance is insurance. There are economic reasons for buying insurance, but economic analyses do not account for anomalies in people's willingness to pay for insurance (McClelland, Schilze, & Coursey, 1993). Economics rationally dictates that insurance should be purchased as a function of the value and probability of its payoff, yet recent studies find that Americans overpay for insurance in cases in which the object (or person) being insured is of high sentimental value. The extant explanation is that purchasers are not just interested in the financial payoff; they want to spare their future self the pain of regret by taking whatever control they can. Some evidence for this process of empathizing with the future self is that overpurchasing is more likely when the object is of high sentimental value, holding constant its financial value and the possibility of replacing it (Hsee & Kunreuther, 2000; Slovic, Finucane, Peters, & MacGregor, 2002). Hence, insurance purchasing in some cases is another means of feeling in control of the uncontrollable, and it is a strategy that results from an intentional stance toward one's future self combined with a penchant for seeking person control.

The design stance engenders a view that coping with risks should be like manipulating a device or maneuvering a bureaucracy based on an understanding of the function for which it was designed. When the mechanistic workings of the device or apparatus are too opaque to understand, individuals may cope by looking to experts to make predictions about the complex, inner workings and potential outcomes of the system. By consulting experts in order to tap their privileged insight, one may adjust future actions to mitigate losses. Similarly, ritual superstitions in daily life assume that a mechanism that is more proximal to the individual can be manipulated. Regarding both divination and ritual superstitions, the individual is adjusting his or her behaviors to minimize conflicts with the design of destiny or more local systems.

To test general differences in preference for these strategies, we presented participants with a list of concrete examples of prayer, divination, insurance, and superstitious strategies. The items varied in life domains such as sports, business, academics; some were oriented around increasing future gains, and others were about avoiding future losses. A list of the items under each category is shown in Table 14.1.

Respondents answered three questions about each item. To assess whether the practice was normative, participants rated their impressions of others who engaged in each practice—on a scale ranging from weird/odd versus reasonable/sensible. In addition, participants rated their personal willingness to use the practice and their inclination to avoid a person or group who used the practice.

We predicted and found a cultural pattern in which Americans are more likely to use petitionary prayer and insurance whereas Hindus more likely to use divination and ritual. Subsequent mediation analyses confirm that perceived social norms mediated the relationship between culture and these two practices for handling anxieties about the future.

A Crucial Test: Insurance and Sentimental Value

TABLE 14.1. Ways of Coping with Risk: Four Strategies with Examples

Petition
- If your business is going bankrupt, pray.
- If you are student, pray to make good things to happen in the future.
- If you are an athlete, pray that no team members get hurt.
- If you are worker in a factory, pray that no accidents will occur.
- If your child is seriously ill, pray that the disease recedes.

Divination
- If you are getting married, choose a date based on horoscopes.
- If you are developing a new hotel, consult an expert about how to position the rooms.
- If you are a shopkeeper, consult a palm reader before making an important decision.
- If you are a businessman, see a psychic to foresee future disasters.

Insurance
- If you manage a museum, insure its artifacts against theft.
- If you own a building, buy fire insurance.
- If you own a car, buy insurance to cover the cost of damage to others in accidents.
- If you are a leader of a temple, insure the artwork against damages by natural disaster.

Alignment magic
- If you are a gambler and want to leave behind bad luck, change the way you pronounce your name.
- If your family wants to bring good fortune to a new home, hold a ritual.
- If you are a movie producer and you have signed several bad deals, change the style of your signature.
- If your family wants to avoid negative energy in the home, carefully plan the arrangement of the furniture.

We have argued that a focus on the intentional stance is associated with increased attention to the potential consequences for future selves and could affect insurance purchases; people who have greater cultural emphasis on seeing intentional agency may be more prone to buying insurance to stave off regret after misfortune falls. To gather more evidence for this argument, we investigated decisions to insuring objects in one's personal life that have sentimental value but cannot be replaced. Hsee and Kunreuther (2000) have found that people pay more when the insurance policy is for an object that has personal sentimental value. We predicted that this effect should be stronger for Americans than for Hindus (Young et al., 2003).

Participants in both cultural settings read vignettes like those in Hsee and Kunreuther (2000), where they imagined that they were facing a decision to buy insurance for an object; the monetary value of the object did not vary across conditions but the sentimental value of it did. Confirming our hypotheses and replicating Hsee and Kunreuther's (2000) original findings, Americans were more sensitive to the changes in severity of consequences for their future self; they were willing to pay for insurance when the object was of high rather than low sentimental value. Hindu respondents were not likely to pay for more insurance when the object was described as having high sentimental value than when it was low in sentimental value. Hindus behaved in the "economically rational" manner whereas Americans did not.

WAYS OF EXPLAINING MISFORTUNES

Witnessing our own or others' misfortunes is ripe occasion for being reminded of the possibility that we are all subject to randomness. However, individuals may avoid these opportunities to be reminded "chance happens" by seeing a contingency between action and outcome—and hence seeing deservedness in life outcomes. In this way, individuals make meaning out of misfortunes that are otherwise causally difficult to explain.

An examination of the word *karma* could provide insight into this process of making meaning in moral judgments. *Karma* became established in English in the mid-19th century as a substitute for prior notions such as just deserts, and in both American and Hindu cultures, it is used to indicate supernatural moral compensation—a relationship between previous actions as causes and subsequent outcomes as effects. Yet karmic explanations may be applied differently owing to different cultural understandings of supernatural influence—that is, *who* or *what* delivers the appropriate rewards or punishments? We submit that intentional and design stances underlie the application of the term *karma* in Hindu and American cultural settings.

Karma for Hindus works primarily through the reincarnation of souls across lifetimes (although some ethnographers document that in particular parts of India, *karma* is used to explain causes and effects within the same lifetime [see Babb, 1983; Daniel, 1983; Keyes & Daniel, 1983]). Individuals are thought to accumulate good and bad karma through their works in one lifetime, and the totality of one's karmic energies determines status and outcomes in the next lifetime. Therefore, Hindus can apply karmic explanations by inferring unobserved transgressions from a previous life. For Americans, karma is understood implicitly within Judeo-Christian assumptions of a watchful, reactive deity who rewards and punishes within a single lifetime. Granted, the notions that karmic compensation can be delivered in a single lifetime or across lifetimes are available—if not equally accessible—in both Hindu and American cultures. In general, however, we hypothesized that moral compensation for deeds is thought to be delivered more expediently in the American setting than it is in the Hindu setting.

In our studies (Young et al., 2003), participants read vignettes of someone who had severe misfortune. Half the participants also read that the focal actor had behaved hurtfully toward others before their own misfortune took place. We hypothesized and found that Americans apply karmic explanation for misfortune only when they know of misdeeds within the target person's lifetime, whereas Hindus apply karmic explanations without having evidence of misdeeds. A severely negative event may elicit karmic inferences in Hindu culture, especially because of the potential of an unseen event in the actor's previous lifetime. It is worthy to note that our measure does not require belief in reincarnation—only a sense that misfortune struck because the person was doomed without evidence of prior misdeeds. Although American participants could have inferred past misdeeds (even within the focal actor's lifetime), no such inferences were made among American participants who read about the misfortune without the precursor event.[2]

Although our findings indicate that *karma* is applied differently as an explanation for misfortune across cultures, it is an open question about how blameworthy the actor is seen to be when karmic explanations are used. Certainly, using the term *karma* links the actor to the event, but it is conceivable that Hindus use *karma* to indicate "destiny," whereas the American usage connotes "just deserts." It may be that Americans used the term *karma* to morally blame the actor, and they see the misfortune as an appropriate punishment, whereas Hindus have other connotations of the term; it could be used to pardon the individual, if he or she is seen as a victim of fixed circumstance.

THE BIAS OF PREDICTING MISFORTUNE FOR THOSE WHO "TEMPT FATE"

The belief that reactive, supernatural agents intervene to reward humans for their good or bad deeds (Gilbert, Brown, Pinel, & Wilson, 2000) seems clearly related to the tendency to ascribe prior misdeeds to victims in order to see their suffering as deserved (Hafer, 2000; Lerner & Miller, 1978). As the belief is related to judgments about existing misfortunes, so it might be related to the tendency to forecast imminent misfortune for those who transgress standards of humility or morality. Folk beliefs about witchcraft in many cultures have this form; transgressors are judged to be doomed, likely targets for disease, accidents, and other unpredictable harms; also these transgressors are avoided by all who wish to avoid sharing in their fate (Evans-Pritchard, 1937). Thus, we propose that striving to see a moral order manifests in forecasts of future events as well as in explanations of past events. We investigated one particular form of the notion that future outcomes are contingent upon current actions: "tempting fate" superstitions or fears that one's missteps will attract the attention of, offend, and solicit punishments from a reactive, supernatural agent.

To check our reasoning, we conducted a study comparing Americans and Nepalese in their judgments of a miscreant's immediate fate (Young et al., 2003). This contrast pits the cultural meaning system prediction (Americans > Nepalese) against the prediction that superstitious thinking tends to be higher among peoples in less modern or less predictable environments (Zusne & Jones, 1989). Searching news articles to find the domains in which this bias appears, we uncovered headlines such as the following: "Local drivers tempt fate during vintage car race," "Drivers tempt fate at flooded crossing," "Fat, Lazy, and Tempting Fate," "Scientists at a . . . fertility clinic tempt fate," "Many young people tempt fate by not having a will."

The bias seems to focus on those who take unnecessary risks (hubris, disdain for safety, impervious). Although some domains differ incommensurably as a function of the lifestyles and economic conditions of American and Nepalese, a domain that is similar for both cultures is risk taking with minor health problems. We created a vignette, with details appropriate to both samples, about a traveler who "tempts fate" by neglecting to bring a large bottle of symptom-alleviating medicine on a trip. The person in the vignette knew that he would be traveling through a remote region in which travelers sometimes fall unpredictably ill.

In the control version of the story, the traveler packs the bulky container of medicine to be prepared. We measured whether participants forecasted that immediate misfortune would ensue for the character (predicted number of days that the illness would strike on the trip) and also measured avoidance (their unwillingness/willingness to work on a team with this character). Results showed that American participants were more likely to avoid working with the traveler when he neglected to pack the medicine than when he packed it (took the precaution). The avoidance reaction was not significant among Nepalese.

Participants in both cultures predicted approximately 30% more days sick for the traveler who did not pack the medicine. Of course, forecasts of misfortune might follow from a rational prediction based on a trait ascription—in this case, a reckless person may be more likely to enter dangerous regions. To distinguish the processes through which participants made their forecasts, we measured their ratings of the character as doomed and as reckless. Americans saw the target person as more doomed, but Nepali's forecasts were based on inferences of character recklessness. We submit that this pattern of predicting misfortune and the tempting fate phenomenon arises from the intentional stance in supernatural control, such that individuals are wary that their actions are deemed reprehensible from a reactive agent; after acting in a way that could offend the supernatural agent, these individuals predict more imminent misfortunes as punishments.

TOPICS FOR FUTURE RESEARCH

We have argued that asserting one's personal control is not the only way in which individuals everywhere strive to make meaning in life; supernatural control concepts that vary in emphasis by culture are also fundamental tools for coping with an uncertain future and making meaning of past outcomes. We have explored control beliefs in Hindu and Judeo-Christian cultural contexts and their associated beliefs and practices related to coping with risk, making moral judgments, and purchasing insurance. In contrast to previous arguments in the locus of control research tradition, we have argued that even traditional *external* control beliefs are accompanied by attempts to maintain some control. We asserted that employing an intentional stance toward supernatural control promotes practices such as praying and buying insurance, whereas a design stance is associated with attempts to divine the future or engage in ritual superstitions. Further, we have outlined that an understanding of types of external control beliefs is needed to understand moral judgments when making sense of our own and others' life outcomes, or predicting future misfortunes from "tempting fate."

Although research on personal control conceptions rarely mentions the ways in which "external" agency beliefs can be beneficial, future research may delve further into the positive psychological effects of seeing life outcomes as a negotiation between the self and a supernatural, intentional being. For example, an investigation by Archer (1997) provides a dramatic example of an attempt to make meaning from a traumatic life event and to grapple with an uncertain future by invoking the concept of a reactive, intentional entity. His article titled "Tornadoes, boys, and superheroes: Externalizing conversations in the wake of a natural disaster," outlines a coping strategy that allowed a 7-year-old boy to recover from the trauma of surviving a tornado. The therapist encouraged the boy to join forces with a "superhero team" in his fight to reclaim control and to cope with feelings of vulnerability. Conceptualizing future outcomes as in the "hands" of superheroes was the most effective coping strategy for the young American boy.

Traditional control research has also been relatively silent about the potential benefits of perceiving predetermined outcomes in life—a single path rather than many. There is research, however, about instances in which individuals relinquish control. For example, individuals gladly avoid having control when tragedy is seen to be inevitable (Burger, 1989). Similarly, after tragedy has struck, it can be comforting to consider a negative outcome as predetermined—that we could not have done anything to prevent it. Belief in predetermination may not alleviate negative feelings from observing a tragedy, but it may absolve one from feeling morally responsible for the event.

Future studies may also examine the relationship between personal control beliefs and anxiety about the consequences of current decisions. As mentioned previously, individuals who are high in personal control may be prone to seeing their decisions as crucial turning points, and thus their decisions may weigh more heavily as they attempt to make the "right" decision while avoiding the "wrong" ones. This focus on the potential consequences of one's decisions can lead to greatly different choices—a phenomenon that researchers have dubbed *anticipatory regret* (Miller & Taylor, 1995). To the extent that personal control orientation highlights potential misjudgments, it may be associated with differential decision making.

Thinking that something is predetermined by a system can also lead to adaptive behaviors; when pursuing a life goal, for example, it may be motivating to think that our direction is prescripted—that we are following our "calling" in life. In this way, negative feedback and setbacks may be interpreted as mere bobbles in living out what is ultimately meant to be, and the individual may persevere far beyond the point where he or she would otherwise have given up the cause

NOTES

1. This is not to say that the elements of cultures that we find today should be understood as functional with regard to their environments. Once a culture becomes institutionalized, tremendous inertial forces work toward its perpetuation (Cohen, 2001). Just as every skier down a slalom course deepens the ruts, every time an individual acts publicly in a way that is guided by cultural structures this perpetuates the structures as future constraints on their own behavior and others' actions.
2. Although the word *karma* was borrowed from Sanskrit to English, our findings indicate that it is applied to specific situations and has a circumscribed meaning among Americans. Further, Americans and Hindus did not differ in their mean propensity to apply the term when the focal actor had previous misdeeds.

REFERENCES

Archer, R. (1997). Tornadoes, boys, and superheroes: Externalizing conversations in the wake of a natural disaster. *Journal of Systemic Therapies, 16,* 73–82.

Babb, L. A. (1983). Destiny and responsibility: Karma in popular Hinduism. In C. F. Keyes & E. V. Daniel (Eds.), *Karma: An anthropological inquiry* (pp. 163–181). Berkeley: University of California Press.

Bandura, A. (1977). *Self-efficacy: The exercise of control.* New York: Freeman.

Boyer, P. (2001). *Religion explained: The human instincts that fashion gods, spirits and ancestors.* London: Basic Books.

Cohen, D. (2001). Cultural variation: Considerations and implications. *Psychological Bulletin, 127*(4), 451–471.

Daniel, S. B. (1983). The tool box approach of the Tamil to the issues of moral responsibility and human destiny. In C. F. Keyes & E. V. Daniel (Eds.), *Karma: An anthropological inquiry* (pp. 27–62). Berkeley: University of California Press.

Dennett, D. (1987). *The intentional stance.* Cambridge, MA: MIT Press.

Dyal, J. A. (1984). Cross-cultural research with the locus of control construct. In H. Lefcourt (Ed.), *Research with the locus of control construct* (Vol. 3, pp. 209–306). New York: Academic Press.

Earley, C. P. (1993). East meets West meets Mideast: Further explorations of collectivistic and individualistic work groups. *Academy of Management Journal, 36*(2), 319–348.

Evans-Pritchard, E. E. (1937). *Witchcraft, oracles and magic among the Azande.* London, Oxford University Press.

Frankl, V. (1963). *Man's search for meaning.* New York: Simon & Schuster.

Fromm, E. (1942). *The fear of freedom.* London: Routledge & Kegan Paul.

Geertz, C. (1966). Religion as a cultural system. In M. Banton (Ed.), *Anthropological approaches to the study of religion* (pp. 1–46). London: Tavistock.

Gilbert, D. T., Brown, R. P., Pinel, E. C., & Wilson, T. D. (2000). The illusion of external agency. *Journal of Personality and Social Psychology, 79*(5), 690–700.

Greenberg, J., Arndt, J., Simon, L., Pyszczynski, T., & Solomon, S. (2000). Proximal and distal defenses in response to reminders of one's mortality: Evidence of a temporal sequence. *Personality and Social Psychology Bulletin, 26*(1), 91–99.

Gurin, P., Gurin, G., & Morrison, B. M. (1978). Personal and ideological aspects of internal and external control. *Social Psychology, 41*(4), 275–296.

Hafer, C. L. (2000). Do innocent victims threaten the belief in a just world? Evidence from a modified Stroop task. *Journal of Personality and Social Psychology, 79*(2), 165–173.

Heine, S. J., & Lehman, D. R. (1995). Cultural variation in unrealistic optimism: Does the West feel more vulnerable than the East? *Journal of Personality and Social Psychology, 68*(4), 595–607.

Heine, S. J., Lehman, D. R., Markus, H. R., & Kitayama, S. (1999). Is there a universal need for positive self-regard? *Psychological Review, 106*(4), 766–794.

Hsee, C. K., & Kunreuther, H. C. (2000). The affection effect in insurance decisions. *Journal of Risk and Uncertainty, 20*(2), 141–159.

Kapp, K. W. (1963). *Hindu culture, economic development and social planning in India.* New York: Asia Publishing House.

Keyes, C. F., & Daniel, E. V. (Eds.). (1983). *Karma: An anthropological inquiry.* Berkeley: University of California Press.

Kitayama, S., Markus, H. R., Matsumoto, H., & Norasakkunkit, V. (1997). Individual and collective processes in the construction of the self: Self-enhancement in the United States and self-criticism in Japan. *Journal of Personality and Social Psychology, 72*(6), 1245–1267.

Langer, E. J. (1975). The illusion of control. *Journal of Personality and Social Psychology, 32,* 311–328.

Langer, E. J., & Rodin, J. (1976). The effects of choice and enhanced personal responsibility for the aged: A field experiment in an institutional setting. *Journal of Personality and Social Psychology, 34*(2), 191–198.

Lefcourt, H. M. (1982). *Locus of control: Current trends in theory and research.* Hillsdale, NJ: Erlbaum.

Lerner, M. J., & Miller, D. T. (1978). Just world research and the attribution process: Looking back and looking ahead. *Psychological Bulletin, 85,* 1030–1050.

Levenson, H. (1981). Differentiating among internality, powerful others, and chance. In H. M. Lefcourt (Ed.), *Research with the locus of control construct* (pp. 15–63). New York: Academic Press.

McClelland, G. H., Schulze, W. D., & Coursey, D. L. (1993). Insurance for low-probability hazards: A bimodal response to unlikely events. *Journal of Risk and Uncertainty*, 7, 95–116.

Miller, D. T., & Taylor, B. R. (1995). Counterfactual thought, regret, and superstition: How to avoid kicking yourself. In N. J. Roese & J. M. Olson (Eds.), *What might have been: The social psychology of counterfactual thinking* (pp. 305–331). Hillsdale, NJ: Erlbaum.

Morling, B., Kitayama, S., & Miyamoto, Y. (2002). Cultural practices emphasize influence in the United States and adjustment in Japan. *Personality and Social Psychology Bulletin*, 28, 311–323.

Morris, M. W., Menon, T., & Ames, D. R. (2001). Culturally conferred conceptions of agency: A key to social perception of persons, groups, and other actors. *Personality and Social Psychology Review*, 5(2), 169–182.

Myrdal, G. (1968). *The Asian drama: An inquiry into poverty of nations*. New York: Pantheon.

Peterson, C., & Seligman, M. (1983). Learned helplessness and victimization. *Journal of Social Issues*, 2, 103–116.

Peterson, C., & Seligman, M. E. P. (1984). Causal explanations as a risk factor for depression: Theory and evidence. *Psychological Review*, 91(3), 347–374.

Roth, N. (1978). Fear of death in the aging. *American Journal of Psychotherapy*, 32, 552–560.

Rothbart, M., & Snyder, M. (1970). Confidence in the prediction and postdiction of an uncertain event. *Canadian Journal of Behavioral Sciences*, 2, 38–43.

Rotter, J. B. (1966). Generalized expectancies for internal versus external control of reinforcement. *Psychological Monographs*, 80(1), 609.

Sartre, J.-P. (1951). *The devil and the good lord*. Paris: Gallimard.

Seligman, M. (1975). *Helplessness: On depression, development, and death*. Oxford, UK: Freeman.

Slovic, P., Finucane, M., Peters, E., & MacGregor, D. G. (2002). The affect heuristic. In T. Gilovich, D. Griffin, & D. Kahneman (Eds.), *Heuristics and biases: The psychology of intuitive judgment* (pp. 397–420). New York: Cambridge University Press.

Smith, P. B., Trompenaars, F., & Dugan, S. (1995). The Rotter locus of control scale in 42 countries: A test of cultural relativity. *International Journal of Psychology*, 30(3), 377–400.

Sperber, D. (1994). The modularity of thought and the epidemiology of representations. In L. A. Hirschfeld & S. A. Gelman (Eds.), *Mapping the mind: Domain specificity in cognition and culture* (pp. 39–67). New York: Cambridge University Press.

Taylor, S. E. (2000). Psychological resources, positive illusions, and health. *American Psychologist*, 55(1), 99–109.

Taylor, S. E., & Brown, J. D. (1999). Illusion and well-being: A social psychological perspective on mental health. In R. F. Baumeister (Ed.), *The self in social psychology* (pp. 43–68). Philadelphia: Psychology Press.

Taylor, S. E., Lichtman, R. R., & Wood, J. V. (1984). Attributions, beliefs about control, and adjustment to breast cancer. *Journal of Personality and Social Psychology*, 46, 489–502.

Wellman, H. M., & Gelman, S. A. (1992). Cognitive development: Foundational theories of core domains. *Annual Review of Psychology*, 43, 337–375.

Wilson, T. D. (2002). *Strangers to ourselves: Discovering the adaptive unconscious*. Cambridge, MA: Harvard University Press.

Yamaguchi, S. (2001). Culture and control orientations. In D. Matsumoto (Ed.), *Handbook of culture and psychology* (pp. 223–243). New York: Oxford University Press.

Young, M. J., Morris, M. W., Krishnan, L., & Regmi, M. P. (2003). *Controlled by higher powers: Fatalistic thoughts and practices in Judeo-Christian and Hindu cultures*. Manuscript submitted for publication.

Zusne, L., & Jones, W. H. (1989). *Anomalistic psychology: A study of magical thinking*. Hillsdale, NJ: Erlbaum.

Chapter 15

Cultural Trauma and Recovery

Cultural Meaning, Self-Esteem, and the Reconstruction of the Cultural Anxiety Buffer

MICHAEL B. SALZMAN
MICHAEL J. HALLORAN

There is compelling evidence from a broad range of indicators to demonstrate that the indigenous peoples of the world experience a state of living and health that is well below acceptable standards. In most cases where this situation exists, the cause is attributed to the impact of colonization and its ongoing effects (e.g., Blaisdell, 1996; Ober, Peeters, Archer, & Kelly, 2000). Although such a view is clearly justified, the complexity and prevalence of psychological and well-being problems suffered by indigenous people today require deeper analysis. Consistent with the existential perspective taken in this book, we suggest that colonization brought about deep suffering for indigenous people due to the subsequent destruction of their culture, a vital source of existential meaning.

In this chapter, we consider the human need for meaning in the context of the consequences of the traumatic disruption of culture and the resultant breakdown of systems of meaning and value for human beings. The experiences of cultural disruption of three groups of genetically distinct and geographically dispersed indigenous peoples will be examined from the existential framework provided by terror management theory (TMT) and research (Becker, 1971; Greenberg, Solomon & Pyszczynski, 1997). Specifically, we use a TMT analysis to help comprehend the psychodynamics of what has been described as cultural trauma (Salzman, 2001) and the motive of genetically diverse and geographically dispersed peoples to recover, reconstruct, and apply traditional culture to current realities.

CULTURE AS A PSYCHOLOGICAL DEFENSE AGAINST THE TERROR INHERENT IN HUMAN EXISTENCE: THE CULTURAL ANXIETY BUFFER

TMT suggests that cultures serve as an essential psychological defense against the terror that is inherent in human existence (Becker, 1971; Greenberg et al., 1997; Pyszczynski, Greenberg, & Solomon, 1997). In particular, culture offers people a means to deny the reality that personal annihilation (mortality) is our inevitable destiny. Cultural conceptions of reality evolved, in part, to provide protection against this most basic of all human fears. At the most fundamental level, these conceptions of reality provide people with a sense of meaning, that life is significant and permanent and consists of more than taking in food, expelling waste, and temporarily clinging to survival on a clump of dirt and rock hurtling through space (Jonas, Schimel, Greenberg, & Pyszczynski, 2002). Thus, in providing meaning and value to life, culture can be seen as an anxiety buffer against the terror intrinsic to human life.

The cultural anxiety buffer consists of a worldview that one has faith in and culturally prescribed standards of being and acting in the world that, if achieved, provide self-esteem and the conviction that one is indeed of value in a meaningful world. An essential function of culture, then, is to make continued self-esteem accessible and possible so anxiety-prone humans can obtain a state of relative equanimity in a terrifying existence where annihilation is the only certainty. Thus, TMT proposes that culture and self-esteem form a dual-component anxiety buffer; because the cultural worldview and self-esteem provide a sense of meaning and value, respectively, they are viewed as adaptations to the problem of existential anxiety. However, as self-esteem is contingent upon an individual meeting culturally prescribed standards of value, the cultural worldview is considered to serve the most basic anxiety-buffering role.

The empirical confirmation of the predictions of TMT (e.g., Greenberg et al., 1997; Rosenblatt, Greenberg, Solomon, Pyszczynski, & Lyon, 1989; Greenberg, Simon, Porteus, Pyszczynski, & Solomon, 1995; Schimel et al., 1999) provides strong support to the notion that the cultural worldview is a central mechanism for buffering human existential anxiety. An implication of this perspective is that if people have little faith in, or connection with, the cultural worldview, they are likely to be susceptible to anxiety and related symptoms. Indeed, TMT research has generated indirect support for this assumption by showing that depressed individuals show even stronger defensive reactions to mortality salience, and when given the opportunity to defend their worldview, they report greater meaningfulness in life (see Simon, Arndt, Greenberg, Pyszczynski, & Solomon, 1998). But, when the structure of the cultural worldview is severely compromised, as in the case of cultural trauma experienced by the people of indigenous cultures, TMT predicts that it would lead to dire psychological and behavioral effects—a point we develop further in the next section of this chapter.

CULTURAL TRAUMA AND INDIGENOUS PEOPLES

Indigenous peoples and the cultural worldviews that have psychologically supported them have been traumatized as a result of contact with European peoples (Salzman, 2001). This contact and its attendant assaults by disease, military conquest, and economic and cultural disruption have produced similar consequences across vast distances and genetic inheritance. The devastating loss of population due to disease resulting from contact with Europeans was experienced throughout indigenous America and the Pacific (Bushnell, 1993; Butlin, 1983; Farnsworth, 1997; Napoleon, 1996). Peoples as genetically dissimilar as Yup'ik Eskimos, Navajos and Athabaskan Indians, Hawaiian Natives, and Australian Aboriginals have experienced similar physical, social, behavioral, and psychological symptomologies (e.g., high rates of suicide, alcoholism, and accidental deaths) as a consequence of contact with Europeans (Brave Heart & DeBruyn, 1995; Bushnell, 1993; Farnsworth, 1997; Napoleon, 1996; Indian Health Service, 1995; Ober et al., 2000). The enduring severity of these symptomologies invites a reconceptualization of the dynamics that produced them in order to provide new insight and inform treatment.

There is evidence that anxiety may be a potent factor underlying many of the negative health statistics associated with Native peoples. For example, Duran (1999) found that 58% of Native American clients at a Native American Health Center had anxiety disorders, and he suggested that anxiety underlies all other problems that Indians are experiencing regardless of whether there was a concurrent substance abuse disorder. Manson et al. (1996) also noted high rates of anxiety in American Indian populations across tribe and region. If culture serves as a psychological defense against anxiety, then its traumatic disruption would subject culturally traumatized people to unmediated existential terror producing the motive to manage that terror by any means available.

To illustrate the aforementioned points further, the cultural trauma experienced at different times by genetically different and geographically distant indigenous populations are considered now through the application of TMT to three naturalistic settings. In the first case, we review the effects of cultural trauma through the eyes of a Native Alaskan. We then consider the progress of white settlement in Hawaii and its effects on indigenous culture. Finally, the health and social problems of indigenous Australians that illustrate the relationship between anxiety and cultural trauma are discussed.

Cultural Trauma in Alaska

Napoleon (1996) vividly describes the trauma experienced by the Native peoples of Alaska as a result of their contact with Europeans and colonization. He depicts a world of meaning shattered by disease and sudden death where the solutions offered by traditional culture (e.g., shamanic interventions) proved incapable of mediating the horror that affected Native populations. In "Yu Yu Raq: The Way of the Human Being," Napoleon's description of how the Yu'pik (Eskimo) world of meaning collapsed as a result of the social consequences of the cultural trauma resulting from the "Great Death" is consistent with the anxiety-buffer hypothesis of TMT:

> Prior to the arrival of Western people, the Yup'ik were alone in their riverine and Bering Sea homeland—they and the spirit beings that made things the way they were. They were ruled by the customs, traditions, and spiritual beliefs of their people, and shaped by these and their environment: the tundra, the river and the Bering Sea. . . . They called it *Yuuyaraq*, the way of being a human being. Although unwritten, this way can be compared to Mosaic law because it governed all aspects of a human being's life. . . . It defined acceptable behavior for all members of the community. (p. 4)

In this description, one can see references to clear prescriptions for being and living in the world. Anxiety-buffering self-esteem would be attained if the individual sees him- or herself as living up to those standards. If one lived up to those standards, one would be rewarded with plenty, health, and even immortality because the individual's spirit was immortal and would be "reborn when its name was given to a newborn" (Napoleon, 1996, p. 7). Napoleon (1996) then goes on to describe the effects of white settlement on the culture of his people:

> When the first white men arrived in the Yup'ik villages, the people did not immediately abandon their old ways . . . but resistance to Western rule would crumble, Yuuyaraq would be abandoned, and the spirit world would be displaced by Christianity. . . . The change was brought about as a result of the introduction of diseases that had been born in the slums of Europe. . . . To these diseases the Yup'ik and other Native tribes had no immunity, and to these they would lose up to 60% of their people. As a result of the epidemics, the Yup'ik world would go upside down; it would end. (pp. 9–10)

> The suffering, the despair, the heartbreak, the desperation, and confusion these survivors lived through is unimaginable. People watched helplessly as their mothers, fathers, brothers, and sisters grew ill, the efforts of the *angalkuq* [medicine men] failing. . . . Whether the survivors knew or understood, they had witnessed the fatal wounding of *Yuuraraq* and the old Yup'ik culture. . . . The Yup'ik world was turned upside down, literally overnight. Out of the suffering, in confusion, desperation, heartbreak, and trauma was born a new generation of Yup'ik people. They were born into shock. They woke to a world in shambles, many of their people and their beliefs strewn around them, dead. Their medicines and their medicine men and women had proven useless. Everything they had believed in had failed. Their ancient world had collapsed. . . . The world the survivors woke to was without anchor. They woke up in shock, listless, confused, bewildered, heartbroken, and afraid. (pp. 10–11)

In the Yup'ik world, imbued with meaning and correct standards of behavior, one had a compass and map to live by in an extremely harsh and dangerous environment. What was required to achieve the anxiety buffer was to believe in the description of reality (faith in the cultural worldview) and to see oneself as living up to its prescribed standards of behavior and being. The individual, with cultural anxiety buffer intact and self-esteem accessed, could then navigate in a dangerous world with anxiety managed sufficiently to enable adaptive action. As shown in the descriptions by Napoleon (1996), white settlement and its effects brought about severe disruption to the Yup'ik worldview, and thus the means for individuals to secure psychological equanimity, was severely compromised. A similar trauma occurred in Hawaii and across the Pacific.

Cultural Trauma in Hawaii

Contact between Hawaii and the Western world began in 1798 with the arrival of Captain James Cook and his crew. Cook's crewmen introduced gonorrhea, syphilis, tuberculosis, and possibly viral hepatitis (Blaisdell, 1989; Stannard, 1989). In a little over 100 years, the Hawaiian community experienced massive depopulation. Numbered at approximately 400,000 to 800,000 in 1778, the Hawaiian community dropped under 40,000 by the 1890s (Hammond, 1988; Stannard, 1989). "This is a population collapse vastly more destructive than the one suffered by medieval Europeans at the hands of the Black Death" (Stannard, 1989, p. 45).

Through contact with the Europeans, Hawaiians gradually lost their socioeconomic and political independence. In 1819, the overthrow of the *Kapu* system, the laws that governed all aspects of Hawaiian culture, led to numerous disenfranchised and culturally disillusioned Hawaiians (Crabbe, 1991). Also, the theft of native lands, called the Māhele of 1848, left Hawaiians with less than 10% of their land (Blaisdell, 1989; Faludi, 1991). Further assaults to the Hawaiian way of life occurred when the monarchy was overthrown in 1893 and the United States forcibly annexed Hawaii in 1898 (Blaisdell, 1989; Marsella, Oliveira, Plummer, & Crabbe, 1995; Trask, 1995). This was indeed a tragic time for the Hawaiian people as "the monarchy represented the last and best hope that somehow the Native Hawaiian people could reestablish themselves and reassert their identity" (Marsella et al., 1995, p. 99). Without the *Kapu* system and monarchy to guide them, Hawaiians eventually gave in to constant pressure to assimilate into an anti-Hawaiian, Western way of living.

Currently, Hawaiians have the worst health profile of any group in the state of Hawaii (Blaisdell, 1989; Marsella et al., 1995). Compared to other ethnic groups in Hawaii, indigenous Hawaiians have the highest rates for cancer deaths, diabetes, high blood pressure, gout, bronchitis, asthma, emphysema, and obesity. They also have the shortest life expectancy, higher rates of infant mortality, congenital diseases, sudden infant death syndrome, and rate of suicide. Hawaiians also show numerous psychological and social well-being problems (Blaisdell, 1989; Hammond, 1988; Marsella et al., 1995; Mokuau, 1990). Hawaiians comprise 40% of the state of Hawaii's prison population, although only 12% of the general population, and have the highest rates of smoking, substance abuse, and teenage and unmarried pregnancies. Exept for Samoans, Hawaiians have the highest rates of child abuse and neglect. Hawaiians also have the highest rates of antisocial behavior, family and school problems, demoralization, alienation, and low self-esteem.

This incomprehensible set of circumstances can be understood in the same way as the Yup'ik Great Death. Old Hawaiian customs previously bonded together by ancient Polynesian beliefs, now fractured by the overthrow of the traditional religion, collapsed at all levels. The worldview was shattered and invalidated and, in TMT terms, anxiety-buffering self-esteem was inaccessible, leaving Hawaiians to cope with these aversive conditions by whatever means were accessible; anxiety-related behaviors would be expected to increase under such conditions. A third example of what may be considered external validation of TMT hypotheses is the experience of Australian Aboriginal people as a result of contact with Europeans and the resultant trauma and its consequences.

Cultural Trauma of Aboriginal Australians

Prior to white colonial settlement in 1788, there were some 500 indigenous tribal groups in Australia, each with distinct language and cultural practices. Nevertheless, common to all indigenous Australian groups was the centrality of the land, law, family and kin relationships, and spirituality to their cultural worldviews (Christie, 1988; Coombs, Brandl, & Snowdon, 1983; Harris, 1990). A close interrelationship between these and many other aspects of life is also a distinctive feature of Aboriginal cultures. By a range of means and interventions, colonization lcd to these elements of the cultural worldview being severely undermined.

The history of white settlement in Australia is plagued with its intervention into Aboriginal life and culture (see Ober et al., 2000). In the first century of settlement, these included land dispossession by force, theft of women, slavery and war, introduced diseases, and the missionary zeal for conversion of Aboriginal people and rejection of Aboriginal spiritual concepts such as the dreaming, a sacred, heroic time, long ago, when humans and nature came to be (Stanner, 1979). Moreover, settlement brought with it the assertion of the British legal system, which effectively extinguished indigenous customary law. In the 20th century, further intervention into Aboriginal culture and life was evidenced in the government's White Australia Policy and a general strategy of indigenous assimilation through forced removal of children from their family of origin and placement with Europeans, which undermined Aboriginal social structures. Altogether, such interventions into Aboriginal life have been argued to represent a not too subtle form of cultural genocide (Human Rights and Equal Opportunity Commission, 1997). At the very least, the destruction of Aboriginal law, spirituality, and social structure and the possession of their land are widely regarded to have severely subverted their traditional cultural worldview (e.g., Ober et al., 2000; Wessells & Bretherton, 2000).

From the terror management perspective, the interventions into indigenous Australian cultural life are likely to completely undermine the effectiveness of their cultural worldview as an anxiety buffer and lead to anxiety-related cognitions and behaviors. In fact, regardless of the criteria used to measure them, anxiety-related cognitions and behavior are prevalent among the indigenous people of Australia and have been likened to the symptomatology of posttraumatic stress syndrome (Ober et al., 2000). For instance, there are disturbingly higher reported proportions of indigenous imprisonment, infant mortality, suicide, drug dependence and substance abuse, and general medical conditions (see Hogg, 1994; Hunter, 1995; Perkins, Sanson-Fisher, Blunden, & Lunnay, 1994; Swann & Raphael, 1995). Indigenous people also show very high levels and rates of self-reported hopelessness, helplessness, and disorientation as well as anxiety, irritability, and insomnia (e.g., Eckermann et al., 1992; Koolmartie & Williams, 2000) and are five times more likely than the Australian population, in total, to die from the consequences of a mental disorder (Bhatia & Anderson, 1995). In addition, due to the low social status and poor living conditions of the indigenous peoples of Australia, they rely on economic assistance from the government, which has exacerbated their perception of dependence and feelings of helplessness (Pearson, 2000).

Altogether the experiences and the state of Aboriginal life in Australia are not dissimilar to those evidenced with indigenous peoples in other parts of the world. In each case we have previously described, we can see cultural destruction and trauma alongside prevalent anxiety-related cognitions and behaviors. We assert that it is the fundamental breakdown in terror management processes that link these two phenomena and give meaning to the complexity of problems experienced by culturally traumatized peoples. Specifically, the cultural destruction and trauma experienced by First Nation indigenous peoples has undermined their basis of existential meaning and value to the extent that they have little protection from basic human anxiety, which has become manifest in the extent and prevalence of the psychological ill health and poor well-being they suffer. Such an analysis, though, suggests that cultural restoration and recovery would go along way toward addressing the dynamics of this set of circumstances. The next section describes the efforts in this direction as well as other expressions of how indigenous peoples have recreated a world of meaning and value.

CULTURAL RECOVERY AND THE RECONSTRUCTION OF A CULTURAL ANXIETY BUFFER

Indigenous people throughout the world, having suffered trauma and an inculcated sense of inferiority supported by oppressive colonial systems, are seeking their traditional cultural worldviews and resurrecting the ontological prescriptions and standards embedded in those worldviews. How can we understand this motive? TMT offers a clear explanation. For many indigenous people, the Western worldview, while overwhelming, was never compelling enough to attract the faith required to establish an adequate cultural anxiety buffer. For others, the overwhelming power of the colonizers may have made its worldview compelling, but racism and other structural barriers made the achievement of its standards extremely difficult. The result in both cases is anxiety.

While maladaptive anxiety reduction strategies may have momentary desired effects, they serve to produce additional sources of grief, pain, and tragedy (Department of Education, 1993). From a TMT perspective, efforts toward cultural recovery and a reconstitution of a world of meaning in which to act represent an important step toward the restoration of the essential psychological prerequisites for adaptive action. Indigenous people with similar histories of traumatic cultural disruption are seeking to identify and operationalize bedrock principles and values that define their being and guide their action. The movement toward cultural recovery is happening across vast distances in geography and genetic inheritance. This section explores the efforts of Native Hawaiians, Alaskans, and Australians to restore the cultural foundations of life and to adapt them to current conditions.

The Hawaiian Renaissance

A cultural revival that began in Hawaii in the late 1960s took off tremendously in the 1970s and continues to influence generations of Hawaiians today (Kanahele, 1982). During the Hawaiian renaissance period, Hawaiians' interest in almost all aspects of Hawaiian culture, including music, hula, art, language, crafts, literature, religion, and politics, increased immensely. Kanahele (1982) writes:

> Like a dormant volcano coming to life again, the Hawaiians are erupting with all the pent-up energy and frustrations of a people on the "make." This great happening has been called a "psychological renewal," a "reaffirmation," a "revival," and a "renaissance." No matter what you call it, it is the most significant chapter in 20th century Hawaiian history. Why? Because it has reversed years of cultural decline; it has created a new kind of Hawaiian consciousness; it has inspired greater pride in being Hawaiian; it has led to bold and imaginative ways of reasserting our identity; it has led to a new political awareness; and it has had and will continue to have a positive impact on the economic and social uplifting of the Hawaiian community. (p. 10)

A focus for Hawaiian cultural reconstruction ("Astonishing cultural revival," 2002) was the construction and navigation by traditional methods of the double-hulled voyaging canoe called the Hokle'a. This effort established routes and methods that ancient Hawaiians used to settle the islands. It helped recover history, culture, and a sense pride and dignity that had been damaged by trauma and colonization. The positive effects of the Hawaiian renaissance are still evident in the 21st century. Hawaiians as a people continue to thrive in traditional and modern evolutions of Hawaiian culture. Despite numerous disparaging statistics resulting from an imposed, Western colonial system, Hawaiians, by participating in *Nä Mea Hawaii,* or "Things Hawaiian," have gained a stronger identity and self-worth. They continue to strive for sovereignty, self-determination, and the ability to define who they are as a nation (Trask, 1995).

Cultural renaissance is also reflected in the recovery of traditional rituals and ceremonies. For example, the ancient Hawaiian healing concept of Ho'oponopono is currently being used to restore and maintain good relationships among family, and the family and supernatural powers (Shook, 1985). Part of Ho'oponopono addresses internalized negative evaluations of being Hawaiian and works to eliminate shame while promoting the acquisition of traditional concepts of healthy relationships and pride in Hawaiian culture. Ho'oponopono has a spiritual aspect through the use of prayers and a process of *mihi* and *kala* or forgiveness and the unbinding of the *hala* or fault. In the Hawaiian worldview, the family is seen as a complex set of relationships where any disturbance in one part of the net will affect the rest of system, thus Ho'oponopono reinforces Hawaiian philosophy and its emphasis on the interrelatedness of all things. Similar cultural revival has occurred with the reestablishment of the "uniki" ceremony that selected the Kahuna (spiritual leaders) of the people ("Alumni keep," 2003).

The positive effects of the cultural renaissance are manifest in the success of efforts to incorporate traditional culture and its resonant meanings into educational practice. Students attending Halau Ku Mana, a charter school at the University of Hawaii, Manoa–Center for Hawaiian Studies, are involved in culture-based education. These students, who had been truant and unsuccessful in the public school system, built a double-hulled Hawaiian canoe and launched it with the support of traditional chanting and blessings calling for wisdom and guidance for the young voyagers ("Canoe embodies," 2002). As evidence of the success of this program, the students achieved a 98% attendance rate and are meeting or exceeding Hawaii State Department of Education standards across the board.

The Hawaiian Immersion School movement is a further example of the positive effects of cultural revival on the general well-being of Hawaiians (Slaughter, 1997). The aim of this program is to incorporate Hawaiian culture and language into the educational experiences of Hawaiian children. Indigenous students in this program would have been considered part of an at-risk group for low school achievement and special education; however, with participation in the immersion program they have shown relatively significant educational achievement. For example, at the end of the sixth grade, one cohort of students displayed an unusual level of fluency in oral Hawaiian and were able to read and comprehend in English on a standardized measure of sixth-grade and junior high school reading ability. Further, of the approximately 100 students who will have graduated from immersion programs by this year, over 80% have been accepted into college, with two accepted into Stanford University ("Hawaiians back," 2003). Moreover, the program has led to increased parental involvement in their children's education, a key element of successful education and community building yet, until recently, less evident with historically marginalized Hawaiians.

From the viewpoint of TMT, the process of recovering and reconstructing Hawaiian culture is a psychological renewal, and the revalidation of one's culture and its standards for being and living in the world serves to strengthen the essential anxiety-buffering function of the culture. The revival of hula, language and culture study, music, and traditional forms of healing such as Ho'oponopono serve to reconstruct a world of meaning for people to act in and achieve anxiety-buffering self-esteem through the meeting of standards of value defined by a worldview infused with new belief. This type of revival makes adaptive action more probable in a wide variety of contexts, including those imposed by the effects of colonization suffered by native Hawaiians.

Cultural Recovery in Alaska

Inupiat Ilitqusiat is a social movement that became institutionalized in northwestern Alaska during the 1980s. This term roughly translates as the "wisdom and lessons of Inupiaq people (McNabb, 1991, p. 63). The movement identified values that define the "Inupiaq Way." These include such core values as sharing, respect for elders, cooperation, respect for others, knowledge of language, love of children, hard work, avoidance of conflict, respect for nature, spirituality, humor, hunter success, and humility.

Efforts to recover core values and essential ontological guidance for living and being in the world are also taking place in the rugged ecology of the Aleutians. In the Unangan region of Alaska rules for living are based on identified Unangan/Unangas values (Carlson, 2003). Twenty-seven "simple instructions" based on identified core cultural values were developed as "The Right Way to Live as an Unangax." These "simple instructions" as translated from the Native language, include the following: share, listen, don't be boastful, be kind to other people, help others, take care of the land, do not do anything to excess, respect elders, respect your peers, don't be envious of what belongs to another, admire one who does well by honest means, don't talk bad about the weather, don't slander another person, subsistence, don't forget your Unangan language.

These values serve as ontological prescriptions for those who identify and have faith in the cultural worldview from which they are derived. They provide people with the possibility of meeting (in TMT terms) the standards of value prescribed by the culture, thereby making a functional cultural anxiety buffer accessible to those who identify with and believe in the cultural worldview.

Cultural Recovery in Aboriginal Australia

Like other similar contexts, the Australian approach to the indigenous psychological and ill-health problems has only recently shifted to one that focuses on culturally relevant methods and practices. Prior to the recognition of cultural factors in Aboriginal health, Western-style approaches to health intervention were prominent. According to Ober et al. (2000), in most cases, these approaches were largely ineffective and served to undermine indigenous culture further, as it focused on diagnosis and cure of disorders, which "had the effect of individualizing and pathologizing what are complex social and historical issues" (p. 248). Nevertheless, of late, Australian recognition of the importance of culture to indigenous health has developed at the highest levels of Australian society, as evidenced by a recent report issued by the Parliament of Australia (2000) that states:

> It is very clear to the Committee that the issue of culture and its importance to Indigenous Australians is a key matter in the planning and delivery of services, if those services are going to be used by, and meet the needs of, Indigenous Australians. (p. 7)

Although it is not possible to conclude with any surety the effectiveness of a cultural recovery and recognition approach to the improvement of Australian indigenous health due to the lack of relevant program review, research activity, and investment in this approach that has occurred thus far, available evidence supports our contention that rebuilding a world of indigenous cultural meaning and relevance goes toward addressing poor health and ill-being problems.

Cultural recognition and recovery are central to the approach of the We Al-Li program, which focuses on strategies to heal pain and trauma of indigenous Australians through the use of traditional ceremonies of healing (Atkinson & Ober, 1995). We Al-Li (the Woppaburra term for fire and water), uses a supportive social context and traditional practices in places of cultural significance for the expression of anger and sorrow. With this method, the program participants report deep emotional healing and moving from victim self-perceptions to those of a survivor. Other programs, such as an Aboriginal Empowerment Program in the Northern Territory (Tsey & Every, 2000), which focuses on family well-being, have also shown promising indications of the value of culturally minded programs to the improvement of indigenous health and well-being (see Swann & Raphael, 1995, for a more extensive review of indigenous mental health programs).

More general health programs also show the positive impact of cultural recognition and rebuilding with indigenous Australians. The Belyuen Health Centre (see Coombs et al., 1983) showed significant improvements in health outcomes of indigenous people by taking into account aspects of Aboriginality, such as social kin relationships and responsibilities, methods of time keeping, gender issues, and the use of traditional healers and language. Furthermore, the Strong Women, Strong Babies, Strong Culture Program led to marked improvements in the health and well-being of pregnant women when cultural factors were taken in account (Fejo & Rae, 1996). This initiative involved participants undertaking traditional food collection to increase exercise and traditional pregnancy practices, such as the smoking ceremony. The program has demonstrated its success with a significant decrease in the rate of low birthweights and preterm births among participants.

While there is lack of strong evidence at this stage, there is substance to the claim that health and well-being programs with indigenous Australians that adopt a strategy consistent with the aims of cultural recognition, maintenance, and regeneration are likely to be more successful than the alternatives. The case of Aboriginal Australians is a demonstration of the implication in TMT that culture, through its provision of a world of existential meaning and value, protects people from basic anxiety. Indigenous Australians are likely to find greater psychological harmony to the extent that there is an investment in their cultural recovery.

Cultural Recovery and Bicultural Adaptation

As a consequence of European settlement, indigenous people have lived with and been exposed to an alternative cultural worldview to their traditional culture. From the perspective of cultural dynamics (e.g., Hong, Chiu, & Kung, 1997; Kashima, 2001), people who are repeatedly exposed to an alternative culture are likely to develop bicultural knowledge and identity. In other words, over time, people who are members of distinct collectives develop distinct networks of cultural meanings to adapt to their different cultural contexts. The TMT approach would suggest that bicultural adaptation is a means of cultural redefinition and recovery.

In the case of contemporary Aboriginal Australians, it is generally believed that they possess two distinct cultural identities: Aboriginal and Australian (Christie, 1988; Clark, 2000). Further, the Aboriginal and Australian cultural worldviews show distinct differences: collectivistic and relational tendencies are a central feature of traditional Aboriginal culture, whereas individualistic tendencies are a characteristic of Australian mainstream culture (Davidson & Reser, 1996; Fogarty & White, 1994; Kashima et al., 1995; Triandis, 1995). Thus, because Aboriginal Australians maintain such distinct sets of cultural knowledge, they are endowed with *bicultural competence* (see LaFromboise, Coleman, & Gerton, 1993), which is the capacity to switch between different cultural frameworks as a function of which identity is activated in the ongoing social context.

On the surface, the adaptation to different cultural realities by indigenous people through maintenance of a bicultural identity appears to contradict the TMT assumption that people find alternative worldviews threatening (Becker, 1971). Nevertheless, Halloran and Kashima (in press) have recently reported evidence that bicultural individuals show endorsement of alternative worldviews as a function of their exposure to distinct social contexts. In their study, bicultural indigenous Australians participants were asked to report their support for collectivism, relationism, and individualism values when asked to contemplate their own mortality under conditions that activated either their Aboriginal or their Australian identity. The findings showed that collectivistic and relational tendencies were stronger when participants defined themselves in Aboriginal terms, and support for individualism was higher when their Australian identity was activated. Moreover, these tendencies were emphasized when mortality was salient and suggest that alternative meaning systems held by bicultural individuals do not necessarily pose them a threat, as they are not likely to be activated in the same context.

Although bicultural individuals have adapted to different cultural realities with the ability to switch between identity-specific cultural meaning systems, they still continue to suffer. We suspect that the low status and prejudice that indigenous people continue to experience is likely to have undermined any positive effects such an adaptation might deliver. While one can envisage that cultural hybrids offering a more flexible meaning system might develop from bicultural competence, the experiences of indigenous peoples suggest that a supportive environment is a necessary condition for such growth to occur.

DISCUSSION AND IMPLICATIONS

In this chapter, we have reported the experiences of cultural trauma and recovery of indigenous people from Alaska, Hawaii, and Australia. There is little doubt that there is an overrepresentation of anxiety and related behavior among these people. Despite their distinct genetic, geographical, and cultural backgrounds, the commonly acknowledged precursor to this situation is the impact of colonization on indigenous people and its subsequent effects on their lives and livelihood. The high prevalence of existential anxiety among indigenous people indicates their deep psychological suffering, which we contend is due in part to the destruction and trauma to indigenous culture. A TMT account of cultural trauma suggests that a range of intrusions into indigenous culture has severely undermined their source of existential meaning and value, which provides protection from basic human anxieties, such as mortality awareness. The evidence presented in this chapter suggests a strong association between the cultural destruction and existential anxiety experienced by indigenous people and preliminary support for the contention that indigenous cultural recovery leads directly to improvement in their health and well-being.

The common link between the damage inflicted on the world's indigenous cultures and the abysmal state of health and psychological well-being suffered by indigenous peoples is suggestive of a general phenomenon we have referred to as cultural trauma. Brave Heart and DeBruyn (1995) refer to cultural trauma as the product of a legacy of chronic trauma and unresolved grief across generations originating from stunning loss of lives, lands, and vital aspects of Native cultures resulting from contact with Europeans. Although cultural trauma shares some etiological similarity with posttraumatic stress disorder, it is clearly distinct, as cultural trauma stems from damage inflicted to a group's rather than an individual's psychological defensive system. Thus, the recent assertion that one can classify indigenous people's suffering as posttraumatic stress disorder is not well founded (see Ober et al., 2000) and, perhaps, further undermines their cultural worldview. From the viewpoint of TMT, our analysis qualifies cultural trauma as a state of emotional anxiety suffered by an individual or group of individuals who have experienced severe compromise to their system of cultural meaning. Specifically, the cultural trauma disruption experienced by indigenous people has severely undermined the capacity of the cultural worldview to meet the need for a world of existential meaning and value and, thus, to minimize basic human anxiety.

Our analysis also suggests that reconstructing a world of meaning and value via cultural recovery is likely to equip indigenous people with the means to achieve greater psychological equanimity than that which they currently experience. Although efforts in this direction are in their infancy, and only one of many possible interventions, the evidence we reviewed indicates that culturally sensitive recovery programs can indeed achieve these ends. The efficacy of traditional ceremonial treatment in addressing the traumatic experiences of Native American people is also noted by Manson et al. (1996), with their comments that the "great relevance for such forms of healing lies in their meaning-making aspects and the co-herence-engendering qualities of the healing ritual" (p. 275). They observe that such rituals are designed to promote a sense of continuity of the community and continuity of the individual in the culture. Nevertheless, the concept and practice of cultural recovery also require clarification, especially as intercultural and tribal difference makes the task of such definition more complicated. In the words of the review conducted by the Parliament of Australia (2000), "Many of the witnesses to the Inquiry, found it difficult to articulate which were the important aspects of culture and how they may be encompassed by health and related services" (p. 70).

The material we have reviewed in this chapter provides some external validity to the claims of terror management theorists. TMT theorists and researchers suggest that self-esteem is a cultural construction that serves the essential function of buffering anxiety-prone humans against the potentially paralyzing terror that may result from an unmediated awareness of mortality (Harmon-Jones et al., 1997). Moreover, if the cultural worldview is threatened or disrupted, anxiety and maladaptive defenses against anxiety are likely to result. As described in this chapter, and in more detail elsewhere in this book, there is compelling experimental evidence to support this claim by showing that people are likely to show anxiety-related behavior through cultural worldview defense when they are threatened. The traumatic disruption of the cultures of genetically diverse indigenous peoples, such as the Alaskan Natives, Australian Aboriginals, and Native Hawaiian, has resulted in similar psychosocial and behavioral consequences, which reflect a breakdown of terror management processes. Specifically, the disruption of the cultural anxiety buffer by Western contact, imported diseases, and colonization has produced similar consequences, therefore suggesting common psychodynamics. Although there is an impressive array of experimental data to provide internal validity to TMT claims, the findings we have reviewed here have been drawn from naturalistic settings with distinct indigenous groups and, thus, provide some important external validity to TMT (see Sue, 1999).

The portrayal of indigenous cultural trauma and recovery we have presented in this chapter raises some specific implications for policy, practice, and research. At one level, our analysis suggests the need to advocate public policy that is responsive to the dynamics of cultural trauma and recovery. While indigenous reconciliation movements in various countries (e.g., Council for Aboriginal Reconciliation, 1996) represent a form of cultural trauma recognition, it can be concluded that the dynamics of cultural trauma suggest the importance of translation of such sentiment into policy toward recovery of indigenous culture (e.g., recognition of indigenous law and land). Although our view is that cultural recovery programs address the effects of cultural trauma most significantly, the political will to support such measures is crucial to their effective implementation.

The dynamics of cultural trauma and revival should also inform the professional areas of practice with indigenous peoples. We suggest that professionals consider the validity of a diagnosis of "cultural trauma syndrome," which we propose to describe as a common cluster of symptoms suffered by people who experience traumatic cultural disruption (see also Salzman, 2001, in press). Furthermore, cultural reconstruction through bicultural adaptation is evidenced as a terror management process with most indigenous peoples and suggests ways that can inform general programs delivered to indigenous people, and in particular, those designed to address the ill-health and well-being problems of indigenous people. Professionals can also assist individuals and communities in the identification of standards and values within the cultural worldview that promote adaptive action in current realities.

Finally, our research in the area of cultural trauma and recovery indicates that there is a lack of quality data to substantiate the effects of cultural trauma and the effectiveness of cultural recovery programs. Although many programs have been developed to implement cultural recovery initiatives, many have lacked funding for their completion, let alone their evaluation. This is perhaps indicative of a lack of the aforementioned political will by national governments to fully recognize the dynamics and effects of their indigenous people's cultural trauma and recovery, despite people's ongoing suffering. Nonetheless, we trust that our analysis provides a credible articulation of the need for such recognition and a potent understanding of why indigenous peoples suffer as they do.

CONCLUSION

The chapter we have presented in this book represents an existential analysis of the effects of cultural trauma and recovery among indigenous people. We conclude, in light of the essential psychological functions of culture in buffering the anxiety inherent in human existence suggested by TMT, that the traumatic disruption of a people's culture is likely to result in unmanageable anxiety requiring compensatory actions which may produce destructive consequences. Therefore, the motive for a people to recover, reconstruct and adapt traditional cultures can be well understood in the context of the essential anxiety-buffering function provided by culture. We also conclude from our analysis of the experiences of three distinct cultural groups that the psychological processes underlying cultural trauma and recovery show clear evidence of the central role of terror management mechanisms in effective human functioning.

ACKNOWLEDGMENT

We wish to acknowledge the contribution of Chris Tanti for providing valuable comments on a draft of this chapter.

REFERENCES

Alumni keep ancient ways alive. (2003, February 23). *Honolulu Advertiser*, p. 17.
Astonishing cultural revival. (2002, December 26). *Honolulu Advertiser*, p. 18.
Atkinson, J., & Ober, C. (1995). We Al-Li 'Fire and Water': A process of healing. In K. M. Hazlehurst (Ed.), *Popular justice and community regeneration: Pathways to indigenous reforms* (pp. 201–218). Westport, CT: Praeger.
Becker, E. (1971). *The birth and death of meaning* (2nd ed.). New York: Free Press.

Bhatia, K., & Anderson, P. (1995). *An overview of Aboriginal and Torres Strait Islander health: Present status and future trends.* Canberra: Australian Government Publishing Service.

Blaisdell, R. K. (1989). Historical and cultural aspects of Native Hawaiian health. *Social Process in Hawaii: The Health of Native Hawaiians, 32,* 1–21.

Blaisdell, R. K. (1996). 1995 update on Kānaka Maoli (Indigenous Hawaiian) health. *Asian American and Pacific Islander Journal of Health, 4*(1–3), 160–165.

Brave Heart, M. Y. H., & DeBruyn, L. M. (1995). The American Indian holocaust: Healing historical unresolved grief. *American Indian and Alaska Native Mental Health Research: The Journal of the National Center, 8,* 56–78.

Bushnell, O. A. (1993). *The gifts of civilization: germs and genocide in Hawaii.* Honolulu: University of Hawaii Press.

Butlin, N. G. (1983). *Our original aggression.* Sydney, Australia: Allen & Unwin.

Canoe embodies school's goals. (2002, December 5). *Honolulu Advertiser,* p. B4.

Carlson, B. (2003). *Sharing our pathways.* Fairbanks, AK: Rural Systemic Initiative.

Christie, M. (1988). The invasion of Aboriginal education. In B. Harvey, & S. McGinty (Eds.), *Learning my way: Papers from the national conference on adult Aboriginal learning* (pp. 5–19). Perth: Australian Government Publishing Service.

Clark, Y. (2000). The construction of Aboriginal identity in people separated from their families, community, and culture: Pieces of the jigsaw [Special issue: Australian indigenous psychologies]. *Australian Psychologist, 35,* 150–157.

Coombs, H. C., Brandl, M. M., & Snowdon, W. E. (1983). *A certain heritage.* Canberra, Australia: ANU Press.

Council for Aboriginal Reconciliation. (1996). *Reconciliation at the crossroads.* Canberra: Australian Government Publishing Service.

Crabbe, K. M. (1991). *Effects of cultural disintegration of Native Hawaiians and mental health.* Unpublished manuscript, University of Hawaii at Mānoa.

Davidson, G., & Reser, J. (1996). Construing and constructs: Personal and cultural? In B. M. Walker, J. Costigan, L. L. Viney, & B. Warren (Eds.), *Personal construct theory: A psychology for the future* (pp. 105–128). Carlton South, Australia: Australian Psychological Society.

Department of Education. (1993). *Hawaii Youth Risk Behaviour Survey report.* Honolulu, HI: Department of Education, Office of Instructional Services/General Education Branch.

Duran, E. (1999). *Aniongwea Native American health center: Original people.* San Francisco: Fast Forward.

Eckermann, A., Dowd, T., Martin, M., Nixon, L., Gray, R., & Choong, E. (1992). *Binan goonj: Bridging cultures in Aboriginal health.* Armidale, New South Wales: University of New England Press

Faludi, S. C. (1991, September 9). Broken promise: Hawaiians wait in vain for their land. *The Wall Street Journal,* pp. A1–A3.

Farnsworth, C. M. (1997, June 8). Australians resist facing up to legacy of parting aborigines from families. *New York Times,* p. 10.

Fejo, L., & Rae, C. (1996). *Report: Strong women, strong babies, strong culture.* Canberra: Australian Government Publishing Service.

Fogarty, G. J., & White, C. (1994). Differences between values of Australian Aboriginal and non-Aboriginal students. *Journal of Cross-Cultural Psychology, 25,* 394–408.

Greenberg, J., Simon, L., Porteus, J., Pyszczynski, T., & Solomon, S. (1995). Evidence of a terror management function of cultural icons: The effects of mortality salience on the inappropriate use of cherished cultural symbols. *Personality and Social Psychology Bulletin, 21,* 1221–1228.

Greenberg, J., Solomon, S., & Pyszczynski, T. (1997). Terror management theory of self-esteem and cultural worldviews: Empirical assessments and conceptual refinements. In M.P. Zanna (Ed.), *Advances in experimental social psychology* (Vol. 29, pp.61–139). San Diego: Academic Press.

Halloran, M. J., & Kashima, E. S. (in press). Cultural validation in social context: The effect of mortality salience on endorsement of cultural values in contexts defined by social identities. *Personality and Social Psychology Bulletin.*

Hammond, O. (1988). Needs assessment and policy development: Native Hawaiians as native Americans. *American Psychologist, 4,* 383–387.

Harmon-Jones, E., Simon, L., Greenberg, J., Solomon, S., Pyszczynski, T., & McGregor, H. (1997). Terror management theory and self-esteem: Evidence that increased self-esteem reduces mortality salience effects, *Journal of Personality and Social Psychology, 72,* 24–36.

Harris, S. (1990). *Two-way Aboriginal schooling: Education and cultural survival.* Canberra, Australia: Aboriginal Studies Press.

Hawaiians back from the brink. (2003, April 24). *Honolulu Advertiser,* p. A12.

Hogg, R. S. (1994). Variability in behavioural risk factors for heart disease in an Australian Aboriginal community. *Journal of Biosocial Science, 26,* 539–551.

Hong, Y., Chiu, C., & Kung, T. M. (1997). Bringing culture out in front: Effects of Cultural meaning activation on social cognition. In K. Leung, Y. Kashima, U. Kim, & S. Yamaguchi (Eds.), *Progress in Asian social psychology* (Vol 1, pp. 135–146). Singapore: Wiley.

Human Rights and Equal Opportunity Commission. (1997). *Bringing them home: Report of the national inquiry into the separation of Aboriginal and Torres Strait Islander children from their families.* Canberra: Australian Government Publishing Service.

Hunter, E. (1995). "Freedom's just another word": Aboriginal youth and mental health. *Australian and New Zealand Journal of Psychiatry, 28,* 374–384.

Indian Health Service. (1995) *Trends in Indian health.* Washington, DC: U.S. Department of health and Human Services.

Jonas, E., Schimel, J., Greenberg, J., & Pyszczynski, T. (2002). The Scrooge effect: Evidence that mortality salience increases prosocial attitudes and behavior. *Personality and Social Psychology Bulletin, 28,* 10, 1342–1353.

Kanahele, G. S. (1982). *Hawaiian renaissance.* Honolulu, HI: Project WAIAHA.

Kashima, Y. (2001). Culture and social cognition: Towards a social psychology of cultural dynamics. In D. Matsumoto (Eds.), *Handbook of culture and psychology* (pp. 325–360). New York: Oxford University Press.

Kashima, Y., Yamaguchi, S., Kim, U., Choi, S., Gelfand, M. J., & Yuki, M. (1995). Culture, Gender, and self: A perspective from individualism-collectivism research. *Journal of Personality and Social Psychology, 69,* 925–937.

Koolmartie, J., & Williams, R. (2000). Unresolved grief and the removal of Indigenous Australian children. *Australian Psychologist, 35,* 158–166.

LaFromboise, T., Coleman, H. L. K., & Gerton, J. (1993). Psychological impact of biculturalism: Evidence and theory. *Psychological Bulletin, 114,* 395–412.

Manson, S., Beals, J., O'Neill, T., Piaseki, J. Bechtold, D., Keane, E., et al. (1996). Wounded spirits, ailing hearts: PTSD and related disorders among American Indians. In A. J. Marsella (Ed.), *Ethnocultural aspects of posttraumatic stress disorder: Issues, research, and clinical application* (pp. 251–282). Washington, DC: American Psychological Association.

Marsella, A. J., Oliveira, J. M., Plummer, C. M., & Crabbe, K. M. (1995). Native Hawaiian (Kanaka Maoli) culture, mind, and well-being. In H. I. McCubbin, E. A. Thompson, A. I. Thompson, & J. E. Fromer (Eds.), *Resiliency in ethnic minority families: Native and immigrant American families* (pp. 93–113). Madison: University of Wisconsin System.

McNabb, S. (1991). Elders, Inupiat, and culture goals in North-West Alaska. *Artic Anthropology, 8,* 63–76.

Mokuau, N. (1990). The impoverishment of Native Hawaiians and the social work challenge. *Health and Social Work, 15,* 235–242.

Napoleon, H. (1996). *Yuuyaraq: The way of the human being.* Fairbanks, AK: University of Alaska.

Ober, C., Peeters, L., Archer, R., & Kelly, K. (2000). Debriefing in different cultural frameworks: Responding to acute trauma in Australian Aboriginal contexts. In B. Raphael & J. P. Wilson (Eds.) *Psychological debriefing: Theory, practice and evidence* (pp. 241–253). Cambridge, UK: Cambridge University Press.

Parliament of Australia. (2000). *Health is life: Report on the inquiry into Indigenous health.* Canberra: Australian Government Publishing Service.

Pearson, N. (2000*). The light on the hill.* Ben Chifley Memorial Lecture, Bathurst Panthers Leagues Club. Melbourne, Australia: The Age.

Perkins, J. J., Sanson-Fisher, R. W., Blunden, S., & Lunnay, D. (1994). The prevalence of drug use in urban Aboriginal communities. *Addiction, 89,* 1319–1331.

Pyszczynski, T., Greenberg, J., & Solomon, S. (1997). Why do we need what we need: A terror management perspective on the roots of human social motivation. *Psychological Inquiry, 8,* 1–20.

Rosenblatt, A., Greenberg, J., Solomon, S., Pyszczynski, T., & Lyon, D. (1989). Evidence for terror management theory I: The effects of mortality salience on reactions to those who violate or uphold cultural values. *Journal of Personality and Social Psychology, 57,* 681–690.

Salzman, M. (2001). Cultural trauma and recovery: Perspectives from terror management theory. *Trauma, Violence and Abuse: A Review Journal, 2,* 172–191.

Salzman, M. (in press). The Dynamics of Cultural Trauma: Implications for the Pacific Nations. In Marsella, A. J., Austin, A., & Grant, B. (eds.). *Social Change and Psychosocial Adaptation in Pacific Island Nations.* New York: Kluwer.

Schimel, J., Simon, L., Greenberg, J., Pyszczynski, T., Solomon, S., Waxmonsky, J., et al. (1999). Stereotypes and terror management: Evidence that mortality salience enhances stereotypic thinking and preferences. *Journal of Personality and Social Psychology, 77,* 905–926.

Shook, V.E. (1985). *Ho'oponopono: Contemporary uses of a Hawaiian problem-solving process.* Honolulu, HI: East-West Center.

Simon, L., Arndt, J., Greenberg, J., Pyszczynski, T., & Solomon, S. (1998). Terror management and meaning: Evidence that the opportunity to defend the worldview in response to mortality salience increases the meaningfulness of life in the mildly depressed. *Journal of Personality and Social Psychology, 66,* 359–382.

Slaughter, H. B. (1997). Indigenous language immersion in Hawaii. In R. K. Johnson & M. Swain, (Eds.), *Immersion education: International perspective* (pp.105–129). London: Cambridge University Press.

Stannard, D. E. (1989). *Before the horror.* Honolulu, HI: Social Science Research Institute, University of Hawaii.

Stanner, W. E. H. (1979). *White man got no dreaming.* Canberra: Australian National University Press.

Sue, S. (1999). Science, ethnicity, and bias: Where have we gone wrong? *American Psychologist, 54,* 1070–1077.

Swann, P., & Raphael, B. (1995). *"Ways Forward" National Consultancy Report on Aboriginal and Torres Strait Islander mental health.* Canberra: Australian Government Publishing Service.

Trask, H. (1995). Native sovereignty: A strategy for Hawaiian family survival. In H. I. McCubbin, E. A. Thompson, A. I. Thompson, & J. E. Fromer (Eds.), *Resiliency in ethnic minority families: Native and immigrant American families* (pp. 133–139). Madison: University of Wisconsin System.

Triandis, H. C. (1995). *Individualism and collectivism.* Boulder, CO: Westview.

Tsey, K., & Every, A. (2000). *Evaluation of an Aboriginal empowerment program.* Canberra: Australian Government Publishing Service.

Wessels, M. G., & Bretherton, D. (2000). Psychological reconciliation: National and international perspectives. *Australian Psychologist, 35,* 109–117.

Chapter 16

Terror's Epistemic Consequences

Existential Threats and the Quest for Certainty and Closure

MARK DECHESNE
ARIE W. KRUGLANSKI

The September 11, 2001, attacks on New York and Washington, DC, in which thousands found their demise, the aftermath of these assaults, and their ripple effects, have altered the world dramatically. The images of planes crashing into the World Trade Center, the collapse of the Twin Towers, and desperate individuals leaping to their death, transmitted by television networks across the globe ushered in an age of existential anxiety of heretofore unknown dimensions. If residents of the most important cities in the most powerful nation on earth cannot be free from the horrors of terrorism, no one, many have felt, can feel safe anymore. The continuous conflicts of ethnic, political, or religious nature combined with the ever-advancing technologies of mass destruction put the specter of annihilation in the forefront of people's awareness the world over and imbued everyday experiences with considerable existential uncertainty. Under these circumstances, the scientific study of existential fears and their implications for social behavior should contribute substantially to the appreciation of the psychology of our time. In the sections that follow, we review recent theoretical analyses and empirical data of considerable relevance to these concerns.

TWO THEORETICAL PERSPECTIVES PERTINENT TO THE PSYCHOLOGY OF TERROR

Over the last 20 years or so, two general perspectives on social behavior have been generating ideas and empirical research relevant to the psychological experience of existential angst:

terror management theory (TMT) and *lay epistemic theory*. TMT (Greenberg, Solomon, & Pyszczynski, 1986; Solomon, Greenberg, & Pyszczynski, 1991; Pyszczynski, Solomon, & Greenberg, 2003) has shown how the state of terror can determine what we do, believe, and feel. Thus, it is directly pertinent to the impact terror may have on people's life experiences. The lay epistemic theory (Kruglanski, 1989a; Kruglanski & Webster, 1996; Webster & Kruglanski, 1998) was designed to come to a general understanding regarding the cognitive and motivational determinants of sociocognitive phenomena such as attitude formation and social judgment. Though it is pitched at a more general level of analysis than the terror management framework, it should intersect with it where the specific motivational forces unleashed by terror are concerned.

The purpose of this chapter is to integrate the two frameworks in an attempt to better understand their interrelations. To do so, we first briefly describe the conceptual and empirical background of effects highlighted by the terror management research program. We subsequently employ the more general framework of the lay epistemic theory to unpack the motivational processes underlying mortality salience effects documented by terror management research and to describe the conditions under which such processes may be activated. The validity of predictions derived from the proposed integrative model are then assessed in light of the relevant research.

EXISTENTIAL QUESTIONS AND THEIR EFFECT
ON SOCIAL BEHAVIOR

TMT stresses the importance of existential motivational processes involved in social phenomena. The theory posits the fear of death figures as a distal cause of a variety of socially significant motives, in particular, those motives that center around finding meaning in reality and value in oneself. Specifically, the theory posits that the juxtaposition of an instinctive drive for self-preservation with the uniquely human cognitive capacity to foresee one's own death has the potential to culminate in a state of overwhelming and paralyzing anxiety when insufficiently managed by adherence to cultural beliefs and a firm sense of symbolic value that are posited to help the individual to maintain a sense of being part of something more significant and enduring than physical existence.

Within the framework of TMT, then, the answers that people find when confronted with the frightening awareness of their own mortality are provided by a particular culture and fall into two broad and interrelated categories: (1) cultural worldviews, defined as socially shared conceptions of reality, provide their adherents a sense of order, stability, and permanence and offer them standards of value and the promise of either literal or symbolic immortality to those who match them and (2) self-esteem, comprising one's sense of living up to these standards, lends one a sense of enduring value and affording, therefore, the feelings of equanimity in the face of mortal danger. Accordingly, TMT predicts that once people become aware of their mortality, they are more likely to confirm their faith in the cultural worldview and to seek to engage in action promising to yield them a positive self-image.

Research findings consistent with the hypotheses that confrontations with mortality lead to cultural-worldview-affirming, and self-esteem-enhancing behaviors are now abundant. Indeed, this volume probably provides the most comprehensive review of mortality salience findings thus far. The general tenet of this research is that reminding people of their mortality enhances the tendencies to like those who share similar opinions, to defend one's position against dissimilarly minded others, and to overestimate the social consensus regarding one's own views (see, e.g., Greenberg, Solomon, & Pyszczynski, 1997, for an overview). Moreover, mortality salience has been shown to enhance one's preferences for actions and identifications having positive benefits for the self (e.g., Taubman - Ben-Ari, Florian, & Mikulincer, 1999; Dechesne, Greenberg, Arndt, & Schimel, 2000).

What Drives These Effects?

One might have thought that for an individual in the relatively artificial context of a laboratory cubicle, death constitutes a remote concept hardly capable of eliciting a direct response. Nonetheless, it does so pervasively and reliably. What might such response consist of? Research on the cognitive underpinnings of mortality salience effects suggests that such responses are primarily instigated by death-related thoughts that escape conscious awareness (see Arndt, Greenberg, Solomon, Pyszczynski, & Simon, 1997; Arndt, Greenberg, Pyszczynski, & Solomon, 1997; see also Pyszcyznski, Greenberg, & Solomon, 1999, for review). Moreover, Greenberg, Pyszczynski, Solomon, Simon, and Breus (1994) demonstrated that the effects of mortality salience on social behavior were appreciably stronger when induced by questions about one's own death relative to question about the death of a friend. This suggests that it is not so much the thought of death per se but, rather, the cognitive linkage between death and self that drives mortality salience effects. Hence, the reminder of mortality appears to require a reaction primarily when it threatens the self.

Death may threaten the self in two distinct ways. First, awareness of the limitations of life may diminish the perceived *significance* of one's existence and activities. In other words, death awareness may make one's investments in the world seem rather insignificant. Consistent with this viewpoint, several experiments have demonstrated that mortality salience decreases self-esteem. Van den Bos (2001), for example, demonstrated that mortality salience led to decreased self-esteem, particularly the esteem derived from one's competencies. Moreover, Koole, Dechesne, and van Knippenberg (2000) demonstrated that mortality salience decreased the preference for the letters of one's own name, an indication of decrease in people's implicit self-evaluations (Pelham, Mirenberg, & Jones, 2002; Koole, Dijksterhuis, & van Knippenberg, 2001; Nuttin, 1985).

Second, and more generally, although death is one of the few certainties of life, the thought of it may induce considerable uncertainty. Indeed, several authors have argued that it is exactly this feeling of uncertainty that mobilizes the defensive responses documented in terror management research (Van den Bos, 2001; McGregor, Zanna, Holmes, & Spencer, 2001). Feelings of uncertainty associated with mortality may stem from the inability to anticipate the time and place of death, the inability to attain an understanding of the state of nonbeing and what happens during the process of dying, and the inability to predict the impact of one's death on the life of others.

In addition, several authors have argued that the self plays a major role in the organization of knowledge (Greenwald, 1980) and serves as a resource for forming opinions and making judgments (Ellis & Kruglanski, 1992). From these perspectives, when the self is threatened, the organizational principle of knowledge and judgment is undermined, potentially culminating in considerable uncertainty. Hence, uncertainty can be assumed to be elicited by reminders of mortality.

As discussed in greater detail later, highlighting the specific concerns elicited by mortality awareness will prove important, because different concerns may have different sociocognitive implications. To extend this point, we now provide a brief overview of the lay epistemic theory.

LAY EPISTEMIC THEORY

The theory of lay epistemics (see Kruglanski, 1989a, 1989b; Kruglanski & Webster, 1996, for overviews) was offered as an integrative analysis of diverse social judgment phenomena, and hence, lay epistemic theory's account of motivational processes underlying human judgment generalizes across the various content domains of social psychology. At its core lies the notion that these phenomena, although differing substantially in content, all involve the use of relevant knowledge that is obtained and maintained through a common process, best described as "naive science" (see Kruglanski, 1989a, for a fuller description). Important for this discussion, the epistemic process is argued to be affected to a great extent by epistemic motivation. People may want to construe and use knowledge quickly, or they may prefer to avoid definite knowledge. Within lay epistemic theory, the former is referred to as a high-need-for-closure and the latter is referred to as high need to avoid closure.

Of particular relevance to the discussion that follows is the distinction between the need for specific and nonspecific closure. When faced with a question, people might want to attain specific knowledge (specific closure) that is pleasing or desirable for them in some sense but may also be willing to accept any knowledge (nonspecific closure) as long as it provides certainty. The idea of a nonspecific closure implies that people are willing to believe, form impressions, and create categories in order to feel sure and avoid ambiguity. Such mental activities provide order, predictability, decisiveness, clarity, and thrift while processing new information, all features contributing to a sense of certainty. To achieve such sense then, people may be quick in their use of information to form knowledge, a tendency referred to as "seizing," and cling onto this knowledge for as long as possible, a tendency referred to as "freezing."

Lay epistemic theory posits that both situational factors and personality features contribute to the strength of the need for nonspecifc closure. Situational circumstances such as time pressure and constraints to cognitive capacity may force an individual to form a decision, impression, or belief quickly, which may often contribute to judgmental errors. Moreover, as Webster and Kruglanski (1994) have noted, individuals differ substantially along a continuum ranging from a high need for nonspecific closure to a high need to avoid nonspecific closure. Individuals high in the need for nonspecifc closure tend to display a rigidity of thought and have a strong aversion toward ambiguity. Individuals low in need for nonspecific closure (or high on the need to avoid nonspecific closure), on the other hand, savor uncertainty and are reluctant to commit to a definite opinion.

The social psychological significance of the need for nonspecific closure has been demonstrated in a variety of social psychological domains. Chronically high and situationally heightened need for nonspecific closure has been found to instigate social behavior conducive of establishing a sense of certainty (e.g., stereotyping, ingroup bias, conservatism, and consensus-seeking) (for reviews see Kruglanski & Webster, 1996; Webster & Kruglanski, 1998).

THEORETICAL INTEGRATION

A lay epistemic perspective may be particularly relevant for describing the motivational components of dealing with existential threat. To do so, however, it is important to recall our previous statement that the thought of death elicits a configuration of concerns, of which self-value and uncertainty are the key components. As we argue next, each of these concerns can be linked to particular type of epistemic motivation. These epistemic motivations, in turn, are predicted to have specific implications for social behavior.

When the analysis of TMT is interpreted within the framework of the lay epistemic theory, some of the described reactions to mortality salience can be characterized as specific closures. That is, answering questions about one's mortality is assumed to evoke the need to affirm one's own significance, a need that is satisfied by specific mechanisms (i.e., the upholding of one's cultural worldviews and self-esteem). The theoretical integration proposed in this chapter assumes, however, that when the specific states of mind evoked by a confrontation with mortality are looked at closely, the need for a nonspecific closure may well be part and parcel of such states alongside the need for specific closure alluded to previously. Specifically, the cognitive and emotional reaction to the threat of one's personal insignificance can be resolved by means of specific closures, namely, via information reflecting positively on the self and hence restoring one's sense of significance. This notion is highly consistent with previous findings showing that mortality salience enhances self-esteem striving (e.g., Taubman - Ben-Ari et al., 1999).

From the lay epistemic perspective, however, the aversive *state of uncertainty* brought on by mortality salience qualitatively differs from concerns about personal insignificance. According to lay epistemic theory, aversive uncertainty constitutes the root cause of the need for nonspecific closure. Hence, the uncertainty associated with the prospect of one's own mortality leads to a broad desire for definiteness in one's beliefs and an aversion toward deviating opinions, people, and beliefs. The integrative model thus suggests that mortality salience is likely to enhance the need for nonspecific closure prompted by the threat of uncertainty, apart from the need for specific closures.

If the notion of death is a source of uncertainty, the lay epistemic theory suggests that individuals with an aversion toward uncertainty are more likely to have negative attitudes toward death. Those who savor uncertainty, on the other hand, may be more at ease when thinking about the prospect of their own mortality. In other words, the uncertainty associated with death should be of greater concern for high-need-for-closure individuals relative to low-need-for-closure individuals, and the solution to this concern (i.e., attainment of a nonspecific closure) should have greater "weight" in the response to mortality salience of individuals high in the need for closure, relative to those low in the need for closure.

In summary, then, the integrative model assumes that the induction of mortality salience elicits a configuration of concerns, of which worries about one's personal insignificance and uncertainty constitute key components. Concerns with insignificance are assumed to enhance the tendency to affirm one's self-value (i.e., to instigate a *need for specific closure*). The state of aversive uncertainty is assumed to enhance a need for firmness in judgments, opinion, and beliefs (i.e., to instigate a need for nonspecific closure). Moreover, tolerance for uncertainty associated with death should vary across individuals. Individuals low in the need for closure are assumed to be less distressed by feelings of uncertainty evoked by thoughts of death, and hence they are *more likely* to exhibit responses indicative of the need for specific closure. Individuals high in the need for nonspecific closure are assumed to be more distressed by feelings of uncertainty than their low-need-for-closure counterparts, and hence they are *less likely* to exhibit responses indicative of the need for specific closure.

We now turn to research evidence relevant to those concerns. Whereas evidence that mortality salience enhances the need for specific closure has been available for some time (cf. Taubman - Ben-Ari et al., 1999), we now review novel evidence that mortality salience is likely to evoke the need for nonspecific closure. This review is followed by evidence that high- and low-need-for-closure individuals react differently to confrontations with the prospect of their own mortality in a manner consistent with the present model.

THE EFFECTS OF MORTALITY SALIENCE ON NEED FOR NONSPECIFIC CLOSURE

Evidence that mortality salience enhances the need for nonspecific closure comes from several separate lines of inquiry. A first source of evidence can be derived from the striking parallels in the social psychological effects of mortality salience and the need for closure. A second source of evidence stems from findings obtained from mortality salience studies that can only be accounted for on the basis lay epistemic theory and studies that directly assessed the effects of mortality salience on the need for (nonspecific) closure.

Parallels between Need for Closure and Mortality Salience Effects

Both TMT and lay epistemic theory have generated a substantial body of research over the past decades. Although the research has been independently conducted, the literatures of TMT and lay epistemic theory show considerable similarities in the phenomena under investigation. Importantly, findings obtained from mortality salience studies also show considerable similarities with the mental and overt reactions associated with high need for nonspecific closure as described in the need-for-closure literature. Moreover, manipulations of the need for nonspecific closure, such as imposed time pressure and ambient noise induction, have been shown to induce responses very similar to responses found under the condition of mortality salience. Indeed, it has been this remarkable parallel between the need-for-closure findings and mortality salience findings that has led Richter and Kruglanski (2004) to conclude that mortality salience may enhance the need for a nonspecific closure.

The similarities between need-for-closure and mortality salience findings center around three themes: (1) both need for closure and mortality salience enhance ingroup bias, (2) both need for closure and mortality salience enhance preference for similar others and an intolerance for dissimilar others, and (3) both need for closure and mortality salience enhance stereotyping.

Shah, Kruglanski, and Thompson (1998) argued that an important function of group affiliation is to provide consensual validation of one's beliefs (cf., e.g., Festinger, Riecken, & Schachter, 1956). Through the process of consensual validation, one's beliefs and perceptions of the world are bolstered and rendered subjectively certain. Hence, consensual validation and the groups that provide it are likely to be particularly attractive to individuals with high-need-for-closure and under circumstances under which closure is desired. Consistent with this hypothesis, Shah et al. (1998) demonstrated in several studies that a heightened need for closure leads to more pronounced ingroup bias.

TAT similarly incorporates consensual validation of one's beliefs as a central tenet in its analysis. According to this theory, consensual validation of one's beliefs is important because it strengthens the conviction that one's worldview constitutes an "absolute representation of reality." At times at which such worldviews increase in pertinence (i.e., when mortality is salient), people are, therefore, expected to exhibit an increased need for consensual validation and are therefore more likely to affiliate with their in groups. Consistent with this particular hypothesis, research has revealed that mortality salience enhances ingroup identification (e.g., Harmon-Jones, Greenberg, Solomon, & Simon, 1996) and enhances the false consensus effect (Pyszczynski et al., 1996).

A related domain wherein need-for-closure effects and mortality salience effects have been found to converge constitutes the evaluation of similar and dissimilar others. Lay epistemic theory posits that the state of high-need-for-closure implies a preference for certainty and aversion toward ambiguity in a variety of domains. Within the domain of social knowledge, the preference for certainty may be expressed in a strong preference for those who are share the same opinion, and a strong aversion toward those who are dissimilar. Indeed, in early work on lay epistemic theory, Kruglanski and Webster (1991) found that the experimental elevation of a need for nonspecific closure (by time pressure and by ambient noise) led to increased rejection of a confederate who confessed to an opinion that differed from that of the remaining participants in his or her group. Similarly, Doherty (1998) found that participants encouraged to reach cognitive closure expressed a more negative attitude toward a woman who deviated from cultural norms than did participants experimentally motivated to avoid closure.

Again, TMT similarly posits that people who are reminded about their own mortality are likely to cling on to their cultural worldviews. Those who threaten the participants cultural worldviews are therefore likely to be evaluated more negatively when mortality concerns are salient. Research suggests, indeed, this to be the case. Rosenblatt, Greenberg, Solomon, Pyszczynski, and Lyon (1989), for example, demonstrated that moral transgressions (i.e., one form of deviancy from consensual norms) were more heavily penalized when participants (both professional judges and students) were reminded about their own mortality.

A final convergence of heightened need-for-closure effects with mortality salience effects can be found in the domain of stereotyping. According to the lay epistemic theory, the state of a high-need-for-closure is associated with a greater need for order and predictability. In this vein, Dijksterhuis, van Knippenberg, Kruglanski, and Schaper (1996) argued that stereotypes allow the individual to perceive the world in an orderly manner, and therefore that stereotypes are more likely to be used by high-need-for-closure individuals compared to their low-need-for-closure counterparts, and conditions of heightened need for closure are likely to lead to increased stereotyping. In their studies, Dijksterhuis et al. (1996) indeed found that high-need-for-closure participants exhibited more stereotypically biased memories of social events than low-need-for-closure participants. Experimentally heightened need for closure was found to have similar effects.

Within the field of TMT, Schimel et al. (1999) similarly argued that stereotypes constitute an important component of a cultural worldview, which provides a sense of order, stability, and permanence in the face of existential threat. If cultural worldviews become more important when people are reminded about mortality, Schimel et al. argued, it follows that mortality salience is also likely to enhance stereotyping. Consistent with this line of reasoning, Schimel et al. (1999) indeed obtained evidence that mortality salience led participants to favor people who behaved in a stereotype-consistent manner, and to disfavor those who behaved in a stereotype-inconsistent manner.

Mortality Salience and the Specificity of Closure

The parallels between mortality salience and need-for-closure effects are striking indeed. And the parallel reaches beyond the effects per se. As illustrated in the previous section, the conceptualization of "cultural worldview" in TMT also converges to a great extent with the conceptualization of "closure" in lay epistemic theory. As outlined previously, however, the conceptualizations of cultural worldview and closure differ in at least one significant respect. Lay epistemic theory suggests that closure motivation as outlined above is nonspecific in nature, whereas TMT suggest that the reaction reviewed earlier reflects specific closures. That is, when people are reminded about their mortality, TMT posits that they will seek out specific information that confirms the beliefs, attitudes, and values inherent to their worldview, or information that confirms their position with their worldview is secured. By contrast, if mortality salience enhances the need for nonspecific closure as outlined in lay epistemic theory, it follows that people reminded about their death should increase (1) their willingness to "seize" and "freeze" on *any* accessible knowledge (e.g., Ford & Kruglanski, 1995), *even if* it is detrimental to dealing with specific concerns about mortality; and (2) tendencies associated with heightened need for nonspecific closure in domains typically unrelated to terror management defenses.

With regard to the former nonspecificity hypothesis, Dechesne and Pyszczynski (2002) recently obtained some intriguing findings suggesting that mortality salience indeed enhances tendencies that fit to a greater extent with the notion of nonspecific closure than with the notion of a specific worldview-defending closure. Participants in the experiment first read an article about the near-death experience, in which half were informed that such experiences provide evidence for an afterlife and the other half that these experiences can be explained as reflecting a physiological reaction to extreme stress. Subsequently, half the participants were led to contemplate their own death, whereas the other half contemplated their feelings and thoughts associated with dental pain. Finally, participants were asked to indicate their belief in an afterlife.

Participants in the mortality salience condition who read the article that defended a spiritual explanation of the near-death experience were found to exhibit a stronger belief in an afterlife compared to participants who read the same article but were not reminded about their death. But far more intriguingly, participants in the mortality salience condition who read the article that defended a physiological explanation exhibited significantly a lower belief in afterlife, presumed to allay concerns about their mortality, compared to participants who read the same article yet who contemplated dental pain rather than mortality. In the dental-pain condition, no differences in belief in afterlife were found between the two article conditions.

To the extent that mortality salience leads exclusively to needs for specific closures, related to defending oneself against the threats inherent in the cessation of being, affirmation that there is an afterlife would have been a particularly likely response to the mortality salience manipulation. However, the findings indicate otherwise. Specifically, under the mortality salience condition, participants were more willing to accept *any* accessible answer to the question about afterlife. Intriguingly, they were even willing to decrease their belief in afterlife when reminded about death after being exposed to (bogus) research findings denying afterlife. These findings suggest that mortality salience manipulations may arouse participants' nonspecific need for closure.

Additional evidence that mortality salience enhances the need for nonspecific closure has been recently obtained by Dechesne and Wigboldus (2001). These investigators argued that the nonspecific closure hypothesis in the context of terror management findings implies that (1) mortality salience enhances the general need to adopt and use cognitive schemas in order to establish a sense of order, predictability, and stability; and (2) this effect applies to any sort of schema, not just culturally shared/meaningful schema such as being Dutch or a belief in heaven.

To examine this hypothesis, Dechesne and Wigboldus (2001) conducted a study wherein mortality salience was induced for half the participants. Subsequently, all participants were asked to recognize as quickly and accurately as possible the letters A and B that were sequentially presented on a computer screen. There were 280 trials of A's and B's, and the participants' reaction times to these stimuli were measured. Importantly, the A's and B's actually appeared in a fixed pattern: ABBABAB. Once participants become aware of this pattern, reaction times should become considerably faster because it allows participants to anticipate the outcome of the next trial. To the extent that mortality awareness increases individuals' need for a nonspecific closure, it should increase participants' motivation to find a connection between the A's and the B's. If so, the mortality reminder manipulation should occasion a speed-up in responding at an earlier stage of the ABBABAB trials compared to circumstances under which this reminder was absent. Analysis of the data revealed that a reminder of mortality, as compared to a reminder of dental pain, indeed led to quicker correct recognition of the A's and B's after several ABBABAB trials, suggesting that participants in the mortality salience condition, but not in the dental-pain condition, developed a cognitive schema in order to predict the outcome of the upcoming letters. These results support the hypothesis that reminders of mortality increase the need for order and predictability, and that this effect is not related to specific contents of schemas and beliefs. This interpretation was further corroborated by a subsequent finding showing parallel effects of need for structure on the development of cognitive schemas, hence suggesting that the development and use of cognitive schemas originate in a desire for order and predictability.

Individual Differences in Need for Closure and Responses to Mortality

If death indeed constitutes a source of uncertainty, individuals who have an aversion toward uncertainty are more likely to have negative attitudes toward death. Those who savor uncertainty, by contrast, may be more at ease when thinking about the prospect of their own mortality. Therefore, high- and low-need-for-closure individuals are likely to respond differently to confrontations with the prospect of their own mortality. Whereas low-need-for-closure individuals may be less concerned with the uncertainty associated with death and may even exhibit some curiosity about the ambiguities associated with death, high-need-for-closure individuals are likely to express discomfort and avoidance behavior when confronted with the prospect of mortality. The results of recent research corroborate these hypotheses.

Need for Closure and Responses to Explicit Confrontation with Mortality

Dechesne (2002) recently examined whether high- and low-need-for-closure participants differed in their direct, verbal answers to questions about mortality. In one study, participants were asked to write down in one sentence the thoughts and feelings that came to their minds when thinking about death. The covariation of need for closure with the amount of distress expressed about the idea of death was striking. Typical answers of low-need-for-closure participants were expressive of acceptance (e.g., "it's something that has to come anyway, it's not something to be afraid of"), and some of these participants even expressed curiosity (i.e., "I am curious what will happen afterwards"). In contrast, high-need-for-closure participants virtually all expressed distress (e.g., "I don't want to die!").

In a separate study, participants were asked two questions about death, instead of one, and were given eight lines to answer each question. These procedural modifications were meant to allow participants to elaborate more on their thoughts and feelings about death. Although the difference in the content of the answers between high- and low-need-for-closure participants was not as striking as with the single-sentence answers, analysis of the time that high- and low-need-for-closure participants had spent on answering the questions revealed a result highly consistent with the hypothesis that individuals high in need for closure are more distressed when thinking about mortality than are low-need-for-closure individuals.

Specifically, low-need-for-closure participants spent almost twice the amount of time that high-need-for-closure participants led to answer the mortality questions. Moreover, high-need-for-closure participants spent significantly less time on their answers to questions about *death* than they did to two parallel questions about *watching television*. In contrast, low-need-for-closure participants spent significantly more time on questions about death compared to questions about watching television. These results suggest that high-need-for-closure individuals attempt to avoid the uncertainties associated with death, whereas low-need-for-closure individuals may actually be intrigued by these uncertainties.

Need for Closure and Social Psychological Reactions to Reminders of Mortality

In TMT, a distinction is drawn between participants' first rational response to a confrontation with mortality and the subsequent experiential and symbolic reaction. Examples of the latter category include increased nationalism, increased intolerance of deviants, increased sensitivity about the appropriate use of cultural icons, and increased awareness of moral virtues. In all cases, TMT conceives of these responses as attempts to either bolster the significance of oneself within one's worldview or to underline and strengthen the validity of the cultural worldview itself. Cultural worldviews are assumed to increase in appeal as people are confronted with mortality, because one of the crucial functions of these worldviews, according to TMT, is to provide the individual a sense of meaning, value, order, and permanence. All these features are assumed to help to manage the affective impact of confrontations with mortality.

Terror management theory thus predicts that people who are reminded about death have a greater need to perceive their convictions as unequivocal and unrivaled. Lay epistemic theory, however, suggests that individuals differ in the extent to which they like their worldview "pure." Specifically, on the basis of lay epistemic theory, it can be predicted that high-need-for-closure individuals, with their greater desire for certainty and aversion toward ambiguity, are more likely to be distressed by deviating people and opinions and will be more favorable toward those who share similar attitudes, values, and beliefs than are low-need-for-closure individuals. In this sense, the lay epistemic theory identifies a moderating condition affecting individuals' reactions to mortality salience.

Consistent with these notions, Schimel et al. (1999) demonstrated that individual differences in need for closure moderated the extent to which people used stereotypical judgments to evaluate a person when confronted with the prospect of their own mortality. Whereas high-need-for-closure participants reminded about their own death became more favorable toward a person who acted in stereotypical fashion compared to a person who did not act in accordance with the stereotype, low-need-for-closure participants did not.

Note that the foregoing findings by Schimel et al. (1999) are open to two alternative interpretations. First, it can be argued that low-need-for-closure participants were *not affected* by the mortality salience manipulation, and, consequently, they had no need to perceive others in a stereotypical way. Alternatively, it can also be argued that enhanced stereotypical judgment does not constitute part of the repertoire from which low-need-for-closure individuals draw. According to this latter hypothesis, low-need-for-closure participants are also likely to be affected by the mortality salience manipulation, but in a different manner than that of high-need-for-closure persons. The model proposed here suggests that low-need-for-closure participants do indeed react to reminders of mortality, but because uncertainty per se is less aversive to these individuals their responses should be more reflective of attempts to deal with the remaining psychological issue aroused by mortality salience, namely, the concern about one's own personal insignificance.

Available research findings are consistent with such a possibility. An early indication to this effect is to be found already in early empirical work on TMT. Specifically, Greenberg, Simon, Solomon, Chatel, and Pyszczynski (1992) demonstrated that a reminder of mortality led participants with a conservative political orientation, a feature linked to high-need-for-closure (cf. Jost, Glaser, Kruglanski, & Sulloway, 2003a, 2003b), to express greater dislike for a person who did not share their political point of view. In contrast, a reminder of mortality led participants with a liberal political orientation to become more tolerant toward a person with different political viewpoints. These findings suggest that whereas high-need-for-closure individuals cling to their worldviews more when reminded of their own mortality, low-need-for-closure individuals may in similar circumstances express their deeply held values (such as tolerance). Clearly, however, this research is only suggestive and rather indirectly related to the need for closure as such. Although authoritarianism and conservatism are somewhat related to the need for closure, there are also considerable differences in the constructs (cf. Jost et al., 2003a, 2003b; Kruglanski & Webster, 1996; Webster & Kruglanski, 1998).

Fortunately research exists that directly examined the moderating role of individual differences in need for closure on various social tendencies. This work has confirmed the notion that both high- and low-need-for-closure individuals are affected by a confrontation with the prospect of their mortality, but they are affected by this circumstance in different ways. Dechesne, Janssen, and van Knippenberg (2000), for example, demonstrated that mortality salience can lead to two qualitatively different reactions. When particular beliefs or group affiliations are threatened, people who are reminded about their mortality can either *derogate* the source of the threat or distance themselves from the belief or group targeted by the threat in order to prevent further harm as a result of the threat. The specific reaction that individuals exhibit, however, was found to depend in part on individual differences in the need for closure.

In the study, half the participants were subliminally primed with the word "death," whereas the other half were subliminally primed with "XXXX." Subsequently all participants were confronted with a negative critique of their home university. After having read the critical comment, participants were asked to evaluate the critic and to rate their degree of identification with the university. It was shown that high-need-for-closure participants under mortality salience manipulation derogated the critic, as attested by increased expressions of dislike toward this person. Low-need-for-closure participants under mortality salience, by contrast, expressed decreased identification with the university when it was being criticized. These findings suggest that whereas high-need-for-closure individuals under mortality tend more to cling to their previous worldviews (identification with their university in this instance), low-need-for-closure individuals are ready to alter those where a need for a specific closure (of agreeing with an "important" person) implies the desirability to do so.

The integrative model outlined in this chapter posits that a confrontation with the notion of mortality would enhance the need for specific closure (i.e., restoration of significance) among low-need-for-closure individuals whereas nonspecific closure concerns (i.e., reestablishing certainty) would predominate the reactions to mortality of high-need-for-closure participants. Whereas the Dechesne, Janssen, & van Knippenberg (2000) research is consistent with this proposition, it is hardly conclusive. Further supportive evidence for this analysis can be derived from a subsequent set of studies by Dechesne, Janssen, and van Knippenberg (2001). In a first study, high- and low-need-for-closure participants were either reminded or not reminded about their death. Subsequently, all participants were either exposed to a very positive or a very negative horoscope. The crucial dependent variable was participants' belief in astrology. If people prefer a positive self-image when reminded about death (reflecting a need for specific closure), they would only increase their belief in astrology as a result of the mortality salience after having read a positive horoscope. In contrast, if people "seize" on any belief-relevant information when reminded about mortality (reflecting a need for a nonspecific closure), they should increase belief in astrology independent of the valence of the horoscope they read prior to indicating their belief.

The results revealed that low-need-for-closure participants only increased belief in astrology after they received a positive horoscope and not when they received a negative horoscope. By contrast, the high-need-for-closure participants who were reminded about their death increased their belief in astrology under both conditions and particularly after they received a negative horoscope. Presumably, the negative horoscope in this case augmented the quest for certainty characteristic of high-need-for-closure individuals. A separate study replicated this effect with emotional intelligence and belief in psychometrics instead of horoscopes and belief in astrology as cover. Low-need-for-closure participants who were reminded about death increased their beliefs in psychometrics only after they were informed that they were highly emotional intelligent, but not after they were informed that they were poor in emotional intelligence. High-need-for-closure participants, by contrast, increased their belief in psychometrics also after they were informed that they had a poorly developed emotional intelligence. In addition, this study also showed that the terror management strategy adopted by high-need-for-closure individuals ultimately had negative repercussions for these persons' self-esteem. Specifically, participants with a high-need-for-closure (but not their low-need-for-closure counterparts) who were both reminded about death and informed about their poor emotional intelligence were found to have lower self-esteem after they increased belief in psychometrics.

Taken as a body, the studies suggest that individual differences in need for closure do not determine *whether* the mortality salience manipulation would lead to defensive reactions but, rather, determine the specific nature of such reactions. In addition, it can be concluded that low-need-for-closure individuals are more likely to adopt flexible, sometimes even pragmatic strategies to manage concerns about mortality, favoring specific (self-esteem enhancing) closures over nonspecific closures. High-need-for-closure individuals, by contrast, are more likely to adopt more rigid strategies, such as hanging on to particular groups or beliefs even if this has negative repercussions for one's self-esteem and subjective well-being, when confronted with the prospect of their own mortality (cf. Dechesne, 2001).

DISCUSSION

The body of research reviewed in this chapter testifies to successful cross-fertilization between the lay epistemic theory and TMT. The principal motivational constructs of lay epistemic theory, namely, the needs for nonspecific and specific closure, have been found to elicit similar psychological reactions from persons as does a reminder of these individuals' own mortality. Furthermore, the needs for specific and nonspecific closure have been found to exert substantial influence on people's first direct reaction to the prospect of their own mortality as well as to their subsequent, more symbolic reactions, also suggesting a conceptual affinity between mortality reminders and the needs for closure. Finally, our evidence suggests that mortality salience may activate both the need for nonspecific closure (a craving for certainty) and the need for a specific closure (the craving for the restoration of one's sense of personal significance), and it may do so differentially as a function of individuals dispositional degree of the need for nonspecific closure.

Although the cross-fertilization of lay epistemic TMT has been successful on the empirical level, these experimental efforts have not heretofore yielded an integrative theoretical statement. In this chapter, we have attempted to provide such a statement. It was suggested that reminders of mortality illicit a configuration of concerns in which threats to significance and certainty play a key role. Application of the lay epistemic perspective to mortality salience effects led to the assumption that mortality salience enhances both the need for specific closure (i.e., to view oneself positively) and the need for nonspecific closure (i.e., the desire for certainty, and aversion to ambiguity). Because the need for nonspecific closure is argued to originate from feelings of uncertainty, for which high-need-for-closure individuals have less tolerance than do low-need-for-closure individuals, responses indicative of the need for nonspecific closure were hypothesized to be found among high-need-for-closure individuals to a greater extent than among their low-need-for-closure counterparts. The research reviewed in this chapter is highly consistent with the model.

Clearly, in our times, insight into the phenomena of "terror," "closure," and their interplay serves a greater purpose than the mere gratification of intellectual interest. Understanding why people cling onto their convictions so fervently and why some people under some circumstances do more than do others, or they themselves in different circumstances, and what influence existential concerns pertaining to insignificance and uncertainty play in the emergence and maintenance of convictions, constitutes not only a pertinent topic for scientific inquiry but also a direly needed area into which insights are needed given the current world's turmoil. Although in this chapter we did not make explicit linkages between the experimental findings and real-world phenomena, we do hope that with the specification of the motivational dynamics involved in dealing with terror, its determinants, and its consequences, the present model can serve as a tool for understanding people's reactions to confrontation with existential terror.

We believe the implications of this model for coping with the current world's terrorism threat are intriguing. First, the present model converges with the original terror management analysis that threats of terror can culminate in ethnocentrism, outgroup derogation, and social judgements based on stereotypes (see Pyszczynski et al., 2003). Moreover, the present model suggests that such tendencies may at least partially reflect people's general increased need for firmness in judgment and beliefs (i.e., their need for nonspecific closure) (see also Landau et al., 2003). In this respect, several additional implications can be outlined, including the notion that existential threat enhances preference for strong leaders and autocratic relationships within a group, a tendency recently linked to the need for nonspecific closure. Indeed, Gordijn and Stapel (personal communication, February 2003) have recently found that terror threat enhances the appeal of charismatic leaders, a finding that echoes similar results obtained by Pierro, Mannetti, DeGrada, Livi, and Kruglanski (2003) with the need for nonspecific closure. It seems important that policymakers be made aware of these and other implications of social psychological research programs on closure and terror management, as the world is attempting to cope with the pervasive menace of terrorism and prospects of mass destruction.

ACKNOWLEDGMENT

This chapter has been written in part during Mark Dechesne's visit to the University of Maryland, College Park, sponsored by the Netherlands Organization for Scientific Research (NWO, Grant No. R 57-213).

REFERENCES

Arndt, J., Greenberg, J., Pyszczynski, T., & Solomon, S. (1997). Subliminal exposure to death-related stimuli increases defense of the cultural worldview. *Psychological Science, 8*, 379–385.

Arndt, J., Greenberg, J., Solomon, S., Pyszczynski, T., & Simon, L. (1997). Suppression, accessibility of death-related thoughts, and cultural worldview defense: Exploring the psychodynamics of terror management. *Journal of Personality and Social Psychology, 73*, 5–18.

Dechesne, M. (2001). *Flexible and rigid reactions to reminders of mortality: Some further explorations of terror management theory.* Doctoral dissertation, University of Nijmegen, The Netherlands.

Dechesne, M. (2002). *Individual differences in terror management research: The case of need for closure.* Manuscript in preparation.

Dechesne, M., Greenberg, J., Arndt, J., & Schimel, J. (2000). Terror management and the vicissitudes of sports fan affiliation: The effects of mortality salience on optimism and fan identification. *European Journal of Social Psychology, 30*, 813–835.

Dechesne, M., Janssen, J., & van Knippenberg, A (2000). Derogation and distancing as terror management strategies: The moderating role of need for closure and permeability of group boundaries. *Journal of Personality and Social Psychology, 79*, 923–932.

Dechesne, M., Janssen, J., & van Knippenberg, A. (2001). *Worldview allegiance vs. egotism in the face of existential threat: Need for closure as moderator of terror management strategies.* Unpublished manuscript.

Dechesne, M., & Pyszczynski, T. (2002). *The effect of evidence of literal immortality and mortality salience on immortality belief.* Unpublished manuscript, University of Nijmegen, The Netherlands.

Dechesne, M., & Wigboldus, D. (2001). *Terror management in a minimal worldview paradigm.* Unpublished data set: University of Nijmegen.

Dijksterhuis, A., van Knippenberg, A., Kruglanski, A., & Schaper, C. (1996). Motivated social cognition: Need for closure effects on memory and judgment. *Journal of Experimental Social Psychology, 32*, 254–270.

Doherty, K. (1998). A mind of her own: Effects of need for closure and gender on reactions to nonconformity. *Sex Roles, 38*, 801–819.

Ellis, S., & Kruglanski, A. (1992). Self as an epistemic authority: Effects on experiential and instructional learning. *Social Cognition, 10*, 357–375.

Festinger, L., Riecken, H., & Schachter, S. (1956). *When prophecy fails.* Minneapolis: University of
   Minnesota Press.

Ford, T., & Kruglanski, A. (1995). Effects of epistemic motivations on the use of accessible constructs
   in social judgement. *Personality and Social Psychology Bulletin, 21*, 950–962.

Greenberg, J., Pyszczynski, T., Solomon, S., Simon, L., & Breus, M. (1994). Role of consciousness and
   accessibility of death-related thoughts in mortality salience effects. *Journal of Personality and Social Psychology, 67*, 627–637.

Greenberg, J., Simon, L., Solomon, S., Chatel, D., & Pyszczynski, T. (1992). Terror management and
   tolerance: Does mortality salience always intensify negative reactions to others who threaten
   one's cultural worldview? *Journal of Personality and Social Psychology, 63*, 212–220.

Greenberg, J., Solomon, S., & Pyszczynski, T. (1986). The causes and consequences of a need for
   self-esteem: A terror management theory. In R. F. Baumeister (Ed.), *Public self and private self*
   (pp. 189–212). New York: Springer-Verlag.

Greenberg, J., Solomon, S., & Pyszczynski, T. (1997). The role of self-esteem and cultural worldviews
   in the management of existential terror. In M. Zanna (Ed.), *Advances in experimental social psychology* (pp. 61–139). New York: Academic Press.

Greenwald, A. (1980). The totalitarian ego: Fabrication and revision of personal history. *American
   Psychologist, 35*, 603–618.

Harmon-Jones, E., Greenberg, J., Solomon, S., & Simon, L. (1996). The effects of mortality salience
   on intergroup bias between minimal groups. *European Journal of Social Psychology, 26*, 677–
   681.

Jost, J., Glaser, J., Kruglanski, A., & Sulloway, F. (2003a). Political conservatism as motivated social
   cognition. *Psychological Bulletin, 129*, 339–375.

Jost, J., Glaser, J., Kruglanski, A., & Sulloway, F. (2003b). Exceptions that prove the rule—Using a
   theory of motivated social cognition to account for ideological incongruities and political anomalies: Reply to Greenberg and Jonas (2003). *Psychological Bulletin, 129*, 383–393.

Koole, S., Dechesne, M., & van Knippenberg, A. (2000). *The sting of death. The effects of mortality
   salience on implicit self-evaluations.* Unpublished Manuscript, University of Nijmegen, The
   Netherlands.

Koole, S., Dijksterhuis, A., & van Knippenberg, A. (2001). What's in a name: Implicit self-esteem and
   the automatic self. *Journal of Personality and Social Psychology, 80*, 669–685.

Kruglanski, A. (1989a). *Lay Epistemics and Human Knowledge: Cognitive and motivational bases.*
   New York: Plenum Press.

Kruglanski, A. (1989b). The psychology of being "right": The problem of accuracy in social perception and cognition. *Psychological Bulletin, 106*, 395–409.

Kruglanski, A., & Webster, D. (1991). Group members' reactions to opinion deviates and conformists
   at varying degrees of proximity to decision deadline and of environmental noise. *Journal of personality and social psychology, 61*, 212–225.

Kruglanski, A., & Webster, D. (1996). Motivated closing of the mind: "Seizing" and "freezing." *Psychological Review, 103*, 263–283.

Landau., M., Johns., M., Greenberg, J., Pyszczynski, T., Goldenberg, J., & Solomon, S. (2003). *Structuring social and non-social information as terror management: Effects of mortality salience on
   primacy, balance, representativeness effects, and fate beliefs.* Unpublished manuscript, University
   of Arizona.

McGregor, I., Zanna, M., Holmes, J., & Spencer, S. (2001). Compensatory conviction in the face of
   personal uncertainty: Going to extremes and being oneself. *Journal of Personality and Social Psychology, 80*, 472–488.

Nuttin, J. (1985). Narcissism beyond Gestalt and awareness: The name letter effect. *European Journal
   of Social Psychology, 15*, 353–361.

Pierro, A., Mannetti, L., De Grada, E., Livi, S., & Kruglanski, A. (2003). Autocracy bias in informal
   groups under need for closure. *Personality and Social Psychology Bulletin, 29*, 405–417.

Pyszczynski, T., Greenberg, J., & Solomon, S. (1999). A dual-process model of defense against conscious and unconscious death-related thoughts: An extension of terror management theory. *Psychological Review, 106,* 835–845.

Pyszczynski, T., Solomon, S., & Greenberg, J. (2003). *In the wake of 9/11: The psychology of terror.* Washington, DC: American Psychological Association.

Pyszczynski, T., Wicklund, R., Floresku, S., Koch, H., Greenberg, J., & Solomon, S. (1996). Whistling in the dark: Exaggerated consensus estimates in response to incidental reminders of mortality. *Psychological Science, 7,* 332–336.

Richter, L., & Kruglanski, A. (2004). Motivated closed mindedness and the emergence of culture. In M. Schaller & C. Crandall (Eds.), *The psychological foundations of culture* (pp. 101–121). Mahwah, NJ: Erlbaum.

Rosenblatt, A., Greenberg, J., Solomon, S., Pyszczynski, T., & Lyon, D. (1989). Evidence for terror management theory I: The effects of mortality salience on reactions to those who violate and uphold cultural values. *Journal of Personality and Social Psychology, 57,* 681–690.

Schimel, J., Simon, L., Greenberg, J., Pyszczynski, T., Solomon, S., Waxmonsky, J., et al. (1999). Stereotypes and terror management: Evidence that mortality salience enhances stereotypic thinking and preferences. *Journal of Personality and Social Psychology, 77,* 905–926.

Shah, J., Kruglanski, A., & Thompson, E. (1998). Membership has its (epistemic) rewards: Need for closure effects on in-group bias. *Journal of Personality and Social Psychology, 75,* 383–393.

Solomon, S., Greenberg, J., & Pyszczynski, T. (1991). A terror management theory of social behavior: On the psychological functions of self-esteem and cultural worldviews. In M. P. Zanna (Ed.), *Advances in experimental social psychology* (Vol. 24, pp. 93–159). San Diego: Academic Press.

Taubman - Ben-Ari, O., Florian, V., & Mikulincer, M. (1999). The impact of mortality salience on reckless driving: A test of terror management mechanisms. *Journal of Personality and Social Psychology, 76,* 35–45.

Van den Bos, K. (2001). Uncertainty management: The influence of uncertainty salience on reactions to perceived procedural fairness. *Journal of Personality and Social Psychology, 80,* 931–941.

Webster, D., & Kruglanski, A. (1998). Cognitive and social consequences of the need for cognitive closure. In W. Stroebe & M. Hewstone (Eds.), *European review of social psychology* (pp. 133–173). New York: Wiley.

Chapter 17

The Ideological Animal

A System Justification View

JOHN T. JOST
GRÁINNE FITZSIMONS
AARON C. KAY

In an interview conducted in Afghanistan, Osama bin Laden (1998) was asked how he could justify the use of terrorist means for achieving political objectives. He replied:

> Every state and every civilization and culture has to resort to terrorism under certain circumstances for the purpose of abolishing tyranny and corruption. Every country in the world has its own security system and its own security forces, its own police and its own army. They are all designed to terrorize whoever even contemplates to attack that country or its citizens. The terrorism we practice is of the commendable kind for it is directed at the tyrants and the aggressors and the enemies of Allah, the tyrants, the traitors who commit acts of treason against their own countries and their own faith and their own prophet and their own nation. Terrorizing those and punishing them are necessary measures to straighten things and to make them right.

Slightly more than 3 years later, bin Laden's terrorist organization was blamed for the most devastating domestic attack in the history of the United States, when four commercial airplanes were hijacked, and two were flown into the World Trade Center in New York City, killing over 3,000 people. In response to these events, President George W. Bush (2002) described his administration's plans for dealing with the threat of terrorism in his famous "axis of evil" speech. He declared, in no uncertain terms:

> Our cause is just, and it continues. Our discoveries in Afghanistan confirmed our worst fears, and showed us the true scope of the task ahead. We have seen the depth of our enemies' hatred in videos, where they laugh about the loss of innocent life.... Thousands of dangerous killers, schooled in the methods of murder, often supported by outlaw regimes, are now spread through-

out the world like ticking time bombs, set to go off without warning. . . . Our nation will continue to be steadfast and patient and persistent in the pursuit of two great objectives. First, we will shut down terrorist camps, disrupt terrorist plans, and bring terrorists to justice. And, second, we must prevent the terrorists and regimes who seek chemical, biological or nuclear weapons from threatening the United States and the world. . . . States like [North Korea, Iran, and Iraq], and their terrorist allies, constitute an axis of evil, arming to threaten the peace of the world. By seeking weapons of mass destruction, these regimes pose a grave and growing danger.

Approximately 1 year later, the Bush administration used this basic rationale to justify its initiation of a preemptive war against Iraq. Although there are obviously many differences between the ideological belief systems held by bin Laden and Bush, a dispassionate observer would also be forced to conclude that there are at least a few key similarities. In the passages just quoted, both speakers profess a deep concern for the principles of justice, a moral obligation to defend their own system against threat, and an unwavering conviction that violence against one's enemies is justifiable, legitimate, and necessary. It is tempting to conclude that ideology, as Eagleton (1991) quipped, is "like halitosis"—something "the other person [or culture] has" (p. 2), but the reality is that ideology is part of what makes us human.

THEORIES OF THE IDEOLOGICAL ANIMAL

Human beings are, of course, animals, but they are decidedly unlike other species in several respects. Ernest Becker (1962/1971), the modern father of terror management theory, invited his readers to: "Try repeating 'man is an animal' a few times, just to notice how unconvincing it sounds" (p. 13). Karl Marx and Friedrich Engels (1845/1976), the chief architects of modern theories of ideology, including system justification theories, wrote that: "Men can be distinguished from animals by consciousness, by religion or by anything else you like" (p. 37), including, presumably, a deep immersion in culture, language, history, politics, ideology, and the accumulation of surplus labor and capital.[1] Social scientists have given many names to *homo sapiens*, including the "political animal" (Lipset, 1959), the "social animal" (Aronson, 1988), the "rationalizing animal" (Aronson, 1973/1989), the "moral animal" (Wright, 1994), and—drawing these themes together—the "ideological animal" (Althusser, 1970/1994). Other primates may be capable of vengeful, even premeditated murder (de Waal, 1989), but only humans can kill or die purely for the sake of an abstract set of ideas (i.e., for ideological reasons).

The Frankfurt School

The 20th century—one of the bloodiest in history—was marked by a dramatic surge in ideological conflict, war, and genocide (e.g., Rummel, 2001). Not by coincidence, this was also the century in which two disparate traditions in philosophy and psychology, namely, existential thought and the critique of ideology, were brought together for the first time. To understand the painful connection between human suffering and institutional attachments, theorists sought to reconcile the intellectual legacies of Marx and Freud, especially in the aftermath of the Nazi Holocaust. This was a primary goal of the members of the Frankfurt School, including Erich Fromm (1941, 1962), Wilhelm Reich (1946/1970), and the authors of *The Authoritarian Personality* (Adorno, Frenkel-Brunswik, Levinson, & Sanford, 1950), as well as Otto Rank (1936/1976) and Ernest Becker (1962/1971, 1968).

Ideology, defined as a set of consensually shared beliefs and doctrines that provide the moral and intellectual basis for a political, economic, or social system, imbues human existence with meaning and inspiration, but it also fosters illusion and threatens individual freedom. On this point (and others), contemporary system justification and terror management researchers are in agreement (see Jost, 1995; Pyszczynski, Solomon, Greenberg, & Stewart-Fouts, 1995). Members of the Frankfurt School and their followers sought to analyze the causes and critique the effects of ideology and false consciousness, thereby contributing to an increase in objective well-being. As Becker (1962/1971) put it, "*serious* social science is an attempt to come to grips with the fictions that constrain human freedom, with the ideas, beliefs, institutions that stifle the intelligent, responsible self-direction of the people . . . the task of social science is nothing less than the uncovering of social illusion" (pp. 158–159). Almost surely, social psychologists have a key role to play in the completion of this task.

Cognitive Dissonance Theory

It has been observed often that certain kinds of ideological beliefs provide excuses and justifications for actions and arrangements that would otherwise seem indefensible, even to the belief holder him- or herself (e.g., Bandura, 1990; Kelman & Hamilton, 1989). Evidence also suggests that ideology serves palliative functions of reducing anxiety, guilt, shame, dissonance, discomfort, and uncertainty (Chen & Tyler, 2001; Jost & Hunyady, 2002; Kluegel & Smith, 1986). For these reasons, one would think that the analysis of ideological thinking would be a cornerstone of psychological investigation. However, few psychological theories, especially in recent years, have done justice to the topic or placed ideology at the center of what makes us human. Festinger's (1957) cognitive dissonance theory was a promising start, stressing the human capacity for justification and rationalization in the social world. Unfortunately, the range of rationalizations studied by dissonance theorists has been limited and tied too narrowly to self-justification for acts of hypocrisy (e.g., Aronson, 1973/1989). Dissonance theory does not say much about the dynamics of complex ideological belief systems (see Jost & Hunyady, 2002) or the tendency to justify the status quo in the absence of personal choice or responsibility (see Jost, Pelham, Sheldon, & Sullivan, 2003; Kay, Jimenez, & Jost, 2002).

Just World Theory

Lerner's (1980) just world theory is perhaps closer than dissonance theory to suggesting a psychological account of ideology, insofar as it postulates that human beings are motivated not merely to achieve attitudinal and behavioral consistency but to preserve the more specific illusion that the world is a just place in which people "get what they deserve and deserve what they get." According to this theory, being confronted with acts of injustice threatens one's worldview and consequently motivates people to restore the belief in a just world (e.g., Hafer, 2000). Research has tended to focus on victim distancing and derogation as strategies for reducing existential anxiety and uncertainty caused by injustice (e.g., Furnham & Gunter, 1984; Lerner & Miller, 1978; Montada & Schneider, 1989; Rubin & Peplau, 1973).[2] Dissociating oneself from innocent victims and blaming them for their own misfortune may indeed preserve the belief in a just world, but research suggests that there is a much wider set of ideological beliefs that serve to justify the status quo. For example, gender inequality may be justified not only by derogating women for occupying an inferior position but also by praising them for their nurturance and moral superiority (e.g., Glick &

Fiske, 2001; Jackman, 1994). Similarly, economic inequality may be justified not only by blaming the poor for their shortcomings but also by fostering the illusion that they are in some ways happier and more virtuous than the rich (see Kay & Jost, 2003; Lane, 1959/2004).

A key assumption of Lerner's (1980) theory is that the belief in a just world follows from universal human needs to predict and control one's environment and to maintain a subjective sense of security. Although we agree that general epistemic motives may underlie ideological beliefs (see Jost, Glaser, Kruglanski, & Sulloway, 2003a, 2003b), this formulation does little to facilitate understanding the sources of variation in political beliefs and their distinctive causes and consequences. In fact, Lerner (1997) has acknowledged that "the phrase 'belief in a just world' originally was intended to provide a useful metaphor rather than a psychological construct" (p. 30). Its explanatory power, therefore, seems limited at best. Another question that arises is whether the belief in a just world is motivated by a deep-seated, genuine commitment to the cause of *justice*, as is increasingly assumed by researchers in this area (e.g., Dalbert, 2001), or whether it is better conceptualized as a defensive form of *justification* on behalf of the existing social and political system (e.g., Jost & Hunyady, 2002).

Terror Management Theory

Terror management theory (TMT) directly addresses the relation between psychology and ideology. According to TMT, people are motivated to defend and justify their cultural worldview—whatever its contents—by venerating those who uphold the worldview and by derogating and punishing those who threaten and challenge it, either symbolically or materially (e.g., Greenberg et al., 1990; Greenberg, Simon, Pyszczynski, Solomon, & Chatel, 1992; McGregor et al., 1998; Rosenblatt, Greenberg, Solomon, Pyszczynski, & Lyon, 1989). Building on the writings of Becker (1962/1971, 1968/1973), terror management theorists propose that these and other defensive responses are instigated by threats to self-esteem and/or reminders of one's mortality (see Pyszczynski, Greenberg, & Solomon, 1997). To cope with the existential anxiety that results from the unique evolutionary combination of an instinct for self-preservation with conscious awareness of the inevitability of death, it is theorized that human beings have developed a buffering system against anxiety that consists of two mutually reinforcing elements: (1) cultural values, norms, and standards that imbue the world with meaning; and (2) a sense of self-esteem that comes from satisfying cultural values, norms, and standards.

To demonstrate the flexibility of motivated responses to sources of existential threat, terror management theorists have repeatedly emphasized that mortality salience does not lead to any specific type of ideological or behavioral response. That is, death primes have been shown to either increase or decrease tolerance of deviants, as a function of one's chronically accessible ideology (Greenberg et al., 1992), to lead people either to derogate or affiliate with others who oppose one's worldview, as a function of whether they are seen as ingroup or outgroup members (Greenberg et al., 1990; Wisman & Koole, 2003), and to either increase or decrease ingroup identification, as a function of whether the group is seen as high or low in social status (Arndt, Greenberg, Schimel, Pyszczynski, & Solomon, 2002; Dechesne, Greenberg, Arndt, & Schimel, 2000; Harmon-Jones, Greenberg, Solomon, & Simon, 1996). Thus, TMT is useful for understanding the myriad ways in which people respond to mortality salience threats, but it takes no position on the unique determinants of specific ideological beliefs (e.g., Greenberg & Jonas, 2003).

System Justification Theory

System justification theory holds that people are motivated to perceive existing social and political arrangements as fair, legitimate, and justifiable (Jost & Banaji, 1994), even sometimes at the *expense* of personal and group interests and esteem (Jost & Burgess, 2000; Jost, Pelham, & Carvallo, 2002; Jost & Thompson, 2000). Threats to the legitimacy or stability of the system—as long as they fall short of toppling and replacing the status quo—should evoke defensive ideological responses, leading people to be even more motivated to justify the system with the use of stereotypes and other ideological devices (see Jost & Hunyady, 2002). According to the most extreme form of the system justification hypothesis, which also draws on the logic of dissonance theory (e.g., Wicklund & Brehm, 1976), people who are most disadvantaged by a given social system should paradoxically be the most likely to provide ideological support for it, insofar as they have the greatest need to justify their suffering. In five national survey studies, Jost et al. (2003c) have found support for this counterintuitive hypothesis.

An important question that arises in attempting to understand system justification effects is *why* people would be motivated to justify the system under which they are living. We have argued that there are several reasons, including preferences for cognitive consistency, uncertainty reduction, conservation of effort and of prior beliefs, fear of equality, illusion of control, belief in a just world, and the need to reduce dissonance associated with inaction and other ways of being complicit in the status quo (see Jost et al., 2002, 2003c). Ideological and structural factors—including political socialization, mass media influences, and the institutional control that dominant groups have over rewards and punishments in society—also affect system justification tendencies. Thus, according to system justification theory, cognitive, motivational, social, and structural factors all contribute to the tendency to explain, justify, and rationalize the way things are.

It should be clear, however, that system justification motives cannot be reduced to standard psychological motives for self-enhancement or ingroup favoritism (Jost & Banaji, 1994; Jost & Hunyady, 2002). Rather, phenomena associated with system justification are guided by specific tendencies to perceive the system as fair, legitimate, valid, meaningful, natural, and predictable. Research examining the theory has suggested the presence of a directional, content-laden motive to preserve the status quo and to subjectively enhance its desirability (e.g., Kay et al., 2002). System-justifying beliefs are therefore conservative in their consequences and may stem at least partially from epistemic and existential needs to manage uncertainty and threat (e.g., Hogg & Mullin, 1999; Jost et al., 2002a; Van den Bos & Lind, 2002). We return to this theme later, but first we flesh out some of the similarities and differences among theories of the ideological animal, focusing especially on terror management and system justification perspectives.

TERROR MANAGEMENT AND SYSTEM JUSTIFICATION: SIMILARITIES AND DIFFERENCES

We have already alluded to the first and most basic similarity between terror management and system justification theories, which is that both perspectives seek to build on the legacy owing to Marx, Freud, Adorno, Reich, Rank, Fromm, Becker, and many others who have sought to understand the relationship between psychology and ideology (Jost & Banaji,

1994; Pyszczynski et al., 1995). A second, related similarity is that both theories stress the social construction of reality and the need for consensual validation of ideological beliefs (Berger & Luckmann, 1966; Greenberg et al., 1990; Jost & Kruglanski, 2002; Pyszczynski et al., 1996; Stangor, Sechrist, & Jost, 2001). A third, more specific similarity is the shared emphasis on the need to defend one's "cultural worldview" or ideological belief system (Greenberg et al., 1990, 1992; Jost & Hunyady, 2002; Rosenblatt et al., 1989). Fourth, both theories have sought to demonstrate that social stereotypes serve the function of justifying and bolstering the status quo (Jost & Banaji, 1994; Kay & Jost, 2003; Schimel et al., 1999). A fifth and final similarity is that research on system justification and terror management has shown that members of disadvantaged groups will engage in ingroup derogation and outgroup favoritism, to the extent that such behavior satisfies existential or ideological needs (Arndt et al., 2002; Jost et al., 2002).

TMT often makes the same empirical predictions as system justification theory, because terror management theorists believe that system justification is one mechanism whereby individuals can reduce death anxiety. The need to justify the system (and, for that matter, to perceive the world as a just and orderly place) is therefore assumed to follow from more fundamental human needs to minimize existential anxiety caused by fear of mortality. Whether system justification motives can be traced (or reduced) to the fear of death is an issue that is open to debate (see also Lerner, 1997).

Not surprisingly, there are also some meaningful differences between system justification and terror management perspectives, and it is useful to clarify these differences in order to understand the proper role of epistemic and existential factors in ideology. One major difference is that terror management theorists accept Becker's (1962/1971) assertion that self-esteem is "the dominant motive of man" (pp. 65–74) and that defending the cultural worldview necessarily increases one's self-esteem, whereas system justification theorists do not.[3] Solomon, Greenberg, and Pyszczynski (1991), for example, proceed from the assumption that "social behavior is primarily directed toward the acquisition and maintenance of self-esteem" (p. 26). Jost and Banaji (1994) argued that motives for self-enhancement and ingroup favoritism are important but do not necessarily trump the motive to rationalize and preserve the status quo. More to the point, perhaps, we have found that among members of disadvantaged groups, ideological support for the status quo is associated with *decreased* rather than increased self-esteem (e.g., Jost et al., 2002; Jost & Thompson, 2000; Quinn & Crocker, 1999).

Another set of issues that arises when one juxtaposes system justification and terror management theories is whether the fear of death is a universal motive that accounts for the emergence of all cultural and ideological forms, as Becker (1968/1973) suggested. In discussing differences between just-world and terror-management perspectives, Pyszczynski et al. (1997) noted that "whereas Lerner et al. view just-world beliefs as providing protection against the general fear that negative things might befall one, TMT posits that this general fear of aversive events is rooted ultimately in the self-preservation instinct and the consequent fear of death" (p. 10). This formulation makes it extremely difficult to empirically distinguish between proximal fears that are related versus unrelated to the fear of death, but research has demonstrated that many of the effects brought about by increased mortality salience are also elicited by heightened levels of uncertainty (e.g., Dechesne, Janssen, & van Knippenberg, 2000; McGregor, Zanna, Holmes, & Spencer, 2001; Van den Bos & Miedema, 2000). Similarly, there is considerable evidence linking political ideologies to uncertainty avoidance and needs for order, structure, and closure, suggesting that ideological belief systems serve many other epistemic and existential functions in addition to repressing death anxiety (e.g., Jost et al., 2003a, 2003b; Sorrentino & Roney, 2000; Wilson, 1973).

Related to this is the question whether all ideologies are equally healthy and adaptive (from both individual and societal points of view) and whether they are equally "caused" by the fear of death and other epistemic and existential variables. While acknowledging that human beings, like other animals, possess a strong (but by no means insurmountable) instinct for survival, we think that it is important to consider variation in the ways in which people cope with existential realities. Postulating a universally shared fear of death does not by itself help to understand or appreciate the heterogeneity of personal and political ideologies.

With regard to personal belief systems, studies have indeed shown variability in the relationship between death acceptance and responses to loss. Bonanno et al. (2002) conducted a prospective study of more than 200 elderly individuals before and after the death of their spouse. The researchers found considerable variation in the degree to which participants held worldviews that were accepting (rather than fearful) of death. Results indicated that the degree to which participants scored high on the acceptance of mortality before their spouses died subsequently predicted more adaptive coping responses (i.e., resilient and depressed-improved bereavement patterns) to the eventual deaths of their spouses. By contrast, participants who tended to fear rather than accept death were more likely to follow maladaptive bereavement patterns (i.e., common grief, chronic grief, and chronic depression).[4] As Freud put it, "If you want to live, you must be prepared for death." Freud's Viennese neighbor, the philosopher Ludwig Wittgenstein (1916/1979), made the point even more starkly: "Fear in the face of death is the best sign of a false, i.e., a bad life" (pp. 74–75; see also Schultz, 1999).

Returning to political belief systems, TMT suggests that all political ideologies are illusory by definition, functionally interchangeable, and equally traceable to an underlying fear of death. As a result, it is difficult to see how any given ideology could be said to be more individually or socially adaptive than its alternatives. Solomon et al. (1991) recognize this problem and address it by suggesting that the *consequences* of different cultural systems can be evaluated according to "reasonably objective standards" (p. 33). Specifically, they argue that "applied social science should be directed toward the development and maintenance of worldviews that maximize the equitable distribution of material resources and development of nondestructive technologies, which emphasize social roles that confer the possibility of acquiring self-esteem to as many people as possible, and which do so at a minimum of expense to others" (p. 35). We are in general agreement with these goals but a deeper and more precise analysis is needed to determine which ideologies will move us closer to achieving these goals, and which ideologies will obstruct them (see also Jost et al., 2003a, 2003b; Pratto, Sidanius, Stallworth, & Malle, 1994).

System justification theory leads us to reject the notion that all ideologies are functionally equivalent. Rather, we suggest that there is utility in distinguishing among different types of ideologies in terms of causes and contents as well as consequences. In addition to highlighting social, cognitive, and motivational tendencies to legitimize the status quo, a system justification perspective can also be used to identify differences in the epistemic and existential bases of different types of political ideologies, including liberalism, conservatism, and other belief systems that can be placed (however imperfectly) on a left–right dimension (Bobbio, 1996). In this sense, system justification theory fills an important gap in explaining the psychological antecedents of specific ideological beliefs. There is an abundance of evidence, as we shall see, that suggests that not all ideologies are the same, psychologically speaking.

CASE STUDY OF A SYSTEM-JUSTIFYING IDEOLOGY:
EPISTEMIC AND EXISTENTIAL BASES
OF POLITICAL CONSERVATISM

Historians and social scientists tend to agree that the core components of right-wing conservative ideology are *resistance to change* and *acceptance of social inequality* (e.g., Huntington, 1957; Kerlinger, 1984; Muller, 2001). Defined in this way, political conservatism is a paradigm case of a system-justifying ideology in that it both preserves the status quo and suggests intellectual and moral rationales for maintaining inequality in society (Jost et al., 2003a, 2003b). To investigate the epistemic and existential roots of political conservatism, therefore, is to investigate (at least partially) the psychological basis of system justification.

Jost et al. (2003a) conducted an extensive meta-analytic review of studies linking psychological variables to the ideology of political conservatism. The original studies, which were conducted between 1958 and 2002, made use of 88 research samples involving 22,818 individual cases, and were carried out in 12 different countries: United States, England, New Zealand, Australia, Poland, Sweden, Germany, Scotland, Israel, Italy, Canada, and South Africa. This body of research made it possible to assess the strength of empirical relations between right-wing conservatism and nine variables pertaining to epistemic and existential functioning: dogmatism/ intolerance of ambiguity; openness to experience; fear of threat and loss; self-esteem; uncertainty avoidance; personal needs for order, structure, and closure; integrative complexity; system instability; and fear of death. These variables were selected on the basis of prior psychological theories of ideology, including right-wing authoritarianism (Adorno et al., 1950; Altemeyer, 1998), dogmatism (Rokeach, 1960), polarity theory (Tomkins, 1963), the dynamic theory of conservatism (Wilson, 1973), TMT (Greenberg et al., 1990), and system justification theory (Jost & Banaji, 1994).

Results of the meta-analysis indicated that all nine of the hypothesized cognitive–motivational variables were indeed significantly related to political conservatism and the holding of right-wing ideological orientations, although the effect sizes for the different variables ranged considerably (see Figure 17.1). The largest effect sizes were obtained for fear of death (and mortality salience) and system instability and threat. Moderate effect sizes were obtained for dogmatism and intolerance of ambiguity, openness to experience, uncertainty avoidance, and personal needs to achieve order, structure, and closure. Weaker effect sizes were obtained for integrative complexity, fear of threat and loss, and self-esteem.

The bulk of the evidence from the meta-analysis by Jost et al. (2003a) supported the notion that there is a "match" between certain epistemic and existential needs and the contents of specific political ideologies. This had been suggested not only by Adorno et al. (1950) but also by Rokeach (1960), who wrote that "if a person's underlying motivations are served by forming a closed belief system, then it is more likely that his motivations can also be served by embracing an ideology that is blatantly anti-equalitarian. If this is so, it would account for the somewhat greater affinity we have observed between authoritarian belief structure and conservatism than between the same belief structure and liberalism" (p. 127). After 50 years of research, the correlational evidence is quite strong that there are a number of consistent psychological differences between proponents of conservative versus liberal ideologies. Specifically, epistemic and existential needs to reduce uncertainty and threat seem to be more acute among people who are drawn to right-wing (vs. left-wing) belief systems, at least in the context of the nontotalitarian political environments investigated by Jost et al. (2003a).

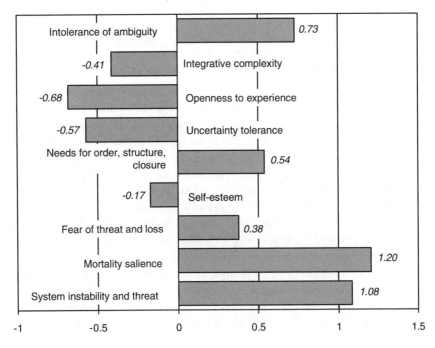

FIGURE 17.1. Epistemic and existential bases of political conservatism: Effect sizes (Cohen's d's) obtained in meta-analysis by Jost, Glaser, Kruglanski, and Sulloway (2003a).

WHY WOULD CERTAIN EPISTEMIC AND EXISTENTIAL NEEDS BE ESPECIALLY WELL SATISFIED BY CONSERVATIVE IDEOLOGIES?

A number of theoretical and empirical considerations led Jost et al. (2003a) to conclude that all nine of the epistemic and existential motives listed in Figure 17.1 originate in psychological attempts to manage *uncertainty* and *threat*. There is also reason to think that the management of uncertainty and threat would be closely linked to the two core components of conservative thought mentioned earlier, namely, resistance to change and acceptance of inequality. This is why we, like Rokeach (1960), argue that there is an especially good *match* between certain epistemic and existential needs and specific ideological contents.

Needs to reduce uncertainty and threat are well served by ideological resistance to change, insofar as change (by its very nature) upsets existing realities and is fraught with epistemic insecurity. As a general rule, the status quo implies less uncertainty and ambiguity than counterfactual alternatives to it. Because certainty, value, and meaning are derived from existing social arrangements and dominant cultural worldviews, fear arising from the possibility of one's own death should similarly induce resistance to change and a rigid rejection of anyone who threatens or deviates from the status quo (e.g., Greenberg et al., 1990). This is why Wicklund (1997) noted several important parallels between the effects of mortality salience and right-wing authoritarianism. Specifically, he concluded:

> The existing research in [the terror management] realm points to a person's guarding and abiding by the established, univocal, ingroup rules; the new, the strange, or the ambiguous is avoided or denigrated. This form of operationalization then obligates further applications of the theory to

define culture in terms of an authoritarian manner of dealing with threats: One's known, trusted position is correct; those who don't abide by that system are excluded (cf. Adorno et al., 1950). (p. 57)

Similarly, heightened sensitivity to uncertainty and threat could be both causes and consequences of embracing inequality in social, economic, and political domains. To the extent that inequality breeds (and perhaps guarantees) competition, dominance struggles, and occasionally even violent strife, it may also lead to an overall increase in fear, anxiety, and suspicion. Fear of the threat posed by competitors, in turn, may lead one to embrace antiegalitarian ideologies even more enthusiastically, in part because these ideologies are particularly useful for justifying the use of force and social control to neutralize one's foes (e.g., Sidanius & Pratto, 1999). For all these reasons, Jost et al. (2003a) argued that psychological needs to manage uncertainty and threat would be especially well satisfied by the core convictions of political conservatives to resist change and justify inequality, especially to the extent that the status quo itself breeds inequality and competition.

The core aspects of conservative ideology should be particularly appealing, therefore, to people who are especially sensitive to fear, uncertainty, and threat for either situational or dispositional reasons (e.g., Wilson, 1973). As Paulhus and Trapnell (1997) put it, "Perhaps conservatives fear both God and death" (p. 43), among other things. A system justification view, as we have shown, is better equipped than a terror management view to account for resonant matches between certain epistemic and existential needs on one hand and specific ideological contents on the other hand.

OBJECTIONS TO DISTINGUISHING BETWEEN PSYCHOLOGICAL ANTECEDENTS OF LIBERAL VERSUS CONSERVATIVE IDEOLOGICAL OPINIONATION

When Adorno et al. (1950) first argued for the existence of a right-wing "authoritarian syndrome" combining ego defensiveness, mental rigidity, intolerance of ambiguity, general ethnocentrism, and a number of other factors, critics objected that Adorno and his colleagues had neglected the phenomenon of left-wing rigidity (e.g., Eysenck, 1954/1999; Rokeach, 1960; Shils, 1954). Specifically, critics denied that there were general cognitive and motivational style variables that were associated with specific ideological positions and argued instead that such variables predicted ideological extremity (dogmatism), regardless of political content. In his 1999 introduction to the revised edition of *The Psychology of Politics*, Eysenck claimed victory for theoretical opponents of work on the authoritarian personality. He stated, for example, that "authoritarianism (tough-mindedness) could appear equally well on the left as on the right," and that "the existence of left-wing fascism [is] as certain as anything in social psychology." Eysenck concluded that based "upon the social experience of the past forty years, as well as upon the many empirical studies published since 1954, I would confidently say that my major thesis is hardly any longer in doubt" (pp. xv–xxi). Indeed, the meta-analysis by Jost et al. (2003a) provides a great deal of evidence to doubt Eysenck's long-held position that there are no epistemic or existential differences that covary with left–right differences in political ideology.

Greenberg and Jonas (2003) echoed many of Eysenck's (1954/1999) objections in critiquing the article by Jost et al. (2003a), arguing that "left-wing ideologies serve these motives [to reduce fear, anxiety, and uncertainty] just as well as right-wing ones" (p. 10).

Consistent with the ideological relativism of TMT, Greenberg and Jonas (2003) flatly rejected the matching hypothesis that specific epistemic and existential needs are more likely to be satisfied by some ideologies than others. They argued that "need for closure, terror management, uncertainty reduction, prevention focus, and system justification are all best served by embracing and rigidly adhering to and defending whatever the prevailing ideology is in one's socio-cultural environment" (p. 10). In responding to this critique, Jost et al. (2003b) suggested that certain epistemic and existential needs could simultaneously increase (1) reliance on culturally available ideologies (i.e., the status quo), and (2) resonance with conservative or right-wing opinions.

STUDIES DIRECTLY PITTING THE MATCHING HYPOTHESIS AGAINST THE EXTREMITY HYPOTHESIS

Jost et al. (2003b) identified 13 individual studies that allowed for a direct test between competing hypotheses. One potential result would be that epistemic and existential needs to reduce uncertainty and threat would increase in a linear fashion from left-wing to right-wing ideologues; this would support the matching hypothesis. Another possibility was that these needs would increase symmetrically with increasing distance from the political center, as suggested by the extremity hypothesis. Finally, a third pattern of results in which *both* effects were present in combination was also considered. Figure 17.2 illustrates these three hypothesized patterns.

In reviewing the 13 most relevant studies, Jost et al. (2003b) found that 7 of them conformed to the linear pattern suggested by the matching hypothesis illustrated in Figure 17.2a. Barker (1963) surveyed student activists in Ohio and found that organized rightists scored significantly higher in dogmatism than did nonorganized students, who scored (nonsignificantly) higher than did organized leftists. Kohn (1974) followed student political groups in Britain and found that Conservatives scored significantly higher than Socialists and Liberals, and they scored marginally higher than Labour Party supporters on intolerance of ambiguity. Studies by Sidanius (1978) in Sweden and Fibert and Ressler (1998) in Israel also investigated relations between political ideology and intolerance of ambiguity. In both studies significant linear effects were observed, and so were quadratic effects in the direction that was opposite to the extremity hypothesis: Intolerance of ambiguity decreased slightly between the center right and the far right. Sidanius (1985) obtained comparable effects for the relation between ideology and cognitive complexity. Studies by Kemmelmeier (1997) in Germany and Chirumbolo (2002) in Italy examined ideological differences related to the need for cognitive closure, and both yielded evidence of significant linear effects (and no evidence of quadratic trends). Thus, most of the evidence unequivocally supported the matching (rigidity-of-the-right) hypothesis against the extremity hypothesis. Similar results were obtained in six different countries and on such convergent measures as dogmatism, intolerance of ambiguity, need for cognitive closure, and integrative complexity.

None of the 13 studies provided exclusive support for the extremity hypothesis depicted in Figure 17.2b. The remaining 6 studies provided evidence that *both* matching and extremity effects were present. McClosky and Chong (1985) found that a preponderance of respondents classified as high on intolerance of ambiguity came from far left and far right groups, as compared with moderates. In all cases, however, the percentage of high scorers from the far right group exceeded the percentage of high scorers from the far left. Although they do not report full data for center left and center right groups, it seems that the

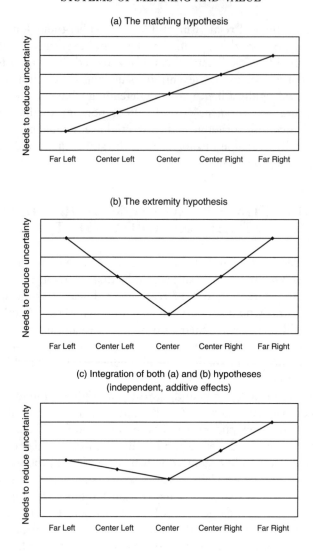

FIGURE 17.2. Patterns of results predicted by competing hypotheses (Jost, Glaser, Kruglanski, & Sulloway, 2003b).

McClosky and Chong data would more closely resemble the combined pattern illustrated in Figure 17.2c than that illustrated in Figure 17.2b.

Five additional studies provide evidence that both rigidity-of-the-right and ideological extremity exert effects, as depicted in Figure 17.2c. Smithers and Lobley's (1978) study of dogmatism and political orientation in Great Britain produced a pattern of results in which "the V-shaped curve did include more of the conservative end of the scale" (p. 135). Tetlock (1983) found that moderates in the U.S. Senate scored non-significantly higher on integrative complexity than did liberals and that both groups scored significantly higher than conservatives. Tetlock, Bernzweig, and Gallant (1985) obtained similar results in their study of U.S. Supreme Court justices' opinions on both economic issues and civil liberties. Tetlock's (1984) study of members of the British House of Commons revealed that the most integratively complex politicians were moderate socialists, who scored significantly higher than extreme socialists, moderate conservatives, and extreme conservatives (who scored lowest in complexity). Finally, Tetlock, Hannum, and Micheletti (1984) found that aggregating across five congressional sessions, conservatives on average scored considerably lower on integrative complexity than did liberals, who scored slightly lower than did moderates. Thus, 6 of the studies provided partial evidence for the ideological extremity hypothesis, and *all* 13 studies provided at least some evidence for the rigidity-of-the-right hypothesis (see Jost et al., 2003b).

AN EXPERIMENTAL STUDY

To further explore the link between existential and ideological factors and to consider the possibility that situational manipulations of mortality salience would affect political conservatism, we conducted an experimental study (Jost, Kay, & Fitzsimons, 2004). With a predominantly liberal university sample, we first measured participants' self-reported political orientations on a liberal–conservative dimension and then evoked either mortality-related or pain-related thoughts. Afterward, participants were asked their opinions about a number of current political issues that were relevant for assessing liberalism and conservatism. This design allowed us to directly pit hypotheses of terror management and system justification theories against one another.

Terror management theorists would predict that liberal participants would become more liberal in their responses to the current political issues following mortality salience, and that conservative participants would become more conservative (an interaction hypothesis). A similar suggestion was made by Paulhus and Trapnell (1997), who wrote that "it is possible that the tendency to defend the worldview in the face of mortality cues is limited to conservatives . . . Thus, the TMT conception and measure of 'worldview' would be more accurately labeled 'conservative worldview.' Liberals may be less responsive to mortality cues or may even act to defend a liberal worldview" (p. 43). Although we agree that there seems to a better *match* between existential fears and conservative ideologies, we do not think that the system-justifying effects of mortality salience would necessarily differ for liberals and conservatives. Specifically, we would predict that both liberal and conservative participants would grow more conservative following mortality salience (a main effect hypothesis). Our situationalist position is closer to that of Wicklund (1997), who observed that "the contents of the death-threatened respondents' worldviews . . . are quite similar to many of the verbalizations of the authoritarian person" (p. 54).

We recruited 56 research participants (31 men and 25 women) from public places on a university campus. Participants were asked to complete a short questionnaire packet that began with demographic information, including self-reported political orientation (with labels ranging from "extremely liberal" to "extremely conservative"). Most of the participants ($N = 36$) identified themselves as liberals. The remainder identified themselves as either moderates ($N = 8$) or conservatives ($N = 12$). The relatively small size of the sample (especially the paucity of conservative and moderate respondents) suggests the need for caution in interpreting the results, but the data from this experimental intervention are instructive nonetheless.

After indicating demographic information, participants completed a word-picture matching task in which seven words on the left side of the page had to be matched with seven corresponding pictures reproduced on the right side of the page. For half of the participants, some of the words and pictures were explicitly related to death (e.g., a funeral hearse, a "dead end" street sign, and the grim reaper), whereas the other half of the participants were exposed to a control group of words and pictures that were related to pain but not to death (e.g., an ambulance, a dentist's chair, and a bee sting). Both sets of materials also included filler items such as a satellite and a dog.

Following the word-picture matching task, participants completed a "current affairs survey" in which they indicated levels of support versus opposition (on 9-point scales) to seven different conservative (vs. liberal) causes, including tighter immigration restrictions, maintaining tax breaks for large corporations, affirmative action policies (reverse-scored), and legalization of same-sex marriages (reverse-scored). Responses on these items were collapsed to form an overall index of conservatism; this index showed adequate reliability (alpha = .62) and correlated with self-reports of political conservatism ($r = .65$, $p < .001$).

To assess the effects of political orientation and mortality salience on conservative responding, a univariate analysis of variance was conducted in which the three levels of political orientation (liberal, moderate, and conservative) and the two levels of priming condition (death vs. pain) were entered as fixed factors, and the overall conservative endorsement index served as the dependent measure, with respondent gender entered as a covariate. The analysis yielded main effects of political orientation and priming condition, but no interaction between these variables (see Jost et al., 2004). As can be seen in Figure 17.3, participants—regardless of political orientation—exhibited a significant tendency to become more conservative following the death primes ($M = 4.64$), as compared with the pain primes ($M = 3.96$).[5] This finding is consistent with system justification theory and supports the contentions of Jost et al. (2003a, 2003b) that specific epistemic and existential variables are associated more with right-wing than left-wing thinking and that temporary directional shifts in political ideology can be brought about experimentally. We are currently seeking to replicate this study using larger sample sizes and more even distributions of liberals and conservatives.

By illustrating that mortality salience increases the attractiveness of politically conservative beliefs, these preliminary data provide additional empirical support for the matching hypothesis by demonstrating that existential threat does not equally or symmetrically rigidify liberal and conservative ideological beliefs. Rather, priming the fear of death exerted a directional effect on ideology, as suggested by system justification theory, leading to an increase in politically conservative responding among self-identified liberals and moderates (as

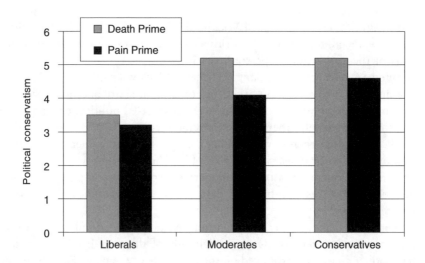

FIGURE 17.3. Political conservatism scores of liberals, moderates, and conservatives following death versus pain primes (Jost, Kay, & Fitzsimons, 2004).

well as conservatives). Furthermore, these data suggest that there is value in examining heterogeneity in the psychological antecedents of different political ideologies, and they question the tempting relativistic assumption that all ideologies serve the same functions and are driven by the same epistemic and existential needs.

CONCLUSION

In this chapter, we have sought to integrate insights from and contribute to the further development of a long and distinguished tradition of analyzing the psychological basis of political ideology. As ideological animals, human beings suffuse the world with socially constructed meanings. The various theories described in this chapter are in general agreement with Marx, Freud, Becker, and many others that meaning systems can be said to reflect underlying need states. In this way, ideologies are socially and psychologically constructed, but they are not constructed arbitrarily (Berger & Luckmann, 1966; Jost & Kruglanski, 2002).

There are a number of contemporary theories—including just-world, terror-management, and system-justification perspectives—that are useful for understanding the role of epistemic and existential variables in the context of political life. Just world theorists were among the first to suggest a motivated psychological account of specific ideological beliefs, namely, that the world is a just and orderly place in which people are deserving of their individual and collective fates (e.g., Lerner & Miller, 1978). Terror management theorists have successfully renewed social psychological interest in the importance of existential motives and their role in supporting ideological belief systems. Dozens of carefully crafted empirical studies in the terror management tradition have convincingly demonstrated the flexibility of cognitive and ideological responses to sources of motivational threat (see Greenberg et al., 1997).

System justification theorists have posited that defensive responses on behalf of the cultural worldview may even supersede self-esteem needs (Jost & Banaji, 1994; Jost & Thompson, 2000). There may be, in other words, general ideological processes that operate in defense of the status quo, even at the expense of individual and collective self-esteem (see Jost & Hunyady, 2002). An examination of these processes, we argue, is needed to explain why "people willingly propagate whole cultural systems that hold them in bondage," as Becker (1962/1971, p. 86) so eloquently put it.

There are reasons to think that system-justifying ideological responses stem from a wide range of epistemic and existential needs and not just the fear of death. One especially common manifestation of system justification—political conservatism—has been linked conclusively to heightened cognitive and motivational needs for order, stability, structure, simplicity, closure, uncertainty avoidance, and ambiguity intolerance, as well as terror management (Jost et al., 2003a, 2003b). The preliminary results of an experimental study we have described also suggest that situationally induced mortality salience leads to a general increase in the endorsement of politically conservative attitudes.

The available evidence to date, therefore, supports the utility of distinguishing among different types of ideological belief systems in terms of how well they satisfy and resonate with a variety of psychological needs pertaining to the management of uncertainty and threat. Ideologies, in this sense, should be judged (at least partially) in terms of how successfully they resolve for their adherents the basic questions and strains of human living. This conclusion parallels in many ways a point made by Marx (1846/1999) in a rare, uncharacteristically existentialist passage: "The classification of the different causes of suicide would be the *classification of the failures of our society itself*" (p. 64).

ACKNOWLEDGMENTS

This chapter was written while John T. Jost held a fellowship at the Radcliffe Institute for Advanced Study at Harvard University, for which we are grateful. We also wish to thank George Bonanno, Orsolya Hunyady, and Tom Pyszczynski for extremely helpful suggestions for revision.

NOTES

1. Becker (1962/1971) also differentiated human beings from other animals on several dimensions, including the fact that man possesses "an unprecedented level of mastery of his world" (p. 12), is "the only time-binding animal" who is aware of his own death (p. 16), "who can dwell on his own experiences and on his fate" (p. 23), and "the only animal in nature who vitally depends on a symbolic constitution of his worth" (p. 67). Solomon, Greenberg, and Pyszczynski (1991) built on this view, noting that "there is a fundamental difference between humans and other living organisms that renders us responsive to different types of reinforcement by virtue of our having different needs (i.e., meaning and value)" (p. 35). Finally, Pyszczynski, Solomon, Greenberg, and Stewart-Fouts (1995) concluded: "What distinguishes humans from other animals . . . is not the existence of a system for the internal control of behavior, but the linguistic capabilities that make an abstract representation of self possible" (p. 360).
2. Just world theory can be distinguished from two other theories we consider later in this chapter, namely, system justification and terror management theories, by considering responses to victims of injustice. Whereas just world theory predicts that people will respond to threat by derogating victims, system justification theory predicts that only when victim blaming serves the higher-order goal of justifying the system will people blame victims for their misfortune. Victim blaming and system justification often do not coincide, such as when victims (like those involved in the 9/11 attacks on the World Trade Center) are symbolic of the cultural meaning systems that people are motivated to defend. In these cases, system justification and terror management theories would predict that people would defend and even lionize the victims and the system to which they belong.
3. Becker (1962/1971) also sought to explain cases of system justification in terms of self-enhancement motives, suggesting, for example, that some people "work out their urge to superiority by . . . being devoted slaves: 'I am a locus of real value because I serve the great man.' Others serve the corporation to get the same feeling, and some serve the war-machines" (p. 71). Jost and Banaji (1994) argue, by contrast, that system justification cannot be reduced to ego justification, and the fact that system justification and self-esteem are negatively correlated among members of disadvantaged groups suggests that the two are separate, distinguishable, and often in opposition (e.g., Jost & Thompson, 2000).
4. Bonanno et al. (2002) also found that endorsement of the belief in a just world was associated with a resilient coping style, whereas rejection of the belief in a just world was associated with patterns of grief and depression following the loss of a spouse.
5. Unfortunately, the sample sizes within each ideological group were too small to test meaningfully for pairwise effects between mortality salience and control conditions.

REFERENCES

Adorno, T. W., Frenkel-Brunswik, E., Levinson, D. J., & Sanford, R. N. (1950). *The authoritarian personality*. New York: Harper.

Altemeyer, B. (1998). The other "authoritarian personality." *Advances in Experimental Social Psychology, 30*, 47–92.

Althusser, L. (1994). Ideology and ideological state apparatuses (Notes towards an investigation). In S. Zizek (Ed.), *Mapping ideology* (pp. 100–140). New York: Verso. (Original work published 1970)

Arndt, J., Greenberg, J., Schimel, J., Pyszczynski, T., & Solomon, S. (2002). To belong or not to belong, that is the question: Terror management and identification with gender and ethnicity. *Journal of Personality and Social Psychology, 83,* 26–43.

Aronson, E. (1988). *The social animal.* New York: Freeman.

Aronson, E. (1989). The rationalizing animal. In H. J. Leavitt, L. R. Pondy, & D. M. Boje (Eds.), *Readings in managerial psychology* (4th ed., pp. 134–144). Chicago: University of Chicago Press. (Original work published 1973)

Bandura, A. (1990). Mechanisms of moral disengagement. In W. Reich (Ed.), *Origins of terrorism: Psychologies, ideologies, theologies, states of mind* (pp. 161–191). Washington, DC: Woodrow Wilson Center Press.

Barker, E. N. (1963). Authoritarianism of the political right, center, and left. *Journal of Social Issues, 19,* 63–74.

Becker, E. (1968). *The structure of evil; an essay on the unification of the science of man.* New York: Braziller.

Becker, E. (1971). *The birth and death of meaning; an interdisciplinary perspective on the problem of man.* New York: Free Press. (Original work published 1962)

Becker, E. (1973). *The denial of death.* New York: Free Press. (Original work published 1968)

Berger, P. L., & Luckmann, T. (1966). *The social construction of reality: A treatise its the sociology of knowledge.* Garden City, New York: Anchor Books.

bin Laden, O. (1998, May). Interview. Retrieved April 21, 2003, from *http://www.pbs.org/wgbh/pages/frontline/shows/binladen/who/interview.html.*

Bobbio, N. (1996). *Left and right: The significance of a political distinction.* Chicago: University of Chicago Press.

Bonanno, G. A., Wortman, C. B., Lehman, D. R., Tweed, R., Haring, M., Sonnega, J., et al. (2002). Resilience to loss and chronic grief: A prospective study from preloss to 18–months postloss. *Journal of Personality and Social Psychology, 83,* 1150–1164.

Bush, G. W. (2002, January 29). The President's State of the Union Address. Retrieved April 24, 2003, from *http://www.whitehouse.gov/news/releases/2002/01/20020129–11.html.*

Chen, E. S., & Tyler, T. R. (2001). Cloaking power: Legitimizing myths and the psychology of the advantaged. In A. Y. Lee-Chai & J. Bargh (Eds.), *The use and abuse of power: Multiple perspectives on the causes of corruption* (pp. 241–261). Philadelphia: Psychology Press.

Chirumbolo, A. (2002). The relationship between need for cognitive closure and political orientation: The mediating role of authoritarianism. *Personality and Individual Differences, 32,* 603–610.

Dalbert, C. (2001). *The justice motive as a personal resource: Dealing with challenges and critical life events.* New York: Plenum Press.

Dechesne, M., Greenberg, J., Arndt, J., & Schimel, J. (2000). Terror management and sports fan affiliation: The effects of mortality salience on fan identification and optimism. *European Journal of Social Psychology, 30,* 813–835.

Dechesne, M., Janssen, J., & van Knippenberg, A. (2000). Derogation and distancing as terror management strategies: The moderating role of need for closure and permeability of group boundaries. *Journal of Personality and Social Psychology, 79,* 923–932.

de Waal, F. (1989). *Peacemaking among primates.* Cambridge, MA: Harvard University Press.

Eagleton, T. (1991). *Ideology: An introduction.* London: Verso.

Eysenck, H. J. (1999). *The psychology of politics.* New Brunswick, NJ: Transaction. (Original work published 1954)

Festinger, L. (1957). *A theory of cognitive dissonance.* Evanston, IL: Row, Peterson.

Fibert, Z., & Ressler, W. H. (1998). Intolerance of ambiguity and political orientation among Israeli university students. *Journal of Social Psychology, 138,* 33–40.

Fromm, E. (1941). *Escape from freedom.* New York: Holt, Rinehart & Winston.

Fromm, E. (1962). *Beyond the chains of illusion: My encounters with Marx and Freud.* New York: Simon & Schuster.

Furnham, A., & Gunter. B. (1984). Just world beliefs and attitudes towards the poor. *British Journal of Social Psychology, 23,* 265–269.

Glick, P., & Fiske, S. T. (2001). An ambivalent alliance: Hostile and benevolent sexism as complementary justifications of gender inequality. *American Psychologist, 56*, 109–118.

Greenberg, J., & Jonas, E. (2003). Psychological motives and political orientation—The left, the right, and the rigid: Comment on Jost et al. (2003). *Psychological Bulletin, 129*, 376–382.

Greenberg, J., Pyszczynski, T., Solomon, S., Rosenblatt, A., Veeder, M., Kirkland, S., et al. (1990). Evidence for terror management theory II: The effects of mortality salience on reactions to those who threaten or bolster the cultural worldview. *Journal of Personality and Social Psychology, 58*, 308–318.

Greenberg, J., Simon, L., Pyszczynski, T., Solomon, S., & Chatel, D. (1992). Terror management and tolerance: Does mortality salience always intensify negative reactions to others who threaten one's worldview? *Journal of Personality and Social Psychology, 63*, 212–220.

Hafer, C. L. (2000). Do innocent victims threaten the belief in a just world? Evidence from a modified Stroop task. *Journal of Personality and Social Psychology, 79*, 165–173.

Harmon-Jones, E., Greenberg, J., Solomon, S., & Simon, L. (1996). The effects of mortality salience on intergroup discrimination between minimal groups. *European Journal of Social Psychology, 26*, 677–681.

Hogg, M. A., & Mullin, B. -A. (1999). Joining groups to reduce uncertainty: Subjective uncertainty reduction and group identification. In D. Abrams & M. A. Hogg (Eds.), *Social identity and social cognition* (pp. 249–279). Oxford, UK: Blackwell.

Huntington, S. (1957). Conservatism as an ideology. *American Political Science Review, 51*, 454–473.

Jackman, M. R. (1994). *The velvet glove: Paternalism and conflict in gender, class, and race relations.* Berkeley: University of California Press.

Jost, J. T. (1995). Negative illusions: Conceptual clarification and psychological evidence concerning false consciousness. *Political Psychology, 16*, 397–424.

Jost, J. T., & Banaji, M. R. (1994). The role of stereotyping in system-justification and the production of false consciousness. *British Journal of Social Psychology, 33*, 1–27.

Jost, J. T., & Burgess, D. (2000). Attitudinal ambivalence and the conflict between group and system justification motives in low status groups. *Personality and Social Psychology Bulletin, 26*, 293–305.

Jost, J. T., Glaser, J., Kruglanski, A. W., & Sulloway, F. (2003a). Political conservatism as motivated social cognition. *Psychological Bulletin, 129*, 339–375.

Jost, J. T., Glaser, J., Kruglanski, A. W., & Sulloway, F. (2003b). Exceptions that prove the rule—Using a theory of motivated social cognition to account for ideological incongruities and political anomalies: Reply to Greenberg and Jonas (2003). *Psychological Bulletin, 129*, 383–393.

Jost, J. T., & Hunyady, O. (2002). The psychology of system justification and the palliative function of ideology. *European Review of Social Psychology, 13*, 111–153.

Jost, J. T., Kay, A. C., & Fitzsimons, G. (2004). Unpublished data, Stanford University.

Jost, J. T., & Kruglanski, A. W. (2002). The estrangement of social constructionism and experimental social psychology: History of the rift and prospects for reconciliation. *Personality and Social Psychology Review, 6*, 168–187.

Jost, J. T., Pelham, B. W., & Carvallo, M. (2002). Non-conscious forms of system justification: Cognitive, affective, and behavioral preferences for higher status groups. *Journal of Experimental Social Psychology, 38*, 586–602.

Jost, J. T., Pelham, B. W., Sheldon, O., & Sullivan, B. N. (2003c). Social inequality and the reduction of ideological dissonance on behalf of the system: Evidence of enhanced system justification among the disadvantaged. *European Journal of Social Psychology, 33*, 13–36.

Jost, J. T., & Thompson, E. P. (2000). Group-based dominance and opposition to equality as independent predictors of self-esteem, ethnocentrism, and social policy attitudes among African Americans and European Americans. *Journal of Experimental Social Psychology, 36*, 209–232.

Kay, A. C., & Jost, J. T. (2003). Complementary justice: Effects of "poor but happy" and "poor but honest" stereotype exemplars on system justification and implicit activation of the justice motive. *Journal of Personality and Social Psychology, 85*, 823–837.

Kay, A., Jimenez, M. C., & Jost, J. T. (2002). Sour grapes, sweet lemons, and the anticipatory rationalization of the status quo. *Personality and Social Psychology Bulletin, 28,* 1300–1312.

Kelman, H. C., & Hamilton, V. L. (1989). *Crimes of obedience: Toward a social psychology of authority and responsibility.* New Haven and London: Yale University Press.

Kemmelmeier, M. (1997). Need for closure and political orientation among German university students. *Journal of Social Psychology, 137,* 787–789.

Kerlinger, F. M. (1984). *Liberalism and conservatism: The nature and structure of social attitudes.* Hillsdale, NJ: Erlbaum.

Kluegel, J. R., & Smith, E. R. (1986). *Beliefs about inequality: Americans' view of what is and what ought to be.* Hawthorne, NJ: Aldine de Gruyter.

Kohn, P. M. (1974). Authoritarianism, rebelliousness, and their correlates among British undergraduates. *British Journal of Social and Clinical Psychology, 13,* 245–255.

Lane, R. E. (2004). The fear of equality. In J. T. Jost & J. Sidanius (Eds.), *Political psychology: Key readings.* New York: Psychology Press/Taylor & Francis. (Original work published 1959)

Lerner, M. J. (1980). *The belief in a just world: A fundamental delusion.* New York: Plenum Press.

Lerner, M. J. (1997). What does the belief in a just world protect us from: The dread of death or the fear of undeserved suffering? *Psychological Inquiry, 8,* 29–32.

Lerner, M. J., & Miller, D. T. (1978). Just world research and the attribution process: Looking back and ahead. *Psychological Bulletin, 85,* 1030–1051.

Lipset, S. (1959). The political animal: Genus Americanus. *Public Opinion Quarterly, 23,* 554–562.

Marx, K. (1999). Peuchet on suicide. In E. A. Plaut & K. Anderson (Eds.), *Marx on suicide* (pp. 43–75). Evanston, IL: Northwestern University Press. (Original work published 1846)

Marx, K., & Engels, F. (1976). *The German ideology.* Moscow: Progress Publishers. (Original work published 1845)

McClosky, H., & Chong, D. (1985). Similarities and differences between left-wing and right-wing radicals. *British Journal of Political Science, 15,* 329–363.

McGregor, H. A., Lieberman, J. D., Greenberg, J., Solomon, S., Arndt, J., Simon, L., et al. (1998). Terror management and aggression: Evidence that mortality salience motivates aggression against worldview-threatening others. *Journal of Personality and Social Psychology, 74,* 590–605.

McGregor, I., Zanna, M. P., Holmes, J. G., & Spencer, S. J. (2001). Compensatory conviction in the face of personal uncertainty: Going to extremes and being oneself. *Journal of Personality and Social Psychology, 80,* 472–488.

Montada, L., & Schneider, A. (1989). Justice and emotional reactions to the disadvantaged. *Social Justice Research, 3,* 313–344.

Muller, J. Z. (2001). Conservatism: Historical aspects. In N. J. Smelser & P. Baltes (Eds.), *International encyclopedia of the social and behavioral sciences* (pp. 2624–2628). Amsterdam: Elsevier.

Paulhus, D. L., & Trapnell, P. D. (1997). Terror management theory: Extended or overextended? *Psychological Inquiry, 8,* 40–43.

Pratto, F., Sidanius, J., Stallworth, L. M., & Malle, B. F. (1994). Social dominance orientation: A personality variable predicting social and political attitudes. *Journal of Personality and Social Psychology, 67,* 741–763.

Pyszczynski, T., Greenberg, J., & Solomon, S. (1997). Why do we need what we need? A terror management perspective on the roots of human social motivation. *Psychological Inquiry, 8,* 1–20.

Pyszczynski, T., Solomon, S., Greenberg, J., & Stewart-Fouts, M. (1995). The liberating and constraining aspects of self: Why the freed bird finds a new cage. In A. Oosterwegel & R. A. Wicklund (Eds.), *The self in European and North American culture: Development and processes.* Dordrecht, Netherlands: Kluwer.

Pyszczynski, T., Wicklund, R., Floresky, S., Gauch, G., Koch, H., Solomon, S., et al. (1996). Whistling in the dark: Exaggerated consensus estimates in response to incidental reminders of mortality. *Psychological Science, 7,* 332–336.

Quinn, D. M., & Crocker, J. (1999). When ideology hurts: Effects of belief in the Protestant Ethic and feeling overweight on the psychological well-being of women. *Journal of Personality and Social Psychology, 77,* 402–414.

Rank, O. (1976). *Will therapy and truth and reality.* New York: A. A. Knopf. (Original work published 1936)

Reich, W. (1970). *The mass psychology of fascism* (V. R. Carfagno, Trans.). New York: Farrar, Straus & Giroux. (Original work published 1946)

Rokeach, M. (1960). *The open and closed mind.* New York: Basic Books.

Rosenblatt, A., Greenberg, J., Solomon, S., Pyszczynski, T., & Lyon, D. (1989). Evidence for terror management theory: I. The effects of mortality salience on reactions to those who violate or uphold cultural values. *Journal of Personality and Social Psychology, 57,* 681–690.

Rubin, Z., & Peplau, L. A. (1973). Belief in a just world and reactions to another's lot: A study of participants in the national draft lottery. *Journal of Social Issues, 29,* 73–93.

Rummel, R. J. (2001). Freedom, democracy, peace; power, democide and war. Retrieved April 24, 2003, from *http://www.mega.nu:8080/ampp/rummel/welcome.html.*

Schimel, J., Simon, L., Greenberg, J., Pyszczynski, T., Solomon, S., Waxmonsky, J., et al. (1999). Stereotypes and terror management: Evidence that mortality salience enhances stereotypic thinking and preferences. *Journal of Personality and Social Psychology, 77,* 905–926.

Schultz, W. (1999). The riddle that doesn't exist: Wittgenstein's transmogrification of death. *Psychoanalytic Review, 86,* 281–303.

Shils, E. A. (1954). Authoritarianism: "right" and "left. " In R. Christie & M. Jahoda (Eds.), *Studies in the scope and method of "The Authoritarian Personality"* (pp. 24–49). Glencoe, IL: Free Press.

Sidanius, J. (1978). Intolerance of ambiguity and socio-politico ideology: A multidimensional analysis. *European Journal of Social Psychology, 8,* 215–235.

Sidanius, J. (1985). Cognitive functioning and sociopolitical ideology revisited. *Political Psychology, 6,* 637–661.

Sidanius, J., & Pratto, F. (1999). *Social dominance: An intergroup theory of social hierarchy and oppression.* New York: Cambridge University Press.

Smithers, A. G., & Lobley, D. M. (1978). Dogmatism, social attitudes and personality. *British Journal of Social and Clinical Psychology, 17,* 135–142.

Solomon, S., Greenberg, J., & Pyszczynski, T. (1991). Terror management theory of self-esteem. In C. R. Snyder & D. Forsyth (Eds.), *Handbook of social and clinical psychology* (pp. 21–40). Elmsford, NY: Pergamon Press.

Sorrentino, R. M., & Roney, C. J. R. (2000). *The uncertain mind: Individual differences in facing the unknown.* Philadelphia: Psychology Press/Taylor & Francis.

Stangor, C., Sechrist, G. B., & Jost, J. T. (2001). Changing racial beliefs by providing consensus information. *Personality and Social Psychology Bulletin, 27,* 486–496.

Tetlock, P. E. (1983). Cognitive style and political ideology. *Journal of Personality and Social Psychology, 45,* 118–126.

Tetlock, P. E. (1984). Cognitive style and political belief systems in the British House of Commons. *Journal of Personality and Social Psychology, 46,* 365–375.

Tetlock, P. E., Bernzweig, J., & Gallant, J. L. (1985). Supreme Court decision making: Cognitive style as a predictor of ideological consistency of voting. *Journal of Personality and Social Psychology, 48,* 1227–1239.

Tetlock, P. E., Hannum, K. A., & Micheletti, P. M. (1984). Stability and change in the complexity of senatorial debate: Testing the cognitive versus rhetorical style hypotheses. *Journal of Personality and Social Psychology, 46,* 979–990.

Tomkins, S. S. (1963). Left and right: A basic dimension of ideology and personality. In R. W. White (Ed.), *The study of lives* (pp. 388–411). Chicago: Atherton.

Van den Bos, K., & Lind, E. A. (2002). Uncertainty management by means of fairness judgments. In M. P. Zanna (Ed.), *Advances in experimental social psychology* (Vol. 34, pp. 1–60). San Diego: Academic Press.

Van den Bos, K., & Miedema, J. (2000). Toward understanding why fairness matters: The influence of mortality salience on reactions to procedural fairness. *Journal of Personality and Social Psychology, 79,* 355–366.

Wicklund, R. A. (1997). Terror management accounts of other theories: Questions for the cultural worldview concept. *Psychological Inquiry, 8,* 54–57.

Wicklund, R. A., & Brehm, J. W. (1976). *Perspectives on cognitive dissonance.* Hillsdale, NJ: Erlbaum.

Wilson, G. D. (Ed.). (1973). *The psychology of conservatism.* London: Academic Press.

Wisman, A., & Koole, S. L. (2003). Hiding in the crowd: Can mortality salience promote affiliation with others who oppose one's worldviews? *Journal of Personality and Social Psychology, 84,* 511–526.

Wittgenstein, L. (1979). *Notebooks: 1914–1916.* Chicago: University of Chicago Press. (Original work published 1916)

Wright, R. (1994). *The moral animal: Evolutionary psychology and everyday life.* New York: Pantheon Books.

Part IV

The Human Connection

Chapter 18

The Terror of Death and the Quest for Love

An Existential Perspective on Close Relationships

MARIO MIKULINCER
VICTOR FLORIAN
GILAD HIRSCHBERGER

The human awareness of personal death is one of the most basic existential concerns that demands the individual to search for means to protect himself or herself from this dreadful awareness. In the last decade, terror management theory (TMT; Greenberg, Pyszczynski, & Solomon, 1997; Pyszczynski, Greenberg, & Solomon, 1999; Solomon, Greenberg, & Pyszczynski, 1991) provides an innovative approach to the understanding of the defensive devices that people use against the awareness of their own mortality. Originally, this theory proposed two psychological mechanisms in dealing with the terror of death awareness—cultural worldview validation and self-esteem enhancement. In this chapter, we want to promote the idea of the existential function of close relationships and review empirical data showing that the quest for love and closeness acts as an additional death-anxiety buffering mechanism.

Based on a comprehensive analysis of the evolutionary, socio-cultural, and personal functions of close relationships, we conclude that one of the major motivations underlying the formation and maintenance of these relationships is the human need to deny the existential threat of one's finitude. As such, the formation and maintenance of close relationships may serve a terror management function. Specifically, we formulate four basic hypotheses. First, reminding people of their own mortality heightens their attempts to form and maintain close relationships in order to mitigate the terror of death awareness. Second, whereas the formation and maintenance of close relationships provide a symbolic shield against death awareness, potential or actual threats to the integrity of close relationships, such as separation or loss, result in an upsurge of the awareness of one's existential plight. Third, the heightening of relational strivings in response to death reminders overrides the activation of other terror management devices. Fourth, the reliance on close relationships as a terror management mechanism depends on a person's inner resources, such as self-esteem and attachment security. In this chapter, we elaborate on the rationale of these hypotheses and review empirical studies from our laboratory delineating the terror management function of close relationships.

THE TERROR MANAGEMENT FUNCTION
OF CLOSE RELATIONSHIPS

Since the late 1980s, TMT (Greenberg et al., 1997; Pyszczynski et al., 1999; Solomon et al., 1991) introduced a fresh and creative approach to social psychology. Based on the global assumption than human beings are motivated to deny the awareness of their finitude, the theory proposes that the exposure to death reminders activate two psychological mechanisms aimed at mitigating mortality concerns—cultural worldview validation and self-esteem enhancement. Cultural worldview validation can minimize the terror of death, because these worldviews imbue the world with order, meaning, and permanence and then provide the promise of protection and death transcendence. By embracing the cultural worldview, people can obtain a sense of continuity of a structure that is greater and more enduring than their own personal existence. The second defensive mechanism consists of cognitive and behavioral efforts aimed at increasing the sense of self-esteem by living up to those standards of value prescribed by the culture. Extensive empirical research has provided ample support to this line of thinking (see Greenberg et al., 1997; Pyszczynski et al., 1999, for reviews).

In spite of the impressive body of empirical evidence supporting the anxiety-buffering function of worldview validation and self-esteem, some critics have claimed that TMT has overlooked basic interpersonal processes, such as mate selection and parenting, which have evolved to promote actual survival and can shield against a wide variety of anxieties (e.g., Baron, 1997; Buss, 1997). We follow this line of thought and propose that the formation and maintenance of close relationships can serve as an additional terror management mechanism. In our view, the human needs for communion, belongingness, affiliation, attachment, togetherness, and intimacy are subordinate components of the fundamental need for self-preservation and then can serve as protective devices against the terror of death awareness. The maintenance of close relationships, which represents both a universal need for bonding to significant others and a culturally valued interpersonal behavior (Baumeister & Leary, 1995), accomplishes major survival functions (Buss & Schmitt, 1993), has basic anxiety-reducing properties (Bowlby, 1969/1982), involves the accomplishment of cultural standards and expectations (Baumeister & Leary, 1995), is a primary source for the construction of a positive sense of self-esteem (Leary & Downs, 1995), and offers the promise of symbolic immortality (Lifton, 1979). As a result, close relationships can be useful tools for mitigating death concerns and protecting the individual from death awareness.

Although TMT has not elaborated on the possible terror management function of close relationships and has not empirically examined the role these relationships play in managing mortality concerns, the idea that close relationships are an important source of protection, meaning, and value can be already found in early writings of Rank and Becker. Rank (1934, 1941), for example, claimed that love relationships provide a basic sense of security and that these relationships are an important means for obtaining a sense of death transcendence. Accordingly, Becker (1962, 1973) wrote about the adult romantic solution, in which the romantic partner is a primary source of meaning, self-worth, and death transcendence. In his view, close relationships are a source of death transcendence in Western culture during the 20th century and they replace the meanings and values that were formerly provided by religion.

In their first presentation of TMT, Greenberg, Pyszczynski, & Solomon (1986) also briefly wrote about the terror management function of close relationships. According to Greenberg et al. (1986), close relationships are a primary source of self-esteem and value and then can protect the person from the terror of death awareness. In Greenberg et al.'s (1986) own words, "in western cultures, love is often lauded as magical, transcendent, and eternal . . . thus making it a particularly suitable basis for minimizing existential terror" (p. 202). Similar statements can be found in Goldenberg, Pyszczynski, Greenberg, and Solomon's (2000) analysis of the problem of human corporeality. In their view, love relationships help people to deny their own creatureliness and elevate them beyond their animal nature to a unique spiritual plane that offers the promise of death transcendence. In love relationships, we "become soul mates with our beloved." (Goldenberg et al., 2000, p. 207).

In our view, six basic properties of close relationships make them an appropriate anxiety-buffering means that can protect the individual from the terror of death. First, close relationships have an evolutionary significance—they are a product of natural and sexual selection processes that have important survival and reproductive benefits (Buss & Schmitt, 1993). Close relationships provide the framework for sexual acts and then increase the chances of reproduction. Close relationships also increase the likelihood of mating, improve the efficiency of resource acquisition (e.g., food), facilitate the exploration of the environment, and increase the chances of bearing offspring that will reach maturity and survive. As a result, we are driven to maintain close relationships because human ancestors who were successful in forming close bonds to others were more likely to survive and reproduce (Buss & Schmitt, 1993). These survival and reproductive benefits of close relationships sustain and enhance life and then can symbolically mitigate death concerns.

Second, close relationships are a source of protection and security during threatening and dangerous circumstances (Bowlby, 1969/1982; Schachter, 1959). According to Bowlby's theory, (1969/1982, 1973, 1980), the formation of close interpersonal bonds accomplishes basic anxiety-reducing functions. Because human infants are born with immature capacities for locomotion, feeding, and defense, they need the care and protection from a relationship partner to survive. As a result, infants are born with an attachment behavioral system that automatically drives them to maintain/restore proximity to protective caregivers in times of stress. In optimal conditions, relationship partners become a *safe haven*, facilitating threat removal and distress alleviation, and a *secure base*, from which the infant can confidently engage in other activities (Bowlby, 1969/1982). Furthermore, proximity maintenance to these supportive others provides comfort and relief, infuses a sense of basic trust and security, and reinforces the individual's confidence in the anxiety-reducing efficiency of close bonds. Mikulincer and Shaver (2003) have shown that the attachment system is active over the entire lifespan and is manifested in thoughts and behaviors related to the formation and maintenance of close relationships. In our view, these anxiety-reducing properties of close relationships also offer protection from the terror of death awareness.

Third, the formation and maintenance of close relationships are culturally valued behaviors. Many social institutions and rituals have been developed to promote and protect one's close relationships with others (Baumeister & Leary, 1995; Goffman, 1972). Moreover, people who fail to form or maintain close relationships are stereotyped as unhappy, problematic, and dysfunctional (e.g., Peplau & Perlman, 1982), and aloneness is viewed as a personal deficiency and a deviant social state (e.g., Horney, 1943; Sullivan, 1953). In most cultures, the formation and maintenance of close relationships seem to be important components of the cultural worldview and basic values that enhance the likelihood and stability of these relationships are transmitted from generation to generation through the process of socialization. Therefore, like other cherished cultural worldviews, the formation and maintenance of close bonds can be a source of meaning, order, and value. Accordingly, hey can be a pathway toward cultural worldview validation and denial of death awareness.

Fourth, close relationships are an important source of self-esteem (e.g., Leary, 1999; Leary & Downs, 1995). According to Leary and his colleagues, self-esteem is strongly affected by information conveying the degree to which one is accepted and valued by other people. That is, self-esteem reflects the extent to which one succeeds or fails to form and maintain satisfactory close relationships. Specifically, high self-esteem connotes a feeling of being accepted and valued by others, whereas low self-esteem is derived from social rejection and the failure to maintain close bonds (e.g., Leary, Tambor, Terdal, & Downs, 1995). Goldenberg et al. (2000) also elaborated on the self-worth significance of close relationships. In their view, being loved provides consensual validation for the view of oneself as valuable (Bowlby, 1973; Walster, 1965). Furthermore, the maintenance of stable, long-term relationships implies that one has so highly valued traits and resources that the partner is willing to forsake other alternatives and commit him- or herself to the relationship (Goldenberg et al., 2000). In our view, the positive impact that the formation and maintenance of close relationships have on the sense of self-esteem represents an additional source of death transcendence that sustains the terror management function of these relationships.

Fifth, close relationships offer a symbolic promise of continuity and lastingness and increase a person's sense of symbolic immortality (Lifton, 1979). Close relationships offer the framework for biological procreation, which allows people to transcend their biological existence and to believe that they will continue to live through their progeny. Such relationships also offer people the opportunity to feel part of a larger symbolic entity (e.g., couple or group) that transcends their biological limitations and expands the boundaries and capacities of their own self (Aron, Aron, & Norman, 2001). Accordingly, close relationships offer people the opportunity to experience passionate love, which can take the form of an intense ecstatic peak experience or a more common feeling of being fully alive. Lifton and Olson (1974) also elaborated on the idea that close relationships are a source of symbolic immortality and emphasized the psychological equation between aloneness and death. In their own words, "We can say that life for the baby means being connected to the source of care and support. Powerful fears and anxiety appear when the child is left alone, separated from the source of nurture. This image of separation is related to an image of death" (p. 46). All these symbolic meaning structures that are derived from close relationships allow people to transcend the self, create a sense of connectedness with the world, and then can assist in denying death awareness.

Sixth, close relationships can directly mitigate basic interpersonal death-related concerns. According to Florian and Kravetz (1983), different people may fear death for different reasons, including intrapersonal worries (e.g., loss of self-fulfillment) and interpersonal concerns (e.g., fear of being forgotten). One of the basic interpersonal death-related concerns is the fear that no one will remember us after death and that we will not leave any impression on the world (Florian and Kravetz's *loss of social identity* factor). In our view, the formation and maintenance of close relationships can mitigate this interpersonal fear. Being engaged in stable and satisfactory close relationships, people can feel confident that their identity will not be lost and that their friends, spouse, and children will remember them after death.

Following this analysis, we can delineate the underlying protective roles of close relationships that can act as a symbolic shield against the terror of death awareness. The formation and maintenance of close relationships offer a sense of security and protection against threatening and dangerous circumstances, including the threat of one's own mortality. This protective role of close relationships is not specific to the terror of death and can be activated by other internal or external sources of threats. However, close relationships also offer the promise of meaning, value, death transcendence, and social identity maintenance after death. All these symbolic promises are specific to death concerns and become highly relevant in a person's attempt to deny death awareness. In this manner, when faced with the awareness of death, people may be motivated to form and maintain close relationships in order to mitigate the terror of death awareness.

In the following sections, we review a series of recent studies conducted in our laboratory that have focused on the terror management function of close relationships. These studies have attempted to implement the basic TMT hypotheses—mortality salience and anxiety-buffering hypotheses—to the study of the existential function of close relationships, and to deal with specific questions that follow the addition of a new terror management mechanism. Specifically, we review studies that examined (1) the effects of reminding people of their own mortality (mortality salience induction) on interpersonal strivings and beliefs as well as on their willingness to form and maintain close relationships, (2) the death-anxiety buffering effects of the maintenance of close relationships and the death-anxiety-arousing effects of the breaking of these relationships, (3) the dynamic interplay between the formation and maintenance of close relationships and the activation of worldview and self-esteem defenses, and (4) the contribution of personal factors (self-esteem, attachment style) to individual variations in the use of close relationships as a terror management device.

THE RELATIONAL EFFECTS OF MORTALITY SALIENCE

One of the basic hypotheses of TMT is the *mortality salience hypothesis*. According to this hypothesis, if a psychological mechanism buffers against thoughts of death, death reminders should increase the activation of that mechanism. Therefore, if the formation and maintenance of close relationships act as a death anxiety buffer, one should expect that making mortality salient increases relational strivings and a person's willingness to form and maintain close relationships. A series of recent studies have followed this reasoning and have examined the effects of typical mortality salience inductions on a wide variety of interpersonal and relational attitudes and behaviors.

In a series of three experimental studies, Taubman - Ben-Ari, Findler, and Mikulincer (2002) examined the impact of death reminders on a person's relational strivings and beliefs. In the first study, Taubman - Ben-Ari et al. (2002) assigned participants to mortality salience or neutral conditions according to Rosenblatt, Greenberg, Solomon, Pyszczynski, and Lyon's (1989) procedure and, after a delay task, asked them to rate their willingness to initiate a variety of social interactions with a hypothetical same-sex target (e.g., asking him or her to study together for an exam). In line with the mortality salience hypothesis, results indicated that a mortality salience induction led participants to report higher willingness to initiate social interactions than a neutral condition.

In the second study, Taubman - Ben-Ari et al. (2002) focused on a cognitive factor that has been found to facilitate the formation of close relationships—the appraisal of one's interpersonal skills and competences (e.g., Buhrmester, 1990; Buhrmester, Furman, Wittenberg, & Reis, 1988). They reasoned that if death reminders increase relational strivings, these reminders would have a positive impact on cognitive factors that facilitate these strivings and then make people more confident on their interpersonal skills and competences. In examining this hypothesis, participants were randomly divided into mortality salience and neutral conditions according to Rosenblatt's et al.'s (1989) procedure, and, then, after a distraction/delay task, they filled out the Interpersonal Competence Questionnaire (Buhrmester et al., 1988). The findings were in line with the predictions: As compared to the neutral condition, making mortality salient led to higher appraisals of interpersonal competences for initiating relationships, disclosing personal information, and making assertive statements to a relationship partner.

In their third study, Taubman - Ben-Ari et al. (2002) examined the effects of death reminder on a cognitive factor that has been found to inhibit the formation of close relationships—rejection sensitivity (e.g., Downey & Feldman, 1996; Downey, Lebolt, Rincon, & Freitas, 1998). They reasoned that if death reminders increase relational strivings, these reminders would have a buffering impact on cognitive factors that inhibit these strivings and then make people less worried of rejection. In examining this hypothesis, participants were randomly divided into mortality salience and neutral conditions according to Rosenblatt's et al.'s (1989) procedure, and, then, after a distraction/delay task, filled out the Rejection Sensitivity Questionnaire (Downey & Feldman, 1996). Findings supported the hypothesis that death reminders weaken cognitive barriers to the formation of close relationships: As compared to the neutral condition, the mortality salience induction led to lower reports of rejection sensitivity. Taken as a whole, Taubman - Ben-Ari et al.'s (2002) findings indicate that the heightening of death awareness promotes a positive motivational and cognitive orientation toward social interactions and interpersonal relationships.

In two recent studies, we examined the effects of mortality salience on a person's attitudes and preferences in romantic love relationships. In the first study, we focused on Lee's (1977) styles of romantic love and examined the impact of mortality salience on a person's preference towards different love styles. Lee (1977) identified three primary love styles—eros (romantic, passionate love), ludus (game-playing, noncommitted love), and storage (friendship, companionate love)—and three secondary styles—mania (possessive, dependent, anxious love), pragma (logical, "shopping-list," social convenient love), and agape (selfless, altruistic, all-giving love). Whereas the adoption of eros and agape styles have been found to positively contribute to the formation and maintenance of romantic relationships, ludus and mania styles have been found to have a negative impact on relationship quality (e.g., Hendrick & Hendrick, 1989; Levy & Davis, 1988). On this basis, we reasoned that if death reminders increase a person's willingness to form stable and satisfactory romantic relationships, these reminders would lead to more positive-approach attitudes toward eros and agape styles and more negative-avoidance attitudes toward ludus and mania styles.

To examine this hypothesis, 33 Israeli undergraduates were randomly assigned to conditions that increased the salience of either mortality or physical pain (according to Rosenblatt et al.'s procedure), and then, following a brief distracting task, they completed Hendrick and Hendrick's (1986) love-style scale. As compared to the physical pain condition, the mortality salience induction (1) led to more positive attitudes toward the eros style, $M = 4.01$ vs. $M = 3.47$, $F(1, 31) = 7.55$, $p < .01$, and the agape style, $M = 4.14$ vs. $M = 3.39$,

$F(1, 31) = 10.08$, $p < .01$, and (2) less positive attitudes toward the ludus style, $M = 2.48$ vs. $M = 2.91$, $F(1, 31) = 3.85$, $p < .05$, and the mania style, $M = 2.68$ vs. $M = 3.15$, $F(1, 31) = 5.96$, $p < .05$. These findings imply that death reminders heighten a positive-approach attitude to love styles that can maintain and enhance the quality and stability of romantic relationships (eros and agape styles).

In the second study, we examined whether the exposure to death reminders affects a person's preferences for romantic partners. Specifically, we asked whether mortality salience would lead people to prefer romantic partners whose love styles facilitate the formation and maintenance of a relationship (eros and agape styles) and to reject partners whose love styles have negative consequences to relationship quality (mania and ludus styles). For this purpose, 67 Israeli undergraduates were exposed to either a mortality salience or a physical pain salience induction according to Rosenblatt et al.'s (1989) procedure, and, then, after a brief distracting task, were presented with six vignettes describing potential romantic partners, each one representing one of the six Lee's love styles. Participants rated the extent to which the described person fitted their expectations for a romantic partner. Findings were consistent with the prediction: As compared to the physical pain salience condition, a mortality salience induction (1) heightened the preference for partners who represented the eros style, $M = 5.76$ vs. $M = 4.59$, $F(1, 65) = 11.31$, $p < .01$, or the agape style, $M = 4.56$ vs. $M = 3.37$, $F(1, 65) = 5.88$, $p < .05$, and (2) lowered the preference for partners who represented the ludus style, $M = 1.19$ vs. $M = 1.66$, $F(1, 65) = 7.07$, $p < .01$.

Taken together, the results of these two studies indicate that mortality salience contributes to the adoption of love styles that foster intimate, committed, and satisfactory romantic relationships. Alternatively, the findings can also imply that mortality salience leads people to a greater desire for forms of love that more closely approximate the romantic ideal—which eros and agape seem to do. In fact, one cannot be sure whether participants' self-reports in the love-style scales reflect what they value in a romantic relationship or what they actually do in such a relationship. Further research should attempt to assess the behavioral manifestations of the various love styles.

Two additional studies have provided further support to the conclusion that death reminders increase a person's strivings for intimate and committed romantic relationships. In one study (Mikulincer & Florian, 2000, Study 5), we examined the effects of mortality salience on a person's desire for romantic intimacy. Specifically, participants were assigned to a mortality salience or neutral condition according to Rosenblatt et al.'s (1989) procedure, and after a distracting task, they completed Sharabany's (1994) intimacy scale tapping the level of intimacy they ideally wanted to have with a romantic partner. Findings clearly showed that the mortality salience induction led to higher reports of desire for romantic intimacy than did the control condition.

In another study (Florian, Mikulincer, & Hirschberger, 2002, Study 1), we examined the effects of mortality salience on the sense of commitment in romantic relationships. Specifically, participants were randomly divided into three conditions according to the type of thoughts that were made salient (mortality, physical pain, neutral). After a distracting task, all the participants completed a shortened version of the Dimensions of Commitment Inventory (Adams & Jones, 1997), which tapped a person's commitment to a romantic partner and moral commitment to the romantic relationship. Overall, the findings indicated that participants in the mortality salience condition reported higher commitment to their romantic partner than did participants in the neutral and physical pain conditions. However, no significant effect of mortality salience was found on moral commitment to the romantic relationship. This finding suggests that mortality reminders increase a sense of love and closeness to a romantic partner but do not affect one's sense of obligation or duty to romantic relationships. Importantly, this effect was not significantly moderated by individual variations in gender and neuroticism and was not significantly mediated by global, death-unrelated aversive feelings.

Beyond the effects of mortality salience on a person's strivings in romantic relationships, a recent study conducted by Yaacovi (2003) revealed theoretically coherent effects of mortality salience on parenting-related strivings and beliefs. In this study, Israeli young adults (married without children) were randomly divided into three conditions according to the type of thoughts that were made salient (mortality, physical pain, neutral). After a distracting task, all the participants completed a 20-item scale assessing their desire to become a parent and the obstacles they perceived in realizing this desire. Findings clearly indicated that participants in the mortality salience condition reported a stronger desire to become a parent and were less likely to perceive parenting-related obstacles than were participants in the physical pain and neutral conditions. That is, heightening death awareness led to a more positive motivational-cognitive orientation toward becoming a parent. It is important to note that these effects of mortality salience were found in both men and women and did not depend on gender differences in parenting-related representations.

Overall, the findings of the reviewed studies provide extensive support for the mortality salience hypothesis and extend this hypothesis to the account of variations in relational strivings following the exposure to death reminders. In other words, these findings are in line with the terror management function of close relationships and suggest that one source of relational strivings in adulthood is derived from the existential encounter with one's vulnerability and finitude.

THE ANXIETY-BUFFERING EFFECTS OF CLOSE RELATIONSHIPS

Another basic hypothesis of TMT is the *anxiety-buffer hypothesis*. According to this hypothesis, if a psychological mechanism buffers death anxiety, then the successful activation of this mechanism following mortality salience should satisfy terror management needs and reduce the need to activate other defensive mechanisms (Greenberg et al., 1997). Another derivate of this hypothesis concerns the arousal of death concerns following the disruption of a terror management mechanism (Greenberg et al., 1997). If a psychological mechanism shields individuals from the awareness of their death, threatening the integrity or functioning of this mechanism should raise the cognitive accessibility of death concerns and then make necessary the activation of other terror management mechanisms in order to mitigate these concerns. Therefore, if the formation and maintenance of close relationships act as death anxiety buffers, success or failure in the accomplishment of these relational tasks should have a strong impact on the accessibility of death-related concerns and the activation of other terror management mechanisms. First, actual or symbolic success in forming and maintaining stable and satisfactory close relationships would assist people in denying death awareness and then reduce the need to activate other terror management devices following the encounter with death reminders. Second, actual or symbolic failure in forming or maintaining close relationships can by itself elicit death concerns, thereby making necessary the activation of alternative terror management mechanisms.

In two independent studies, Florian et al. (2002) tested the anxiety-buffering hypothesis in regard to the possible death-related effects of romantic commitment. In one study (Florian et al., 2002, Study 2), participants, who were randomly assigned to a mortality salience or neutral condition, were randomly divided into two subgroups according to the manipulation of the salience of romantic commitment. Participants in the *romantic-commitment-salience* condition were asked to describe the emotions that commitment to a romantic partner arouses in them and to write about how this commitment is manifested in their romantic relationship. Participants in the *no-commitment-salience* condition were asked similar questions about the neutral topic of hearing radio. Then, all the participants rated the severity of social transgressions in order to examine the activation of a typical worldview validation defense—negative responses against persons who transgress socially accepted norms (Florian & Mikulincer, 1997; Rosenblatt et al., 1989). The finding revealed the anxiety-buffering effects of romantic commitment. Whereas the mortality salience induction led to more severe ratings of social transgressions than did the neutral condition in the no-commitment-salience condition, it had no significant effect on severity ratings when romantic commitment was made salient. That is, asking people to think about their romantic commitment reduced the need to activate another worldview defense following a mortality salience induction.

In the second study (Florian et al., 2002, Study 3), participants were randomly divided into three conditions according to the type of thoughts that were made salient (problems in romantic relationship, academic problems, neutral). Then, all the participants completed a Hebrew version of Greenberg et al's (1994) word completion task, which tapped the accessibility of death-related thoughts. Findings indicated that participants in the "problems in romantic relationship" condition completed more death-related words than did participants in the "academic problems" and neutral conditions. This finding provides strong support for the anxiety-buffering function of close relationships. In fact, thinking about problems in close relationships implies a potential threat to the integrity of this relational defense, which seems to heighten death-thought accessibility.

Following these findings, Mikulincer, Florian, Birnbaum, and Mashlikovitz (2002) reasoned that if close relationships act as a terror management mechanism aimed at mitigating death concerns and denying death awareness, separation from a relationship partner may threaten the integrity of this terror management mechanism and then increase death awareness. That is, separation episodes make us aware of our existential condition as a vulnerable and finite organism.

In examining this line of reasoning, Mikulincer et al. (2002) conducted three independent experiments in which participants were randomly assigned to diverse conditions according to the topics on which they were asked to imagine (a separation from a close relationship partner, neutral topics). Following this procedure, death-thought accessibility was assessed in a Hebrew version of Greenberg, Pyszczynski, Solomon, Simon, and Breus's (1994) word completion task. Findings revealed that asking participants to imagine a separation from a close relationship partner led to higher accessibility of death-related thoughts than did a control condition. However, this effect was moderated by the identity of the partner and the length of the separation. Heightened accessibility of death-related thoughts was found only when the imagined separation was from a close relationship partner but not when the partner was a mere acquaintance. Accordingly, heightened accessibility of death-related thoughts was found when participants were requested to imagine a long-term separation but not when they were asked to imagine a brief separation from their close relationship partner. Overall, these findings imply that the experience of separation per se does not necessarily lead to death awareness. Only when this separation implies a sustained disruption of a meaningful close relationship, the individual feels defenseless to deny the terror of death and then mortality concerns become more accessible.

The blocking of parenting strivings seems to be an additional source of death concerns. In a recent study, Yaacovi (2003) asked Israeli young adults to imagine that they are not able to become a parent or to imagine that they fail important exam. Then, all the participants completed a Hebrew version of Greenberg et al.'s (1994) word completion task in order to assess the accessibility of death-related thought accessibility. Findings revealed that asking participants to think about a possible blocking of their parenting strivings led to higher accessibility of death-related thoughts than did a control condition. Again, the disruption of a relational striving—becoming a parent—seems to leave the person more defenseless against the cognitive activation of death concerns.

Overall, the findings of the reviewed studies provide initial support for the anxiety-buffering hypothesis and extend this hypothesis to the account of the death concerns and terror management processes that follow the successful accomplishment or frustration of a person's relational strivings. These findings suggest that one source of death concerns is derived from the frustration of relational strivings and the breaking of a person's meaningful close relationships.

THE INTERFACE BETWEEN CLOSE RELATIONSHIPS AND OTHER TERROR MANAGEMENT MECHANISMS

Having delineated the terror management function of relational strivings, it is important to elaborate and examine the possible associations between this defense and previously examined terror management mechanisms, such as worldview validation and self-esteem maintenance. One alternative is that close relationships are merely a subcomponent of the cultural worldview and therefore do not constitute a distinct defense from the well-validated defenses of worldview validation and self-esteem maintenance. We agree that relational strivings are influenced to some extent by cultural norms, that close relationships are a source of self-esteem, and then that the defensive properties of these relationships somewhat overlap with other terror management mechanisms. However, like other personality theories (e.g., Bowlby, 1969/1982; Fromm, 1956; Sullivan, 1953), we believe that a person's relational strivings are not merely a derivate of cultural norms and values but are inborn motivational tendencies that appear in the early stages of development before the internalization of cultural worldviews.

We believe that close relationships are a biologically based, evolutionary evolved mechanism that constitutes the most basic form of protection and meaning for a human infant and may precede the symbolic needs of worldview validation and self-esteem maintenance. As a result, the formation and maintenance of meaningful close relationships can be viewed as the default defense against death awareness and can sometimes override the need to engage in worldview validation or self-esteem maintenance. In our terms, the reliance on these culturally derived defenses can result from the failure of close relationships to accomplish their anxiety-buffering goal.

We follow this reasoning in two studies that have examined the activation of relational defenses in conditions than endanger self-esteem maintenance. In one study, Hirschberger, Florian, and Mikulincer (2003) examined participants' need for emotional intimacy and closeness in response to specific relationship contexts that can impair self-esteem—the receipt of manifest expression of complaint or criticism from a partner. If relational defenses override self-esteem maintenance, participants were expected to react to death reminders by searching for emotional intimacy even with complaining, rejecting partners who represent a real threat to their sense of self-worth.

Participants were assigned to a mortality salience or control condition and were asked to imagine having dinner at their partner's parents' home and receiving manifest expressions of either admiration, complaint, or criticism from their partner. Then, after a distracting task, they were asked to rate their willingness to engage in emotionally intimate interactions with the partner in the imagined situation (as assessed by Sharabany's Intimacy scale). Findings revealed that participants exposed to a mortality salience induction reporting more desire for emotional intimacy after the hypothetical situation than did participants in the neutral condition. More important, whereas in the neutral condition, partner's expressions of admiration led to higher desire for intimacy than did partner's expressions of complaint or criticism, this effect was not significant in the mortality salience condition. That is, death reminders heightened desire for emotional intimacy even following partner's expressions of complaint or criticism. This finding implies that the heightening of death awareness makes participants ready to pay the price of losing self-esteem in order to maintain emotional closeness with a romantic partner.

Although Hirschberger et al.'s (2003) findings seem to support the overriding activation of relational defenses, they can still be interpreted as related to self-esteem mechanisms. In fact, the heightened seeking for emotional closeness following mortality salience may reflect a self-esteem striving if one views the self-esteem that one gets from the maintenance of a stable, long-term romantic relationship as especially valuable. Certainly there are many domains in which our attempts to obtain a stable sense of self-esteem expose us to other types of threats to self-esteem. For example, a scientist may promote an idea that he believes will provide much self-esteem even though he expects that doing so will lead to a lot of criticism in the short term. Perhaps romantic partners put up with the threats to their self-esteem that come from daily relational hassles (complaints, criticisms) because of the much stronger boost to self-esteem that comes from the maintenance of a long-term loving relationship. Putting up with criticism and complaining may also be viewed as enduring a threat to relatedness. In this case, mortality salience could lead people to endure threats to relatedness in order to maintain the anxiety-buffering rewards that relatedness can provide.

In another independent study, Hirschberger, Florian, and Mikulincer (2002) focused on the readiness to compromise ideal mate standards following a mortality salience induction. This readiness to compromise has both psychological benefits and costs. On the one hand, it facilitates the formation of romantic relationships and then can serve as a relational defense following mortality salience. On the other hand, it may be particularly aversive due to the negative implications it has on one's self-esteem and on the cultural worldview of ideal mate characteristics. On this basis, heightened readiness to compromise ideal mate standards in response to a mortality salience induction would attest that the need to form close relationships outweighs the significance of self-esteem maintenance or otherwise important cultural values.

Following this reasoning, Hirschberger et al. (2002) instructed participants to complete a scale tapping ideal mate characteristics and assigned them to a mortality salience, physical pain salience, or neutral condition. Then, after a distracting task, all the participants were asked to rate the extent to which they were ready to compromise and deviate from their ideal mate selection standard when considering a potential romantic partner for marriage. As compared to the control and physical pain salience condition, mortality salience led participants to report higher readiness to deviate from their ideal mate selection standards in order to form a long-term relationship. That is, when exposed to death reminders, our participants were prone to form close relationships even at the cost of finding a less than ideal partner.

Again, although these findings support the powerful impact of mortality salience on relational defenses, one should take into account the possible action of other cultural defenses. In fact, one can argue that cultural standards put a high value on having a mate and that mortality salience makes participants more willing to go for a less appealing mate and forego the greater self-esteem that the "perfect mate" would provide in order to get a more obtainable but less desirable mate. That is, being mateless may be so damaging to self-esteem that people are willing to accept less than perfect others for relationships. Alternatively, it may be that there are negative implications for self-esteem of being "too picky" when it comes to choosing a mate, at least in the context of self-reports in psychology studies.

However, Hirschberger et al. (2002) findings on the emotional consequences of compromising in mate selection seem to argue against the foregoing possibility. Hirschberger et al. (2002) assigned another independent sample to either the mortality salience, physical pain salience, or neutral conditions but asked participants to complete a neutral questionnaire instead of the scale assessing their readiness to compromise ideal mate selection standards. These participants were compared with those who completed the readiness-to-compromise scale on the extent to which they felt pride, shame, and guilt during the experimental situation. Findings indicated that mortality salience led participants who completed the readiness-to-compromise scale to report lower levels of pride and higher levels of shame and guilt than the neutral and physical pain conditions. However, these emotional effects of mortality salience were not significant among participants who did not complete the readiness-to-compromise scale. It seems that our participants paid a double price while securing a close relationship following death reminders: Their threshold for mate selection was lowered and they suffered from the arousal of negative emotions.

Interestingly, Wisman and Koole (2003) also reported initial evidence on the interplay between relational defenses and worldview validation. Participants were exposed to either a mortality salience or a neutral condition and then were asked to participate in a group discussion and to choose where to seat in a prearranged room. In this room, participants were asked to choose between sitting alone and defending their worldviews during the discussion or sitting close to other participants and having their worldviews attacked. Findings indicated that a mortality salience induction, as compared to the neutral condition, heightened the preference for sitting close to other participants, even if this seating preference implied exposing their worldviews to potential attack. That is, it seems that heightening death awareness motivates people to affiliate with others to the extent that they are ready to endanger the validity of their cultural worldviews.

Overall, the reviewed findings indicate that reminders of death motivate people to form and secure a close relationship to the extent that they seem to be willing to overlook threats to their worldviews and self-esteem. However, the current findings do not imply that self-esteem can be only achieved in close relationships or that it functions only as an indicator of one's eligibility for social inclusion (as implied in Baumeister & Leary's, 1995, writings). In our view, self-esteem has psychological importance in and of itself and can be maintained or enhanced in nonrelational settings. Moreover, the current findings cannot rule the possibility that self-esteem and cultural worldview are still operating following mortality salience. In fact, as discussed earlier, self-esteem and worldview maintenance are one of the reasons that close relationships serve a terror management functioning, and then they may be involved in the activation of relational defenses. More research should be conducted to delineate the complex interplay between the various terror management mechanisms.

In addition, one should take into account that other studies have shown that self-esteem and worldview validation sometimes override the desire to relate or affiliate. For example, Dechesne, Greenberg, Arndt, and Schimel (2000) showed that mortality salience led to distancing from one's university sports team after it failed, and Arndt, Greenberg, Schimel, Pyszczynski, and Solomon (2002) showed that mortality salience led Hispanics and women to disidentify with their ethnic and gender groups when such identification would be damaging to self-esteem. These findings may suggest some "interchangeability" of the various terror management mechanisms, with some contextual and personality factors making one mechanism preferred over others. It also may be that once a person has defended in one way, the threat is resolved, death access has been reduced, and there is therefore no need to defend in other ways (see findings reported by McGregor et al., 1998, and by Dechesne et al., 2003, that seem to support this view). Further research should attempt to delineate the contextual and personality factors that determine what kind of terror management defense is activated following death reminders.

INDIVIDUAL DIFFERENCES IN THE ACTIVATION OF RELATIONAL DEFENSES

Beyond examining the impact of mortality salience on relational strivings and cognitions, we also delineate the basic individual differences factors that may moderate the use of close relationships as a terror management mechanism. Among these factors, TMT assumes that self-esteem is one of the most basic moderators of mortality salience effects (Greenberg et al., 1997). On this basis, Hirschberger et al. (2002) examined the effects of individual variations in global self-esteem on the willingness to compromise ideal mate standards under a mortality salience condition. The findings of this analysis were at odds with the hypothesized anxiety-buffering function of self-esteem as originally conceptualized by TMT (e.g., Greenberg et al., 1997). Specifically, the effects of mortality salience on compromise in mate selection seemed to be more pronounced among high self-esteem persons. These persons, who exhibited higher mate selection standards than did low self-esteem persons and were less willing to compromise these standards in a neutral condition, dramatically increased their inclination to compromise when exposed to death reminders.

This pattern of finding can be integrated with previous TMT studies. On the one hand, previous studies have shown that high self-esteem persons are less likely to activate worldview validations defenses following death reminders than are low self-esteem persons (e.g., Harmon-Jones et al., 1997). On the other hand, Hirschberger et al. (2002) revealed that high self-esteem persons are more likely to activate relational defenses following a mortality salience induction than are low self-esteem persons. It is possible that persons differing in their global self-esteem rely on different terror management mechanisms. Whereas persons with relatively lower levels of internal resources (i.e., low self-esteem) defend against the terror of death by attempting to validate their cultural worldviews, persons with relatively high levels of internal resources (i.e., high self-esteem) may defend against the terror of death by relying on relational defenses.

Another basic psychological factor that seems to be relevant for explaining individual differences in the reliance on relational defenses is a person's sense of attachment security—the extent to which the person feels comfortable with intimate, close relationships and confident on the partner's availability and responsiveness in times of need (Hazan & Shaver, 1987; Fraley & Shaver, 2000; Mikulincer & Shaver, 2003). Research has shown that the sense of attachment security underlies basic individual differences in the process of coping with internal and external sources of threats (see Mikulincer & Florian, 1998, 2000, for reviews). Specifically, this sense is associated with the appraisal of stressful events in benign terms, positive expectancies of self-efficacy in dealing with these events, the reliance on proximity and support seeking as well as other constructive strategies for coping with threats, and the maintenance of emotional equanimity in times of stress. Attachment-related differences in the process of affect regulation have also been manifested in a person's attitudes toward death. Mikulincer, Florian, and Tolmacz (1990) found that securely attached persons reported less fear of death than more insecure persons, and Florian and Mikulincer (1998) found that the sense of attachment security was associated with a higher sense of continuity and lastingness, as assessed through Lifton's (1973) concept of symbolic immortality.

Following this line of research, Mikulincer and Florian (2000) suggested that attachment-related differences are also manifested in the way people react to the terror of death awareness. Whereas insecurely attached persons may react to mortality salience with defensive attempts to validate their cultural worldview, more securely attached persons would not necessarily activate worldview defenses. Secure persons' adequate coping skills, which allow them to manage distress without defensively distorting their cognitions, can act as a cognitive shield against the terror of death and abolish the need to validate cultural worldviews and derogate persons and opinions that threaten these worldviews. This response resembles the way high-self-esteem persons have been found to react to death reminders. In both cases, having a positive sense of value, people do not need to react to death reminders with increased worldview defense. Indeed, Mikulincer and Florian (2000, Study 1) found that mortality salience activated worldview defenses mainly among insecurely attached persons but not among secure persons.

This finding raised a basic question about the alternative ways securely attached persons defend themselves against the terror of death. Mikulincer and Florian (2000) proposed that these persons rely on close relationships and the search for closeness and intimacy as anxiety-buffering devices. This hypothesis was based on findings that secure persons tend to seek for others' proximity and support in times of need and that this response is a basic affect regulation device that help people in alleviating distress and managing their existential fears (see Mikulincer & Shaver, 2003, for a review). In support of this view, Mikulincer and Florian (2000, Study 5) found that mortality salience led to heightened desire for intimacy in romantic relationships mainly among securely attached persons. That is, secure persons tend to search for intimacy as a defensive means against the awareness of death.

Taubman - Ben-Ari et al. (2002) provided further support for secure persons' reliance on relational defenses. Their findings indicated that heightened willingness to initiate social interactions, lower levels of rejection sensitivity, and more positive appraisals of interpersonal competence following a mortality salience induction were mainly found among persons who hold a relatively high sense of attachment security. Accordingly, Yaacovi (2003) found that heightened positive representations of parenting following a mortality salience induction were mainly found among securely attached persons. Importantly, other personal characteristics, such as social desirability and self-esteem, could not explain the observed attachment-style differences.

These findings imply that variations in the history of interactions with close relationship partners and the resulting sense of attachment security are directly manifested in the way people manage the terror of death awareness. On the one hand, people who hold a sense of attachment security have a history of satisfactory close relationships and hold positive beliefs about the supportiveness and protective function of relationship partners (e.g.,

Collins & Read, 1990; Feeney & Noller, 1990; Hazan & Shaver, 1987). During positive interactions with relationship partners, people learn that they can rely on close relationships as an anxiety-reduction device, and they develop a sense of self-worth and confidence on other's love. In Lifton's (1973) terms, these persons also develop a sense of continuity and connectedness with the world, which are the core components of the sense of symbolic immortality. As a result, securely attached persons can confidently rely on close relationships while coping with death awareness.

On the other hand, people who hold more insecure styles of attachment have a history of frustrating and painful close relationships and hold negative beliefs about relationship partners (e.g., Collins & Read, 1990; Feeney & Noller, 1990; Hazan & Shaver, 1987). When close relationships fail to accomplish their regulatory goal, people develop serious doubts about others' goodwill and their own worth (Bowlby, 1988). These negative interactions also thwart a person's sense of security, continuity, and connectedness to the world and foster the development of alternative regulatory strategies that replace the primary strategy of proximity seeking (Bowlby, 1988; Lifton, 1973). Therefore, following the heightening of death awareness, these persons are not able or willing to rely on close relationships in order to mitigate mortality concerns. These relationships have failed to provide a sense of continuity and connectedness—the core components of the sense of death transcendence—and they cannot be used as a reliable death-anxiety buffer. As a result, these persons attempt to adhere to cultural worldviews as a means to enhance their impoverished self-esteem and to achieve some value and meaning that can distally protect them from death awareness.

CONCLUSIONS

In this chapter, we review recent evidence on the terror management function of close relationships. The findings clearly indicate that close relationships serve as a fundamental buffer of existential anxieties. First, death reminders have been found to heighten the motivation to form and maintain close relationships. Second, whereas the successful accomplishment of relational tasks tend to buffer death concerns and make the activation of other defenses less necessary, the potential disruption of close relationships lead to an upsurge of death awareness. Third, the activation of relational defenses in response to death reminders tends to override other culturally derived defenses and people seem to be ready to pay the psychological price of securing close relationships. Fourth, theoretically coherent individual differences have been found in the reliance on relational defenses. Overall, these variations imply that the use of close relationships as a terror management mechanism is characteristic of persons who have developed a strong sense of self-worth and connectedness to the world. We believe that these findings can open new avenues of research on the existential functions of close relationships and deepen our understanding of basic existential concerns about love and death.

ACKNOWLEDGMENT

This chapter was completed near the time of Victor Florian's death. He contributed a great deal to the ideas and research summarized herein.

REFERENCES

Adams, J. M., & Jones, W. H. (1997). The conceptualization of marital commitment: An integrative analysis. *Journal of Personality and Social Psychology, 72,* 1177–1196.

Arndt, J., Greenberg, J., Schimel, J., Pyszczynski, T., & Solomon, S. (2002). To belong or not to belong, that is the question: Terror management and identification with gender and ethnicity. *Journal of Personality and Social Psychology, 83,* 26–43.

Aron, A., Aron, E. N., & Norman, C. (2001). Self-expansion model of motivation and cognition in close relationships and beyond. In Fletcher, G. J. O., & Clark, M. S. (eds.), *Blackwell handbook of social psychology: Interpersonal processes* (pp. 478–501). Malden, MA: Blackwell.

Baron, R. M. (1997). On making terror management theory less motivational and more social. *Psychological Inquiry, 8,* 21–22.

Baumeister, R. F., & Leary, M. R. (1995). The need to belong: Desire for interpersonal attachments as a fundamental human motivation. *Psychological Bulletin, 117,* 497–529.

Becker, E. (1962). *The birth and death of meaning.* New York: Free Press.

Becker, E. (1973). *The denial of death.* New York: Free Press.

Bowlby, J. (1973). *Attachment and loss: Separation, anxiety and anger.* New York: Basic Books.

Bowlby, J. (1980). *Attachment and loss: Sadness and depression.* New York: Basic Books.

Bowlby, J. (1982). *Attachment and loss: Attachment.* New York: Basic Books. (Original work published 1969)

Bowlby, J. (1988). *A secure base: Clinical application of attachment theory.* London: Routledge.

Buhrmester, D. (1990). Intimacy of friendship, interpersonal competence, and adjustment during preadolescence and adolescence. *Child Development, 61,* 1101–1111.

Buhrmester, D., Furman, W., Wittenberg, M. T., & Reis, H. T. (1988). Five domains of interpersonal competence in peer relationships. *Journal of Personality and Social Psychology, 55,* 991–1008.

Buss, D. M. (1997). Human social motivation in evolutionary perspective: Grounding terror management theory. *Psychological Inquiry, 8,* 22–26.

Buss, D. M., & Schmitt, D. P. (1993). Sexual strategies theory—An evolutionary perspective on human mating. *Psychological Review, 100,* 204–232.

Collins, N. L., & Read, S. J. (1990). Adult attachment, working models, and relationship quality in dating couples. *Journal of Personality and Social Psychology, 58,* 644–663.

Dechesne, M., Greenberg, J., Arndt, J., & Schimel, J. (2000). Terror management and the vicissitudes of sports fan affiliation: The effects of mortality salience on optimism and fan identification. *European Journal of Social Psychology, 30,* 813–835.

Dechesne, M., Pyszczynski, T., Arndt, J., Ransom, S., Sheldon, K. M., van Knippenberg, A., et al. (2003). Literal and symbolic immortality: The effect of evidence of literal immortality of self-esteem striving in response to mortality salience. *Journal of Personality and Social Psychology, 84,* 722–737.

Downey, G., & Feldman, S. I. (1996). Implications of rejection sensitivity for intimate relationships. *Journal of Personality and Social Psychology, 70,* 1327–1343.

Downey, G., Lebolt, A., Rincon, C., & Freitas, A. L. (1998). Rejection sensitivity and children's interpersonal difficulties. *Child Development, 69,* 1074–1091.

Feeney, J. A., & Noller, P. (1990). Attachment style as a predictor of adult romantic relationships. *Journal of Personality and Social Psychology, 58,* 281–291.

Florian, V., & Kravetz, S. (1983). Fear of personal death: attribution, structure, and relation to religious belief. *Journal of Personality and Social Psychology, 44,* 600–607.

Florian, V., & Mikulincer, M. (1997). Fear of death and the judgment of social transgressions: A multidimensional test of terror management theory. *Journal of Personality and Social Psychology, 73,* 369–380.

Florian, V., & Mikulincer, M. (1998). Symbolic immortality and the management of the terror of death—The moderating role of attachment style. *Journal of Personality and Social Psychology, 74,* 725–734.

Florian, V., Mikulincer, M., & Hirschberger, G. (2002). The anxiety buffering function of close relationships: Evidence that relationship commitment acts as a terror management mechanism. *Journal of Personality and Social Psychology, 82,* 527–542.

Fraley, R. C., & Shaver, P. R. (2000). Adult romantic attachment: Theoretical developments, emerging controversies, and unanswered questions. *Review of General Psychology, 4,* 132–154.

Fromm, E. (1956). *The art of loving.* New York: HarperCollins.

Goffman, E. (1972). *Strategic Interaction.* New York: Ballantine.

Goldenberg, J. L., Pyszczynski, T., Greenberg, J., & Solomon, S. (2000). Fleeing the body: A terror management perspective of the problem of human corporeality. *Personality and Social Psychology Review, 4,* 200–218.

Greenberg, J., Pyszczynski, T., & Solomon, S. (1986). The causes and consequences of a need for self-esteem. A terror management theory. In R. F. Baumeister (Ed.), *Public and private self* (pp. 189–192). New York: Springer-Verlag.

Greenberg, J., Pyszczynski, T., & Solomon, S. (1997). Terror management theory of self-esteem and cultural worldviews: Empirical assessments and conceptual refinements. In M. P. Zanna (Ed.), *Advances in experimental social psychology* (Vol. 29, pp. 61–141). San Diego: Academic Press.

Greenberg, J., Pyszczynski, T., Solomon, S., Simon, L., & Breus, M. (1994). The role of consciousness and accessibility of death related thoughts in mortality salience effects. *Journal of Personality and Social Psychology, 67,* 627–637.

Harmon-Jones, E., Simon, L., Greenberg, J., Pyszczynski, T., Solomon, S., & McGregor, H. A. (1997). Terror management theory and self-esteem: Evidence that increased self-esteem reduces mortality salience effects. *Journal of Personality and Social Psychology, 72,* 24–36.

Hazan, C., & Shaver, P. R. (1987). Romantic love conceptualized as an attachment process. *Journal of Personality and Social Psychology, 52,* 511–524.

Hendrick, C., & Hendrick, S. S. (1986). A theory and method of love. *Journal of Personality and Social Psychology, 50,* 392–402.

Hendrick, C., & Hendrick, S. S. (1989). Research on love: Does it measure up? *Journal of Personality and Social Psychology, 56,* 784–794.

Hirschberger, G., Florian, V., & Mikulincer, M. (2002). The anxiety buffering function of close relationships: Mortality salience effects on the willingness to compromise mate selection standards. *European Journal of Social Psychology, 32,* 609–625.

Hirschberger, G., Florian, V., & Mikulincer, M. (2003). Strivings for romantic intimacy following partner complaint or partner criticism—A terror management perspective. *Journal of Social and Personal Relationships, 20,* 675–688.

Horney, K. (1943). *Our inner conflicts: A constructive theory of neurosis.* New York: Norton.

Leary, M. R. (1999). Making sense of self-esteem. *Current Directions in Psychological Science, 8,* 32–35.

Leary, M. R., & Downs, D. L. (1995). Interpersonal functions of the self-esteem motive: The self-esteem system as a sociometer. In M. H. Kernis (Ed.), *Efficacy, agency and self-esteem* (pp. 123–144). New York: Plenum Press.

Leary, M. R., Tambour, E. S., Terdal, S. K., Downs, D. L. (1995). Self-esteem as an interpersonal monitor: The sociometer hypothesis. *Journal of Personality and Social Psychology, 68,* 518–530.

Lee, J. A. (1977). A typology of styles of loving. *Personality and Social Psychology Bulletin, 3,* 173–182.

Levy, M. B., & Davis, K. E. (1988). Lovestyles and attachment styles compared: Their relations to each other and to various relationship characteristics. *Journal of Social and Personal Relationships, 5,* 439–471.

Lifton, R. J. (1973). The sense of immortality: On death and the continuity of life. *American Journal of Psychoanalysis, 33,* 3–15.

Lifton, R. J. (1979). *The broken connection.* New York: Simon & Schuster.

Lifton R. J., & Olson, E. (1974). *Living and dying.* New York: Praeger.

McGregor, H., Leiberman, J., Greenberg, J., Solomon, S., Arndt, J., Simon, L., et al. (1998). Terror management and aggression: Evidence that mortality salience promotes aggression against worldview-threatening individuals. *Journal of Personality and Social Psychology, 74,* 590–605.

Mikulincer, M., & Florian, V. (1998). The relationship between adult attachment styles and emotional and cognitive reactions to stressful events. In J. A. Simpson & W. S. Rholes (Eds.), *Attachment theory and close relationships* (pp. 143–165). New York: Guilford Press.

Mikulincer, M., & Florian, V. (2000). Exploring individual differences in reactions to mortality salience—Does attachment style regulate terror management mechanisms? *Journal of Personality and Social Psychology, 79*, 260–273.

Mikulincer, M., Florian, V., Birnbaum, G., & Mashlikovitz S. (2002). The death-anxiety buffering function of close relationships: Exploring the effects of separation reminders on death-thought accessibility. *Personality and Social Psychology Bulletin, 28*, 287–299.

Mikulincer, M., Florian, V., & Tolmacz, R. (1990). Attachment styles and fear of personal death: A case study of affect regulation. *Journal of Personality and Social Psychology, 58*, 273–280.

Mikulincer, M., & Shaver, P. R. (2003). The attachment behavioral system in adulthood: Activation, psychodynamics, and interpersonal processes. In M. P. Zanna (ed.), *Advances in experimental social psychology* (Vol. 35). New York: Academic Press.

Peplau, L. A., & Perlman, D. (Eds.). (1982). *Loneliness: A sourcebook of current theory, research, and therapy.* New York: Wiley.

Pyszczynski, T., Greenberg, J., & Solomon, S. (1999). A dual process model of defense against conscious and unconscious death-related thoughts: An extension of terror management theory. *Psychological Review, 106*, 835–845.

Rank, O. (1934). *Psychology and the soul.* New York: Dover.

Rank, O. (1941). *Beyond psychology.* New York: Dover.

Rosenblatt, A., Greenberg, J., Solomon, S., Pyszczynski, T., & Lyon, D. (1989). Evidence for terror management theory I: The effects of mortality salience on reactions to those who violate or uphold cultural values. *Journal of Personality and Social Psychology, 57*, 681–690.

Schachter, S. (1959). *The psychology of affiliation.* Stanford, CA: Stanford University Press.

Sharabany, R. (1994). Intimacy friendship scale: Conceptual underpinnings, psychometric properties, and construct validity. *Journal of Social and Personal Relationships, 11*, 449–469.

Solomon, S., Greenberg, J., Pyszczynski, T. (1991). A terror management theory of social behavior: The psychological functions of self-esteem and cultural worldviews. In L. Berkowitz (Ed.), *Advances in experimental social psychology* (Vol. 24, pp. 93–159). New York: Academic Press.

Sullivan, H. S. (1953). *The interpersonal theory of psychiatry.* New York: Norton.

Taubman - Ben-Ari, O., Findler, L., & Mikulincer, M. (2002). The effects of mortality salience on relationship strivings and beliefs—The moderating role of attachment style. *British Journal of Social Psychology, 41*, 419–441.

Walster, E. (1965). The effects of self-esteem on romantic liking. *Journal of Experimental Social Psychology, 1*, 184–197.

Wisman, A., & Koole, S. L. (2003). Hiding in the crowd: Can mortality salience promote affiliation with others who oppose one's worldview. *Journal of Personality and Social Psychology, 84*, 511–527.

Yaacovi, E. (2003). *A terror management perspective of parenting strivings and representations.* Unpublished Ph.D. dissertation, Bar-Ilan University, Ramat Gan, Israel.

Chapter 19

Transcending Oneself through Social Identification

EMANUELE CASTANO
VINCENT YZERBYT
MARIA-PAOLA PALADINO

To deny one's mortal nature is the whole point of being different from animals, contends *White Noise* character Murray (Delillo, 1984). And the history of humanity confirms this insight, so filled with very many strategies that have been deployed to this end. Spatially separating the living from the dead can be considered the most straightforward of all strategies. Alas, it turns out to be too simplistic to fool the intelligent beings we claim to be (see Hallam, Hockey, & Howarth, 1999). Another interesting approach consists in claiming that death is not what it looks like; it is not the end of the story. Being is eternal, and life and death are just two forms of existence, the Hindus tradition suggests. Alternatively, one can distinguish between a perishable body and an immortal soul, as became fashionable in the Hellenistic era. For Plato, the human soul (*psyche*) is made of the same stuff of the cosmos, and it is therefore eternal. This same idea is of course central to Christianity, and it is argued that it is at the core of the formidable success of this religion.

According to Ulansey (2000), in the pre-Hellenistic era, the local and timeless community around which life was organized provided its members with a corporate identity which was central to their self-understanding. The meaningful entity was the community, not the individual, and the former was not threatened by physical decay. This order of things is endangered with the conquests of Alexander the Great (4th century), with whom "begins man as an individual" (Tarn, 1974; quoted in Ulansey, 2000, p. 217). The new order brought about by Alexander changed the imagined world of these individuals, destroying their local corporate identity and with it their unproblematic relationship with death. It is because of this uncertainty, Ulansey (2000) claims, that the Christian movement spread with such remarkable success. Indeed, it provided a new order which no longer needed local identifications but built on the distinction between the body and the soul, the latter being the repository of transcendence (Ulansey, 2000).

In more recent times, elements of the above-mentioned strategies have been successfully synthesized in the ideology of the nation state (Anderson, 1991). Independently from the very many forms it can take, the immortality of the *folk* is the recurrent theme and in its narrative the citizen/subject/national can transcend her mortal self by participating into the immortal (national) community. As it has been elegantly summarized by Smith (1995): "Over and beyond any political and economical benefits that ethnic nationalism can confer, it is this promise of collective and terrestrial immortality, outfacing death and oblivion, that has helped to sustain so many nations and national states in an era of unprecedented social change" (p. 160).

This brief survey of life strategies suggests that a recurrent theme in human beings' struggle with the unbearable finitude of being is the reliance on a community, be it local or imagined. [1] In this chapter we elaborate on this thesis from a social psychological perspective and argue that affiliation to and, more crucially, identification with social groups is ranked high in the repertoire of strategies that human beings use to transcend themselves. Specifically, we contend that through social identification, individuals expand their sense of self in space and time, thus participating in a larger, immaterial, and therefore immortal entity. The development of these ideas is grounded in social identity theory and terror management theory. We begin by outlining the main concepts of these theoretical perspectives before presenting some empirical evidence in support of our thesis.

SOCIAL IDENTITY AND TRANSCENDENCE

One of the most thoroughly investigated topics in social psychology is certainly intergroup relations. This is not surprising if we consider that these relations are often conflictual, and that so much of the suffering and violence in the world has an intergroup character (Brown, 2000). The contributions of Allport (1954) and Sherif (1967) have proven seminal for our understanding of this phenomenon, and so is the work of Henri Tajfel who in the late 1970s elaborated his social identity theory (SIT; Tajfel, 1972, 1978a; Tajfel & Turner, 1979).

Tajfel set out to identify the minimal conditions under which individuals start discriminating between the ingroup and the outgroup, notably by reserving more positive treatments to the former than to the latter. With his colleagues, he began by dividing participants in a laboratory study into two groups, on minimal bases (like their preference for one of two abstract painters). The idea was to add other factors to whatever this minimal criterion and to assess when discrimination would appear (e.g., Tajfel, Billig, Bundy, & Flament, 1971). Indeed, "it was hoped that from this situation in which no discrimination would appear, others could then be constructed in which (they) could assess the relative impact of various theoretically selected variables on the development of discrimination. Nothing of the kind happened; in one study after another, the 'minimal' situations threw up findings of intergroup discrimination . . . " (Tajfel, 1978a, pp. 10–11). In other words, the conditions set out in what became to known as the *minimal group paradigm* proved sufficient to trigger ingroup favoritism (see Brewer, 1979). Tajfel (1981) argued that such a basic process of social categorization required the establishment of a distinct and positively valued social identity and defined social identity as "that part of an individual's self-concept which derives from his knowledge of his membership in a social group (or groups) together with the value and emotional significance attached to that membership" (p. 255).

Not only did the framework put forth by Tajfel provide an explanation for intergroup discrimination in the absence of conflict about actual resources (Sherif, 1967), but it also considered the joint impact of cognitive and motivational factors and supplied a unique understanding of the interplay between the individual and the group (see Capozza & Brown, 2000). As a result of this, SIT and its most prominent theoretical and empirical successor, self-categorization theory (Turner, Hogg, Oakes, Reicher, & Wheterel, 1987), have been most successful in inspiring a host of theoretical developments (Brewer, 1991; Hogg, 2003) and a new understanding of several phenomena such as stereotyping (e.g., Spears, Oakes, Ellemers, & Haslam, 1997) and group dynamics (e.g., Hogg & Abrams, 1993). It has also proven useful in applied settings dealing with the reduction of prejudice (Hewstone & Brown, 1986), the understanding of the psychology of organizations (Haslam, 2001), and the analysis of political identities (Brewer, 2002; Castano, 2003a, in press-a; Castano, Yzerbyt, & Bourguignon, 2003; Herrmann, Brewer, & Risse, in press; Huddy, 2001, 2002; Oakes, 2002).

Central to SIT and especially self-categorization theory is the concept of depersonalization: the process by which individuals shift from their personal identity as unique individuals to their social identity. The shift leads to a change in individuals' (now group members) perception of the social world and the norms that regulate it, thus prompting forms of behavior that are very different from the behavior emerging in situations in which personal identity is salient (cf. the interpersonal–intergroup continuum, Tajfel, 1978b).

The cognitive underpinnings of the depersonalization process have been the target of considerable empirical research, notably by self-categorization theorists (Turner et al., 1987), but research stemming from SIT has only recently moved on from what has long been considered the key motivational basis of social identification, namely self-esteem, to investigate other potential function served by group membership (cf. Abrams & Hogg, 1988). A multiplicity of needs such as self-knowledge, meaning, and balance have been proposed by social identity theorists as possible, complementary accounts for why it is that individuals identify with social groups and led to the proposition that social identification reduces the uncertainty about the social world (Hogg & Abrams, 1993). A different perspective was adopted by Brewer (1991) who, in her optimal distinctiveness theory, proposes that individuals hold two competing needs, of assimilation and differentiation, and that social identification can contribute to maintaining a dynamic equilibrium between the two.[2] Recent empirical research has aimed at investigating the functions that individuals spontaneously attach to their membership to social groups (e.g., Deaux, Reid, Mizrahi, & Cotting, 1999) and a portion of these efforts relate these functions directly to human evolutionary history (Brewer & Caporael, 1990; Caporael, 1995, 1997; Caporael & Brewer, 1995; Stevens & Fiske, 1995).

In this chapter, we propose that social identity may serve another function, one largely neglected by social psychologists. Indeed, we argue that social identity provides individuals with a different level of existence that is immune to the mortal fate of personal identity, thus possibly contributing to alleviate existential concerns. The idea that social identity operates as a buffer to human beings' existential concerns can already be found in the writings of sociologists (e.g., Berger & Luckmann, 1967) and psychoanalysts (Freud, 1933/1965). A similar idea has been developed within a fully fledged theory of the human condition by Ernst Becker (1973). More recently, this work has undergone further theoretical development and rigorous scientific testing within the framework of terror management theory (TMT; Greenberg, Pyszczynski, & Solomon, 1986). Based on the insights of Ernst Becker on human beings' problematic relationship with death (1973), the basic tenet of TMT is that two mechanisms have developed for human beings to cope with the formidable anxiety that de-rives from the awareness of the inevitability of death: self-esteem and cultural worldviews. Support for this hypothesis comes from a vast amount of empirical studies, which demon-strate that self-esteem is negatively related to anxiety and that making people thinking of their own death leads them to hold to their cultural worldview more strongly (for a review, see Solomon, Greenberg, & Pyszczynski, Chapter 2, this volume).

TMT recognizes the intrinsically social dimension of self-esteem and, of course, of cul-tural worldviews. In fact, to be effective, the latter need to be socially shared and can only be established and maintained within a social group. Accordingly, Greenberg, Solomon, and Pyszczynski (1997) suggest that "symbolic immortality is provided through identification with entities larger and longer-lasting than the self" (p. 65). They also argue, however, that when it comes to defend against the anxiety of death, it is not membership per se which mat-ters but, rather, the consensual validation implied by membership in social groups (Greenberg et al., 1990).

Despite sharing many similarities with TMT at the conceptual level and being based on research which makes use of the same experimental paradigm, our perspective on the func-tion of social identity in managing human beings' existential concerns differs in significant ways from the one found in TMT. To appreciate this difference it is important to focus on the distinction between personal and social identity. *Personal identity* is finite, restricted in space by the very skin of our body. It is also restricted in time. Although we Westerners pride ourselves of the longevity that we can attain in our societies, the increase in lifespan looks still as a Phyrrus's victory: Death is around the corner, and we know it.

Social identity, on the contrary, extends beyond the physical experience of the individ-ual being to comprise others, and it thus does not suffer from the same sense of finitude that personal identity does. The infinite character of social identity is even more palpable on the time dimension. Although groups can and sometimes do dissolve more quickly than individ-uals die, they usually far outlive individuals. Furthermore, large social entities such as ethnic groups, nations, or ideological categories (e.g., the socialist international) enjoy some sort of built-in immortality. Indeed, they were there well before our birth and, presumably, will stick around for long after our death.

Because of these characteristics, social identity seems particularly well suited to satisfy this crucial need of human beings: the need to transcend their mortal fate. Confronted with the awareness of a fatal destiny human beings invest in the social groups to which they be-long, which are larger and more long-lasting than their individual self, in a desperate at-tempt to transcend the latter. Social identity, in this perspective, does not buffer existential concerns exclusively by providing self-esteem or as a consequence of being the repository of cultural worldviews. It may well do so simply by virtue of extending the sense of self, or, metaphorically, its proprioception. Rather than concentrating on the issue of *better*, ours is a perspective that focuses on *more, larger*.

We thus anticipated that when reminded of their mortality, individuals would focus on their social identity, oftentimes more so than on their personal identity. Also, individuals will more tenaciously defend the symbolic existence of the groups they belong to and go to great lengths to guarantee its actual survival. When embarking on a long car journey, we routinely check our automobile to ensure it will take us where we want to go. If groups are vehicles for transcendence, individuals will take care of the social entities they belong to, notably by paying attention to whom is included in its ranks, so as to ensure the group integrity.

For groups to fulfill the transcendental function one expects from them, we also argued that they would need to be reified. In the language of modern social psychology, this means that groups need to be high in entitativity—the extent to which the group is perceived as a real entity (Campbell, 1958). Only to the extent that groups are seen to be real entities will people be willing to make a deposit of their identification assets. Empirical evidence showing that increased levels of entitativity of the ingroup triggers higher identification (Castano et al., 2003) is consistent with this idea (see Castano, 2003b).

Our rationale concerning the function of the social identification process leads us to the formulation of several hypotheses. As a matter of fact, we would expect that heightened existential concerns will lead individuals to more strongly identify with their own ingroup, to perceive such an ingroup as more entitative, and to defend its integrity more vigorously. These straightforward hypotheses were tested across a series of experiments in which individuals were asked to think of their own death or were subliminally primed with death-related words. We then assessed the effects of these manipulations on the variables outlined above. It is to the presentation of the results emerging from this work that we now turn.

TESTING THE EXISTENTIAL VALUE OF SOCIAL IDENTIFICATION

A straightforward test of the first hypothesis consists in making people think about their own death, and subsequently observing whether their social identity is in some way affected. According to the present rationale, people's social identity should become a more important part of their self-definition. This means that we would expect people to see themselves more readily as members of different social groups or that people should feel and report more commitment to the particular social group that happens to be salient in the situation. Our initial empirical test of such a hypothesis was conducted using Belgian and Italian students as participants and used the "who-am-I?" task (Castano & Sacchi, 1999). The dependent variable consisted simply in seeing how many social identities (male/female, Belgian/Italian, student, etc.) participants listed. Prior to this task, participants completed a first questionnaire that varied depending on the condition. Participants in the mortality salient condition were first asked to write a short paragraph describing the emotions that the thought of their death aroused in them (cf. Greenberg et al., 1990). Control participants were asked to engage in a parallel writing task—they were asked to write a short paragraph describing the emotions that arise in them when reading a book. Consistent with expectations, participants in the mortality salient condition listed a greater number of social identities than did those in the control condition.

A further, more thorough test of our hypothesis was conducted in a second study (Castano, Yzerbyt, Paladino, & Sacchi, 2002). Participants to this study were Italian students at the University of Padova, Italy. The study allegedly consisted of two parts. In the first part, participants were randomly assigned to one of two conditions. They either were asked to write about their death (mortality salient condition) or to write about reading a book (control condition). After a brief delay, in what was presented to them as the second, unrelated part of the study, participants were requested to fill out another questionnaire, the focus of which was Italy and Italians.

This second questionnaire, which was identical in the mortality salient and control conditions, included measures of ingroup entitativity, ingroup identification, and ingroup bias. The entitativity of the ingroup (i.e., Italians) was assessed by means of a modified version of the entitativity scale developed by Castano, Yzerbyt, and Bourguignon (1999) (e.g., "Italians have many characteristics in common," "Italians have a sense of common fate," "Italy has real existence as a group"). The identification measure consisted of a six-item identification scale (e.g., "I identify with Italians," "Being Italian has nothing to do with my identity"). The ingroup bias measure consisted of having participants rate Italians and Germans (i.e., the outgroup) on 10 traits (e.g., gourmet, warm, and hard working). The order of presentation of the target group was counterbalanced.

After ensuring the internal consistency of the entitativity and identification scale as well as the scales on which the ingroup and the outgroup were judged, we compared the means for each of these variables in the two conditions. Results showed that in the mortality salient condition, participants, Italian students, identified more strongly with Italy, perceived Italy as more entitative, and judged Italians, but not Germans, more positively. Table 19.1 presents the means.

Further analyses showed that the impact of our manipulation on ingroup bias (ingroup ratings minus outgroup ratings) was mediated by the enhanced perception of entitativity and by the increased identification with the ingroup in the mortality salient condition. This result allows bringing together previous research showing the impact of mortality salience on ingroup bias (Harmon-Jones, Greenberg, Solomon, & Simon, 1996) and the work on the impact of entitativity on ingroup bias (Gaertner & Schopler, 1998).

The results of the aforementioned study focused on a national group. A national group is a kind of group that has elements of immortality built in in its constitutive narrative. We thus turned to test our hypothesis on a different kind of group, namely, common-bond groups (Prentice, Miller, & Lightdale, 1994). In this experiment (Yzerbyt, Castano, & Vermeulen, 1999), a sample of Belgian undergraduates at the Catholic university of Louvain at Louvain-la-Neuve were approached and asked to take part in a study that consisted of two separate parts. The first part consisted of a mortality salience manipulation similar to the one used in the study described earlier. After a delay, participants underwent the second part of the study consisting in conveying their opinion with respect to their group of friends. Specifically, they were presented with a series of circles that represented the participant him- or herself and his or her friends. Six different diagrams were proposed, in which the circles could vary in the extent to which they overlapped with each other, going from no overlap at all to an important overlap. This measure, first developed by Aron, Aron, and Smollan (1992) to study interpersonal relationships, has also been used in social psychology to measure the level of perceived entitativity in small groups (e.g., Gaertner & Schopler, 1998). In line with expectations, we observed a higher perception of entitativity of the group of friends in the mortality salient condition, suggesting that the effect of mortality salience on the tendency of individuals to cling to the ingroup is not only restricted to large social categories but extends to common-bond groups.

The pattern emerging from these studies is consistent with our claim concerning the role of group-derived social identities in providing individuals with a sense of transcendence. A question, however, emerges with respect to the specific mechanism that brings about this

TABLE 19.1. Entitativity, Identification, Ingroup, Outgroup, and Ingroup Bias (Ingroup–Outgroup Rating) Scores as a Function of the Experimental Condition (Mortality Salient vs. Control)

Experimental condition	Entitativity	Identification	Ingroup	Outgroup	N
Mortality salient	5.4	6.19	6.7	5.69	24
Control	4.77	5.09	5.88	5.43	24

Note. Adapted from Castano, Yzerbyt, Paladino, and Sacchi (2002).

effect. Is this effect a conscious, deliberate choice of the individuals? Are participants thinking that they are better off seeing themselves as Italians or as part of an entity because they realize that as single individuals their existence is threatened, or are they largely unaware of the reasons underlying their reactions? [3]

Two routes can be followed in order to disentangle these alternative explanations. One can either capitalize on some modification of the independent variable or rely on some change in the dependent variable. Turning to the independent variables first, subliminal priming of death can be used, as has been done in previous TMT research (e.g., Arndt, Greenberg, Pyszczynski, & Solomon, 1997). If participants are not aware that death-related thoughts have been activated in their mind, any observed effect cannot follow from a deliberate response. Second, one could try to avoid the issue of controlled answers in the dependent measures. This means that one should strive to measure the degree to which people cling to the ingroup using more indirect measures than what has previously been done.

Social psychological research indicates that group members go a long way to protect their ingroup (for reviews, see Castano, 1999, 2003b; Yzerbyt, Castano, Leyens, & Paladino, 2000). An important form of ingroup protection consists of being very careful when including a target person in the ingroup category. Research has shown that individuals request more information before categorizing an individual target as an ingroup rather than an outgroup member (Leyens & Yzerbyt, 1992) and commit more mistakes selecting ingroup members than outgroup members, thus placing fewer targets in the ingroup category (Yzerbyt, Leyens, & Bellour, 1995). The latter tendency also seems to be moderated by ingroup identification (Castano, Yzerbyt, Bourguignon, & Seron, 2002), further supporting the interpretation of this ingroup overexclusion effect as a group-defense mechanism (for a review, see Yzerbyt et al., 2000).

The interest of the ingroup–outgroup categorization task rests on its implicit character with respect to the facet of entitativity. We believe that decisions pertaining to group membership, and especially the latency for such decisions (Castano, Yzerbyt, et al., 2002), are not as overt measures of ingroup-clinging reactions as traditional, questionnaire-based, identification measures. It follows that effects observed on these measures should not be considered as consequences of a deliberate strategy adopted by participants. For this reason, the categorization measure was used in an experiment in which participants were subliminally primed with the word "death" or "field" (Castano, in press-b).

In this study, Scottish students were called to the laboratory allegedly to take part in a study on their national identity. Upon their arrival, they were explained that there were two portions in the study, and that a word association task preceded a study on national identity. The word association task allowed for the subliminal manipulation to be implemented (see Arndt et al., 1997, for details about the procedure). Following this manipulation, participants were presented with 30 pictures of males that were randomly selected from a larger pool of 50 pictures and asked to indicate, for each of them, whether the person was a Scottish (ingroup) or an English (outgroup). The software recorded participants' categorization decisions (dichotomous) along with their response latency.

Because previous research indicates that the ingroup–outgroup categorization task is jointly affected by group members' motivation and the characteristic of the stimuli, the pictures used in this experiment had been carefully pretested. A sample of 35 Scottish students were asked to indicated on a 7-point scale to what extent each picture represented an English (1) or a Scottish man (7). On the bases of their answers, pictures were divided into five levels representing various degrees of "ingroupness," from 1 (English, or very low ingroupness) to 5 (Scottish, or very high ingroupness).

A score for each participant for each of these five levels was obtained by separately averaging answers within the five levels of ingroupness. Whereas categorization of the target as an outgroup was given a value of 1, categorization of the target as an ingroup was given a value of 0. In other words, scores could vary between 0 and 1, with high values meaning categorization of the targets as English, the outgroup. The latencies for categorization were also averaged separately for the five different degrees of ingroupness.

Consistent with previous findings (e.g., Castano, Yzerbyt, Bourguignon, & Seron, 2002), people showed a clear tendency to categorize more targets as outgroup than as ingroup members. More important, however, our subliminal manipulation of mortality salience interacted with the within-subjects factor "ingroupness" to predict participants' categorization.

As can be seen in Figure 19.1, a linear trend emerged in the control condition between the factor ingroupness and the categorization decision, showing that the more the pictures were associated with ingroupness, the less likely it was for participants to categorize these pictures as depicting outgroup members. This trend simply shows that pretest and experimental participants agreed in their classification of pictures. Most interestingly, however, this trend was exacerbated in the mortality salient condition. At lower levels of ingroupness, participants in the mortality salient condition excluded the targets from the ingroup even more than participants in the control condition. A reverse pattern emerged for targets at higher levels of ingroupness, showing a tendency toward more inclusion of targets who looked very much like ingroup members.

The same analytical strategy was used for the response latencies. Here, again, we found a very interesting pattern of results. The time participants took to reach a decision increased as a linear function of the ingroupness of the target among participants in the mortality salient condition. In other words, the more the target looked like an ingroup, the longer it

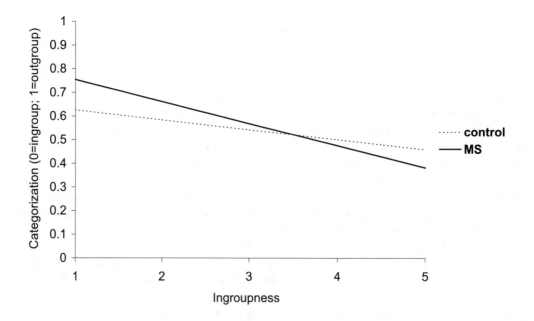

FIGURE 19.1. Ingroup–outgroup categorization as a function of ingroupness and of the experimental condition. Adapted from Castano (in press-b).

took to be categorized. In the mortality salient condition, a quadratic trend also emerged, indicating that at the highest levels of ingroupness, participants in the mortality salient condition more quickly categorized targets. This is hardly surprising, because self-evident outgroup and self-evident ingroup members should take less time to be categorized. However, the presence of a linear trend suggests that the effect due to the degree of ambiguity of the target is not symmetrical: Participants took significantly longer to categorize pictures at higher, compared to lower, levels of ingroupness.

The results of this study provide suggestive evidence that subliminal priming of death thoughts leads to the same increased ingroup attachment that has been observed with supraliminal manipulations. Furthermore, the measure of ingroup attachment was much more implicit than traditional measures of the importance of the ingroup (e.g., ingroup identification). In other words, it is reasonable to assume that when they were doing the categorization task, participants were not fully aware that they were expressing their attachment to their ingroup.

A further test of the hypothesis that the enhanced importance of social identities follows from unconscious reactions to death-related stimuli was conducted in a study that used a supraliminal manipulation of death, but the measure of the importance of social identity was again very much implicit (Yzerbyt, Carnaghi, & Castano, 2003).

Participants to this study were psychology students at the Catholic University of Louvain at Louvain-la-Neuve, and the ingroup of reference were psychologists. Participation involved answering to three separate questionnaires: The first was a self-description in which participants were asked to describe themselves by means of a series of personality traits. Specifically, the list of traits comprised, among filler traits, six traits that pretest work had revealed were stereotypical of psychologists, three positive (empathic, understanding, sensitive) and three negative (disorganized, messy, disordered). Participants rated the extent to which each trait was characteristic of the "self" on a 9-point Likert-type scale ranging from 1 (= not at all characteristic of myself) to 9 (= very characteristic of myself). The questionnaire differed depending on the experimental conditions. Half of the participants were instructed to write a short paragraph describing the emotion that the thought of their own death aroused in them (mortality salience condition). The remaining participants were asked to write a short paragraph describing the emotion aroused by the thought of leaving their parental house in order to live alone (control condition). Finally, in a third questionnaire, they were asked to think about psychologists as a group and describe them by means of a list of traits associated with a 9-point Likert-type scale ranging from 1 (= not at all characteristic of psychologists) to 9 (= very characteristic of psychologists). This list of traits included the same items that participants had seen in the first questionnaire albeit in a different order.

To test whether the representation of participants' ingroup was more likely to be based on the representation of their self in the case of mortality salience than in the control condition, we calculated a d-square score for each one of the stereotypical traits. When averaged across a series of answers, this measure indicates the degree of similarity between two profiles (in this case the self and the ingroup). As it happens, it has been used in an increasing number of social psychological studies (e.g., Cadinu & Rothbart, 1996) because it reflects similarity in terms of elevation, scatter, and shape between profiles (Cronbach & Gleser, 1953). The lower the d-square, the higher the degree of overlap between the self and the ingroup.

The d scores were averaged across the three positive traits and across the three negative traits to obtain two indices of self-group similarity. Analysis carried out on these scores re-

vealed two main effects. Not surprisingly, the overlap was stronger for positive than for negative traits. More important, mortality salient participants showed a stronger overlap than
did control participants. The interaction was also significant, revealing that making mortality salience dramatically increased the self-ingroup overlap, as compared to the control condition, but that this was the case only for the negative traits. The absence of effects of the
manipulation on the positive traits was most likely due to a ceiling effect, as the self-ingroup
overlap was clearly very high in both conditions.

The pattern that emerged from this study is consistent with our hypothesis about the increased importance of the ingroup under mortality salient conditions. Because of the use of
an implicit measure of social identification (the ingroup–self overlap measure), the results of
this study should be interpreted as reflecting spontaneous processes, akin to those of the
study where we relied on subliminal priming of death (Castano, in press-b). Furthermore,
the fact that individuals under mortality salience showed a greater degree of overlap between the self and the ingroup on the negative traits suggests that they were not driven by
self-serving considerations but, rather, by social identification per se.

DISCUSSION

Social groups undoubtedly fulfill a variety of needs for human beings. Research suggests
that they satisfy the need of assimilation and the need of self-definition. Smaller groups have
been said to satisfy a need for intimacy as well as a need for achievement. In this chapter, we
argued that social groups do serve yet another important function. They provide individuals
with a *social identity* that allows for an extension of the self in space and time; it is abstract,
intangible, and therefore everlasting. Social identity, we argue, is human beings' vehicle for
transcendence.

For certain social groups, the claim that membership provides individuals with some
form of transcendence is obviously a central part of their narratives. As we noted previously,
nation-states are prototypical in this respect (Smith, 1995). The very way in which they have
been and continue to be promoted is supposed to instigate among their members the feeling
that they, as individuals, may die (notably in war to preserve the nation-state) but that they
will somehow live forever because their nation will do so. If individual immortality is not
within reach, individuals may well settle for collective immortality.

The data we collected on our Italian and Scottish participants give credence to the foregoing conjecture regarding the role of national identification. Italian participants increased
their level of identification with their country, Italy, and reified the national group more
when they had been previously thinking about their own death. Incidentally, they also saw
Italians, but not Germans, in a more positive light. Similarly, when asked to classify pictures
of young males as Scottish or English, Scottish participants differed in how they approached
the task depending on whether they had or had not previously been primed with the word
"death". Those participants who had been subliminally exposed to the idea of death took
longer to categorize individuals who (because of their looks) were more likely to be Scottish.
They also showed a tendency to include them more in the ingroup. This tendency was coupled with a definite response, compared to participants in the control condition, to exclude
those individuals who were less likely to be Scottish. All in all, death-primed participants
seemed much more concerned with the group boundaries than did their control
counterparts.

As a set, these results strongly suggest that individuals do indeed cling to their nation when the idea of death, and in particular the perspective of their own finitude, is made salient. Importantly, our participants display a set of reactions generally associated with strong group identification when the idea of death has been brought by means of an explicit request to think about it as well as when the activation takes place via subliminal priming, thereby preventing any conscious evocation on the part of participants.

The nation's built-in promise of immortality does not appear, however, as a necessary element to explain this pattern of result. Additional experimental evidence emerging from our experiments shows that making mortality salient leads individuals to list a greater number of social identities (Castano & Sacchi, 1999), to see themselves more embedded into their group of friends (Yzerbyt et al., 1999), and to see a greater overlap between the self and their own professional group (Yzerbyt et al., 2003).

Taken together, the evidence emerging from our program of research is consistent with our claim that social identity allows for an extension of the self in space and time, thus providing the human beings with a different level of existence that is not threatened by the fate of their finite personal identity (Castano, Yzerbyt, Paladino, & Sacchi, 2002). Two caveats need be mentioned, however, with respect to this conclusion. They both come from research stemming from TMT. As suggested earlier, TMT postulates that self-esteem and cultural worldviews serve as two buffers against the anxiety of death. At present, our work has not addressed the relationship between these two anxiety-buffer mechanisms and social identification. Although this is definitely an important goal for future research, we may offer some speculations.

SOCIAL IDENTITY, SELF-ESTEEM AND CULTURAL WORLDVIEWS

One interesting line of research has explored the idea that the anxiety-buffer role of social identity may depend on whether it boosts or threatens individuals' self-esteem. This hypothesis has found support in a series of studies by Dechesne and his colleagues, showing that when social identities are presented in a negative light, individuals tend to distance from the relevant groups (Dechesne, Greenberg, Arndt, & Schimel, 2000; Dechesne, Janssen, & van Knippenberg, 2000). In these studies, the groups that were used were, among others, university affiliation or sports team fans. Except for a minority of people, such groups are often unlikely to provide individuals with a strong sense of identity. Indeed, a recently proposed taxonomy of groups (Lickel et al., 2000) would include these groups under the category of "loose associations." Groups such as these are moderately entitative at best. This is an interesting aspect, because entitativity is a characteristic that we deemed important for a proper fulfillment of the transcendental functions of social identification.

Other groups that serve more of an identity function for individuals may be less likely to induce deidentification among death-primed individuals when they may contribute to negative self-esteem. An obvious example are national groups which, as indicated previously, provide individuals with precisely that kind of existence that would constitute an anxiety buffer. National groups are also generally unlikely to induce negative self-esteem in their members. When the value of our national identity is threatened in the individual's eye because a corrupt or arrogant government is ruling the country, subtyping processes are likely to occur precisely to maintain a positive image of the group as a whole (e.g., Kunda & Oleson, 1995; Hewstone, 1994). Research has also shown that group members are very apt indeed in exercising social creativity and focusing on positive aspects of their ingroup identity (Hinkle, Taylor, Fox-Cardamone, & Ely, 1998; Simon, Glaessner-Bayerl, & Stratenwerth, 1991). Finally, national groups are far less permeable than "loose associations," and this factor may also account for the different ways in which they serve as anxiety buffers. Consistent with this reasoning, Dechesne et al. (2000b) found that when permeability was reduced (Study 2), and among individuals who have a tendency to "fight rather than switch" (Study 1), lower ingroup status did not produce a reduction in identification with the group when death was made salient.

In line with the results obtained by Dechesne and colleagues, Arndt, Greenberg, Schimel, Pyszczynski and Solomon (2002) found that members of ethnic minorities in the United States primed with negative characteristics of their group distanced themselves from their fellow group members more when they had been thinking of their own death. Because ethnic groups do certainly fulfill an identity function for their members and tend to be perceived as highly entitative, these results may be interpreted as shifting the balance in favor of a self-esteem interpretation of the role of social identification. However, these results emerged only among stigmatized groups and in contexts in which individuals may switch to a more inclusive social identity (e.g., American). Also, the fact that they emerged on measures of distancing from ingroup members as opposed to direct group identification measures, makes a straightforward comparison with other available evidence difficult.

Yet another way in which social identities may become of great importance when mortality is salient is through their link with cultural worldviews. Social identities are derived from group membership, and groups are the milieu where worldviews are created and maintained. A large amount of evidence exists in support of the anxiety-buffer role of cultural worldviews, and it may thus be that social identities are important because, or to the extent to which, they are the repository of such worldviews (Greenberg et al., 1990). Our understanding of the precise role of social identity in buffering anxiety will be enhanced by research that tests the competing hypotheses within the same experimental design. To our knowledge, the only evidence of this kind available to date comes from a series of experiments by Wisman and Koole (2003). In one of these experiments each participant was confronted with the dilemma of choosing between sitting alone and defending his or her own worldviews or sitting in a group and assuming the group's worldviews, which opposed those held by the participant. The results clearly indicated that participants in the mortality salient condition were more likely to resolve the dilemma by choosing the latter over the former strategy. It thus seems that affiliation may, under certain circumstances, be more important as an anxiety-buffer mechanism than the defense of one's cultural worldviews.

Earlier in this chapter we pointed to the difference that we see between a TMT interpretation of the function of social identification and our own perspective. We believe that this is a conceptually important distinction, that may well have an impact on the way in which social psychologists use these theoretical framework to influence policy and more generally to inform social intervention (e.g., Pyszczynski, Solomon, & Greenberg, 2002). However, we also believe that these two perspectives are highly compatible and one needs not choose between them. The mechanisms through which the transcendental need of human beings is satisfied are unlikely, to borrow the theological formulation, to be *Uno* or even *Trino*. Although the quest has a long history, it is clear that, from a psychological standpoint, we are only at the beginning. And it is only with the advent of TMT that rigorous attempts have begun to tackle the question empirically. Our hope is that the present ideas will have some heuristic power, and that research into this fascinating issue will flourish in the years to come.

CONCLUSION

All the authors of this chapter share a profound interest in group phenomena. We are particularly motivated to gain a better understanding of the causes and consequences of social identification (Castano, 2003b; Yzerbyt et al., 2000). We also are European, and thus perhaps somewhat more prone to communitarian, rather than liberal–individualistic conceptions of the human being. The emphasis we place on social identification as a mechanism through which human beings can transcend themselves may thus come as no surprise. We think, however, that the ideas expressed here are grounded on more than ingroup bias.

We believe that important insights can be gained by looking at the very different ways in which human beings have attempted to come to terms with the inconvenience of death in various points in time. As suggested by Ulansey (2000), collective identities have provided anxiety-buffer mechanisms at various points in the history of civilization, and collective-identity crises seem to correspond to period of increased anxiety and quest for alternative forms of symbolic or literal immortality. In recent times, the promise of collective immortality of the nation-state is perhaps the best example of social identification as a means to transcend oneself. It is not, however, the only one. In this chapter, we argued that social identities grounded in any group that meets certain criteria of entitativity have the potential to provide individuals with a sense of transcendence, and not only national groups. The empirical evidence we presented indicates that this conjecture is in fact borne out.

Because of our focus on the characteristics of social identities in providing a shield against existential terror, we believe that important insights in this respect will have to be gathered from research in cultures in which the self is structured differently, notably more interdependent and collective (Markus & Kitayama, 1991). Preliminary research suggests that some of the effects observed in Western societies replicate in Japan (Heine, Harihara, & Niiya, 2002) and among Australian Aboriginals (Halloran, 2001) but future research will need to look at the extent to which and the conditions under which the use of the reviewed anxiety-buffer mechanisms differs across cultures (see Salzman & Halloran, Chapter 15, this volume).

In this chapter we confer a function to social identity that is not strictly dependent on its ability to provide individuals with high levels of self-esteem. In other words, the issue is not simply how much of a positive view of the self people can derive from their group membership. Ours is perhaps a less utilitarian view of the link between the individual and the group than is usually presented in the psychological literature and more broadly in social and behavioral sciences (cf. Caporael, 1995). However, our perspective still takes for granted that social identification is a function of *individual* motives: the individual remains prior to the social. Recent years have witnessed the emergence of a challenge to this view, one that implicitly underlies most if not all social psychological research. The dissidence has been brought forward by Caporael (1997), who proposes a model of human evolution in which sociality is a constitutive part rather than a consequence of individually evolved beings. In Caporael's perspective, the relationship between social identification and the need to buffer the anxiety deriving from a newly acquired self-awareness may emerge as more complex than is currently theorized. Consistent with the concept of downward causation (Campbell, 1974), her analysis proposes that group life should not be simply considered as one of the consequences of human cognition but that the latter may have been shaped by the social conditions. As an emergent property of increased cognitive complexity, self-awareness and the associated anxiety may have appeared in parallel with the mechanisms that allow us to cope with them: self-esteem, cultural worldviews, and social identification. To be sure, the empirical data we presented in this chapter do not allow to sanction one or the other approaches. Still, they may usefully contribute to fuel the debate regarding these important issues and, ideally, help us to better understand the factors underlying the complex relations between individuals and groups.

NOTES

1. Immortality, of course, is not everybody's main concern. Our friend B. S., for instance, notes "What's the point of immortality if one looks like hell!"
2. Coming from an interpersonal perspective, Baumeister and Leary (1995) also propose the need to belong as a fundamental human motivation.
3. Although stronger identification with the ingroup can emerge as a deliberate strategy used by individuals when reminded of their own death, because it bears no direct relationship with death, we do not refer to it as a proximal defense mechanism (as opposed to a distal defense mechanism; see Pyszczynski, Greenberg, & Solomon, 1999).

REFERENCES

Abrams, D., & Hogg, M. A. (1988). Comments on the motivational status of self-esteem in social identity and intergroup discrimination. *European Journal of Social Psychology, 18*, 317–334.

Allport, G. W. (1954). *The nature of prejudice*. Reading, MA: Addison-Wesley.

Anderson, B. (1991). *Imagined communities. Reflections on the origin and spread of nationalism.* London, UK: Verso.

Arndt, J., Greenberg, J., Pyszczynski, T., & Solomon, S. (1997). Subliminal exposure to death-related stimuli increases defense of the cultural worldview. *Psychological Science, 8*, 379–385.

Arndt, J., Greenberg, J., Schimel, J., Pyszczynski, T., & Solomon, S. (2002). To belong or not to belong, that is the question: Terror management and identification with gender and ethnicity. *Journal of Personality and Social Psychology, 83*, 26–43.

Aron, A., Aron, E. N., & Smollan, D. (1992). Inclusion of Other in the Self Scale and the structure of interpersonal closeness. *Journal of Personality and Social Psychology, 63*, 596–612.

Baumeister, R. F., & Leary, M. R. (1995). The need to belong: Desire for interpersonal attachments as a fundamental human motivation. *Psychological Bulletin,117*, 497–529.

Berger, P. L., & Luckmann, T. (1967). *The social construction of reality: a treatise in the sociology of knowledge.* Garden City, NY: Anchor Books

Becker, E. (1973). *The denial of death*. New York: Free Press.

Brewer, M. B. (1991). The social self: On being the same and different at the same time. *Personality and Social Psychology Bulletin, 17*, 475–482.

Brewer, M. B. (2002). The many faces of social identity: Implications for political psychology. *Political Psychology, 23*, 39–58.

Brewer, M. B., & Caporael, L. R. (1990). Selfish genes vs. selfish people: Sociobiology as origin myth. *Motivation and emotion, 14*, 237–243.

Brown, R. J. (2000). *Group processes: Dynamics within and between groups* (2nd ed.). Oxford, UK: Blackwell.

Cadinu, M. R., & Rothbart, M. (1996). Self-anchoring and differentiation processes in the minimal group setting. *Journal of Personality and Social Psychology, 70*, 661–677.

Campbell, D. T. (1958). Common fate, similarity, and other indices of the status of aggregates of person as social entities. *Behavioural Science, 3*, 14–25.

Campbell D. T. (1974): "Downward causation" in hierarchically organized biological systems. In F. J. Ayala & T. Dobzhansky (Ed.), *Studies in the philosophy of biology* (pp. 179–186). Berkeley: University of California Press.

Caporael, L. R. (1995). Sociality: Coordinating bodies, minds and groups. *Psycholoquy* [On-line serial], 6(1). Available at: *http://www.cogsci.soton.ac.uk/cgi/psyc/newpsy?6.01*.

Caporael, L. R. (1997). The evolution of truly social cognition: The core configurations model. *Personality and Social Psychology Review. 4*, 276–298.

Caporael, L. R., & Brewer, M. B. (1995). Reviving evolutionary psychology: Biology meets society. *Journal of Social Issues, 47,*187–195.

Capozza, D., & Brown, R. (Eds.). (2000). *Social identity processes.* London: Sage.

Castano, E. (1999). *The phenomenology of the ingroup: Entitativity and identification.* Unpublished doctoral dissertation, Catholic University of Louvain, Louvain-la-Neuve, Belgium.

Castano, E. (2003a). Ethos, demos and project: Is it possible to construct a common identity even in the absence of a European "people"? *European Synthesis.* Available at: *http://www.europeansynthesis.org/n1/articolo08.htm*.

Castano, E. (2003b). On the advantages of reifying the ingroup. In V. Y. Yzerbyt, C. M. Judd, & O. Corneille (Eds.), *The psychology of group perception: Contributions to the study of homogeneity, entitivity, and essentialism* (pp. 381–400). Philadelphia: Psychology Press.

Castano, E. (in press-a). European identity: A social psychological perspective. In R. H. Herrmann, M. B. Brewer, & T. Risse (Eds.), *Identities in Europe and the institutions of the European Union.* Lanham, MD: Rowman & Littlefield.

Castano, E. (in press-b). In case of death, cling to the ingroup. *European Journal of Social Psychology.*

Castano, E., & Sacchi, S. (1999). *The effect of mortality salience on self-definition.* Unpublished raw data.

Castano, E., Yzerbyt, V. Y., & Bourguignon, D. (1999). *Measuring entitativity.* Unpublished manuscript, Catholic University of Louvain, Louvain-La-Neuve, Belgium.

Castano, E., Yzerbyt, V. Y., & Bourguignon, D. (2003). We are one and I like it: The impact of entitativity on social identification. *European Journal of Social Psychology, 33,* 735–754.

Castano, E., Yzerbyt, V. Y., Bourguignon, D., & Seron, E. (2002). Who may come in? The impact of ingroup identification on ingroup–outgroup categorization. *Journal of Experimental Social Psychology, 38,* 315–322.

Castano, E., Yzerbyt, V. Y., Paladino, M.-P., & Sacchi, S. (2002). I belong therefore I exist: Ingroup identification, ingroup entitativity, and ingroup bias. *Personality and Social Psychology Bulletin, 28,* 135–143.

Cronbach, L. J., & Gleser, C. G. (1953). Assessing similarity between profiles. *Psychological Bulletin, 50,* 456–473.

Deaux, K., Reid, A., Mizrahi, K., & Rotting, D. (1999). Connecting the person to the social: The functions of social identification. In T. R. Tyler, R. Kramer, M. Roderick, et al. (Eds.), *The psychology of the social self: Applied social research* (pp. 91–113). Mahwah, NJ: Erlbaum.

Dechesne, M., Greenberg, J., Arndt, J., & Schimel, J. (2000). Terror management and the vicissitudes of sports fan affiliation: the effects of mortality salience on optimism and fan identification. *European Journal of Social Psychology, 30,* 813–835.

Dechesne, M., Janssen, J., & van Knippenberg, A. (2000). Derogation and distancing as terror management strategies: The moderating role of need for closure and permeability of group boundaries. *Journal of Personality and Social Psychology, 79,* 923–932.

Delillo, D. (1984). *White noise.* New York: Viking Press.

Freud, S. (1965). *New introductory lectures on psychoanalysis.* New York: Norton. (Original work published 1933)

Gaertner, L., & Schopler, H. (1998). Perceived ingroup entitativity and intergroup bias: An interconnection of self and others. *European Journal of Social Psychology, 28,* 963–980.

Greenberg, J., Pyszczynski, T., & Solomon, S. (1986). The causes and consequences of the need for self-esteem: A terror management theory. In R. F. Baumeister (Ed.), *Public self and private self* (pp. 198–212). New York: Springer-Verlag.

Greenberg, J., Pyszczynski, T., Solomon, S., Rosenblatt, A., Veeder, M., Kirkland, S., et al. (1990). Evidence for terror management theory II: The effects of mortality salience reactions to those who threaten or bolster the cultural worldview. *Journal of Personality and Social Psychology, 58,* 308–318.

Greenberg, J., Solomon, S., & Pyszczynski, T. (1997). Terror management theory of self-esteem and cultural world views: Empirical assessments and conceptual refinements. In P. M. Zanna (Ed.), *Advances in experimental social psychology* (Vol. 29, pp. 61–139). San Diego: Academic Press.

Hallam, E., Hockey, J. L., & Howarth, G. (1999). *Beyond the body: Death and social identity.* London: Routledge.

Halloran, M. (2001). *Cultural validation in social context: The effect of mortality salience on endorsement of cultural values in contexts defined by social identities.* Unpublished doctoral dissertation, Swinburne University, Victoria, Australia.

Harmon-Jones, E., Greenberg, S., Solomon, S., & Simon L. (1996). The effects of mortality salience on intergroup bias between minimal groups. *European Journal of Social Psychology, 26,* 677–681.

Haslam, S. A. (2001). *Psychology in organizations: The social identity approach.* London, UK & Thousand Oaks, CA: Sage.

Heine, S. J., Harihara, M., & Niiya, Y. (2002). Terror management in Japan. *Asian Journal of Social Psychology, 5,* 187–196.

Herrmann, R. H. Brewer, M. B., & Risse, T. (Eds.). (in press). *Identities in Europe and the institutions of the European Union.* Lanham, MD: Rowman & Littlefield.

Hewstone, M. (1994). Revision and change of stereotypic beliefs: In search of the elusive subtyping model. In M. Hewstone & W. Stroebe (Eds.), *European review of social psychology* (Vol. 5, pp. 69–109). Chichester, UK: Wiley.

Hewstone, M., & Brown, R. J. (1986). Contact is not enough: An intergroup perspective on the contact hypothesis. In M. Hewstone & R. J. Brown (Eds.), *Contact and conflict in intergroup discrimination* (pp. 1–44). Oxford, UK: Blackwell.

Hinkle, S., Taylor, L. A., Fox-Cardamone, L., & Ely, P. G. (1998). Social identity and aspects of social creativity: Shifting to new dimensions of intergroup comparison. In S. Worchel, J. Francis Morales, D. Paez, & J.-C. Deschamps (Eds.), *Social identity: International perspectives* (pp. 166–179). Thousand Oaks, CA: Sage.

Hogg, M. A. (2003). Uncertainty and extremism: Identification with high entitative groups under conditions of uncertainty. In V. Y. Yzerbyt, C. M. Judd, & O. Corneille (Eds.), *The psychology of group perception: Contributions to the study of homogeneity, entitivity, and essentialism* (pp. 401–418). Philadelphia: Psychology Press.

Hogg, M. A., & Abrams, D. (1993). Towards a single-process uncertainty-reduction model of social motivation in groups. In M. A. Hogg & D. Abrams (Eds.), *Group motivation: Social psychological perspectives* (pp. 173–190). Hemel Hempstead, UK: Harvester Wheatsheaf; New York: Prentice-Hall.

Huddy, L. (2001). From social to political identity: A critical examination of social identity theory. *Political Psychology, 22,* 127–156

Huddy, L. (2002). Context and meaning in social identity theory: A response to Oakes. *Political Psychology, 23,* 825–838

Kunda, Z., & Oleson, K. C. (1995). Maintaining stereotypes in the face of disconfirmation: Constructing grounds for subtyping deviants. *Journal of Personality and Social Psychology, 68,* 565–579.

Leyens, J.-P., & Yzerbyt, V. Y. (1992). The ingroup overexclusion effect. Impact of valence and confirmation on stereotypical information search. *European Journal of Social Psychology, 22,* 549–569.

Lickel, B., Hamilton, D. L., Wieczorkowska, G., Lewis, A., Sherman, S. J., & Uhles, A. N. (2000). Varieties of groups and the perception of group entitativity. *Journal of Personality and Social Psychology, 78,* 223–246.

Markus, H. R., Kitayama, S. (1991). Culture and the self: Implications for cognition, emotion, and motivation. *Psychological Review, 98,* 224–253.

Oakes, P. (2002). Psychological groups and political psychology: A response to Huddy's "Critical examination of social identity theory." *Political Psychology, 23,* 809–824

Prentice, D. A., Miller, D. T., & Lightdale, J. R. (1994). Asymmetries in attachments to groups and to their members. Distinguishing between common-identity and common-bond groups. *Personality and Social Psychology Bulletin, 20,* 484–493.

Pyszczynski, T., Greenberg, J., & Solomon, S. (1999). A dual-process model of defense against conscious and unconscious death-related thoughts: An extension of terror management theory. *Psychological Review, 106*, 835–845.

Pyszczynski, T., Solomon, S., & Greenberg, J. (2002). *In the wake of 9/11: The psychology of terror.* Washington, DC: American Psychological Association.

Sherif, M. (1967). *Group conflict and cooperation: Their social psychology.* London: Routledge & Kegan Paul.

Simon, B., Glaessner-Bayerl, B., & Stratenwerth, I. (1991). Stereotyping and self-stereotyping in a natural intergroup context: The case of heterosexual and homosexual men. *Social Psychology Quarterly, 54*, 252–266.

Smith, A. D. (1995). *Nations and nationalism in a global era.* Oxford, UK: Blackwell.

Spears R., Oakes, P. J., Ellemers, N., & Haslam, S. A. (1997). *The social psychology of stereotyping and group life.* Oxford, UK: Blackwell.

Stevens, L. E., & Fiske, S. T. (1995). Motivation and cognition in social life: A social survival perspective. *Social Cognition, 13*, 189–214.

Tajfel, H. (1972). La catégorisation sociale. In S. Moscovici (Ed.), *Introduction à la psychologie sociale* (pp. 272–302). Paris: Larousse.

Tajfel, H. (1978a). *Differentiation between social groups: Studies in the social psychology of intergroup relations.* London, Academic Press.

Tajfel, H. (1978b). Interindividual behaviour and intergroup behaviour. In H. Tajfel (Ed.), *Differentiation between social groups: Studies in the social psychology of intergroup relations* (pp. 27–60). London: Academic Press.

Tajfel, H. (1981). *Human groups and social categories.* Cambridge, UK: Cambridge University Press.

Tajfel, H., Billig, M., Bundy, R., & Flament, C. (1971). Social categorization and intergroup behavior. *European Journal of Social Psychology, 1*, 149–178.

Tajfel, H., & Turner, J. C. (1979). An integrative theory of intergroup relations. In W. G. Austin & S. Worchel (Eds.), *Psychology of intergroup relations* (pp. 33–47). Monterey, CA: Brooks-Cole.

Turner, J. C., Hogg, M. A., Oakes, P. J., Reicher, S. D., & Wheterel, M. S. (1987). *Rediscovering the social group: A self-categorization theory.* Oxford, UK: Blackwell.

Ulansey, D. (2000). Cultural transition and spiritual transformation: from Alexander the Great to cyberspace. In T. Singer (Ed.), *The vision thing: Myth, politics, and psyche in the world* (pp. 213–231). New York: Routledge.

Wisman, A., & Koole, S. L. (2003). Hiding in the crowd: Can mortality salience promote affiliation with others who oppose one's worldviews? *Journal of Personality and Social Psychology, 84*, 511–526.

Yzerbyt, V. Y., Carnaghi, A., & Castano, E. (2003). *The impact of mortality salience on self-ingroup overlapping.* Manuscript in preparation.

Yzerbyt, V. Y., Castano, E., Leyens, J.-P., & Paladino, M.-P. (2000). The primacy of the ingroup: The interplay of identification and entitativity. In W. Stroebe & M. Hewstone (Eds.), *European review of social psychology* (Vol. 11, pp. 258–295). Chichester, UK: Wiley.

Yzerbyt, V. Y., Castano, E., & Vermeulen, J. (1999). *The impact of mortality salience on ingroup entitativity.* Unpublished raw data.

Yzerbyt, V. Y., Leyens, J.-P., & Bellour, F. (1995). The ingroup overexclusion effect. Identity concerns in decisions about group membership. *European Journal of Social Psychology, 25*, 1–16.

Chapter 20

Moral Amplification and the Emotions That Attach Us to Saints and Demons

JONATHAN HAIDT
SARA ALGOE

...and God divided the light from the darkness. And God called the light Day, and the darkness he called Night.

—GENESIS, 1: 4–5

When love and hate are both absent everything becomes clear and undisguised. Make the smallest distinction, however, and heaven and earth are set infinitely far apart. If you wish to see the truth then hold no opinions for or against anything. To set up what you like against what you dislike is the disease of the mind.

—BUDDHA, *The Dhammapada*

astern and Western religions point to the act of separating opposites as the beginning of the drama of life. Whether these opposites are night and day, man and woman, or good and evil, it is commonly thought that one cannot exist without the other. In the Bible, the act of separation is a wondrous act, done by God in order to create the physical world. But Hindu and Buddhist scriptures more frequently discuss the acts of separation that we all do in our daily lives and warn that such separations blind us to truth and bind us to the material world and its passions.

In this chapter we examine this separation of good and evil from a psychological perspective. We suggest that an important part of social cognition is the separation and amplification of good and evil in our judgments of others. People seem to want to live in a world full of saints and demons. They want their saints saintly and their demons demonic. However, one of the most basic lessons of social psychology is that good and bad behaviors do not spring entirely, or even primarily, from the goodness or badness of individuals. In the

322

first part of this chapter we explore a few of the mechanisms that underlie moral appraisals and their amplifications. Next, we suggest that moral appraisals can be partially understood by positing three dimensions of social cognition, including a vertical dimension running from divinity/purity/goodness above to animality/pollution/evil below. In the third part of the chapter we examine a few of the emotions that play out along these dimensions: disgust and anger toward demons and villains and elevation and admiration toward saints and heros. Throughout the chapter we suggest that the exaggerated separation of good and evil—what Buddha called "the disease of the mind"—is one of the ways that people find meaning in life and solidarity with others.

MORAL AMPLIFICATION

In the wake of the September 11 terrorist attacks, Americans quickly developed a kind of moral bipolar condition. The first-order effect was a separation of the many people involved into heros and villains, or saints and demons. This first separation was straightforward: 19 men had killed thousands of innocent people, including hundreds of firefighters and other rescue workers who died trying to save innocent lives. For Americans, as for most people in other countries, the terrorists were bad and the rescue workers were good. But as time went on it became clear that these separations were driven not just by appraisals of the facts, but by a hunger for purity: the perfect separation of good and evil, such that the villains ended up with only evil traits and motives while the heros ended up with only good traits and motives. President Bush declared that the terrorists were "cowards" who acted because they "hate our freedom." Because freedom is a foundational moral good for Americans, anyone who would sacrifice his or her life to strike at a moral good must be monumentally evil. Conversely, firefighters all over America were lionized and showered with flowers and money.

But the second-order moral effects were more interesting. Americans did not just want a perfect separation of good and evil; they reacted angrily to anyone who questioned the purity of the separation. For example, the comedian Bill Maher pointed out that the word "coward" did not apply to the terrorists. Agreeing with a comment from a guest on his television talk show, he said: "We have been the cowards. Lobbing cruise missiles from two thousand miles away. That's cowardly. Staying in the airplane when it hits the building, say what you want about it, not cowardly." An uproar ensued, and many stations stopped broadcasting Maher's program. Maher's use of the word "coward" was certainly more semantically correct than Bush's, but Maher had violated both halves of the moral purity process: America was not perfectly virtuous, and the terrorists were not perfectly craven. Similar condemnation was heaped on anyone else who suggested that American foreign policy played some role in causing the attacks. This second-order process—punishing people who fail to vilify consensually shared demons, or who impugn the perfect motives of consensually shared saints—is sometimes seen in other contexts in which groups come together to fight what they see as evil. Whether the villain is homosexuals or homophobes, African Americans or racists, once a group or movement is formed, any acknowledgment of virtue in the enemy is seen as a kind of treason.

Moral amplification can be defined as *the motivated separation and exaggeration of good and evil in the explanation of behavior.* Moral amplification is a way of stating in psychological terms what was known in history as the doctrine of Manichaeism: the belief that the visible world is a product of an eternal struggle between the forces of good/God/light and the forces of evil/Satan/darkness. Humanity and the material world were created when the forces of darkness penetrated the world of light. People are therefore a mixture of good and evil, and their goal in life should be to work to purify themselves and the world, restoring the perfect separation of good and evil that was the original state of the universe (Wilson, 1967). Manichaeism emanated from Babylonia in the third century and spread widely in the ancient world. While it was eventually ruled to be a heresy in Christianity, it attracted many Christians, including St. Augustine. Part of its appeal, like that of later dualist doctrines in Christianity, was that it helped to reconcile the belief in a just and loving God with the obvious existence of evil in the world. Evil is not God's fault, it is the Devil's, and God needs our help (Russell, 1988).

Moral amplification clearly involves several well-known social–cognitive mechanisms. For example, the fundamental attribution error (Ross, 1977) states that people overascribe both good and bad behaviors of other people to traits rather than taking situational constraints into account. This bias on its own would be sufficient to make people see an illusory Manichaean world full of good and bad people. We can add to this the problem of "naive realism" (Robinson, Keltner, Ward, & Ross, 1995), in which people underestimate the difficulty and ambiguity of the construal process. People believe that they see the facts of a situation as they truly are and have based their judgments on those facts. If the facts are so obvious, then it follows that the other side in a dispute must see the same set of facts, and their disagreement must reflect a radically different and frightening set of values (e.g., a rejection of the value of life, or of autonomy, in the abortion debate). The result is that small differences between groups get amplified into the perception of major and unbridgeable differences.

Once a disagreement is seen as a fight between opposing worldviews, people have a motivation to engage in motivated reasoning (Kunda, 1990; Pyszczynski & Greenberg, 1987). People have already chosen the conclusion they wish to reach, and they search only for evidence that will support that conclusion. Haidt (2001) has recently argued that nearly all moral reasoning is motivated reasoning—at least, in real-life situations in which one cares about the outcome, in contrast to the disembodied hypothetical cases that have been used to elicit moral reasoning in research studies. Thus once a disagreement becomes a moral disagreement, reasoning becomes part of the "war effort," devoted to supporting both the defense (of one's own side) and the offense (criticism of the other side).

The process of purifying good and evil has been described in perhaps the greatest detail by Roy Baumeister. Baumeister (1997) analyzed portrayals of evil in literature and movies, and in laypeople's conceptions, and integrated them all into what he called "the myth of pure evil." The myth has several parts to it, but the three most important parts for our purposes are (1) denying the motivations of the "evildoer"—that is, people resist seeing any coherent reasons for the perpetrators action, beyond sadism (the enjoyment of doing evil things) and greed (the desire for money and power); (2) denying the participation of the victim—that is, people see evil as falling out of the sky onto innocent victims, and they resist the idea that the victims shared any portion of blame; (3) evil is the outsider—that is, the conflict of good versus evil is assimilated to a perceived conflict of ingroup versus outgroup. Cartoon villains, for example, often speak with a foreign accent.

Baumeister's analysis of portrayals of evil fits with his own empirical findings. Baumeister, Stillwell, and Wotman (1990) collected "micronarratives" of real-life conflicts, including both those in which the participant was a victim and those in which the same participant had been the perpetrator of harm. The accounts differed in many ways that can help us to understand the origins and escalations of conflicts. For example, perpetrators were likely to report mitigating circumstances and reasons for having committed the harm, even though they often acknowledged that they were not fully justified. Victims were much less likely to talk about such factors, if they even knew of them in the first place. Conversely, victims were more likely to describe a string of provocations, the last of which was the trigger for an emotional outburst. Perpetrators, however, saw shorter histories, and often saw the victims reactions as overreactions.

It is interesting to note that Americans and the Muslim minority that supported the September 11 attacks use differing time perspectives that allow each to claim the morally righteous role of victim. For Americans the story begins on September 11 when evil fell, literally, out of a clear blue sky onto 3,000 innocent victims. The wars in Afghanistan and Iraq are, for some Americans, the justified responses to those attacks. For those who sympathize with al Qaeda, however, the story begins long ago, with a series of Western provocations and humiliations of Arab peoples. The September 11 attacks are framed as David finally and heroically standing up to Goliath. (Note: Because of the moral amplification processes still operating in the United States, the authors feel compelled to state that they themselves do not endorse al Qaeda's framing of the attacks.) There are many differences between secular Western morality and fundamentalist Islam, but those differences appear much larger than they are when both sides use the myth of pure evil to view the events of September 11.

WHY AMPLIFY?

Why do people systematically misunderstand their social worlds, amplifying small differences into large ones? Why do people seem to *like* the myth of pure evil? It is obvious that victims benefit from the "myth" because it frees them from blame, while amplifying the call to arms from potential allies in the struggle against the perpetrator. But it is more difficult to explain why people are drawn to the myth to explain other people's misfortunes. After all, the existence of free-floating evil preying on perfectly innocent victims is an unsettling threat to people's belief in a just world (Lerner & Miller, 1978). Furthermore, listening to the exaggerated claims of others may lead us astray and decrease our chances of forming relationships with ethical people. Perhaps there are other psychological or material benefits to employing the myth of pure evil and exaggerating the separation of good and evil?

The Intuitive Theologian

Tetlock, Kristel, Elson, Green, and Lerner (2000) examined two functionalist frameworks that people are often said to adopt in the judgment and choice literature: the framework of the intuitive scientist, striving to maximize accuracy, and the framework of the intuitive economist, striving to maximize utility. In a series of studies he and his colleagues have demonstrated that these two utilitarian frameworks cannot account for a variety of phenomena in which people seem to be working to satisfy more existential needs. He argues that we sometimes work within the social-functionalist framework of the *intuitive theologian*, which strives to protect sacred values against secular encroachment. For example, Tetlock et al. (2000) asked people to contemplate policies that would create legal commercial markets for body parts, sex, orphans, and other things that are thought by most Americans to be off limits for purchase. Not surprisingly, most people were against such policies. More interestingly, people (particularly political liberals) reported that they would feel high levels of moral outrage toward anyone who favored such policies, or who even contemplated making such "taboo trade-offs." Similarly, Tetlock et al. (2000) showed that religious Christians resisted even considering a set of "heretical counterfactuals," such as "what if Joseph had not believed that Mary was pregnant via the holy ghost and had therefore abandoned her. Jesus would then have grown up in a single-parent household, and would have turned out differently." And across several studies, participants who were forced by the experiment simply to contemplate taboo trade-offs or heretical counterfactuals were more likely to avail themselves of opportunities for "moral cleansing," such as volunteering for organizations dedicated to defending the challenged values.

Tetlock organizes his findings in terms of the "sacred value protection model," which posits that people respond with outrage, disgust, harsh attributions, and enthusiastic support for punishment toward people who are willing even to entertain thoughts that challenge or threaten the collective conscience. In other words, not only do people easily separate the world into a battle of good versus evil, but they readily judge others in terms of whether they are right-thinking or wrong-thinking people. But this is not a final answer, as we can still ask: Why do we need to protect sacred values?

Terror Management Theory

Terror management theory (TMT; see Solomon, Greenberg, & Pyszczynski, Chapter 2, this volume) draws on the work of Becker (1973) to explain the motivation behind moral amplification. Because people know that they will die, they have a continual need ward off or repress a ubiquitous fear of death and insignificance. People do this in part by creating and clinging to heroic narratives. By believing that one is part of a team fighting for virtue and against evil, one attains both a meaningful worldview and a valued place within that worldview. Becker drew on the Freudian notion of transference to explain our attachment to heroes. In transference, a patient transfers the feelings she had toward her parents as a child onto the therapist. She blows the therapist up larger than life to create a powerful figure on whom she can become dependent. Becker suggests that we do the same thing with heroes, all in an attempt to avoid the existential threats of mortality and insignificance. Becker goes further, suggesting that negative or "hate transference" helps to explain our attachment to villains as well:

> It helps us to fix ourselves in the world, to create a target for our own feelings even though those feelings are destructive. We can establish our basic organismic footing with hate as well as by submission. In fact, hate enlivens us more, which is why we see more intense hate in the weaker ego states. The only thing is that hate, too, blows the other person up larger than he deserves. (1973, p. 144)

By continually projecting our childhood feelings of love and hate onto people in our adult world, we can create a rich Manichaean world in which our lives are bound to have meaning.

Whatever one thinks of the psychoanalytic emphasis on childhood, Becker's general claim that fear of death leads to both love and hate has received strong empirical support. The original empirical finding of TMT was in fact moral amplification: After thinking about their own death, participants were more critical of people who violated cultural norms or who were outgroup members, while being more praising of people who upheld group norms (Rosenblatt, Greenberg, Solomon, Pyszczynski, & Lyon, 1989). Even more to the point, Greenberg et al. (1990; expt. 3) found that mortality salience amplified Americans' liking and disliking of people who wrote essays for and against the American system. TMT works particularly well in understanding the moral amplification that occurred after September 11, when Americans were forced to confront their own vulnerability to death on a scale never before seen so directly (see Pyszczynski, Solomon, & Greenberg, 2003).

DIMENSIONS OF SOCIAL COGNITION: HIERARCHY, SOLIDARITY, AND DIVINITY

The theories just described can help us understand the ubiquitous phenomenon of moral amplification. People seem to want to live in a world of saints and demons, but because moral reality is so muddy they resort to a variety of mechanisms to separate the light from the darkness and amplify the difference between good and bad. In this section we propose an additional mechanism that complements those described so far. We suggest that human social cognition is designed to view the social world as being spread out along at least three dimensions of social space, one of which is a specifically moral dimension.

As people interact with each other, they effortlessly and automatically make several absolute appraisals about each other, such as the sex and race of the person. But several other appraisals are relative appraisals, about where the other stands in relation to the self. Social theorists have most often talked about two such dimensions (Brown & Gilman, 1960; Hamilton & Sanders, 1981; Sahlins, 1965), each of which is clearly visible in the lives of other primates (de Waal, 1996). The first is a horizontal dimension sometimes labeled "solidarity" or "closeness," which refers to the fact that in any group, some people are felt to be closer or more allied to the self than are others. Friendship and alliance seem to be universally present features of human and chimpanzee life (Brown, 1991; de Waal, 1996). The second dimension is variously labeled "hierarchy" or "status," and it refers to the fact that individuals in a society usually vary on power or rank. Human societies are quite variable on this dimension, ranging from rigidly structured military orders and caste-based cultures through adamantly egalitarian bands of hunter–gatherers. However, even among egalitarians, there is a cognitive preparedness for life in hierarchies, which is only held in abeyance by chronic vigilance against those who would seize power (Boehm, 1999). The societies of other primates are also quite variable but also generally hierarchically structured (de Waal, 1996; Boehm, 1999).

The human mind seems therefore to be designed to play out its social life along these two dimensions, which can be crossed to create a Cartesian space (see Figure 20.1). As Brown and Gilman (1960) showed, many languages (such as French and German) encode both of these dimensions into their forms of address (e.g., *tu* versus *vous* to connote both familiarity and lower status of the addressee). More interestingly, even in languages such as English, which lack such explicit pronoun coding, speakers find ways to mark the same two dimensions (e.g., using first name, as opposed to title plus last name, to connote both familiarity and lower status of the addressee). These dimensions also correspond to the two dimensions of valence and power that Osgood (1962) found were used in most forms of human appraisal. However there are reasons to believe that there is (at least) one more dimension at work.

Haidt (2000, 2003b) argued that in many cultures people and other social entities are arranged along a vertical dimension that runs from Gods, angels, and saints above down through animals and demons below. This dimension may be labeled "elevation" versus "degradation," "purity" versus "pollution," or, most generally, "divinity" versus

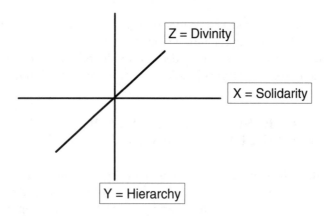

FIGURE 20.1. The three dimensions of social cognition and interaction.

"animality." Such a *scala naturae* or "chain of being" was originally formulated by Plato and Aristotle as a description of the degree of perfection of everything in creation, running from God at the top down through spirits, man, the lower animals, plants, rocks, and finally formless matter. The *scala naturae* was not exactly a moral dimension, for rocks and dirt are not less good than plants and butterflies. But Aristotle's other writings reveal an explicitly vertical moral dimension in which human beings occupy the middle ground between the gods above and the brutes below. He cites the contemporary idea that "an excess of virtue can change a man into a god" (*Nicomachean Ethics*, Bk. VI, 1145a) and he discusses numerous examples of "brutish" behavior found particularly among barbarians. For example:

> . . . the female who is said to rip open pregnant women and devour the infants; or what is related about some of the savage tribes near the black sea, that they delight in eating raw meat of human flesh, and that some of them lend each other their children for a feast. (Bk. VI, 1148b)

It is noteworthy that Aristotle chose examples that blended two types of disgust—physical and moral. The idea that people of "lower" races and castes are polluted both by their physical activities and by their lack of ethics has been found in many parts of the world (e.g., in Nazi attitudes about Jews and in American segregationist attitudes about blacks). In both cases the response by the "superior" group was separation (to guard physical, sexual, and moral purity) and cruelty (justified by the "inhuman" conduct of the "lower" group).

As Christianity grew in the ancient world it brought with it ideas from the Near East about evil and the devil. In the new cosmology, some of the angels on high had sinned and "fallen" down below, converting the *scala naturae* into a truly moral dimension with perfect goodness at the top (the Greek gods had never been perfectly good), and perfect evil at the bottom (Russell, 1988). Human beings were again seen to inhabit a middle region, and to contain elements of both good and evil.

In Hinduism and Buddhism a similar idea appears: that all beings can be placed onto a great vertical line, and that, at least for human beings in the middle regions of this line, one rises and falls based on the virtue of one's deeds (karma) in this life. Doing good works in this life adds to one's karmic bank account, and one comes back at a higher position in the next life. Doing bad deeds subtracts from one's account, making one come back as a lower being the next time around. Hindu conceptions of this vertical dimension differ in important ways from Christian conceptions—for example, the ultimate goal in Hinduism is not to make it to the top but to get off of the line by breaking all attachments, including attachments to good and evil (Klostermaier, 1989). Yet despite these differences, the frequency with which cultures equate up with moral goodness and down with vice or badness suggests that the human mind is predisposed to take verticality as a source domain in our physical embodiment and then use it as a metaphor to structure our social and moral embodiment (Lakoff, 1987). There is even a recent finding that people are quicker to judge the valence of words when good words are presented at the top of a computer screen and bad words on the bottom than when they are presented in reversed positions (Meier & Robinson, in press).

Hinduism also draws our attention to an aspect of verticality that is clear in many world religions: the equation of up with physical purity and down with physical pollution. The daily practice of Hinduism requires great attention to the regulation of one's bodily purity. Events such as defecating, menstruating, or having sex taint a person with a physical essence of corporeality that is seen to be incompatible with approaching God (Fuller, 1992). Hinduism (like Islam, Judaism, and many other religions) prescribes methods of cleansing and purifying the body before one should approach God in prayer or by physically entering holy places. The link between divinity and physical purity may sound odd to modern Christians, who are not required to bathe before entering a church. But in earlier times Cotton Mather's idea that "cleanliness is next to Godliness" may have sounded like a self-evident truth. Even into the 20th century a language of purity and pollution was quite common in Christian writings. For example, one author of advice books for young men (Stall, 1904) urged his readers to bear in mind that "God gave him a moral sense and a spiritual nature, and these elevate him immeasurably above all other creatures of God's hand" (p. 29). To be worthy of this elevated position, Stall urged his readers to guard their personal purity by avoiding polluting practices such as masturbation, eating pork, and reading novels.

Haidt (2003b) has argued that this linkage of divinity, morality, and physical purity is an easy one for human beings to develop because we are all built with a pair of related emotions—disgust and elevation—which will be described in detail later. For now the important point is that people, or cultures, seem predisposed (though not pre-ordained) to interpret their social worlds in terms of a vertical dimension in which divinity, virtue, and physical purity are up, and bestiality, vice, and physical pollution are down.

THE EMOTIONS THAT TELL US ABOUT SAINTS AND DEMONS

Many approaches to emotion have focused on the valenced appraisals that trigger subsequent changes in cognition, motivation, and behavior (Frijda, 1986; Schwarz & Clore, 1996). If we limit ourselves to those appraisals that judge a person's actions against standards or expectations, we can create a 2 x 2 table, crossing positive versus negative evaluation with evaluation of self versus other. Table 1 shows these four cells, with the principal emotions labeled in each cell (following Ortony, Clore, & Collins, 1988, with some updates from Haidt, 2003a). The numbers after each emotion show the number of records found in a PsycInfo search on that term, limited to the title and key phrase fields of all references posted as of March 2003.

Table 20.1 shows a severe imbalance, with far more research done on the negative or blaming emotions than on the positive or praising emotions. Table 20.1 also shows that there has been a moderate amount of work on the "self-praising" emotions such as pride,

TABLE 20.1. Emotions That Judge Agents, and the Number of Articles in PsycINFO for Each Emotion

	Praiseworthy		Blameworthy	
Self	Pride	246	Guilt	2,144
	Self-satisfaction	60	Shame	1,242
Other	Gratitude	60	Anger	3,341
	Admiration	20	Disgust	146
	Elevation[a]	2	Contempt	45

[a]The term "elevation" returned 465 hits, but only two of these referred to elevation as an emotion; the rest referred to the increase in some physical substance such as a hormone.

but that there has been very little work on the "other-praising" emotions, that is, the positive emotions that people feel when other people do good things. In our own research (Algoe & Haidt, 2003) we have begun studying these emotions by asking people to tell us stories about times when they have seen everyday saints and demons. We asked the following specific questions to elicit these stories:

1. Please think of a specific time when you saw someone demonstrating humanity's higher or better nature. Please pick a situation in which you were not the beneficiary, that is, you saw someone doing something good, honorable, or charitable *for someone else.*
2. Please think of a specific time when you saw someone demonstrating humanity's lower or worse nature. Please pick a situation in which you were not the victim, that is, you saw someone do something bad, dishonorable, or sleazy *to someone else.*

We then asked participants to write out their stories and to answer a series of open-ended and rating questions designed to measure the various components of the emotions they remembered feeling, if any. As a control group, we asked a third group of participants to write about a situation we expected to elicit simple happiness. Specifically, we asked people to tell us about a time when "a really good thing happened to you. Please pick a situation in which something that you had really been hoping for, or wanting to happen, finally happened." We used happiness as a comparison because it is the "standard" positive emotion, and we wanted to determine whether responses to good deeds were anything other than simple happiness.

Table 20.2 shows a summary of some of the main findings. As expected, in the Good Event condition people reported feeling happy, wanting to celebrate, and wanting to tell others about their good fortune, or good feelings. In the Good Deed condition, the most commonly reported word is also happiness, but we do not believe participants here are reporting the same kind of happiness as in the Good Event condition. In fact, we believe it is a different positive emotion, which we call elevation. Elevation is a member of the broader emotion family of awe, specifically, awe at a display of moral beauty (Haidt, 2003b; Keltner & Haidt, 2003). The motivations reported in the Good Deed condition suggest the operation of a moral emotion, that is, an emotion that makes people care about the state of the social world, and makes them want to do something to improve it (Haidt, 2003a). Participants reported wanting to do good deeds themselves and wanting to tell other people about the good-deed doer.

Conversely, the Bad Deed condition produced a mix of self-labeled anger and disgust, with motivations that were generally the opposite of the Good Deed condition: to tell others

TABLE 20.2. Summary of Recall Study of Good and Bad Deeds

Elicitor	Good event (something positive happens to you)	Good deed (Someone does something good for another)	Bad deed (someone does something bad to another)
Reported emotion word[a]	• Happy (84%)	• Happy (40%) • Awe/admiration (20%)	• Anger (32%) • Disgust (21%)
Motivations	• Celebrate • Tell others about positive feelings	• Tell others about good person • Praise good person • Be prosocial/emulate	• Tell others about bad person • Chastise bad person
Relationship considerations	• Wanted to spend time with the person who made them feel good	• Gained respect and appreciation for other • Emphasized strengthening/stronger relationship with other	• Lost respect and appreciation for other • Emphasized weakening or distancing selves from relationship with other

[a]The five emotion word clusters listed represent all word clusters that were listed by at least 10% of the sample, and they account for over 60% of participant responses. There were many other idiosyncratic emotion and nonemotion words.

about the bad person and to directly chastise or criticize the person. It is interesting to note that participants in these two conditions often reported updating their degree of respect, admiration, or appreciation for the people in their social worlds. Our hypothesized vertical dimension of divinity is all about maintaining a running balance or scorecard about the virtue of other people. The good and bad deeds that people do cause us to change their scores on this dimension, and each time we make a change, we feel something. These feelings are a kind of information (Schwarz & Clore, 1996) that helps us modify our desires for interaction. For example, when asked if the action changed how the participant felt toward the other, two participants in the Good Deed condition said:

"Yes, it did change the way I think about him. Before this, he was my best friend but after that I even looked up to him as someone with qualities worth emulating."

"The act was completely selfless. The act made me feel very good about human nature for that one instant and I looked up to my classmate as a role model."

In the Bad Deed condition, two participants said:

"I thought he was even more of a weasel."

"The actions of his mother represent the basest nature of man because she was his mother and refused to protect him like a mother should."

Importantly, people experiencing these emotions did their part to amplify the distinctions between good and bad through their behaviors and motivations. Not only did they want to praise or vilify the other publically, they thought about their relationships with the others in new ways. Good deeds often gave rise to a desire for stronger relationships with the virtuous other, while bad deeds did the opposite. If we assume that people sometimes do act on these motivations, at least by gossiping, then we can see how emotions such as elevation, admiration, disgust, and anger help to churn the waters of social relationships, encouraging those who did not witness the original act to choose sides and update their moral registers for the people involved.

These findings fit with an earlier study by Rozin, Lowery, Imada, and Haidt (1999) on the "CAD triad hypothesis." The CAD hypothesis states that the three "other-critical" emotions of contempt, anger, and disgust are linked to the ethics of community, autonomy, and divinity proposed by Shweder, Much, Mahapatra, and Park (1997). These three ethics can be thought of as clusters of moral concerns or goals that vary in strength across cultures. Descriptions of the three ethics that were actually given to participants by Rozin et al. (1999) are as follows:

1. (The ethics of Autonomy). Individual freedom/rights violations. In these cases an action is wrong because it directly hurts another person, or infringes upon his/her rights or freedoms as an individual. To decide if an action is wrong, you think about things like harm, rights, justice, freedom fairness, individualism, and the importance of individual choice and liberty.
2. (The ethics of Community). Community/hierarchy violations. In these cases an action is wrong because a person fails to carry out his or her duties within a community, or to the social hierarchy within the community. To decide if an action is wrong, you think about things like duty, role-obligation, respect for authority, loyalty, group honor, interdependence, and the preservation of the community.
3. (The ethics of Divinity). Divinity/Purity Violations. In these cases a person disrespects the sacredness of God, or causes impurity or degradation to himself/herself, or to others. To decide if an action is wrong, you think about things like sin, the natural order of things, sanctity, and the protection of the soul or the world from degradation and spiritual defilement. (pp. 575–576)

Rozin et al. generated a corpus of 27 situations that were a priori violations of one of the three ethics and then asked participants in the United States and Japan to match the situations to the emotion words "contempt," "anger," and "disgust" (Study 1a); photographs of people making facial expressions of contempt, anger, and disgust (Study 1b); and descriptions of the three ethics, as given previously (Study 2). In an additional study participants were asked to create the facial expression they would make if they actually saw each of the 27 situations occurring. Across all studies and both cultures, a strong relationship was found: violations of the ethics of community were linked with contempt, violations of the ethics of autonomy were linked with anger, and violations of the ethics of divinity were linked with disgust. (The odds of achieving such a neat match of first letters, when no etymological roots are shared, is less than 1 in 10,000.)

The CAD study demonstrates that there is emotional order in the moral world, and that the emotions of contempt, anger, and disgust are common responses to certain classes of violations. Both the CAD study and the Algoe and Haidt study show that anger is the most common emotional response to everyday violations of rights, but that disgust is often triggered in a subclass of cases where people's actions are perceived to be degrading or sleazy.

FUTURE DIRECTIONS FOR THE EXISTENTIAL PSYCHOLOGY OF MORALITY

The creation of a moral world, full of saints and demons, heros and villains, seems to be an important part of the human reaction to existential concerns. Processes such as moral amplification may help to give people a sense that they are part of a larger cosmic struggle, and that they have an important role to play. Morality may therefore be an important area for the future of experimental existential psychology. While work in TMT has already begun to demonstrate both prosocial (Jonas, Schimel, Greenberg, & Pyszczynski, 2003) and antisocial effects of mortality salience (McGregor et al., 1998), we suggest that existential psychology might profitably look to two new sources for inspiration and hypotheses.

First, just as Freud looked to the myths and practices of other cultures, existential psychology should forge links with cultural psychology and psychological anthropology. Mental processes are more clear, vivid, and available for inspection in some cultures than in others. For example, processes related to purity and pollution, hierarchy, and caste divisions (which are based on hierarchy as well as purity) have been extensively described by anthropologists in India, and these psychosocial facts seem to play an important role in providing Indians with a sense of meaning and belonging. Yet many of the same processes seem to be at work in modern Western cultures, although people have much more difficulty talking about them because such issues are politically unacceptable in a democratic society. For example, the emergence of "cooties" (invisible contagion from children of the opposite sex, or from unpopular children) among American children in elementary school seems quite puzzling, unless one views cooties as the emergence of the mental machinery of purity and pollution, which is then left relatively unsupported by a somewhat egalitarian culture (Haidt, 2001).

Second, just as psychology is currently experiencing a (re)birth of positive psychology, existential psychologists might profitably think about whether there is such a thing as existential positive psychology. The origins of existential psychology in the work of Freud and Becker guarantees that constructs such as fear of death, anxiety, isolation, and the search for meaning in an intrinsically meaningless world will be at the heart of the field. But experimental existential psychologists should be careful about automatically assuming that the positive parts of life (e.g., love, parenting, altruism, creativity, and productive work) are always driven by or reactions to fear, loneliness, and alienation. As humanistic psychology argued (Maslow, 1970), there may be some more thoroughly positive and growth oriented processes and motives at work as well. The positive emotions, such as elevation and awe, offer one possible starting point (Fredrickson, 1998; Keltner & Haidt, 2003). Existential psychology and positive psychology may each help the other to avoid lying down in a Procrustean bed.

William James (1902/1961) said "Mankind's common instinct for reality . . . has always held the world to be essentially a theater for heroism" (quoted by Becker, 1973, p. 1). If so, then moral amplification and moral emotions such as elevation and disgust help set the stage.

REFERENCES

Algoe, S. B., & Haidt, J. (2003). *Witnessing virtue in others: Evidence for distinct positive emotions.* Unpublished manuscript, University of Virginia.

Aristotle (1941). Nichomachean ethics (W. D. Ross, Trans.). In R. McKeon (Ed.), *The basic works of Aristotle* (pp. 927–1112). New York: Random House.

Baumeister, R. F. (1997). *Evil: Inside human cruelty and violence.* New York: Freeman.

Baumeister, R. F., Stillwell, A., & Wotman, S. R. (1990). Victim and perpetrator accounts of interpersonal conflict: Autobiographical narratives about anger. *Journal of Personality and Social Psychology, 59,* 994–1005.

Becker, E. (1973). *The denial of death.* New York: Free Press.

Boehm, C. (1999). *Hierarchy in the forest: The evolution of egalitarian behavior.* Cambridge, MA: Harvard University Press.

Brown, D. E. (1991). *Human universals.* Philadelphia: Temple University Press.

Brown, R., & Gilman, A. (1960). The pronouns of power and solidarity. In T. A. Sebeok (Ed.), *Style in language* (pp. 253–276). Cambridge, MA: MIT Press.

de Waal, F. (1996). *Good natured: The origins of right and wrong in humans and other animals.* Cambridge, MA: Harvard University Press.

Dhammapada: The sayings of the Buddha (T. Byrom, Trans.) (1993). Boston: Shambhala.

Fredrickson, B. L. (1998). What good are positive emotions? *Review of General Psychology, 2,* 300–319.

Frijda, N. (1986). *The emotions.* Cambridge, UK: Cambridge University Press.

Fuller, C. J. (1992). *The camphor flame: Popular Hinduism and society in India.* Princeton, NJ: Princeton University Press.

Greenberg, J., Pyszczynski, T., Solomon, S., Rosenblatt, A. V., M., Kirkland, S., & Lyon, D. (1990). Evidence for terror management theory II: The effects of mortality salience on reactions to those who threaten or bolster the cultural worldview. *Journal of Personality and Social Psychology, 58,* 308–318.

Haidt, J. (2000). The positive emotion of elevation. *Prevention and Treatment, 3,* n.p.

Haidt, J. (2001). The emotional dog and its rational tail: A social intuitionist approach to moral judgment. *Psychological Review, 108,* 814–834.

Haidt, J. (2003a). The moral emotions. In R. J. Davidson, K. R. Scherer & H. H. Goldsmith (Eds.), *Handbook of affective sciences* (pp. 852–870). Oxford, UK: Oxford University Press.

Haidt, J. (2003b). Elevation and the positive psychology of morality. In C. L. M. Keyes & J. Haidt (Eds.), *Flourishing: Positive psychology and the life well-lived* (pp. 275–289). Washington, DC: American Psychological Association.

Hamilton, V. L., & Sanders, J. (1981). The effects of roles and deeds on responsibility judgements: The normative structure of wrongdoing. *Social Psychology Quarterly, 44,* 237–254.

James, W. (1961). *The varieties of religious experience.* New York: Macmillan. (Original work published 1902)

Jefferson, T. (1975). Letter to Robert Skipwith. In M. D. Peterson (Ed.), *The portable Thomas Jefferson* (pp. 349–351). New York: Penguin.

Jonas, E., Schimel, J., Greenberg, J., & Pyszczynski, T. (2003). The Scrooge effect: Evidence that mortality salience increases prosocial attitudes and behavior. *Personality and Social Psychology Bulletin, 28,* 1342–1353.

Keltner, D., & Haidt, J. (2003). Approaching awe, a moral, spiritual, and aesthetic emotion. *Cognition and Emotion, 17,* 297–314.

Klostermaier, K. (1989). *A survey of Hinduism.* Albany: State University of New York Press.

Kunda, Z. (1990). The case for motivated reasoning. *Psychological Bulletin, 108,* 480–498.

Lakoff, G. (1987). *Women, fire, and dangerous things.* Chicago: University of Chicago Press.

Lerner, M. J., & Miller, D. T. (1978). Just world research and the attribution process: Looking back and ahead. *Psychological Bulletin, 85,* 1030–1051.

Maslow, A. H. (1970). *Motivation and personality* (2nd ed.). New York: Harper & Row.

McGregor, H., Lieberman, J., Greenberg, J., Solomon, S., Arndt, J., Simon, L., et al. (1998). Terror management and aggression: Evidence that mortality salience promotes aggression toward worldview-threatening individuals. *Journal of Personality and Social Psychology, 74,* 590–605.

Meier, B. P., & Robinson, M. D. (in press). Why the sunny side is up: Automatic inferences about stimulus valence based on vertical position. *Psychological Science.*

Ortony, A., Clore, G. L., & Collins, A. (1988). *The cognitive structure of the emotions.* Cambridge, UK: Cambridge University Press.

Osgood, C. E. (1962). Studies on the generality of affective meaning systems. *American Psychologist 17,* 10–28.

Pyszczynski, T., & Greenberg, J. (1987). Toward an integration of cognitive and motivational perspectives on social inference: A biased hypothesis-testing model. *Advances in Experimental Social Psychology, 20,* 297–340.

Pyszczynski, T., Solomon, S., & Greenberg, J. (2003). *In the wake of 9/11: The psychology of terror.* Washington, DC: American Psychological Association.

Robinson, R. J., Keltner, D., Ward, A., & Ross, L. (1995). Actual versus assumed differences in construal: "Naive realism" in intergroup perception and conflict. *Journal of Personality and Social Psychology, 68,* 404–417.

Rosenblatt, A., Greenberg, J., Solomon, S., Pyszczynski, T., & Lyon, D. (1989). Evidence for terror management theory: I. The effects of mortality salience on reactions to those who violate or uphold cultural values. *Journal of Personality and Social Psychology, 57,* 681–690.

Ross, L. (1977). The intuitive psychologist and his shortcomings: Distortions in the attribution process. In L. Berkowitz, (Ed.), *Advances in experimental social psychology* (Vol. 10, pp. 174–214). New York: Academic Press.

Rozin, P., Lowery, L., Imada, S., & Haidt, J. (1999). The CAD triad hypothesis: A mapping between three moral emotions (contempt, anger, disgust) and three moral codes (community, autonomy, divinity). *Journal of Personality and Social Psychology, 76,* 574–586.

Russell, J. B. (1988). *The prince of darkness: Radical evil and the power of good in history.* Ithaca, NY: Cornell University Press.

Sahlins, M. (1965). On the sociology of primitive exchange. In M. Banton (Ed.), *The relevance of models for social anthropology* (pp. 139–236). London: Tavistock.

Schwarz, N., & Clore, G. L. (1996). Feelings and phenomenal experiences. In E. T. Higgins & A. W. Kruglanski (Eds.), *Social psychology: Handbook of basic principles* (pp. 433–465). New York: Guilford Press.

Shweder, R. A., Much, N. C., Mahapatra, M., & Park, L. (1997). The "big three" of morality (autonomy, community, and divinity), and the "big three" explanations of suffering. In A. Brandt & P. Rozin (Eds.), *Morality and health* (pp. 119–169). New York: Routledge.

Stall, S. (1904). *What a young man ought to know.* London: Vir.

Tetlock, P. E., Kristel, O. V., Elson, B., Green, M., & Lerner, J. (2000). The psychology of the unthinkable: Taboo trade-offs, forbidden base rates, and heretical counterfactuals. *Journal of Personality and Social Psychology, 78,* 853–870.

Wilson, R. M. (1967). Mani and Manichaeism. In P. Edwards (Ed.) *The encyclopedia of philosophy* (Vols. 5–6, pp. 149–150). New York: Macmillan.

Chapter 21

Ostracism

A Metaphor for Death

TREVOR I. CASE
KIPLING D. WILLIAMS

> If no one turned round when we entered, answered when we spoke, or minded what we did, but if every person we met 'cut us dead,' and acted as if we were non-existing things, a kind of rage and impotent despair would ere long well up in us, from which the cruelest bodily tortures would be a relief; for these would make us feel that, however bad might be our plight, we had not sunk to such a depth as to be unworthy of attention at all.
> —WILLIAM JAMES, *The Principles of Psychology* (1890/1950, pp. 293–294)

This quote from James's classic, *The Principles of Psychology*, encapsulates the necessity of social recognition and inclusion for the definition and survival of the social self. The social self is created and reflected in the presence of others (Mead, 1934), but, we would argue, only when those present take notice of the individual. It flourishes in positive social interaction, is wounded in negative interaction, but resides in psychological limbo when there is no interaction whatsoever. So desperate is our need to be woven into the tapestry of social life, it is hardly surprising that we might prefer physical assault to being ignored or excluded. In this sense, being shunned by our social network is tantamount to social death.

Since James's insightful observation over a century ago there has been renewed interest in psychology on the topic of social ostracism, social exclusion, and rejection[1] (see Williams, 2001, for review). In keeping with the overarching theme of this book, we report research that has used experimental methods to investigate the human struggle to come to terms with one of life's basic realities—the inevitable occurrence of being ignored and excluded. In this chapter, we describe the central tenets of a theoretical model of social ostracism and review research that casts light on the predictions of this model. We go on to examine the consequences of social ostracism and conclude by discussing the parallels between ostracism and reminders of death.

WHAT IS OSTRACISM?

Ostracism occurs when an individual or a group excludes or ignores other individuals or groups (Williams, 1997). It is a pervasive and powerfully aversive social phenomena, cutting across all cultures and reported throughout history (Gruter & Masters, 1986). The term "ostracism" derives from the ancient Greek practice (488 B.C.) of voting to exile individuals with political ambitions, where citizens of Athens would cast their vote using shards of pottery called *ostraca* (Zippelius, 1986). The many everyday terms used to refer to ostracism, such as "the silent treatment," "the cold shoulder," "time out" and "shunning," reflect the ubiquity of this social phenomenon. In fact, a representative U.S. survey of over 2,000 people revealed that 67% admitted to using the silent treatment on a loved one and 75% reported that the silent treatment had been used on them by a loved one (Faulkner, Williams, Sherman, & Williams, 1997). Although these figures are high, the general tendency to underreport behaviors that are not socially desirable (Krosnick, 1999) suggests that these actually underestimate the true incidence of ostracism.

Ostracism is used by institutions (e.g., governments and religions), small groups (employees in the workplace, tribal groups), and individuals (spouse, parent) in response to unacceptable behavior (Williams, 2001). In this sense, ostracism may often signal that the target of ostracism has transgressed and, as a consequence, the lifeline to his or her social network has been severed. For example, in one case study a class of preschoolers successfully controlled the bullying behavior of one student by spontaneously ignoring him and excluding him from games (Barner-Barry, 1986). What greater punishment can members of a social network bring to bear on one of their kind than to deny his or her social existence?

However, ostracism is not always used as a punitive measure. There are also many occasions where it occurs because the target is not considered worthy of attention. In Wertmüller's film *Swept Away* (Cardarelli & Wertmüller, 1975), the lower-class protagonist, Gennarino, finds work on a luxury yacht in view of a beautiful and rich woman, Rafaella, who is sunbathing in the nude. Gennarino later reveals that her lack of modesty reflected that he was no more important to her than an animal. Similarly, Muzafir Sherif posed as a janitor in the famous "Robbers Cave" experiments, so that he could be in the social presence of the boys while not inhibiting their conversations and behaviors. He reasoned that as a janitor, he would be ignored by the children. Like Ralph Ellison's (1952) *Invisible Man*, Sherif took advantage of his invisibility. In such situations the target is not being punished; rather, because of his or her perceived lowly status, race, or religion, others are oblivious to him or her—it would not matter if he or she existed or not (Williams, 1997; 2001). Thus, ostracism may reflect an unworthiness of attention rather than a deliberate act to punish. We believe that Sherif and Ellison notwithstanding, given the choice, most people would prefer punitive ostracism over oblivious ostracism. Consistent with James's reasoning in the opening quote, at least when ostracism is perceived to be punitive, the target of the ostracism feels worthy of others' deliberate and effortful inattention.

One of the most extraordinary accounts of the dire consequences of being cut off from one's social network comes from the early anthropological literature. The belief that death can result from magical rituals, incantations, and curses has been common among many tribal peoples of Africa, South America, Australia, New Zealand, and the Pacific Islands

(Zusne & Jones, 1989). Generally referred to as voodoo death after the Haitian form of the phenomenon, belief in the witchdoctor's death spell has the effect of bringing about the victim's own demise. However, for a group of Aboriginal people from the Northern Territory of Australia, a crucial component of voodoo death is the withdrawal of all social support once the spell has been cast (Cannon, 1942). The collectivist nature of Aboriginal culture only underlines the importance Aborigines place on social connections. Believing that their fate has been sealed by the death spell and with the addition of being ostracized by family and friends, the unfortunate individual often perished (Cannon, 1942).

Equally remarkable are the few people who suffer from Cotard's delusion (Langdon & Coltheart, 2000). These individuals have the belief that they are dead, nonexisting entities. To make sense of their ability to reflect on their own death, they often reason that this is what death must be like: These individuals can watch others with whom they used to be familiar as they carry on with their lives, but notably, the typical affective sense of familiarity is gone. Thus, individuals with Cotard's delusion deduces they have no feelings because they are dead. Although hallucinations such as rotting skin or gums may or may not accompany this startling delusion, depression is *always* associated with it.

From our description thus far, ostracism would appear to be a higher-order complex social behavior. However, it is not exclusive to humans. Instinctive behaviors that ward off intruders from a designated territory and thus exclude others from food and opportunities to mate are common to many animals (Kurzban & Leary, 2001). Furthermore, status hierarchies present in such species as birds, lions, and primates, render those occupying the lowest ranks ostracized and deprived of access to resources (Kurban & Leary, 2001). In addition, primates ostracize group members who have made unsuccessful leadership attempts, or who are ill or behaving abnormally (de Waal, 1986; Goodall, 1986). To the extent that such animal behavior parallels human behaviors, ostracism may represent a deep and primitive response that serves a similar adaptive function across many species. Nonetheless, human ostracism occurs within the context of a uniquely rich and complex social world and the reasons for ostracism and its consequences reflect this complexity. Thus ostracism in humans is not confined to territoriality, status transgressions, or the ill. Therefore, its interpretation and meaning go beyond attributions of territory invasion, hierarchy struggles, and fitness. Because humans have the capacity to consider and reflect on their own mortality, ostracism also presents a powerful and palpable mortality metaphor. In effect, being subjected to ostracism is experiencing what life would be like if one was dead. This observation that depression would follow from feelings of nonexistence foreshadows our predictions of the consequences of long-term ostracism, to which we return later.

Most everyday instances of ostracism comprise short-term episodes where the target is ignored for a brief interval and is then, after some suffering, reincluded (Williams, Wheeler, & Harvey (2001). When a friend doesn't reply to your e-mail, your superior fails to acknowledge your greeting, or your spouse gives you the silent treatment after an argument, the episode of ostracism may last anywhere from a few minutes to a couple of days. By far, the majority of research on ostracism concerns these type of short-term episodes because they can be ethically and easily investigated in the laboratory. However, for many people, episodes of ostracism endure for months or years, often leading to helplessness, despair, and depression (Faulkner & Williams, 1995; Williams & Zadro, 1999, 2001). In an interview study on long-term ostracism, Faulkner and Williams report the tragic account of "Lee," who was ostracized by her late husband for the last 40 years of his life. For 40 years Lee and her husband never ate at the same table, nor did he speak or make eye contact with her, even during sex! Ironically, after the torment of almost a lifetime of ostracism, Lee could not even remember why it began in the first place. In her 70s at the time of interview, Lee reflected, "I wish he would've beaten me instead of giving me the silent treatment, because at least it would have been a response. This has ruined my life—I have no chance for happiness now . . . " (Williams, 1997, p.17).

Although the preponderance of literature focuses on short-term ostracism, there is some evidence to suggest that, at least initially, similar processes underlie both short- and long-term ostracism (see Williams, 1997, 2001). Accordingly, our laboratory investigations, which typically invoke episodes of ostracism as short as 5 minutes, also provide insight into the nature of more enduring ostracism. We now go on to review this literature on ostracism and discuss Williams's (1997, 2001) model of social ostracism. In this review we also draw on relevant findings from the related literature on social exclusion (exclusion without specific reference to ignoring) and rejection (expelling, often accompanied by derogation).

A NEEDS-THREAT MODEL OF OSTRACISM

Based on existing social psychological theory and empirical findings from the literature on ostracism, Williams (1997, 2001) advanced a model of ostracism. This model is intended to provide a framework for which systematic and theory-driven investigations could proceed. Williams's model details taxonomic dimensions, antecedent conditions, variables that moderate and mediate ostracism, and reactions to ostracism (see Williams, 2001, for a detailed discussion of all aspects of the model). Within the taxonomic dimensions lies one distinction that we think is pertinent to existential psychology. Whereas most motives of ostracism (by those who are ostracizing, and perceived by those who are ostracized) are intentional and punitive, two are not: role-prescribed and oblivious. When these motives are operating or perceived, they imply that the target of ostracism is not worthy of attention. From the perspective of the ostracizers, the targets are not on their "radar." When role-prescribed, it is because the cultural norms dictate that acknowledging the existence of another is unnecessary or even inappropriate, as when elevator riders look up and forward, not acknowledging the presence of their co-riders. When oblivious, however, a more sinister attribution can be made, that despite being in a situation in which the cultural norms would encourage recognition of others, the target goes about unnoticed. This, we argue, suggests to the targets that they are so unworthy of attention; it is as though they do not exist at all.

The consequences of ostracism signaling punishment or lack of worth play out in the core of the model, that ostracism individually and simultaneously threatens four basic needs.

Threatened Needs

When targets are excluded or ignored their needs for belonging, self-esteem, control, and meaningful existence are threatened. There is much evidence to suggest that these needs are each fundamental to human well-being and that they underlie most social behavior (e.g., Smith & Mackie, 1995). Accordingly, we do not suggest that they are only affected by ostracism. Nor do we argue that the four needs are mutually exclusive; there is evidence to suggest that each need might subsume the others. For example, according to the sociometer hypothesis, self-esteem might serve as an indicator when the need for belonging is threatened (Leary, Tambor, Terdal, & Downs, 1995). Furthermore, self-esteem has been implicated to play a critical role in buffering people from reminders of the meaninglessness of

existence (Solomon, Greenberg, & Pyszczynski, Chapter 2, this volume). Having acknowledged these caveats, the model holds that ostracism threatens these four needs and that
reactions to ostracism reflect attempts to restore threatened needs.

Belonging

As we described in the introduction, ostracism threatens our need for frequent, positive, and
stable connections with others—the need for belonging (see also Pinel, Long, Landau, &
Pyszczynski, Chapter 22, this volume). In their review of the literature on intimacy and
affiliation, Baumeister and Leary (1995) maintain that the need to belong is important for
emotional stability and eroded need for belonging is associated with a range of negative psychological and physical consequences such as depression, anxiety, and mental illness (see
also Shaver & Mikulincer, 2003, for the relatedness between belonging and attachment
styles). Moreover, those who do not enjoy close interpersonal connections also tend to be
more likely to engage in criminal and antisocial behavior than those who are part of a close
social network (Baumeister & Leary, 1995). In terms of evolution, coexisting with others in
social groups would confer the advantage of increasing opportunities for reproduction and
other resources (see Buss, 1990). Compared to other forms of rejection, ostracism may pose
a particularly powerful threat to the need for belonging because it represents the severing of
social contact with the target. Other forms of verbal and physical aggression, although
likely to trigger rejection fears, still acknowledge the target's existence and as such the target
maintains a social attachment with the source.

Self-Esteem

The need to maintain a high self-esteem is another vital need that is threatened by ostracism.
Maintaining high self-esteem is both adaptive and necessary for psychological well-being
(Greenberg et al., 1992; Steele, 1988; Tesser, 1988). Being rejected by others as unworthy of
attention or acknowledgment is enough, in itself, to threaten a target's self-esteem. However,
when the reasons for ostracism are unclear, targets are prompted to search for reasons *why*
they are being ostracized. Unfortunately, such a search often yields self-depreciating justifications for this treatment, further lowering self-esteem. In a related vein, Sommer and
Baumeister (2002) demonstrated that those with low self-esteem might be particularly prone
to self-deprecation and giving up when they are ostracized.

Control

Another basic need suggested by Williams's (1997, 2001) model to be threatened by ostracism is to perceive one has a sufficient level of control over one's social environment. The
need for control has long been identified as a basic human motivation in the psychological
literature (e.g., deCharms, 1968; White, 1959). People attempt to control their environment
to attain positive outcomes and avoid negative outcomes, suggesting that the existence of a
need for control has considerable adaptive value. Furthermore, even the mere perception of
control is associated with psychological and physical well-being (e.g., Taylor & Brown,
1988), whereas undermined perceptions of control are associated with reactance (Wortman
& Brehm, (1975), followed by helplessness and other negative consequences (Abramson,
Seligman, & Teasdale, 1978; Seligman, 1975). Ostracism poses a direct threat to the target's
ability to control the social interaction and often leaves him or her feeling frustrated and

helpless: It is imposed upon the target and there is little the target can do to affect outcomes in the conflict.

Meaningful Existence

Central to the theme of this book, the final need proposed to be threatened by ostracism is the need for meaningful existence. The empirical evidence from the extensive terror management literature points to the fact that people constantly attempt to buffer themselves from the terror that derives from acknowledging the inherent meaninglessness of existence and the inevitability of their own mortality (for a review see Solomon, Greenberg, & Pyszczynski, Chapter 2, this volume). Ostracism, more than any other form of interpersonal conflict, involves cutting off targets from their social network. Effectively, the target ceases to exist as a social being. In a vivid example of this social death, Sudnow (1967) described accounts of hospital staff ignoring terminally ill patients and pushing their eyelids shut before they were clinically dead. More horrifying, two physicians even discussed a dying patient's forthcoming autopsy, at the bedside.

To assert their presence and establish their social existence, targets of ostracism may attempt to seize attention, even negative attention. Furthermore, the withdrawal of attention and recognition that characterizes ostracism may remind targets of their fragile and temporary existence, and its lack of meaning and worth. Relegated to a position of impotence and invisibility, it is hardly surprising that targets of ostracism often report questioning their own existence (e.g., Williams, Shore, & Grahe, 1998).

Reactions to Ostracism

Williams's model suggests that the inescapable and automatic initial response to ostracism is reacting with negative affect, hurt feelings, and physiological arousal. However, after this automatic response, targets are expected to engage in behaviorally, emotionally, or cognitively controlled acts to repair their threatened needs. This assumed direct relationship between need deprivation and need fulfillment is consistent with the research on needs for belonging (Baumeister & Leary, 1995), self-esteem (Steele, 1988), control (Friedland, Keinan, & Regev, 1992) and meaningful existence (Greenberg et al., 1990). Attempts to repair threatened needs are expected to be confined to the consequences of short-term and infrequent acts of ostracism. In cases of chronic or long-term ostracism, depleted coping resources may eventually give way to alienation, despair, and depression. We now go on to review some of the empirical evidence for Williams's (1997, 2001) model of ostracism, focusing specifically on the key element of the model that reactions to short-term ostracism reflect attempts to regain threatened needs for belonging, self-esteem, control and meaningful existence.

RESEARCH ON OSTRACISM AND NEEDS THREAT

Improving Inclusionary Status

Targets of ostracism may restore threatened needs either by reestablishing social ties with those who are ostracizing them or by affiliating with others. Prosocial behavior such as apologizing or attempting to conform should be motivated principally by needs to fulfill belonging (affiliation with others) and self-esteem (reinclusion implies positive evaluation).

Following successful reinclusion, needs for control (agency over the interaction) and meaningful existence (recognition and attention; affirmation of social existence) should also be fulfilled.

To test the assumptions of the model, Williams developed a minimal ostracism paradigm (see Williams, 1997; Williams & Sommer, 1997). In this procedure, two carefully trained confederates of the experimenter either include or exclude an unsuspecting participant in an incidental game of catch whilst in a waiting room. After receiving the ball for 1 minute, those in the ostracism condition are cut out of the game by the two confederates, who proceed to throw the ball only to each other. Furthermore, the confederates even cut off all eye contact with the participant and ignore any attempts to be reincluded. In short, the confederates behave as if the participant is not there. In contrast, the remaining participants are included throughout the game. After 5 minutes of ball tossing, the experimenter returns to the waiting room to commence the experimental session. This method of inducing ostracism reliably increases ratings of feelings of being ignored and excluded and has been demonstrated to threaten each of the four needs as measured by self report rating (e.g., see Williams, Case, & Govan, 2003, Study 1).

After manipulating ostracism using this ball-tossing paradigm, Williams and Sommer (1997) had participants generate as many uses for an object as possible. Importantly, the participants performed this task either collectively (where only the group performance counted) or coactively (where individual performances were compared within the group). They found that female participants performed much better when they are required to complete this task collectively than when they completed it coactively. Consistent with the idea that threatened belonging would motivated attempts to be reincluded, it appeared that these participants were socially compensating in a prosocial attempt to appease the confederates who had just ostracized them. The failure to detect any differences for males may have reflected an overriding tendency of males to engage in social loafing in the collective task.

In another study using the same ball-tossing paradigm, participants were shown a recruitment videotape for either a reputable or a dubious student group after they were included or ostracized (Wheaton, 2002, reported in Williams et al., 2003, Study 1). In the reputable group condition, a smart, casually dressed spokesperson described the activities of his group as focusing on improving study habits, helping members to chose their best career path, and increasing communication skills. In contrast, the spokesperson for the dubious group was dressed in tie-dyed garments and described the activities of his group as learning how to harness personal psychic energies. The results showed that ostracized participants were more attracted to the spokesperson than were included participants, regardless of whether they saw the reputable or the dubious videotape. Again, this suggests that ostracized participants attempt to refortify threatened needs by forming bonds with others—even with those who were not involved in the episode of ostracism.

In an Internet version of the ball-tossing paradigm, called Cyberball, Williams, Cheung, and Choi (2000) had participants engage in a virtual game of catch with two other online participants as part of mental visualization task. In fact, the two online participants were computer controlled and after an initial phase of inclusion participants were randomly allocated to an inclusion or exclusion condition. Like the ball-tossing paradigm, Cyberball, has proved to be an effective way of manipulating ostracism and has reliable effects on self-report needs threat (Williams et al., 2002). After completing the Cyberball phase of the experiment, participants were reassigned to a new six-person group in which they completed an Asch-type social conformity task. Ostracized participants demonstrated greater conformity than included participants, again suggesting that prosocial attempts to be reincluded may also be directed beyond the sources of ostracism.

Such prosocial responses to ostracism may reflect an increased tendency to focus on social information when belonging is threatened. Gardner, Pickett, and Brewer (2000) found that participants who were excluded from a chat room discussion subsequently demonstrated enhanced memory of social information presented in a diary. Moreover, they suggest that this focus on social information represents a desire to refortify the need for belonging, threatened by rejection. Together with research using other paradigms to induce ostracism, such as the conversation paradigm and role-play paradigms (see Williams, 2001), ostracism often results in prosocial attempts to refortify threatened needs.

Asserting Control and Demanding Attention

We have argued that prosocial reactions to ostracism such as conformity and increased effort in cooperative tasks may reflect attempts to improve inclusionary status (belonging) and to be positively evaluated (self-esteem). However, attempts to refortify needs for control and meaningful existence may actually thwart the targets chances of being reincluded. In terms of control, one way a target can overcome the frustration associated with being powerless over the course of the interaction or associated with the overall threat to belonging, self-esteem, and meaningful existence is to respond aggressively. Likewise, threats to meaningful existence may be associated with desperate attempts to seize attention and recognition, which may result in behavior that is provocative, antisocial, or aggressive.

In a first attempt to investigate the relationship between ostracism and a behavioral measure of control, Lawson-Williams and Williams (1998) either ostracized or included participants using the ball-tossing paradigm described earlier. However, the two confederates either posed as friends with each other or as strangers. After the ball-tossing task, apparently as part of a nonverbal messages study, participants were given the task of identifying a concealed card that another participant (a third confederate) was looking at. They were informed that research has shown that each side of a person's face reveals different types of nonverbal cues and that to determine the identity of the concealed card, they should request "head turns" of the card holder. Targets who were ostracized by two friends made more head-turn requests than did included participants. In a follow-up study, targets who were ostracized by friends also indicated greater desire for control on a state form of the Desire for Control scale (Burger, 1992). These findings provided evidence that ostracism increases the need for control and that, if the opportunity presents itself, targets will attempt to regain this lost control even if it means gaining control in an unrelated situation. Moreover, the findings suggest that frustration associated with being powerless over the course of the interaction might be particularly salient when the target is faced with the futility of interacting with people who already share close personal connections.

Attempts to regain control or recognition (and we believe recognition to be a precursor to meaningful existence) in response to ostracism may also manifest as antisocial or aggressive acts. Targets of ostracism have been found to retaliate against sources (Thompson & Richardson, 1983) and rate them as less likeable and interpersonally attractive (Insko & Wilson, 1977). Moreover, in their review of 15 school shootings, Leary, Kowalski, Smith, and Phillips (2003) revealed that 13 of the cases were associated with some form of ostracism, bullying, or romantic rejection, although other risk factors such as depression and interest in firearms were also present. Interestingly, targets of ostracism may experience conflicting motivations: On the one hand they are motivated to enhance their inclusionary status, driven by needs for belonging and self-esteem. On the other hand, attempts to assert control and seize attention may have the effect of repelling others. The result of these conflicting motivations may be that attempts to improve inclusionary status typically emerge as overt attitudes and behaviors, while antisocial urges are kept under wraps.

To explore this idea, Govan, Case, and Williams (2002) used the Cyberball paradigm to manipulate ostracism. They then gave participants an implicit association test (IAT; Greenwald, McGee, & Schwartz, 1998) designed to assess attitudes toward Aboriginal and Europeans, using Sydney train station names of either Aboriginal or European origin. The IAT has been used to assess a variety of socially sensitive attitudes including racial attitudes (e.g., Dasgupta, McGee, Greenwald, & Banaji, 2000). In our study, the IAT was not used as an absolute diagnosis of prejudice (a prospect debated by many) but, rather, as a dependent variable that we hypothesized would indicate stronger negative associations with Aboriginals following ostracism. The advantage of using the IAT to measure attitudes toward race is that it circumvents socially desirable responding and explicit attempts to impression manage. In addition to obtaining an implicit measure of racial attitudes, Govan et al. also obtained an explicit measure of prejudice towards Aboriginals, by administering a racism scale (Pedersen & Walker, 1997). The findings revealed that ostracized targets had stronger negative associations with Aboriginal people on the IAT than did included targets. Yet, there were no differences between the ostracized and included targets on the explicit measure of racism. This finding provides support for the idea that negative sentiment below the surface may coexist with prosocial attempts to improve exclusionary status.

Antisocial responses to ostracism have also been observed in series of studies by Twenge, Baumeister, Tice, and Stucke (2001). In these experiments, social exclusion was manipulated by informing targets that they had been rejected by other participants or by providing false personality feedback indicating that they would end up having a life alone. Participants were then give the opportunity to aggress against another person who had just insulted them. As expected, excluded targets gave more negative job evaluations and blasted this person with higher levels of white noise during a competitive computer game. Furthermore, excluded targets even blasted an innocent stranger (who had offered no insult) with higher levels of white noise, compared to those who were included. However, if the stranger offered praise, excluded targets were not more aggressive. Praise may have had the effect of restoring self-esteem and belonging, which may have, in turn, diminished the needs to assert control.

In an attempt to investigate the role of control in aggressive responding to ostracism more closely, Warburton (2002) exposed targets of ostracism to either controlled or uncontrolled aversive stimuli and then gave the them the opportunity to aggress. After completing an initial ball-tossing phase, participants were subjected to uncontrolled bursts of aversive noise or were given personal control over the onset of each noise burst. The final phase of the experiment comprised Lieberman, Solomon, Greenberg, and McGregor's (1999) aggression measure where, participants were given the opportunity to assist the experimenter by anonymously allocating a taste sample to another (unknown) participant. In all cases, the food sample was hot chili sauce, and the amount of chili sauce allocated by participants served as the measure of aggression. The results showed that ostracism did increase aggressive responding (chili sauce allocation), but only for those targets who were exposed to uncontrolled aversive noise. Importantly, targets of ostracism who were given the opportunity to restore a sense of personal control (controlling the aversive noise) were no more likely to aggress than were included participants.

Together this research suggests that in the attempt to restore threatened needs, targets often attempt to reinstate their social ties by behaving prosocially. However, threatened needs for control and meaningful existence may result in behavior that is counterproductive to the goal of reinclusion. As such, provocative and aggressive responses to threatened control and meaningful existence are usually covert.

Other Findings to Emerge from Experimental Investigations

Regardless of whether the consequences of ostracism are prosocial or antisocial, one robust finding to emerge from this literature is that the effects of ostracism cannot be accounted for by negative affect. That is, although ostracism typically increases negative affect, mood does not meditate the relationship between ostracism and its consequences (e.g., Twenge et al., 2001; Williams et al., 2000), which suggests that ostracism poses a very basic and unique threat to the individual. This depth and primitiveness of the response to ostracism is illustrated by two studies using the Cyberball paradigm (Zadro, Williams, & Richardson, 2003). In Study 1, participants were told they were playing Cyberball with two other participants at nearby universities, or that they were playing the computer. Half of the participants were included and half were ostracized. Self-reported levels of the four needs (belonging, control, self-esteem, and meaningful existence) and mood were measured. Not surprisingly, all four needs and mood dropped significantly when the individual was ostracized; surprisingly, it did not matter whether the individual was ostracized by people or by the computer. In Study 2, Zadro et al. (2003) crossed the aforementioned manipulations with whether individuals believed the others (or the computer) were scripted to do what they did or whether it was under their (or the computer's) control. Again, significant drops in need levels and mood occurred for those who were ostracized, but whether they were playing people or the computer and whether or not the people or computer were scripted to ostracize made no difference. We believe these results suggest that even a "whiff of ostracism" is enough to trigger automatic responses that signal needs threat. These automatic responses would seem to be evolutionarily adaptive: Threats to these needs have very real implications for social and physical survival.

To summarize, the research on ostracism has resulted in the development of several experimental paradigms that can be effectively used to investigate short-term ostracism. The results of the many experimental investigations using various ostracism paradigms have provided support for the key assumption of Williams's (1997, 2001) model and suggest that sensitivity to being ostracized is a basic and low-level process.

OSTRACISM AND SOCIAL DEATH

Our experimental investigations have determined that ostracism powerfully threatens needs for belonging, self-esteem, control, and meaningful existence. Furthermore, we have provided behavioral evidence that ostracized targets attempt to restore belonging and self-esteem (e.g., cooperating, conforming, and affiliating) and control (aggression). As is the case for control, attempts to restore meaningful existence may also result in antisocial or aggressive behavior. However, evidence of the relationship between meaningful existence and ostracism has thus far been based on self-report ratings of items given to participants after they have been ostracized ("I felt invisible, I felt meaningless, I felt nonexistent") and qualitative studies of ostracism (e.g., Sommer, Williams, Ciarocco, & Baumeister, 2001; Williams et al., 1998).

Terror Management Theory

As we discussed earlier, ostracism serves as a reminder of what life would be like if we did not exist. In this sense, ostracism may have the effect of making mortality salient to the target. The large body of research on terror management has revealed that mortality salience has reliable and predictable effects on judgments and attitudes (for a review see Solomon, Greenberg, & Pyszczynski, Chapter 2, this volume). According to terror management theory, our beliefs and values—cultural worldviews—provide us with a sense that life is significant, permanent, and meaningful and, thus, protects us from the paralyzing terror that results from contemplating death.

In line with this formulation, mortality salience has consistently been shown to enhance the favorability of those who support the individual's worldview and increase derogation toward those who challenge it (e.g., Greenberg, Pyszczynski, Solomon, Simon, & Breus, 1994). Such attempts to bolster cultural worldview in response to mortality salience occurs for a diverse range of human behavior including ingroup bias and prejudice (e.g., Greenberg et al., 1990), false consensus (Pyszczynski et al., 1996) and violating cultural norms (Greenberg, Porteus, Simon, Pyszczynski, & Solomon, 1995).

Ostracism and Cultural Worldview

Like other mortality salience inductions such as writing about one's death or walking by a funeral home, ostracism may provoke attempts by targets to increase faith in their cultural worldview. Several findings to emerge from our ostracism experiments are sympathetic to this interpretation (see also Pinel, Long, Landau, & Pyszczynski, Chapter 22, this volume).

Prejudice

Most obviously, the finding that ostracism increases (implicit) racism (Govan et al., 2002), described earlier, supports the notion of cultural worldview defense. The mere existence of other worldviews is threatening because to accept them is to undermine one's own worldview (Greenberg, Solomon, & Pyszczynski, 1997). Thus, by dismissing other worldviews or derogating those who hold them, we can bolster faith in our own worldview. Consistent with this account, reminders of death associated with being ostracized may have been responsible for increased negativity toward Aboriginal concepts and increased positivity toward European concepts, in our non-Aboriginal participants.

Social Consensus

Pyszczynski et al.'s (1996) finding that people overestimate consensus with their minority views in response to mortality salience has also been obtained in response to ostracism. After manipulating ostracism, Zadro and Williams (see Williams, 2001) asked participants about whether they were in favor of Australia becoming a republic or remaining a monarchy (a controversial topic at the time). In addition, participants estimated how many people in general would agree with their particular position. Overall estimates accurately reflected the clear bias toward favoring a republic. However, those ostracized targets who held the minority position (favoring a monarchy) overestimated the amount of agreement with their position in the population. Overestimating the consensus of their minority opinion served to validate their worldview and thus buffer the anxiety of the mortality reminder brought about by being ignored.

Ingroup Rejection

In Williams et al.'s (2000) ostracism and conformity study, described earlier, a condition was included in which targets were ostracised by either an outgroup, an ingroup, or a mixed group. The strength of the social ties between the target and the sources of ostracism was expected to affect the impact of being ignored, such that ostracism by outgroup members would affect targets less than ostracism by ingroup members. Notwithstanding, ostracism increased conformity on a second task, regardless of the group membership of the sources of ostracism. However, two curious results did emerge. First, of all the experimental conditions, only one group inaccurately reported how often they received the Cyberball: Targets ostracized by ingroup members vastly inflated their estimates of how often they had received the ball. In fact, these targets estimated that they received the ball as often as included participants. Second, ostracism threatened self-reported belonging except in those who were ostracized by ingroup members. Again, they reported similar levels of belonging to included participants.

These two similar patterns obtained for the targets ostracized by ingroup members are at odds with finding that these same participants conformed more then their included counterparts. In particular, their estimates of inclusion and ratings of belonging suggest ostracism had no effect. Yet, these targets conformed more than did included participants, suggesting the ostracism manipulation was successful. Williams et al. (2000) suggested that one explanation for this inconsistency is that targets who were ostracized by ingroup members were adversely affected by the ostracism but did not want to admit it—perhaps even to themselves. It would be particularly difficult for targets to maintain faith in their cultural worldview while being ostracized by those who are like minded. Moreover, it is when they are ostracized that targets desperately need to maintain faith in their cultural worldviews to assuage the anxiety associated with this reminder of social death. Accordingly, the least painful solution may have been for targets to deny that they were being ostracized by their ingroup in order to preserve faith in their cultural worldview.

Self-Esteem

According to terror management theory, self-esteem is the perception that one is a valuable member of a meaningful universe, and it is the primary means by which cultural worldviews perform anxiety buffing (Greenberg et al., 1997). In a series of studies that compared the effects of primed concepts of acceptance, rejection, and other aversive outcomes, Sommer and Baumeister (2002) found that rejection primes led individuals low in trait self-esteem to make negative self appraisals, give up sooner, and perform poorly. For those with high self-esteem, rejection primes might be expected to have little (detrimental) impact compared to other primes. However, rejection primes appeared to actually enhance efforts to maximize performance in those high self-esteem. This suggests that due to their high self-esteem, these individuals had the capacity and motivation to defend against rejection threat through improving effort and performance. As is the case for mortality salience, these findings implicate self-esteem as playing a crucial role in defending against threats of rejection.

These studies provide converging evidence to suggest that, like other mortality salience inductions, ostracism may trigger cultural worldview defense. Obviously, demonstrating that ostracism and mortality salience have similar consequences is far from establishing that ostracism *is* a mortality salience induction. Such consequences may reflect the operation of entirely different motivational processes for ostracism (e.g., attempts to refortify belonging or control). Nonetheless, these findings provide the first step in investigating the relationship between ostracism and mortality salience.

Future Research Directions

Whereas the self-report ratings and qualitative data suggest that ostracism is associated with thoughts of death and meaninglessness, the next step is to investigate whether ostracism actually does serve as mortality salience induction. We are currently attempting to directly investigate this by measuring the accessibility of death-related concepts in ostracized and included participants. The measure of accessibility of death-related concepts comprises a word-stem completion task that has been used by Greenberg and his colleagues (e.g., Arndt, Greenberg, Pyszczynski, & Solomon, 1997) to validate their mortality salience inductions.

On a theoretical level, it may be that a deeply rooted concern with existential isolation is an additional threat of ostracism. The existential therapist Irvin Yalom (1980) discusses the fundamental human fear that one experiences when one realizes the unbridgeable gulf between oneself and any other being. Ostracism, therefore, could serve as a very frequent and potent reminder of the deeper anxieties that people have about their existential isolation from others (Pinel, Long, Landau, & Pyszczynski, Chapter 22, this volume). While this fear may be related conceptually to loss of belonging (perhaps accompanied by self-awareness that inevitably one is distinct and separate from others), it may also be a separate fear that future ostracism research could attempt to establish and distinguish. It may be that certain motives are necessary for ostracism to provoke reminders of death. For example, when the motive for complete ostracism is oblivious, targets may be prone to ask "Am I here?" or "Do I really exist?" (indeed, some of our experimental participants have been observed to pinch themselves while the two confederates gleefully toss the ball to each other). If we establish that ostracism does make mortality salient, it will then be important to distinguish between effects that result from mortality salience and attempts to refortify the other needs. In any case, we believe that establishing that ostracism represents social death is a fruitful avenue of future investigation.

CONCLUSION

In summary, we have reported on our experimental investigations of the powerful and aversive social phenomenon of ostracism. Using a series of paradigms, these investigations have demonstrated that ostracism threatens the need for belonging, self-esteem, control, and meaningful existence. With occasional and infrequent exposure to ostracism episode, the reactions, whether they be prosocial or antisocial, reflect attempts to fulfill these threatened needs. We presented evidence to suggest that ostracism may have the effect of making mortality salient and consequently provoke similar cultural worldview defenses as other mortality salience cues. We also discussed the long-term consequences of ostracism, which can lead to alienation, helplessness, depression, and feelings of worthlessness. Like individuals with Cotard's delusion, feeling nonexistent inevitably leads to a lack of will, purpose, and meaning. And, like James's eloquent statement with which we opened our chapter, both rage, in the short term, and impotent (existential) despair, in the long term, will invade the mind of the ostracized.

NOTE

1. Although ostracism, social exclusion, and rejection may have unique aspects, the psychological distinctiveness of these three concepts has not yet been uncovered; thus we use the terms interchangeably throughout this chapter.

REFERENCES

Abramson, L. Y., Seligman, M. E., & Teasdale, J. D. (1978). Learned helplessness in humans: Critique and reformulation. *Journal of Abnormal Psychology, 87,* 49–74.

Arndt, J., Greenberg, J., Pyszczynski, T., & Solomon, S. (1997). Subliminal exposure to death-related stimuli increases defense of the cultural worldview. *Psychological Science, 8,* 379–385.

Barner-Barry, C. (1986). Rob: Children's tacit use of peer ostracism to control aggressive behavior. *Ethology and Sociobiology, 7,* 281–293.

Baumeister, R. F., & Leary, M. R. (1995). The need to belong: Desire for interpersonal attachments as a fundamental human motivation. *Psychological Bulletin, 117,* 497–529.

Burger, J. M. (1992). *Desire for control: Personality, social, and clinical perspectives.* New York: Plenum Press.

Buss, D. M. (1990). The evolution of anxiety and social exclusion. *Journal of Social and Clinical Psychology, 9,* 196–201.

Cannon, W. (1942). "Voodoo" death. *American Anthropologist, 44,* 169–181.

Cardarelli, R. (Producer), & Wertmüller, L. (Director). (1975). *Swept away . . . by an unusual destiny in the blue sea of August* [Film]. Available from Fox Lorber, Inc., Los Angeles, CA.

Dasgupta, N., McGhee, D. E., Greenwald, A. G., & Banaji, M. R. (2000). Automatic preference for White Americans: Ruling out the familiarity effect. *Journal of Experimental Social Psychology, 36,* 316–328.

de Waal, F. B. (1986). The brutal elimination of a rival among captive male chimpanzees. *Ethology and Sociobiology, 7,* 237–251.

deCharms, R. (1968). *Personal causation: The internal affective determinants of behavior.* New York: Academic Press.

Ellison, R. (1952). *Invisible man.* New York: Quality Paperback Book Club.

Faulkner, S., & Williams, K. D. (1995, May). *The causes and consequences of social ostracism: A qualitative analysis.* Paper presented at the 67th annual Midwestern Psychological Association, Chicago.

Faulkner, S., Williams, K. D., Sherman, B., & Williams, E. (1997, May). *The "silent treatment:" Its incidence and impact.* Paper presented at the 69th annual Midwestern Psychological Association, Chicago.

Friedland, N., Keinan, G., & Regev, Y. (1992). Controlling the uncontrollable: Effects of stress on illusory perceptions of controllability. *Journal of Personality and Social Psychology, 63,* 923–931.

Gardner, W. L., Pickett, C. L., & Brewer, M. B. (2000). Social exclusion and selective memory: How the need to belong influences memory for social events. *Personality and Social Psychology Bulletin, 26,* 486–496.

Goodall, J. (1986). Social rejection, exclusion, and shunning among the Gombe chimpanzees. *Ethology and Sociobiology, 7,* 227–236.

Govan, C., Case, T. I., & Williams, K. D. (2002). Implicit and explicit responses to ostracism: Social judgments of Aboriginal and white Australians. *Australian Journal of Psychology, 54*(Suppl.), 118.

Greenberg, J., Porteus, J., Simon, L., Pyszczynski, T., & Solomon, S. (1995). Evidence of a terror management function of cultural icons: The effects of mortality salience on the inappropriate use of cherished cultural symbols. *Personality and Social Psychology Bulletin, 21,* 1221–1228.

Greenberg, J., Pyszczynski, T., Solomon, S., Rosenblatt, A., Veeder, M., Kirkland, S., et al. (1990). Evidence for terror management theory II: The effects of mortality salience on reactions to those who threaten or bolster the cultural worldview. *Journal of Personality and Social Psychology, 58,* 308–318.

Greenberg, J., Pyszczynski, T., Solomon, S., Simon, L., & Breus, M. (1994). Role of consciousness and accessibility of death-related thoughts in mortality salience effects. *Journal of Personality and Social Psychology, 67,* 627–637.

Greenberg, J., Solomon, S., & Pyszczynski, T. (1997). Terror management theory of self-esteem and cultural worldviews: Empirical assessments and conceptual refinements. *Advances in Experimental Social Psychology, 29,* 61–139.

Greenberg, J., Solomon, S., Pyszczynski, T., Rosenblatt, A., Burling, J., Lyon, D., et al. (1992). Why do people need self-esteem? Converging evidence that self-esteem serves an anxiety-buffering function. *Journal of Personality and Social Psychology, 63,* 913–922.

Greenwald, A. G., McGhee, D. E., & Schwartz, J. L. K. (1998). Measuring individual differences in implicit cognition: The implicit association test. *Journal of Personality and Social Psychology, 74,* 1022–1038.

Gruter, M., & Masters, R. D. (1986). Ostracism as a social and biological phenomenon: An introduction. *Ethology and Sociobiology, 7,* 149–158.

Insko, C. A., & Wilson, M. (1977). Interpersonal attraction as a function of social interaction. *Journal of Personality and Social Psychology, 35,* 903–911.

James, W. (1950). *The principles of psychology* (Vol. 1). New York: Dover. (Original work published 1890)

Krosnick, J. A. (1999). Survey research. *Annual Review of Psychology, 50,* 537–567.

Kurzban, R., & Leary, M. R. (2001). Evolutionary origins of stigmatization: The functions of social exclusion. *Psychological Bulletin, 127,* 187–208.

Langdon, R., & Coltheart, M. (2000). The cognitive neuropsychology of delusions. *Mind and Language, 15,* 184–218.

Lawson-Williams, H., & Williams, K. D. (1998, April). *Effects of social ostracism on desire for control.* Paper presented at the meeting of the Society for Australasian Social Psychology, Christchurch, New Zealand.

Leary, M., Kowalski, R. M., Smith, L., & Phillips, S. (2003). Teasing, rejection and violence: Case studies of the school shootings. *Aggressive Behavior, 29,* 202–214.

Leary, M. R., Tambor, E. S., Terdal, S. K., & Downs, D. L. (1995). Self-esteem as an interpersonal monitor: The sociometer hypothesis. *Journal of Personality and Social Psychology, 68,* 518–530.

Lieberman, J. D., Solomon, S., Greenberg, J., & McGregor, H. A. (1999). A hot new way to measure aggression: Hot sauce allocation. *Aggressive Behavior, 25,* 331–348.

Mead, G. H. (1934). *Mind, self and society.* Chicago: University of Chicago Press.

Pedersen, A., & Walker, I. (1997). Prejudice against Australian Aborigines: Old fashioned and modern forms. *European Journal of Social Psychology, 27,* 561–587.

Pyszczynski, T., Wicklund, R. A., Floresku, S., Koch, H., Gauch, G., Solomon, S., et al. (1996). Whistling in the dark: Exaggerated consensus estimates in response to incidental reminders of mortality. *Psychological Science, 7,* 332–336.

Seligman, M. (1975). *Helplessness: On depression, development, and death.* San Francisco: Freeman.

Shaver, P. R., & Mikulincer, M. (2003). The psychodynamics of social judgments: An attachment theory perspective. In J. P. Forgas, K. D. Williams & W. von Hippel (Eds.), *Responding to the social world: Implicit and explicit processes in social judgments and decisions* (pp. 85–114). New York: Cambridge University Press.

Smith, E. R., & Mackie, D. M. (1995). *Social psychology.* New York: Worth.

Sommer, K. L., & Baumeister, R. F. (2002). Self-evaluation, persistence, and performance following implicit rejection: The role of trait self-esteem. *Personality and Social Psychology Bulletin, 28,* 926–938.

Sommer, K. L., Williams, K. D., Ciarocco, N. J., & Baumeister, R. F. (2001). When silence speaks louder than words: Explorations into the intrapsychic and interpersonal consequences of social ostracism. *Basic and Applied Social Psychology, 23,* 225–243.

Steele, C. M. (1988). The psychology of self-affirmation: Sustaining the integrity of the self. In L. Berkowitz (Ed.), *Advances in experimental social psychology: Social psychological studies of the self: Perspectives and programs* (Vol. 21, pp. 261–302). San Diego: Academic Press.

Sudnow, D. (1967). *Passing on: The social organization of dying.* Englewood Cliffs, NJ: Prentice-Hall.

Taylor, S. E., & Brown, J. D. (1988). Illusion and well-being: A social psychological perspective on mental health. *Psychological Bulletin, 103*, 193–210.

Tesser, A. (1988). Toward a self-evaluation maintenance model of social behavior. In L. Berkowitz (Ed.), *Advances in experimental social psychology: Social psychological studies of the self: Perspectives and programs* (Vol. 21, pp. 181–227). San Diego: Academic Press.

Thompson. H. L., & Richardson, D. R. (1983). The Rooster effect: Same-sex rivalry and inequity as a factors in retaliate aggression. *Personality and Social Psychology Bulletin, 9*, 415–425.

Twenge, J. M., Baumeister, R. F., Tice, D. M., & Stucke, T. S. (2001). If you can't join them, beat them: Effects of social exclusion on aggressive behavior. *Journal of Personality and Social Psychology, 81*, 1058–1069.

Warburton, W. A. (2002). *Aggressive responding to ostracism: The moderating role of control motivation and narcissistic vulnerability, and the mediating role of negative affect.* Unpublished honors thesis, Macquarie University, Sydney Australia.

White, R. W. (1959). Motivation reconsidered: The concept of competence. *Psychological Review, 66*, 297–333.

Williams, K. D. (1997). Social ostracism. In R. M. Kowalski (Ed.), *Aversive interpersonal behaviors: The Plenum series in social/clinical psychology* (pp. 133–170). New York: Plenum Press.

Williams, K. D. (2001). *Ostracism: The power of silence.* New York: Guilford Press.

Williams, K. D., Case, T. I., & Govan, C. (2003). Impact of ostracism on social judgments and decisions: Explicit and implicit responses. In J. P. Forgas, K. D. Williams & W. von Hippel (Eds.), *Responding to the social world: Implicit and explicit processes in social judgments and decisions* (pp. 325–342). New York: Cambridge University Press.

Williams, K. D., Cheung, C. K., & Choi, W. (2000). Cyberostracism: Effects of being ignored over the Internet. *Journal of Personality and Social Psychology, 79*, 748–762.

Williams, K. D., Govan, C. L., Croker, V., Tynan, D., Cruickshank, M., & Lam, A. (2002). Investigations into differences between social- and cyberostracism. *Group Dynamics: Theory, Research, and Practice, 6*, 65–77.

Williams, K. D., Shore, W. J., & Grahe, J. E. (1998). The silent treatment: Perceptions of its behaviors and associated feelings. *Group Processes and Intergroup Relations, 1*, 117–141.

Williams, K. D., & Sommer, K. L. (1997). Social ostracism by coworkers: Does rejection lead to loafing or compensation? *Personality and Social Psychology Bulletin, 23*, 693–706.

Williams, K. D., Wheeler, L., & Harvey, J. (2001). Inside the social mind of the ostracizer. In J. Forgas, K. Williams, & L. Wheeler (Eds.), *The social mind: Cognitive and motivational aspects of interpersonal behavior* (pp. 294– 320). New York: Cambridge University Press.

Williams, K. D., & Zadro, L. (1999, April). *Forty years of solitude: Effects of long-term use of the silent treatment.* Paper presented at the 71st annual Midwestern Psychological Association, Chicago.

Williams, K. D., & Zadro, L. (2001). Ostracism: On being ignored, excluded, and rejected. In M. R. Leary (Ed.), *Interpersonal rejection* (pp. 21–53). New York: Oxford University Press.

Wortman, C. B., & Brehm, J. W. (1975). Responses to uncontrollable outcomes: An integration of reactance theory and the learned helplessness model. In L. Berkowitz (Ed.), *Advances in experimental social psychology* (Vol. 8, pp. 277–336). San Diego: Academic Press.

Yalom, I. D. (1980). *Existential psychotherapy.* New York: Basic Books.

Zadro, L., Williams, K. D., & Richardson, R. (2003). *How low can you go?: Ostracism by a computer lowers belonging, control, self-esteem, and meaningful existence.* Unpublished manuscript, University of New South Wales, Sydney Australia.

Zippelius, R. (1986). Exclusion and shunning as legal and social sanctions. *Ethology and Sociobiology, 7*, 159–166.

Zusne, L., & Jones, W. H. (1989). *Anomalistic psychology: A study of magical thinking* (2nd ed.). Hillsdale, NJ: Erlbaum.

Chapter 22

I-Sharing, the Problem of Existential Isolation, and Their Implications for Interpersonal and Intergroup Phenomena

ELIZABETH C. PINEL
ANSON E. LONG
MARK J. LANDAU
TOM PYSZCZYNSKI

[It is impossible] that our senses can ever reveal to us the true nature and essence of the material world.
—JOHANNES MUELLER, *Elements of Physiology* (1834–1840/ 1912, p. 541)

When Mueller observed the impossibility of our senses ever revealing the true nature of reality, he did more than summarize the limits of human knowledge. He also identified the precursor to feelings of existential isolation, feelings that result from the realization that we cannot ever know phenomenologically how another person experiences the world (see Yalom, 1980). To experience any stimulus—simple or complex, significant or trivial, short-lived or enduring—we must filter that stimulus (consciously and preconsciously) through our own sense organs and higher-level perceptual apparatti and schemata. We cannot borrow people's optical or olfactory or auditory nerves to know what something looks like or smells like or sounds like to them, nor can we lend them ours for a peek at the world through our senses. We can turn to others for evidence that they share our experiences, but we cannot get inside their minds to know for sure, nor can they step inside ours.

These limitations in our ability to share our phenomenological experiences with others render us *existentially isolated*. Our experience of the world resides entirely within ourselves, and we can never share those experiences directly with another person, nor can other people directly share their experiences with us. Yalom (1980) distinguished this form of isolation from two other psychologically significant forms: interpersonal and intrapersonal isolation. Interpersonal isolation results from literal separation from others, such as when a person has limited social contacts or does not receive an invitation to a broadly attended gathering (see also Case & Williams, Chapter 21, this volume). Although interpersonal isolation could certainly trigger feelings of existential isolation, people can feel existentially isolated even when surrounded by friends and family. Intrapersonal isolation—which results when people lose touch with their own private experiences (as sometimes occurs among victims of early childhood trauma)—also differs from existential isolation. After all, one can feel very alone in one's experiences without disassociating, and one can disassociate without feeling existentially alone.

Although we recognize that individual differences exist with regard to the frequency and salience of people's feelings of existential isolation, we propose that existential isolation factors into virtually everyone's life in the context of their dealings with others. Specifically, we propose that people like those who keep their feelings of existential isolation at bay and dislike those who stir up their feelings of existential isolation. Our reasoning comes from the observation that existential isolation makes it difficult for people to satisfy two fundamental needs: the need to know (Dechesne & Kruglanski, Chapter 16, this volume; Festinger, 1954; Greenberg, Pyszczynski, & Solomon, 1986; Solomon, Greenberg, & Pyszczynski, Chapter 2, this volume; Swann, 1996; Trope, 1983)[1] and the need for interpersonal connectedness (Baumeister & Leary, 1995; Bowlby, 1969; Brewer, 1991; Florian, Mikulincer, & Hirschberger, 2002).[2]

Here we propose that the potential for existential isolation to thwart our needs to know and to feel connected to others underlies our tendency to gravitate toward people who make us feel existentially connected—*I-sharers*—and to steer clear of those who make us feel existentially isolated—*non-I-sharers*. To make our case, we begin with an introduction of the construct of I-sharing and follow this up with a review of recent findings that highlight the powerful role I-sharing plays in interpersonal and intergroup liking.

THE DUAL SELF

The term "I-sharing" comes from James's (1890/1918) partition of the self into two aspects: the Me and the I. The Me consists of our representation of ourselves, our self-concept. It includes anything pertaining to what we call ours, what we think of ourselves, how we feel about ourselves, what we know about our behaviors, our memories, etc. If we look in a mirror, the Me would represent the reflection we see in that mirror.

In contrast to the Me, the I refers to the agentic part of the self, or the self-as-subject. It represents that aspect of our self that, at any given moment perceives, reacts, interprets, in short, experiences. If we look in a mirror, the I represents the part of us that sees the reflection. Whereas the Me tends toward stability, changing only insofar as people add to their representations of self, the I takes on a fleeting nature; it changes from one moment to the next, and leaves what James dubbed a "stream of consciousness" in its wake.

Although research on the self—including the self as it pertains to relationships—has proliferated over the past few decades, the vast majority of this research concentrates on the Me. This emphasis on the Me stems, at least partly, from the difficulties associated with empirically studying the I. The fleeting nature of the I makes it difficult to capture with standard psychological measures (e.g., pencil-and-paper measures). Moreover, we cannot ask people to describe their I because, by definition, the I refers to the part of the self that *does* the describing.[3] Considerations such as these led James to suggest that psychologists focus their attention on understanding the Me, leaving the I to the realm of philosophers and theologians, a bit of advice that the psychological community seems to have taken to heart.

If the nature of the I poses methodological challenges for researchers interested in the self, it also explains why people are vulnerable to feelings of existential isolation (Yalom, 1980). Because people can never get inside the minds of others, they are essentially alone when it comes to their experience of the world. We propose that the problem of existential isolation provides the major impetus behind people's desire to share their subjective world with others and explains why I-sharing moments can have such a profound effect on people's feelings toward others.

I-Sharing

Literally speaking, I-sharing refers to those moments when people feel as though their self-as-subject merges with that of at least one other person. When people I-share, they believe that they and at least one other person are having the same experience in a given moment. Whatever one person experiences at a given moment—whether it be the bitter taste of unsweetened chocolate or the mind-numbing challenge of a zen *koan*—the person whom she will come to consider an I-sharer is presumed to be experiencing as well.

We hasten to add that the impossibility of being able to experience the world as another subject means that conclusions about I-sharing could be wrong. For this reason, I-sharing refers to a subjective sense that one or more people have experienced a given moment identically; whether or not they actually have is another matter altogether and beyond the scope of this chapter. For our purposes here, we consider any time people perceive that they and at least one other person have an identical experience in a given moment as an instance of I-sharing, regardless of whether or not their experiences actually are the same. More important, we maintain that I-sharing experiences—whether objectively true or not—provide people with the closest approximation of existential connectedness possible. Although people may erroneously conclude that they experienced a given moment identically to another person, the perception of having I-shared eliminates the feeling of being alone in one's own experience of the world.[4] In so doing, I-sharing eliminates the threat to the needs for belief validation and connectedness posed by feelings of existential isolation.

What causes people to believe that they have I-shared with another person (or several other people)? We argue that the most convincing evidence of I-sharing occurs when people perceive that someone else *simultaneously* reacts to some stimulus or event *identically* to the way they themselves are reacting. When two or more people simultaneously laugh in response to the same joke, cry in response to the same sad song, say the word "antidisestabishmentarianism" in response to a request for a word that starts with "a," or erupt into a frenzied polka upon receiving a reminder of the approach of Octoberfest, they believe that they have experienced a moment identically, that they have I-shared.

As implied in the discussion so far, I-sharing can happen among more than two people. Large groups of people can I-share when they laugh at a comedian's antics, or when they sing their national anthem, when they combine forces to fight for a common cause, or when they undergo a tragedy that affects all of them. For ease of presentation, throughout the remainder of this chapter, when we discuss I-sharing, we typically refer to two-person I-sharing. Nonetheless, we ask that the reader keep in mind that I-sharing experiences are not restricted to dyadic interactions.

Note that the recognition that one has or has not I-shared with one or more people necessarily comes after the fact, when one reflects on the moment. Several factors should moderate the extent to which one will reflect on the moment in this way. As we noted earlier, people no doubt vary with regard to their dispositional feelings of existential isolation and these individual differences should influence the extent to which people attend to I-sharing moments or do not. Similarly, certain situations (e.g., situations that make one feel like an outcast) make the fact of our existential isolation more salient than others; when in those existentially isolating situations, people will evince a greater tendency to look for I-sharing than when in more neutral situations (for a similar argument regarding reactions to ostracism, see Case & Williams, Chapter 21, this volume). In a related vein, people might feel more existentially isolated with regard to distinctive aspects of their I than with regard to less distinctive aspects. A person who has always recognized that her sensitivity to barometric pressure distinguishes her from other people will look for I-sharing on this dimension; someone who has never given barometric pressure a moment's thought will not. In short, although people can I-share about just about anything, their sensitivity to I-sharing experiences may depend on their dispositional level of existential isolation, the situation in which they find themselves, and the I-sharing dimension in question.

Although the most convincing evidence of I-sharing occurs when two people respond identically and simultaneously to the same stimulus, we argue that people have strong opinions about the extent to which they I-share with other individuals and that they arrive at these opinions on the basis of a diverse set of information. Most commonly, people tend to believe that people with whom they share important aspects of their Me (e.g., race, age, career aspirations, political ideology, and life experiences) will I-share with them at important moments. From this perspective, people like people who share their Me's because similarity of the Me serves as a proxy for similarity of the I. If so, then we would expect to see people favoring people with whom they share aspects of their Me over those with whom they do not, *unless* they receive more compelling evidence that they do not actually share I's with a Me-sharer. We tested this reasoning in several of our preliminary studies on the link between I-sharing and liking. Before discussing this research, however, we turn to a discussion of the power for I-sharing to satisfy the needs for belief validation and connectedness.

Existential Isolation, I-Sharing, and the Need for Belief Validation

> Reality is that which, when you stop believing in it, doesn't go away.
> —PHILLIP K. DICK (1985, p. 4)

If all we can know is the state of our own nervous system (Mueller, 1834–1840/1912), and reality is that which doesn't go away when we stop believing in it, we can never really get at the "truth" of things. How can we determine what is real if we cannot get outside our own heads and verify that something exists outside our experience of it? Existential isolation renders us vulnerable to doubts about what is real and what is merely a product of our own creative minds. This state of affairs can serve as a great source of distress for members of a species with a strong drive to know the true nature of reality.

Given their existential isolation, how do people satisfactorily convince themselves that they can and do know anything at all? Previous researchers and theorists have proposed that other people help us to accomplish this goal: to the extent that others agree with our conceptions of ourselves and the world around us, we feel certain of knowing (Festinger, 1954; Kelly, 1955; Swann, 1996). Following in this tradition, we propose that people seek out and gravitate toward evidence that others *subjectively* experience reality in the same way that they themselves do. Such information provides consensual validation for people's experiences, providing much-needed evidence that the world really is as they perceive it and that their more personal and subjective experiences make sense in a given context. Although existential isolation precludes us from arriving at this evidence through firsthand knowledge of another person's subjective experience, we feel like we *do* have this firsthand knowledge when we I-share with someone. When people I-share, they believe that the other person experiences reality identically to them; thus, although they cannot get inside the mind of the other person, they can presume to know what they would find out if they could. As such, I-sharing provides people with the best evidence they can find that the other person had the same experience that they did and therefore provides satisfaction for our need to know.

As some have noted before us, the identification of similar others can serve this same function. For example, when we find people who see us similarly to how we see ourselves, we gain confidence in the validity of our self-conceptions (Pinel & Constantino, 2003; Swann, 1996). Likewise, when we discover a group of individuals who all share our worldview or standards for behavior, we bask in the heightened sense that we understand reality as it "really is" and know the "right" way to live our lives (Greenberg et al., 1986; Solomon, Greenberg, & Pyszczynski, 1991; Solomon et al., Chapter 2, this volume). Although we agree that finding people who share our conceptions of ourselves and the world around us can satisfy our need to know, we maintain that these routes to feelings of knowing promote more powerful feelings of attraction to and communion with the other partly because such shared beliefs serve as a proxy for I-sharing.

Existential Isolation, I-Sharing, and Feelings of Connectedness

> Jack Kerouac sat beside me on a busted rusted iron pole. Companion,
> we thought the same thoughts of the soul.
>
> —ALLEN GINSBERG, *The Sunflower Sutra* (1956, p. 35)

In addition to playing a key role in satisfying our need to know, we argue that I-sharing plays a key role in satisfying our need to feel interpersonally connected. Typically, when researchers talk about interpersonal connectedness, they concentrate on being liked or accepted by one or more individuals (e.g., Baumeister & Leary, 1995; Leary, Tambor, Terdal, & Downs, 1995) or simply on being a member of a group (e.g., Brewer, 1991). We maintain that regardless of how many people claim to "accept us" and how many groups to which we belong, others can help satisfy our need for connectedness only insofar as we feel existentially connected to them. Indeed, being with several other people who make us feel existentially isolated could trigger greater feelings of loneliness than actually being alone (see Yalom, 1980).

As a case in point, consider the participants in Asch's (1951, 1956) conformity study. Recall that these participants indicated which of three lines most closely approximated the length of a target line. To create a situation replete with conformity pressures, Asch instructed confederates to give the (obviously) wrong answer trial after trial. Imagine how existentially isolated this procedure must have left participants feeling. Suddenly they found themselves in an experiment in which everyone, save them, seemed to perceive reality identi-cally. Although participants clearly had interpersonal contact with other people, this proce-dure must have left them feeling terribly alone. Perhaps for this reason, those participants in a version of the study in which one confederate answered identically to them exhibited palpable feelings of connection to that confederate.

In short, we propose that, in addition to threatening our need to know, existential isola-tion threatens our need to feel interpersonally connected. As such, just as I-sharing satisfies our need to know by bringing us as close as we can get to experiencing reality through the eyes of another person, so too does I-sharing satisfy our need for connectedness. When we sense that someone experiences a moment in the same way we do, we believe that person understands us at our core, at the level of how we experience the world. Such I-sharing ex-periences satisfy the need for interpersonal connectedness by creating feelings of existential connectedness. These feelings, in turn, foster a sense that the positive regard that people shower on us reflects genuine liking for us and not for some erroneous understanding or im-age of us. I-sharing also satisfies the need for interpersonal connectedness because when someone shares our "I", it turns that "I" into a "We" (Wegner, 1987).

Summary

We have argued that existential isolation threatens people's need to know and to feel con-nected, and that I-sharing satisfies these needs because it represents the closest we can get to feeling existentially connected to another person. It follows that people should seek out and like I-sharers—who make them feel existentially connected—and avoid and dislike non-I-sharers—who make them feel existentially isolated. We test this reasoning in the stud-ies described in the next section.

I-SHARING AND LIKING: ESTABLISHING THE PHENOMENON

To date, we have conducted seven studies to establish the basic phenomenon that I-sharing contributes to liking for others. In designing these studies, we took special care to differenti-ate I-sharing from other forms of similarity, namely, similarity of the Me. A long tradition of social psychological research documents the contribution that perceived similarity makes to liking, and we want to clarify the distinction between predictions generated from this past research versus predictions generated from our current analysis of I-sharing. To this end, we begin this section with a brief review of this past research and how it fits in with the current analysis.

Similarity All Over Again?

Like seeks out like. We see this principle manifest itself on several different levels, but no-where does this preference for similarity seem more ubiquitous than in the psychology of human interaction (for a review, see Berscheid & Reis, 1998). Indeed, it is a theme uniting seemingly distinct research traditions, such as work on similarity and attraction (Byrne, 1971; Newcomb, 1961), stereotyping and prejudice (Allport, 1954; Tajfel & Turner, 1986), balance (Heider, 1958), self-verification (Swann, 1996), and terror management (Greenberg et al., 1986; Solomon et al., 1991). Collectively, this work has shown that people prefer oth-ers who share their background (Newcomb, 1961), race and ethnicity (Allport, 1954), friends (Heider, 1958), physical appearance and manner of dress (Berscheid, Dion, Walster, & Walster, 1971), values (Rokeach, 1960), and even bogus characteristics that they just learned describe them (Tajfel, Billig, Bundy, & Flament, 1971). In addition, people prefer people who share their viewpoints on a vast array of topics ranging from what movie should win the Oscar this year to what kind of person we are (Byrne, 1971; Swann, 1996). The relationship between similarity and liking works in the reverse direction as well; not only does similarity lead to liking, liking also leads to assumptions about similarity (e.g., Murray, Holmes, Bellavia, Griffin, & Dolderman, 2002).

Unfortunately, this robust preference for similarity does not merely reflect an innocuous desire to surround ourselves with the familiar, it can also underlie long-standing intergroup rivalries, including ones that cost lives (e.g., Greenberg, Simon, Solomon, Chatel, & Pyszczynski, 1992; Pyszczynski, Solomon, & Greenberg, 2003). Thus it behooves us to identify the reasons we seem so enamored with similarity. Over the years, researchers and theorists have proffered a wide range of answers to this question. People who are similar to us are familiar (Allport, 1954; Zajonc, 1968); they like us back (Aronson & Worchel, 1966; Condon & Crano, 1988). They tend to be near us geographically, or they tend to be in the same groups as us and this proximity makes it more likely that we'll get to know them in the first place (Segal, 1974). They confirm our conceptions of ourselves (Swann, 1996) and the world around us (Greenberg et al., 1986); they are like us but better and therefore help us transform our ideal selves into reality (Wetzel & Insko, 1982).

Each of these explanations contributes to our understanding of the link between similarity and liking, and yet each and every one of them rests on the assumption that similarity with respect to one's self-as-object (or Me-sharing) drives similarity effects.[5] According to this perspective, we like people who drive the same cars as us or who vote for the same candidates we vote for or who have the same color skin as us because they are similar to us with regard to these aspects of our Me. Such objective similarity—what we refer to as Me-sharing—implies that our objective traits, features, and characteristics are reasonable and desirable, at least to those who are similar to us on these dimensions, and thus provide a boost to our sense of self-esteem or personal value. This certainly constitutes an important part of why people like similar others; after all, people seem to care a great deal about their Me's. Consider the growing popularity in the United States of cosmetic plastic surgery; people will go into considerable debt and even risk their lives to undergo these procedures, presumably because people care so much about themselves as objects (see also Fredrickson & Roberts, 1997; Frederickson, Roberts, Noll, Quinn, & Twenge, 1998; Goldenberg & Roberts, Chapter 5, this volume). Trends toward consumerism lead us to a similar conclusion (Kasser & Ahuvia, 2002; Kasser & Ryan, 1996).

These examples notwithstanding, we also have good reason to believe that people consider themselves to be more than an amalgamation of what they look like, where they are from, to whom they are related, and the traits that describe them. Targets of widespread stereotypes file discrimination suits, immigrants reject the language of their homeland, and sons and daughters turn down the chance to inherit the family business, all because of the unease that results from being reduced to an object. Indeed, research from several different traditions points to the pitfalls of focusing too much on one's self as an object. Consider work on objective self-awareness theory (Duval & Wicklund, 1972; Wicklund, 1975) and the more recent self-objectification theory (Fredrickson & Roberts, 1997; Frederickson et al., 1998; Goldenberg & Roberts, Chapter 5, this volume), the results of which indicate that focusing on oneself as an object can have deleterious consequences, both affective and cognitive. Similarly, research on consumerism indicates that equating one's possessions with one's self-worth can be bad for one's mental health and general well-being (Kasser &

Ahuvia, 2002). It also appears that people report being the happiest when they are not focusing on themselves as objects but instead are in a state of flow, completely immersed in a task (Csikszentmihalyi, 1997).

Although people clearly pursue the validation of their self-concept (or Me) and feel attracted to those who provide such validation, we suggest that the validation of people's subjective experience (or I) may serve as an even more powerful source of interpersonal attraction. Indeed, we propose that people like those who share their Me's, in part, because of what they assume similarity with respect to the Me says about similarity with respect to the I. From this perspective, we like people who share our taste in cars and political candidates and who have the same skin color as us, not because we care so much about cars, political candidates, and skin color, per se, but because we believe that people who share these things with us will also share our I's. If we have reason to believe otherwise, we suddenly do not like these people nearly as much.

With the foregoing reasoning in mind, we designed four studies to disentangle the contribution of Me-sharing and I-sharing to interpersonal liking. We describe these studies next.

Studies 1–3: First Impressions

Using a scenario-based methodology, Studies 1 through 3 examine whether I-sharing moderates people's liking for a Me-sharer versus someone who does not share his or her Me. We reasoned that if people infer I-sharing based on Me-sharing, their preference for Me-sharers would depend on whether or not they have reason to believe those Me-sharers also share their I's. Because we used the same basic design for each study, we will describe Study 1 in detail and then note where Studies 2 and 3 deviate from this basic design.

Participants read a description of a scenario with which college students have a lot of experience: the first day of class. Specifically, while reading the scenario, participants imagine that it is the first day of class and that the professor invites the students to introduce and say something about themselves. Participants receive information about two students: specifically, they learn that one student (of their gender) comes from their hometown and thus is a Me-sharer, and they learn that another student (also of their gender) comes from another country and thus is a non-Me-sharer. Participants also receive information about the extent to which these two students share their I. This variable gets manipulated next in the scenario, when participants read about a third student (of their same gender) who describes him- or herself as a fan of a band that the participants either love or hate. Participants go on to read that the facial expressions of the Me-sharer and non-Me-sharer indicate either that the Me-sharer loves the band and the non-Me-sharer hates the band or that the Me-sharer hates the band and the non-Me-sharer loves the band. Thus, when participants hate the band, whoever else hates the band constitutes the I-sharer and when participants love the band, whoever else loves the band constitutes the I-sharer. We next measured participants' liking for the Me-sharer and the non-Me-sharer. Thus, Study 1 employed a 2 (I-sharing dimension: love band, hate band) x 2 (I-sharer: Me-sharer, non-Me-sharer) x 2 (Liking: for Me-sharer, for non-Me-sharer) design. As expected, we observed an interaction between I-sharing and Liking. When the I-sharer was a Me-sharer, participants preferred the Me-sharer to the non-Me-sharer. However, when the I-sharer is a non-Me-sharer, participants preferred the non-Me-sharer to the Me-sharer. Put succinctly, participants liking for the people in the scenario depended on whether they I-shared with those people and not on whether they Me-shared with those people.

Importantly, these preferences for the I-sharer over the non-I-sharer emerged despite the tendency for participants to indicate that they place more importance on their hometown than on their taste in music. That is, in Study 1, in addition to measuring participants' liking for the target individuals, we asked participants to indicate the value they place on their hometown and their taste in music. Analysis of these importance ratings indicated that participants regarded their hometown as more important than their taste in music, suggesting that our findings did not stem from a tendency for people to place more importance on their taste in music than on their hometown. To explore the relation between our findings and perceived importance further, we calculated a difference score representing the relative importance participants placed on their taste in music versus their hometown and reran our analysis using this difference score as a covariate. If anything, the inclusion of this *increased* the effect of the I-sharer x liking interaction, again suggesting that a difference in the importance people place on their taste in music and their hometown did not mediate our effects. Finally, we also divided our participants into three groups—those who place more importance on their hometown than on music, those who equally weight their hometown and music, and those who place more importance on music than on their hometown—and we entered this new variable (called "relative importance") into our analyses. Results indicated the same I-sharer x liking interaction described earlier, and relative importance did *not* moderate this effect. These findings make the critical point that importance of domain cannot account for the impact of I-sharing on interpersonal liking.

Of course, one might argue that the I-sharing dimension used in Study 1 implicates people's Me just as much as it implicates the I. Although one's taste in music provides information about how one might react to musical stimuli (and thus the I), it also can represent an important part of how people see themselves (as in "I am a Dylan fan"). If so, perhaps the results of Study 1 say more about the extent to which music tastes pervade both the Me and the I than they do about a preference for I-sharers over non-I-sharers.

To address this issue, we conducted a second study that focused on a more in-the-moment form of I-sharing: giggling (or not giggling) immediately upon hearing someone speak. As in Study 1, we asked participants to imagine the first day of class and, further, that a Me-sharer (i.e., someone from their hometown) and a non-Me-sharer (i.e., someone from another country) introduce themselves. Next, participants imagine that a third person introduces him- or herself in a voice that either does or does not make participants giggle. Sometimes the Me-sharer giggles at the same time as the participants; sometimes the non-Me-sharer does. Thus, when participants giggle, whoever giggles constitutes the I-sharer, but when participants do not giggle, whoever does *not* giggle in the scenario constitutes the I-sharer. In short, Study 2 employed a 2 (I-sharing dimension: giggle, no giggle) x 2 (I-sharer: Me-sharer, non-Me-sharer) x 2 (liking: for Me-sharer, for non-Me-sharer) design.

Results replicated the findings of Study 1. Specifically, we observed an I-sharer x liking interaction such that people liked the Me-sharer more when the Me-sharer shared his or her I but the non-Me-sharer more when the non-Me-sharer shared his or her I and the Me-sharer did *not*. Also, as in Study 1, the I-sharing dimension (in this case whether the participant giggled or did not giggle) did not moderate this effect. Finally, when we asked participants in Study 2 to report the extent to which their sense of humor and hometown reflect on their Me (i.e., their background, race/ethnicity, age, social class, and family structure) and their I (i.e., how they perceive, think about, react to, and interpret the world), participants said that their sense of humor said more about their I than their Me and that their hometown said more about their Me than their I. This latter finding adds to our confidence that our results reflect the role that I-sharing plays in people's liking for others.

A final scenario study that used the same methodology of Studies 1 and 2 explored the importance of context in the way I-sharing influences attraction. Specifically, we wondered whether people's preference for I-sharers would depend on the normativeness of their sub-jective reactions to the social situation. To this end, we replicated Study 2 but added a ma-nipulation of the normativeness of the participant's response context. Specifically, we told some participants to imagine that the rest of the class giggled in response to the third stu-dent's voice and others to imagine that the rest of the class did not giggle in response to the third student's voice. Thus, we conducted a 2 (I-sharing dimension: giggle, no giggle) x 2 (I-sharer: Me-sharer, non-Me-sharer) x 2 (liking: for Me-sharer, for non-Me-sharer) x 2 (normative response: to giggle giggling, not to giggle) design. Results indicated that this ad-ditional independent variable—the normativeness of the response—made no difference with regard to our results. As in Study 2, we observed a Me-sharer x I-sharer interaction such that people liked the Me-sharer more when the Me-sharer shared his or her I but the non-Me-sharer more when the non-Me-sharer shared his or her I and the Me-sharer did not. Whether or not participants viewed giggling or the absence of giggling as the norm made no difference in people's preferences for the targets.

Studies 4 and 5: The Role of Assumed I-sharing in Ingroup Bias

We have argued that people like others who share their Me's because of what Me-sharing implies about I-sharing. We get at this issue from a different angle in Studies 4 and 5 by ex-ploring the extent to which assumptions about I-sharing underlie people's liking for mem-bers of their ingroup. Given the importance people place on their social identities (Brewer, 1979), as well as their willingness to favor their ingroup under even the most minimal cir-cumstances (e.g., Tajfel et al., 1971), we reasoned that belonging to the same ingroup may constitute a particularly profound form of Me-sharing. We further reasoned that if Me-sharing serves as a proxy for I-sharing, and if I-sharing promotes liking, assumptions about I-sharing with ingroup members should underlie people's preferences for members of their ingroup.

To test this reasoning, we asked participants to indicate the extent to which their social identity (their race, in Study 4; their gender, in Study 5) represents an important part of their self-definition. In addition, participants indicated the extent to which they believed they share I's with members of their ingroup. Specifically, they rated the extent to which they and a member of their ingroup would feel hurt by the same remark, feel the same way about things, say the same thing at the same time, react similarly to music, like or dislike the same foods, and so on (we included a total of 15 such questions and averaged them to form a composite score; alpha's = .94; .93). Finally, participants indicated the extent to which they like and are friends with members of their ingroup.

Results indicated that as importance of one's social identity to one's self-definition in-creased, so too did one's preference for ingroup members. Importance of social identity to self-definition also predicted assumed I-sharing such that as importance of social identity in-creased, so did the perception that one I-shares with people with the same social identity. In addition, assumed I-sharing predicted liking for ingroup members such that the more people believed they I-shared with ingroup members, the more they liked ingroup members. Most important, mediational tests indicated that assumptions about I-sharing entirely mediated this effect. Specifically, when we entered assumptions about I-sharing into a regression equa-tion along with importance of social identity, the link between social identity and liking disappeared (see Figures 22.1 and 22.2).

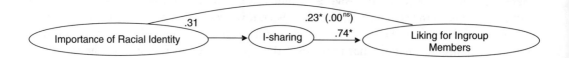

FIGURE 22.1. Mediational model illustrating how I-sharing mediates the relationship between the importance of race and liking for ingroup members. All values represent standardized beta weights; $*p < .05$.

Study 6: Online I-Sharing through Free Associations

Although the results of Studies 1 through 5 generally support our claim that I-sharing promotes liking, we wanted to test this idea in the context of a more involving, realistic "online" interaction with another person. In addition, we wanted to begin our exploration of the role that existential isolation—or personality variables related to existential isolation—plays in people's preferences for I-sharers. To this end, we conducted a laboratory investigation in which participants interacted with an ostensible other at either the Me or I level. Prior to the interaction, we administered a measure of emotional reliance in order to assess its moderating effect on I-sharing and liking. Specifically, we hypothesized that people high in emotional reliance, as compared to those low in emotional reliance, have an insatiable thirst for interpersonal closeness, depend more on others for confirmation of their conception of reality, and thus feel less attracted to someone with a discrepant I and more attracted to an I-sharer.

After completing the measure of emotional reliance, participants began an interactive computer task described as part of a study of how people form relationships through e-mail, Internet chat rooms, and so on. While completing this task, participants believed that they and another participant (who, in reality, did not exist) would exchange information over the computer. Some participants provided and received Me-information; others provided and received I-information. In the Me-information condition, participants completed a series of "I am . . . " statements describing aspects of their selves. In the I-information condition, participants provided their free associations to a series of word-stem completions. We modeled this latter condition after the I-sharing experiences that occur when people simultaneously make the same pun, come up with the same nonintuitive answer to a question, or otherwise indicate that they are "on the same wavelength."

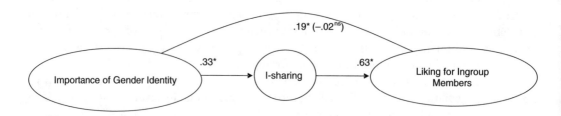

FIGURE 22.2. Mediational model illustrating how I-sharing mediates the relationship between the importance of gender and liking for ingroup members. All values represent standardized beta weights; $*p < .05$.

Almost immediately after completing each "I am . . . " statement or providing a word association, participants viewed the response that their partner ostensibly provided to the same exact item (generated, of course, by the program itself). Some participants discovered that their partner responded identically to them 70% of the time (similar condition); others discovered that their partner responded identically to them only 30% of the time (dissimilar condition). After receiving this information, participants indicated their liking for their communication partner.

The results revealed a significant three-way interaction between emotional reliance, type of information, and similarity (see Figure 22.3, panels *a* and *b*). The nature of this interaction was such that similarity and emotional reliance (ER) had no effect on liking among those who received Me-information. These people showed equal levels of liking across all conditions. Among those who received I-information, however, we observed an interaction between emotional reliance and similarity. When they had provided and received I-information, low-ER participants exhibited equal levels of liking for their partner across both similarity conditions. In contrast, when high ER participants had provided and received I-information, they liked the similar partner significantly more than the dissimilar one. Indeed, compared to all other groups, high-ER participants exposed to a partner who did *not* share their I exhibited the least amount of liking for their partner, suggesting that a lack of I-sharing proves especially distasteful to those especially likely to depend on others for feelings of closeness and for validation of their beliefs (i.e., those high in emotional reliance).

Study 7: Existential Isolation Increases the Appeal of I-Sharing

Our most recent study took a more direct approach to examining the role of existential isolation in producing attraction to those with whom we I-share. Specifically, we manipulated existential isolation by having participants engage in a "lucid memory" task that we described as an assessment of their ability to "mentally relive past experiences when you recall

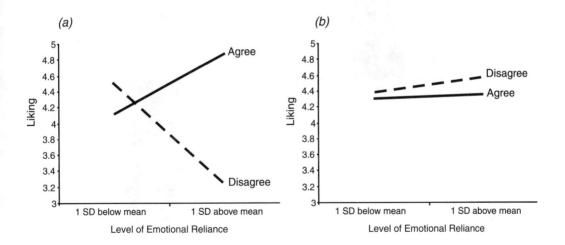

FIGURE 22.3. Liking for partner as a function of agreement and emotional reliance in (*a*) I-information condition, and (*b*) Me-information condition.

them." While completing this task, participants attempted to recall vividly one of three types of memories: (1) a time when they felt out of touch with those around them or felt "alone in a crowd"; (2) a time when they felt bored; or (3) their morning routine. We had participants recall these three different types of memories to create an existential isolation condition, a negative control condition, and a neutral control condition respectively. After this lucid memory task, participants engaged in the same online communication task described earlier, in which they exchanged information with an ostensible partner about which traits describe them or the first word that comes to mind when they hear a particular word.

As may be seen in Figure 22.4, the data revealed that participants primed with feelings of existential isolation exhibited greater levels of liking for the I-sharer than for the Me-sharer. Importantly, participants in the remaining two priming conditions (those in the negative and neutral conditions) tended to prefer the Me-sharer over the I-sharer. Thus, taken together, the findings of Studies 6 and 7 show that both dispositional levels of emotional reliance and priming of memories of past instances of existential isolation make I-sharers particularly appealing. As such, these results support our contention that I-sharing leads to feelings of closeness to others because it relieves feelings of existential isolation.

DISCUSSION

Across seven separate studies we have seen how I-sharing factors into people's liking for others. Consider the results of Studies 1 through 3, which suggest that assumptions about I-sharing may at least partially account for people's preference for similar others (i.e., Me-sharers, according to our analysis). Specifically, when participants received information about

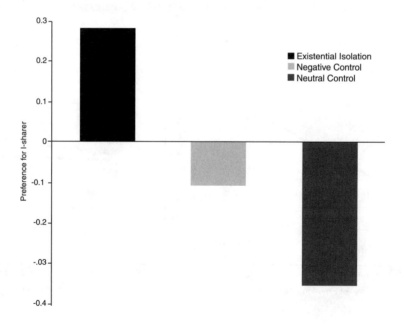

FIGURE 22.4. Preference for I-sharer as a function of feelings of existential isolation.

the extent to which someone from their hometown (i.e., a Me-sharer) or another country (i.e., a non-Me-sharer) also shared their I, they preferred the Me-sharer to the non-Me-sharer when the Me-sharer shared their I. This effect completely reversed itself under conditions when the non-Me-sharer turned out to share the participants' I and suggests that Me-sharing may often serve as a proxy for I-sharing. Having established this basic effect, in Studies 4 and 5, we concentrated on the role of I-sharing in intergroup processes. The findings indicate that assumptions about I-sharing underlie people's preference for people with whom they share important social identities (e.g., aspects of their Me). Study 6 looked at the relative effects of Me-sharing and I-sharing on liking in the context of online interactions. In addition, in Study 6 we looked at a potential moderator of I-sharing. The results indicate that whereas people low in emotional reliance show no preference for an I-sharer over a non-I-sharer, people high in emotional reliance favor people with whom they share I's. Finally, Study 7 provides the strongest evidence to date of the proposed link between I-sharing and existential isolation by showing that priming participants with memories of past instances of existential isolation leads to increased attraction to an I-sharer.

Evidence that I-sharing fosters liking offers a new perspective from which to view seemingly distinct sets of research findings. As noted earlier, we suspect that assumptions about I-sharing can account for the robust tendency for people to prefer similar others. From our perspective, people prefer similar others largely because similarity with respect to the Me signals the potential for I-sharing. Once people learn that a Me-sharer does not experience a stimulus identically to them, however, this preference for the Me-sharer seems to disappear. Thus, when the sole female in an otherwise all male organization hears of a new, female hire, she might initially feel thrilled, thinking that finally someone will validate her perceptions of the discrimination that regularly occurs at work. Imagine her surprise when in the company of the new hire, she encounters what she perceives as discrimination and learns that the new hire disagrees! Such an experience should indicate to her that, despite sharing Me's with the new hire (i.e., gender), she does not share I's with this person. The consequence? All that initial excitement and liking for the new hire becomes a thing of the past.

The possibility that I-sharing underlies people's preferences for similar others (i.e., Me-sharers) suggests new avenues for research on interpersonal and intergroup processes. Those interested in improving interpersonal and intergroup relationships could create situations that foster I-sharing experiences between people. Indeed, we believe that some previous attempts at reducing intergroup tension may have been successful precisely for this reason. Consider the Robbers Cave study (Sherif, Harvey, White, Hood, & Sherif, 1961), in which Sherif and colleagues created and then attempted to undo intergroup rivalry among a group of young boys. These researchers noted that the only successful strategy for undoing the rivalry consisted of providing the boys with superordinate goals, goals that the boys could meet only with everyone's cooperation. Aronson made a similar claim based on his research on the Jigsaw Classroom (Aronson, Blaney, Stephan, Sikes, & Snapp, 1978). We propose that superordinate goals can effectively ease intergroup tension precisely because goal sharing constitutes a form of I-sharing. Viewed from this perspective, Antoine de St. Exupery's suggestion that "Love is not looking at one another, but looking out in the same direction" takes on a whole new meaning.

More generally, our work on I-sharing, however, suggests a very new and potentially important way in which our selves enter into our relationships with others, through a process of sharing our subjective experience of the world. Whereas previous work on the self and relationships has focused almost exclusively on people's representations of self (i.e., the Me), the I-sharing perspective focuses on the role that the self-as-subject (i.e., the I) plays in people's relationships. In so doing, the I-sharing perspective points to the importance of studying the self-as-subject more generally.

Not only could a newfound emphasis on the "I" add to the field's theoretical sophistication, it could also yield important insights in the applied realm. For example, existentially oriented clinical psychologists have long recognized the problem of existential isolation (Laing, 1971; Schneider & May, 1995; Yalom, 1980), and they view it as one of the major challenges that people have to confront in life. To the extent that I-sharing experiences provide an antidote to feelings of existential isolation, clinical psychologists might find value in developing ways to reach their clients at the level of subjective experience.

CONCLUSION

As if death, freedom, and meaninglessness were not enough, we humans also have to deal with the reality of our existential isolation. Here we identify one way in which existential isolation factors into our lives, through our interpersonal dealings with others. Because our existential isolation poses threats to our need to know and our need for interpersonal connectedness, we develop a special fondness for people whom we believe experience a moment in the same way that we do, for I-sharers. I-sharing has this effect because, although we can never really know phenomenologically how another person experiences reality, I-sharing gives us the sense that we can. We may never experience existential connectedness in a literal sense, but I-sharing brings us breathtakingly close.

NOTES

1. Some researchers have made a distinction between the motive to acquire information (e.g., the self-assessment motive; Trope, 1983) and the motive to confirm the validity of information that one has already acquired (e.g., the self-verification motive; Swann, 1996). Because we believe that these two motives stem from the same, overarching drive to know, we combine them in our analysis.
2. Although differences of opinion exist with regard to whether this need for connectedness constitutes a fundamental motive or is derived from more basic needs, few people would deny its existence.
3. In many ways, these characteristics of the "I" have a lot in common with *implicit* components of the self. Nonetheless, an important distinction exists between the I and the implicit self: Whereas people *can* describe their I after the fact, by definition, the implicit self refers to those aspects of the self that remain below conscious awareness.
4. It seems likely that certain hazards might be unique to the erroneous (as opposed to the accurate) belief that one I-shares with one or more people. For instance, when two people involved in a relationship erroneously believe that they I-share, they could neglect their partner out of a belief that they know him or her all too well. As such, they could make faulty decisions or arrive at faulty conclusions about their partner's preferences, wishes, and so on, and this could create problems for the relationship (see Buber, 1923/1958, Wicklund & Vida-Grim, Chapter 23, this volume).
5. To be sure, some of these explanations—such as those pertaining to belief-validation—pertain to aspects of the Me that presumably have close ties to the I. To our knowledge, however, no one has described these findings from an I-sharing perspective as of yet.

REFERENCES

Allport, G. W. (1954). *The nature of prejudice*. Reading, MA: Addison-Wesley.

Aronson, E., Blaney, N., Stephan, C., Sikes, J., & Snapp, M. (1978). *The jigsaw classroom*. Beverly Hills, CA: Sage.

Aronson, E., & Worchel, P. (1966). Similarity versus liking as determinants of interpersonal attractiveness. *Psychonomic Science, 5,* 157–158.

Asch, S. E. (1951). Effects of group pressure upon the modification and distortion of judgments. In H. Guetzkow (Ed.), *Groups, leadership, and men*. Pittsburgh, PA: Carnegie Press.

Asch, S. E. (1956). Studies of independence and conformity: A minority of one against a unanimous majority. *Psychological Monographs, 70,* 416.

Baumeister, R., & Leary, M. (1995). The need to belong: Desire for interpersonal attachments as a fundamental human motivation. *Psychological Bulletin, 117,* 497–529.

Berscheid, E., Dion, K., Walster, E., & Walster, G. W. (1971). Physical attractiveness and dating choice: A test of the matching hypothesis. *Journal of Experimental Social Psychology, 7,* 173–189.

Berscheid, E., & Reis, H. T. (1998). Attraction and close relationships. In D. T. Gilbert, S. T. Fiske, & G. Lindsey (Eds.), *Handbook of social psychology: Vol. 2* (4th ed., pp. 193–281). New York: McGraw-Hill.

Bowlby, J. (1969). *Attachment and loss*. New York: Basic Books.

Brewer, M. B. (1979). In-group bias in the minimal intergroup situation: A cognitive-motivational analysis. *Psychological Bulletin, 86,* 307–324.

Brewer, M. B. (1991). The social self: On being the same and different at the same time. *Personality and Social Psychology Bulletin, 17,* 475–482.

Buber, M. (1958). *I and thou* (2nd ed.; R. G. Smith, Trans.). New York: Charles Scribner's Sons. (Original work published 1923)

Byrne, D. (1971). *The attraction paradigm*. New York and London: Academic Press.

Condon, J. W., & Crano, W. D. (1988). Inferred evaluation and the relation between attitude similarity and interpersonal attraction. *Journal of Personality and Social Psychology, 54,* 789–797.

Csikszentmihalyi, M. (1997). *Finding flow*. New York: Basic Books.

Dick, P. K. (1985). How to build a universe that doesn't fall apart three days later. In M. Hurst & P. Williams (Eds.), *I hope I shall arrive soon* (pp. 1–26). New York: St. Martin's Press.

Duval, S., & Wicklund, R. A. (1972). *A theory of objective self-awareness*. New York: Academic Press.

Festinger, L. (1954). A theory of social comparison processes. *Human Relations, 7,* 117–140.

Florian, V., Mikulincer, M., & Hirschberger, G. (2002). The anxiety-buffering function of close relationships: Evidence that relationship commitment acts as a terror management mechanism. *Journal of Personality and Social Psychology, 82,* 527–542.

Fredrickson, B. L., & Roberts, T. (1997). Objectification theory: Toward understanding women's lived experiences and mental health risks. *Psychology of Women Quarterly, 21,* 173–206.

Fredrickson, B. L., Roberts, T., Noll, S. M., Quinn, D. M., & Twenge, J. M. (1998). That swimsuit becomes you: Sex differences in self-objectification, restrained eating, and math performance. *Journal of Personality and Social Psychology, 75,* 269–284.

Ginsberg, A. (1956). The sunflower sutra. In *Howl and other poems* (pp. 35–38). San Francisco: City Lights Books.

Greenberg, J., Pyszczynski, T., & Solomon, S. (1986). The causes and consequences of a need for self-esteem: A terror management theory. In R. Baumeister (Ed.), *Public self and private self* (pp. 189–212). New York: Springer-Verlag.

Greenberg, J., Simon, L., Solomon, S., Chatel, D., & Pyszczynski, T. (1992). Terror management and tolerance: Does mortality salience always intensify negative reactions to others who threaten the worldview. *Journal of Personality and Social Psychology, 63,* 212–220.

Heider, F. (1958). *The psychology of interpersonal relations*. New York: Wiley.

James, W. (1918). *Principles of psychology*. Toronto: General Publishing. (Original work published 1890)

Kasser, T., & Ahuvia, A. (2002). Materialistic values and well-being in business students. *European Journal of Social Psychology, 32,* 137–146.

Kasser, T., & Ryan, R. M. (1996). Further examining the American dream: Well-being correlates of intrinsic and extrinsic goals. *Personality and Social Psychology Bulletin, 22,* 281–288.

Kelly, G. A. (1955). *The psychology of personal constructs.* New York: Norton.

Laing, R. D. (1971). *Self and others.* Oxford, UK: Penguin Books.

Leary, M. R., Tambor, E. S., Terdal, S. K., & Downs, D. L. (1995). Self-esteem as an interpersonal monitor: The sociometer hypothesis. *Journal of Personality and Social Psychology, 68,* 518–530.

Mueller, J. (1912). Elements of physiology. (W. Baly, Trans.). In B. Rand (Ed.), *The classical psychologists: Selections illustrating psychology from Anaxagoras to Wundt* (pp. 530–544). London: Constable. (Original work published 1834–1840)

Murray, S. L., Holmes, J. G., Bellavia, G., Griffin, D. W., & Dolderman, D. (2002). Kindred spirits? The benefits of egocentrism in close relationships. *Journal of Personality and Social Psychology, 82,* 563–581.

Newcomb, T. (1961). *The acquaintance process.* New York: Holt, Rinehart & Winston.

Pinel, E. C., & Constantino, M. J. (2003). Putting self psychology to good use: When social and clinical psychologists unite. *Journal of Psychotherapy Integration, 13,* 9–32.

Pyszczynski, T., Solomon, S., & Greenberg, J. (2003). *In the wake of 9/11: The psychology of terror.* Washington, DC: American Psychological Association.

Rokeach, M. (1960). *The open and closed mind.* New York: Basic Books.

Schneider, K. J., & May, R. (1995). *The psychology of existence: An integrative, clinical perspective.* New York: McGraw-Hill.

Segal, M. W. (1974). Alphabet and attraction: An unobtrusive measure of the effect of propinquity in a field setting. *Journal of Personality and Social Psychology, 30,* 654–657.

Sherif, M., Harvey, L. J., White, B. J., Hood, W. R., & Sherif, C. W. (1961). *The Robbers Cave experiment: Intergroup conflict and cooperation.* Middletown, CT: Wesleyan University Press. (Reprinted in 1988)

Solomon, S., Greenberg, J., & Pyszczynski, T. (1991). Terror management theory of self-esteem. In C. R. Snyder & D. R. Forsyth (Eds.), *Handbook of social and clinical psychology: The health perspective* (Vol. 162, pp. 21–40). New York: Pergamon Press.

Swann, W. B., Jr. (1996). *Self-traps: The elusive quest for self-esteem.* New York: Freeman.

Tajfel, H., Billig, M. G., Bundy, R. P., & Flament, C. (1971). Social categorization and intergroup behaviour. *European Journal of Social Psychology, 1,* 149–178.

Tajfel, H., & Turner, J. C. (1986). The social identity of intergroup behavior. In S. Worchel & W. G. Austin (Eds.), *Psychology of intergroup relations* (2nd ed., pp. 7–24). Chicago: Nelson-Hall.

Trope, Y. (1983). Self-assessment in achievement behavior. In J. Suls & A. Greenwald (Eds.), *Psychological perspectives on the self* (Vol. 2, pp. 93–121). Hillsdale, NJ: Erlbaum.

Wegner, D. M. (1987). Transactive memory: A contemporary analysis of the group mind. In B. Mullen & G. R. Goethals (Eds.), *Theories of group behavior* (pp. 185–208). New York: Springer-Verlag.

Wetzel, C. G., & Insko, C. A. (1982). The similarity–attraction relationship: Is there an ideal one? *Journal of Experimental Social Psychology, 18,* 253–276.

Wicklund, R. A. (1975). Objective self-awareness. In L. Berkowitz (Ed.), *Advances in experimental social psychology* (Vol. 8, pp. 233–275). New York: Academic Press.

Yalom, I. D. (1980). *Existential psychotherapy.* New York: Basic Books.

Zajonc, R. B. (1968). Attitudinal effects of mere exposure. *Journal of Personality and Social Psychology Monographs, 9* (2, pt. 2), 1–27.

Chapter 23

Bellezza in Interpersonal Relations

ROBERT A. WICKLUND
RENATE VIDA-GRIM

PROLOGUE: SOLIDARITY AS FOUNDED IN SOCIAL EXCHANGE

Interpersonal attraction, seeking of human contact, group formation, and—more generally—solidarity among humans are often viewed as the products of individual needs and need satisfaction. In the classic work of Thibaut and Kelley (1959), for example, the existence of a relation among two or more people is analyzed in terms of the mutual exchange of "points," or rewards. The reward offered by one person can be anything pertinent to the other's individual needs.

Such primitive examples as obtaining food, drink, or shelter from others come to mind, but psychology has also developed frameworks that address the seeking of human contact as a function of more complex individual needs. Festinger (1954) has looked at group formation from the point of view of the individual's need to be certain about evaluations of one's own opinions and abilities. Schachter (1959) has investigated the role of individual fear or anxiety in group formation in that others are sought out as a reaction to states of fear. A major theoretical undertaking called terror management theory deals with existential fears (Greenberg, Solomon, & Pyszczynski, 1997; Pyszczynski, Solomon, Greenberg, & Stewart-Fouts, 1995; Solomon, Greenberg, & Pyszczynski, 1991). The existential fear of not being immortal, often translated into fear of death, is regarded as the basis of a desire for solidarity with similar others and for clinging to the symbolic components of a given culture or value system.

These conceptions have in common a sweeping implication. If each individual carries needs or drives to the interaction, that individual will desire to satisfy the needs quickly. An acute uncertainty about one's abilities or opinions (Festinger, 1954), the existence of strong anxiety (Schachter, 1959), or preoccupation with dying (Greenberg et al., 1997) implies a certain impatience, an orientation toward a solution, and subsequent drive reduction. If such drives can be addressed quickly by a telephone call, or an electronic communication (McKenna & Bargh, 2000; Rheingold, 1993), then the development of an interaction with extensive physical presence would be unnecessary. That is, the motivation for seeking others does not lie within the pleasures of interaction per se, as with Clark and Mills's (1979) notion of communal relationships. Rather, the person approaches the interaction with impatience, looking for relief, satisfaction, oriented toward drive reduction. The solidarities that result stem from using others to move toward drive reduction.

THE SOLIDARITY OF INTERPERSONAL BELLEZZA

Our focus in this chapter is on an entirely different basis for solidarity among interacting humans. This is a solidarity, an attraction to and interest in others, which comes from the mutual offering and receiving of sensations that can be characterized as esthetic, as beautiful, as pleasing to the senses. We are using the term "bellezza" (Wicklund & Vida-Grim, 2001, 2002) to describe the objects that are pleasing to the senses (e.g., recognized art objects, architecture, or nature). Our notion focuses particularly on the visual, acoustical, olfactory, and tactile qualities of other people.

We may begin with a simple example. When two people happen to sit beside one another in an airplane, they may have no immediate basis in their individual drive states for initiating an interaction. That is, neither of them necessarily carries an acute need for certainty, for information, for reassurance, or the like. On the other hand, simply for reasons of politeness, one of them says "Hello" after sitting down. The second person, pleased by the tone of the first person's voice, smiles and says "Hi, it looks like it will be a good flight today." They continue to exchange smiles and brief comments, and each of them enjoys the other's highly presentable physical appearance. The conversation continues intermittently and meanders between joking, expressing opinions about the food, and reacting mutually to the in-flight film.

Just as in an art gallery (see Arnheim, 1971) or a concert hall (Handel, 1989), their mutual presence entails partaking in an esthetic atmosphere. Each person is pleased by the visual and acoustical offerings of the other, and this esthetically based pleasure is the basis for continuing the communication. Thus the motivation for continuing the interaction lies within the interaction itself; the contact is intrinsically motivating (Berlyne, 1957; Csikszentmihalyi, 1975; Deci, 1975).

The emotions associated with experiencing beauty, or bellezza, may be varied. By definition, the sights, sounds, or words basic to an esthetic sensation are experienced as "beautiful," but the emotion is not simply happiness, delight, "I am satisfied," or the like. Sontag (2002) has pointed out that beauty in prose can also set off pathos. A funeral can also be a moment of bellezza for the participants in that they are partaking in shared mutual thoughts regarding the deceased and are also taking in a common, likely well-planned visual and acoustical stimulation. Mutual solidarity should result, just as in a moment of parting between two intimate friends. An object or person who stimulates a sensation of beauty can be associated with a wide range of emotions, which is to say that interpersonal bellezza is not only about contentment or joy. One can be attracted to the beauties of another person's presence and also desire to continue those sensations, even if the corresponding emotions run between happiness, sorrow, elation, and nostalgia.

There is a crucial difference between the experience of art galleries or concert halls and the interpersonal bellezza that we are describing. In the present case the person is not simply a perceiving observer. Each person *offers* bellezza as well, and it is this combination of actively creating something esthetically pleasing for the other, and enjoying the beauty offered by the other, that brings about a growing solidarity.

Mother and Infant

A solidarity with its basis in bellezza does not have to be limited to adults or to interactions dominated by conversation. Even the earliest contact between infant and parent (Shaffer, 1993; Tronick, 1989) can evidence the mutual offering of esthetically pleasing gestures and vocalizations. In the "synchronized routines" described by Tronick, the movements of both infant and mother or father take on the character of a dance. A sound, a single word, or an arm gesture serves to invite the other to take part, to reciprocate, and once these signals and reactions move into a so-called dance form, the interaction is self-perpetuating. Rather than a concrete drive (as anxiety) being reduced, the continuation of the interaction can best be described as each person's enjoyment in the visual, acoustical, or tactile stimulation offered by the other.

The First Romantic Encounter

A bit later in the child's development, toward adolescence, the dance form can be found in romantic flirting and attraction (Wicklund & Vida-Grim, 2001, 2002). For instance, a young man and a young woman, not yet acquainted, notice one another from opposite sides of the street. At first their nonverbal interaction is dominated by visual cues—attention to the other's face, the appearance of various forms of smiling and other inviting expressions, expressions of excitement, and also the mutual stimulation of posture, form of body, and the style and colors of clothing. Each person takes the other's perspective as the ritual develops, and the subtle feedback signals whether or not a given gesture or physical appearance is pleasurable. As they approach one another physically, their words, tone of voice, and perhaps the touch of hands become salient. For the ritual to develop in this fashion each person must be sensitive to what is esthetically pleasing for the other, for without this mutual empathy or perspective taking, the ritual will be cut short.

Further, there must be some similarity of background: If the girl stems from a liberal culture in which the esthetic pleasure is associated with a rapid advance, intimate, provocative glances, scanty clothing, and direct words about the other's physical appeal, the boy from a traditional culture might retreat. For him, much of what she offers will be over stimulation, and will not fit his notions of esthetics in boy–girl relations. Rather than esthetically pleasing, he will find the encounter too direct, offensive, even rude (see Caldwell, 1999), and solidarity will not develop.

But if each person stems from a common background, such that there is a good overlap in terms of the elements and pace of interpersonal bellezza, then the mutual displays will motivate continuation. As the encounter transforms itself into words, it might take the form of "I like your smile," "Your voice is fascinating," "You are beautifully tanned." And as the physical distance is reduced further, body odors, perfume, and aftershave can play into the encounter. Research by Levine and McBurney (1986) shows that the perception of another's smell, for women and men both, often leads to a positive reaction. Thus these repertoires of tone of voice, glances, movements, body, clothing, smell, and touch can all contribute to the "dance" that develops, and in turn, to a feeling of solidarity with the other. The interaction is motivating in and of itself, and the tendency is to continue.

It Is Not a Case of Using the Other

From the standpoint of a classic social psychology (Jones, 1964; Snyder, 1987), it can well happen that a person enters an interaction to satisfy a particular desire. This is the point that we made in the prologue. Someone who urgently needs acceptance by the group, who requires a job or other position, who wants a specified material item or security, or who is seeking an elevated social status (Veblen, 1899; Wicklund & Vandekerckhove, 1999) might think in terms of presenting stimuli that are positive for the other's senses. This implies dressing smartly, visiting the barber beforehand, wearing a perfume or aftershave, and using a strategic verbal repertoire. But all such preparations, in this case, are organized around getting to the individual goal. In turn, this implies an impatient attitude and an orientation of using the particular form of beauty to gain objects, privilege, or power from the other. It is an orientation toward consuming what one needs, and once the consummation takes place, there is little basis for continuing the encounter.

In such a relationship the would-be bellezza is a one-sided affair, in that the person driven by the certain need will not automatically be open to the other's offering of bellezza. In addition, the presence of a drive state will block the person's openness to the other's perspectives (Steins & Wicklund, 1996; Wicklund & Gollwitzer, 1982; Wicklund & Steins, 1996). In turn, the "bellezza" that is offered might be unsuitable for the other's senses. The impatience based in goal orientation and the relative absence of an empathic posture will guarantee that the rituals, dance forms, and solidarity of bellezza will not develop. To be sure, the person's inclination is to reach the goal and end the "relationship" at that point. This is in contrast to the interaction entailing esthetics that is not dominated by acute drive states.

PREREQUISITES FOR THE SOLIDARITY OF BELLEZZA

Exposure and Education

It is conceivable that a certain amount of esthetic appreciation is associated with innate factors underlying perceptual processes. For instance, the child developmental literature indicates that young children are not blind to esthetic considerations. Rather, infants show pleasure when confronted with certain Gestalts. Within the first few weeks after birth, babies show a preference for visual forms of moderate complexity, with strong contrasts, which show movement, and which are not linear (Banks & Ginsburg, 1985; Olson & Sherman, 1983).

Psychology can detail in a precise manner the physical dimensions pertinent to esthetic enjoyment. In discussing visual art, Arnheim (1971) refers to dimensions such as form, balance, growth, light, color, and movement. In a parallel manner it is possible to analyze music in terms of frequency of the sounds, duration, timbre, rhythm, and vibrato (Handel, 1989). But these dimensions, as useful as they might be in analyzing the stimuli underlying esthetic pleasure, tell us neither what an individual will find pleasing nor what esthetic sensations the individual is capable of producing for others.

For this reason it makes sense to talk about *exposure* and *education* with respect to bellezza, within given cultures or subcultures. A person who is exposed adequately to varieties of interpersonal forms within a culture will come to appreciate the nuances, the subtleties (cf. Gibson, 1969), and may also develop an active repertoire of offering these elements to others (Wicklund & Vida-Grim, 2001). Immersed in society, a person will learn by observation and imitation (cf. Bandura, 1977) the nuances of receiving and offering that which is esthetically pleasing.

For instance, just within the visual dimension, there are myriad subtleties that go into the culturally appropriate eye contact, posture, form of body, clothing, style of hair, and the arrangement of one's home, colors, plants, and furnishings. In the acoustical realm, exposure and active practice are required to appreciate and offer a pleasing tone of voice (for the particular culture), the selection of words and phrases that engage others positively. We can take this list further into the sensory dimensions of smell and touch, but the general idea remains the same. A person growing up and living in a deprived environment, as an orphanage or hospital, will not have the full exposure to the interpersonal esthetics of the relevant culture. Correspondingly, that same person will not develop fully the repertoires that are important—within the cultural framework—for offering others pleasing visual, auditory, olfactory, or tactile stimulation. In short, no matter whether through formal education (Piombo, 2001) or by way of informal contact, a person's culture is the source of the individual esthetic repertoire.

How Many Sensory Dimensions?

Not only does the precise form of interpersonal esthetics vary from culture to culture, but there are also wide variations in the focus on one perceptual dimension or another. In a socalled oral culture (Locke, 1998), the spoken word is a dominant feature, and minor acoustical variations and voice quality play a dominant role. In a modern society in which the written word is dominant, esthetics are more confined to the sensations generated by written words. For example, the esthetic properties of a person's handwriting, coupled with the potential of written expressions, contribute to the solidarity of bellezza that is realizable within written communications. And as handwriting becomes obsolete, the parties to a written communication still have the power of expression within the language to produce esthetic stimulation for one another. The point is that an esthetically pleasing interpersonal interaction does not have to entail all possible sensory dimensions simultaneously. Depending on an individual's exposure and training, some dimensions will play a greater role in esthetics than others. At the same time, it seems clear that the varieties of esthetic social experiences and their intensity will be highly constrained if human contact is limited to only the written word, only the voice, or only visual impressions.

Absence of Pressing Drive States

This second prerequisite for the solidarity of bellezza refers to the *absence* of certain psychological states. A person who enters a relation might well be transporting a personal concern, a need, an urgent matter to the interaction. Such a drive state (e.g., severe hunger or anxiety) or preoccupation (e.g., needing to prove one's self-worth) will narrow the person's focus. The person's readiness to perceive or react to complexities and subtleties will be diminished (Easterbrook, 1959; Wicklund & Steins, 1996). Further, a strong drive or preoccupation interferes with attention to the other's mental states, and without taking the other's perspectives, it is difficult to offer fitting esthetic stimulation to the other. The person with preoccupations will miss cues and subtleties requisite to building the ritual—the "dance"—that produces solidarity.

Accordingly, the ideal condition for the emergence of a bellezza-based solidarity is a state of mind unencumbered by strong drives, fears, anxieties, self-esteem needs, and the like. Horney (1945) expressed as much in describing the deficient interpersonal habits of the so-called neurotic.

Preparation for the Other: The Short Term and Long Term

The prerequisites just characterized should enable a person to enter an interaction with an openness to perceiving what the other offers, to enjoy the dimensionality of what the other offers, and to create esthetic sensations for the other. But this latter component, creating bellezza for the other person, demands a kind of preparation. Such preparations can be instantaneous, but then again often entail efforts prior to the interaction.

The Short Term

Many of the gestures offered to the other involve only a shortterm preparation, as in eye contact, appropriate distance, posture, tone of voice, and bodily contact. As long as the person is not beset with pressing needs, and given that the exposure/education has taken place earlier, the person is ready to adjust such aspects as tone of voice in a manner fitting for the other.

For instance, two people who are previously unacquainted strike up a conversation at a coffee bar. They stem from similar cultures and possess comparable repertoires regarding perspective taking and meeting strangers. The first moment of the encounter involves glances, followed by greetings, these carried out immediately without devoting great amounts of time to preparing for the other's perspective. Given that each person senses a pleasure in these first few overtures, the "dance" continues. The physical distance is reduced and the verbal exchanges proceed. Each partner to the encounter takes the other's perspective, drawing on a repertoire that should be esthetically pleasing for the other.

In such everyday encounters there is little that can be said to describe the preparation for the other, as the fine-tuning for the other's perspective is made on the spot during the rapid giveandtake of esthetically pleasing gestures and words. If some of the gestures are off the mark, or go beyond a cultural limit, the flaw can be corrected rapidly. All this assumes that the two partners have comparable prior exposure and education in interpersonal esthetics and that neither person is preoccupied with pressing needs.

The Long Term

How do we talk about preparation in a longterm sense within the confines of a casual meeting at a coffee bar? The long term makes sense if we imagine that the two people agree to see each other on some future occasion. For instance, the man may have sensed that the woman favored sober colors and was also fascinated by expressions in foreign languages. Thinking about her perspective prior to the second meeting, he arrives the second time dressed in dark blue and having reviewed his French. Correspondingly, the woman brings along samples of her short stories, having inferred that the man appreciates a certain kind of fiction.

Clearly such preparations are not confined to adult male/female interactions. The pair in question could be two men, two women, business associates, colleagues, or relatives. The same analysis applies: If the first encounter develops into a solidarity of esthetic impressions, each person will be inclined to prepare for the other's perspective for subsequent encounters. Surely some of the preparations might bypass or even violate the other's receptiveness, as in bright colors carried to extreme, or a perfume whose intensity registers as offensive on the other person. This is a likely characteristic of long-term preparations, as they are carried out without immediate feedback from the other and cannot be coordinated in a fine-tuned manner to the other's training and exposure.

TWO CLASSIC ILLUSTRATIONS OF PREPARATION OVER THE LONG TERM

The Tea Ceremony and the Dinner Table

Far from being a simple drink to awaken one's senses, tea in its classical social contexts is a social ceremony of some duration, full of aspects bearing on bellezza. Kesten (1997), in characterizing the Japanese tea ceremony, points to certain "unseeable" principles of the tea ceremony, including harmony among people, respect and appreciation for others, and the proper use of the tea utensils. In its more elaborate form, a number of physical (seeable) elements accompany and surround the ceremony, such as the landscaped garden, the low entrance to the tea room, placement of flowers, utensils, and color of tea bowls. Kesten refers to these seeable and unseeable components as contributing to the esthetic experience of drinking tea.

The tea ceremony is not a routine that a person indulges in instinctively; the factor of education becomes central in an esthetic exchange of such complexity. For example, there are worldwide centers that educate non-Japanese people in the intricacies of the tea ceremony (Kesten, 1997).

In a parallel manner, almost any classical dinner table—as in France or Italy—entails a set of social repertoires and physical elements that make up the esthetic experience of eating. Each family member or other dinner guest exercises a certain preparation beforehand. This means not "grazing" prior to the dinner, dressing to please the tastes of the others, and being ready to converse with the others. Arriving at the table is not about the consummatory act of chewing and swallowing; it has to do with mutual esthetic perceptions.

An extreme form of the elaborate dinner is the Indian wedding feast, lasting up to 5 days (Kesten, 1997). Quite the opposite of a mere consummatory act, oriented toward drive reduction, a feast of such longevity entails elaborate social rituals, mixtures of verbal expressions, myriad nonverbal communication, elaborate standards for clothing, and the patience to conduct oneself in appropriate ways, day after day.

In a corresponding way, the person responsible for the table and the kitchen carries out a preparation for the potential esthetic enjoyment of the guests at the table. Far from being a substance containing calories to be consumed, the food can be regarded as fine perfume, even as a subtle aphrodisiac (Paolini, 2002). Also on a visual level it is easy to talk about offering forms of art to guests at the table (Gregory, 2002).

The cook is potentially an artist, a person who has thought about the perspectives of the guests, and their readiness to savor the perfumes, the visual contours of the courses, and the atmosphere at the table. If the dinner guests bring along a readiness to enjoy these elements, based on earlier training and lack of current preoccupation with other matters, the dinner can evolve into an interaction of bellezza among all participants. The resulting solidarity should then lead to a tendency to prolong the occasion, just as any other esthetically based interaction.

On the other hand, if the training/exposure are absent, or if the guests arrive in a condition of impatience, the mealtime will be reduced to a consummatory act. The guests will not take note of the potential bellezza being offered and will be oriented primarily toward the act of eating and returning to their urgent preoccupations. An extreme case of bypassing esthetic exchanges during a meal is to be found in *Overcoming Overeating* by Hirschmann and Munter (1988). Central to their notion is the virtue of knowing when we are hungry and appeasing the hunger need promptly. Translated to the operational level, they advocate the person's carrying around a supply of food and "grazing" whenever hunger arises. Such grazing certainly should develop, in one form or another, given a dominance of personal concerns, fears, or deadlines. One such personal concern, made explicit in the Hirschmann and Munter work, is the person's need to control overeating and lose weight.

Body Weight and Figure

This topic is closely related to the issues surrounding the dinner table. As we have looked at the classic eating occasion, a location of esthetically based interactions, the prerequisites are a certain education/exposure that orient people to esthetic facets of eating. For instance, education/exposure can sensitize people to the visual and olfactory elements of a mealtime and corresponding esthetically based interaction. Similarly, when people appear at the dinner table or any other social setting, they may or may not be sensitive to their own bodies as a basis of esthetic pleasure (or disgust) for the others. Education and exposure can be seen as the sources of such a sensitivity. That is, a given culture, subculture, or group will place repeated emphasis on a body weight and form that are esthetically pleasing to others in that culture; frequent contact with others in a face-to-face fashion will provide the exposure necessary to internalize a concept of that culture's ideals regarding body weight and form (Gniech et al., 1999). This means that if a child in Culture X grows up having intense human contact, and if the culture's ideals of body weight and figure are well communicated formally and informally, the child will be attuned to the dimension "body" in social interaction.

The same child, in the course of encounters with others, will come to derive esthetic pleasure from seeing a fine figure—"fine" always through the perspective of that culture's or group's standards. A figure too lean or too overweight will appear to the child as uninteresting or aversive. If such children are not caught up with personal needs, anxieties, preoccupations, and the like, they will take the other's perspective during interaction. In turn, they will be attuned to their own bodies as perceived by the other. They will be sensitized to whether or not their bodies generate a sense of bellezza for the other, or indifference, or perhaps even aversion or disgust. In this manner the body enters into the "dance," the interaction grounded in esthetic impressions.

It should be apparent that this analysis applies equally for all features of one's own person that are carried into an interaction, including manner of speaking, hairstyle, or clothing. Once the individuals are sensitized to a particular dimension (e.g., weight) during cultural training, and if they are indeed attuned to others' perspectives, they will sense whether or not their physical presence is a source of esthetic pleasure or displeasure for the other.

We are concentrating here particularly on *sensitivity* to body weight and form in social settings, and on the person's intentions or efforts to coordinate the body to the esthetics of interpersonal interaction. But it must be noted that the literature on body weight focuses more on the weight fluctuations that do, in fact, take place. And within that context, it is also clear that there are some genetic components in a person's maintenance of a culturally prescribed weight (Smith, 1999). For instance, there is evidence in research comparing identical and fraternal twins that resting metabolic rate is partially under genetic control (Smith, 1999). On the other hand, the relatively recent crescendo in obesity in the United States (Kesten, 1997; Smith, 1999; Stearns, 1997), as well as comparisons between the United States and France (Stearns, 1997), indicate that the researcher has ample liberty to apply social and other environmental factors in analyzing overweight.

The development of a continuing interaction, based in part on participants' esthetically pleasing figures, is to be differentiated from an interaction rooted in a definite need. In the latter case, stereotypical examples come to mind: A woman develops a "perfect" figure in order to gain power or influence among targeted men; a man works out in a fitness studio in order to woo more women into bed for his conquests. By now it is clear that we can differentiate these need- or drive-dominated encounters from an encounter in which both parties offer, and receive, esthetic impressions—the encounter tending to continue and to result in solidarity.

Long-Term Preparation

Body weight cannot be adjusted rapidly, as contrasted with eye contact, interpersonal distance, or facial expressions. Preparing for the other's perspective in the case of body weight means sensing what physical parameters would set off esthetic pleasures in the other, and then commencing to reduce, or gain, weight accordingly. Such preparations are a relatively short-term task when eating habits are controlled externally, as in the French culture, where children's eating routines are monitored with more rigor than in the United States (Stearns, 1997). That is: When the cultural standards for weight are clear and salient, then a person's intense social contact will bring an ample feedback regarding the body. In turn, we should expect that participants in such a culture will be attuned frequently to whether their own bodies tap into the esthetic sensibilities of their associates, and there will be a pronounced tendency to attempt to present a body of potential bellezza to others.

When would such attempted preparation for others not take place? The answer is the same as in our illustrations of the dinner table:

1. If a particular culture places no emphasis on body weight or form as a component of interpersonal esthetics, then the dimension "body" will not enter into the person's preparations for others. In discussing fashion and the body in 19th-century England, Germany, and the United States, Hollander (1994) refers to an emphasis on "sensible" dress for women, such that "Feminine trappings were now seen to hinder the action of female reason, health, morality and intellect . . . " (p. 125). That is, the potential sexual attractiveness of the female body, by this value system, was not regarded as an element to be emphasized in social interaction. A similar theme was struck by McKenna and Bargh (2000). Noting the advantages of electronically mediated contacts with others, they indicate that the actual physical presence of another person, at least during the initial stages of acquaintance, can inhibit coming to know the other person in a deeper manner. In other words, the value system being forwarded by McKenna and Bargh would seem to prescribe the virtue of coming to know the other's personality, character, or interests without the interference of physical attractiveness/unattractiveness, weight, skin quality, posture, or other nonverbal aspects.

2. If there is lacking exposure, meaning an absence of face-to-face social exchange, the salience and possibility of communicating bellezza with the aid of one's body will be attenuated.

3. If a person is momentarily or permanently caught up with personal concerns, then preparing for the other's perspective will be blocked and the body as a source of bellezza for others will be neglected. In like manner, there will be fewer intentions or efforts to bring about a bellezza by means of attending to skin quality, hair, posture, musculature, clothing, odors, and tone or quality of voice.

Body Weight and the Coffee Bar Encounter

What do these three factors look like when applied more concretely to a characteristic scene that makes weight reduction salient? We may return to the example of the first encounter between two people at a coffee bar. The woman finds the man's interest in foreign languages to be interesting; the man finds her literary interests intriguing. These interests spark a mutual desire to meet again, and perhaps also a third or fourth time, and maybe into the future. At the same time, neither of them is dressed with an eye toward fashion or coordination of colors, their clothing does not accentuate the forms of their bodies, and both are overweight. Each of them evidences a body mass index above the 80th percentile.

1. If their particular culture indeed pays little heed to the body as a component in interpersonal esthetics, then each of them will look away from that dimension. They will continue to exchange pleasant words, glances, and touches, and they will continue to think about the other's interests (foreign languages; literature) between encounters. But given that weight and form of body do not figure strongly into the esthetics of interaction, within their particular culture, neither of them will undertake to reduce or to improve muscle tone for the other. Stated in another way: Their culture provides no motive, based in interpersonal interaction, for their focusing on reducing.

2. How about the factor of presence/absence of face-to-face contact? Assuming that their culture *does* emphasize the body in interpersonal attraction, then they will go home and think about "his perception of my body" and "her perception of my body" between encounters. Their interest in one another will imply the initiation of longterm preparations: Trying to slim down, to improve musculature, and to dress more carefully in line with the assumed preferences of the other. But this chain of events, potentially motivating each of them to lose weight, can easily be broken by eliminating face-to-face contact. Suppose, for instance, that the second meeting is only a long telephone call, and that most of the subsequent encounters are carried out by e-mail. Their bodies no longer being salient for one another, any remaining interpersonal bellezza will shift to the level of the exchange of pleasant, elegant, exciting, or erotic words. Preparation for the other with respect to weight and form of body will cease.

3. Even if their cultures emphasize the body in interpersonal attraction, and even if the encounters continue to be at the coffee bar or otherwise face-to-face, it might be that each of them is caught up chronically in preoccupations. These could be based in work, health, children, or any of a number of other standard stress factors. Such needs or preoccupations will keep the stressed person from perceiving that which delights or engages the other, and again, longer-term preparations for esthetic encounters with the other, including weight-reduction, will be attenuated.

It is interesting to note that weight reduction in the United States is almost invariably regarded through the perspective of the oversized person's individual needs—these needs being cast largely as health and medical cost issues. In France, by way of contrast, the esthetic dimension is more likely to figure into recommendations for weight reduction (Stearns, 1997). One culture may have evolved such that the dimension overweight–underweight is defined as an individual health issue (i.e., a personal need, and not a question of the person's bellezza in social relations). Another culture may have evolved in a different manner, whereby personal health becomes secondary to the social–esthetic function of the body.

But aside from such cultural evolutions, our analysis implies that absence of intense face-to-face contact with others, *or* the dominance of personal need states, will tend to eliminate body weight, style and fit of clothing, perfume, posture, and gestures from the salient dimensions involved in interpersonal esthetics. The result is that weight, clothing, posture, skin quality, and musculature will be regarded from the standpoint of the individual's own current needs and practical concerns. Functionality for the individual thereby replaces the involvement of the body in esthetics-based interactions.

DISSOLUTION OF THE CULTURE OF BELLEZZA IN INTERACTION

The reader should not think that we are describing an ideal culture in which every human intention or movement is guided by the desire to spark off esthetic pleasure in the next person. Our purpose is much more to describe the factors that should lead to humans' being motivated to continue interactions on the basis of giving and receiving impulses that set off a sense of esthetics. We have pointed to education/exposure with respect to the many objects and dimensions of beauty within a culture, and to the necessity of *absence* of personal needs, drives, or preoccupations. With this final factor, we are referring to the possibility of the person's being open to others' perspectives, and thus being in a position to act so as to set off esthetic reactions in the other.

Using these concepts to characterize human interaction, one can characterize the flow of an encounter in terms of the mutual offering and receiving of gestures, objects, and words setting off esthetic pleasure in the other person. Much as in the phenomena of curiosity (Berlyne, 1957), intrinsic motivation (Deci, 1975), or the flow experience (Csikszentmihalyi, 1975), the interaction of bellezza will tend toward continuation.

How does it happen, then, that a culture can change? That is, if interpersonal bellezza and the corresponding solidarity dominate a culture, what factors underlie the collapse of this bellezza and solidarity? To address this question we can point toward two elements central in our analysis: exposure and personal needs.

Exposure

A culture rich in interactions guided by subjectively experienced esthetics is also a culture of interpersonal contact. By this, we mean the kind of contact that defines the "oral" culture, in which people have intense visual, auditory, olfactory, and tactile contact. The illustrations of the mother–infant dance, the flirting among adolescents, the casual meeting at the coffee bar, and the French dinner all depend on face-to-face communication.

The collapse of the bellezza-based communication can come about through less exposure to these several sensory dimensions. One author, John Locke (1998), has documented such decreases in exposure in the United States. He points to increments in gated or exclusive communities, one-person households, and impersonal shopping centers, and to varieties of technical developments such as cellular telephones or computer-based communication.

Following Locke's lead, we may suppose that all developments that create distance between individuals (one's own house, one's own cell phone) and abbreviated forms of contact reduce the possibility of bellezza during a social encounter. The reason should be apparent. Each sensory dimension adds to the participants' potential for creating and experiencing esthetic impulses during the interaction, and with the dimensionality greatly reduced, there is not much room left over for exercising esthetically based communications with others. As pointed out by McKenna and Bargh (2000), the Internet eliminates cues as to the other's physical characteristics. The advantage, according to them, is a reduction in fear of taking up contact with others. But at the same time, as we are noting here, the continuation of an interaction guided by physically based bellezza drops to nil. The culture changes.

Personal Needs

While many forms of personal needs can interfere with the perspective taking necessary for interpersonal bellezza, we refer here to two sorts of needs, or preoccupations, that could easily bring about a cultural change.

Anxiety

If an entire culture or large group is beset with threats, as in war, terror, contagious diseases, or criminality, the participants to interactions will carry such preoccupations into their relations with others. Mutually experienced fear, as in wartime, might well create a sense of solidarity and adherence to common values (Greenberg et al., 1997). This is a solidarity deriving from mutual concerns and shared goals and lies outside the idea of solidarity beginning in mutual bellezza. For instance, the members of a persecuted minority or the victims of an epidemic will perhaps experience solidarity, but such a solidarity has to do with the sense of being threatened, and with being oriented toward a common solution.

Achievement Concerns

Another sort of personal preoccupation is akin to achievement motivation (McClelland, Atkinson, Clark, & Lowell, 1953). A society that obligates its workers to focus continuously on their tasks, to work overtime, to be on call, and to work under insecure conditions is also a society that does not grant its members leisure time to focus on the subtleties in interpersonal interaction. Institutions such as the "power lunch" develop (Wicklund & Vida-Grim, 2001), in which a lunch turns into a quick business discussion. In such an achievement-dominated society the preoccupation with work, homework, and meeting deadlines will readily transform encounters at the coffee bar and relations at home into workdominated scenarios. Functionality and efficiency will dominate interactions, leaving little room for participants to enjoy interaction or prepare the potential esthetics of interaction.

It must be noted that people "reach the goal" in cultures that are characterized by higher anxiety levels or a severe work ethic, and certainly there are pleasures to be had by reaching definite goals. This is the message of the psychology of drive reduction and is the sense of our prologue (earlier). But our point is that social interactions dominated by goal-orientation and attempted drive reduction are not self-perpetuating. The individual need comes first, as does its satisfaction, and participation is necessary as long as it serves such drive reduction. By comparison, the pleasures entailed in the interaction of bellezza develop within the interaction itself, implying that participants tend to continue, without an orientation toward getting to the end.

ACKNOWLEDGMENT

We are indebted to Ursula Kaufmann for preparing the manuscript.

REFERENCES

Arnheim, R. (1971). *Art and visual perception: A psychology of the creative eye*. Berkeley, CA: University of California Press.

Bandura, A. (1977). *Social learning theory*. Englewood Cliffs, NJ: Prentice-Hall.

Banks, M. S., & Ginsburg, A. P. (1985). Infant visual preferences: A review and new theoretical treatment. In H. W. Reese (Ed.), *Advances in child development* (Vol. 19). Orlando, FL: Academic Press.

Berlyne, D. E. (1957). Uncertainty and conflict: A point of contact between information theory and behavior theory. *Psychological Review, 64*, 329–339.

Caldwell, M. (1999). *A short history of rudeness*. New York: Picador.

Clark, M. S., & Mills, J. (1979). Interpersonal attraction in exchange and communal relationships. *Journal of Personality and Social Psychology, 37*, 12–24.

Csikszentmihalyi, M. (1975). *Beyond boredom and anxiety*. San Francisco: Jossey-Bass.

Deci, E. L. (1975). *Intrinsic motivation*. New York: Plenum Press.

Easterbrook, J. A. (1959). The effect of emotion on cue utilization of behavior. *Psychological Review, 66*, 183–201.

Festinger, L. (1954). A theory of social comparison processes. *Human Relations, 7*, 117–140.

Gibson, E. J. (1969). *Principles of perceptual learning and development*. East Norwalk, CT: Appleton-Century-Crofts.

Gniech, G., Bölitz, A., Lange, M., Bark-Lenz, G., Harden, J., Lex, B., et al. (1999). *Wonneproppen: Dicke Menschen in "mageren" Zeiten*. Berlin: Pabst.

Greenberg, J., Solomon, S., & Pyszczynski, T. (1997). Terror management theory of self-esteem and cultural worldviews: Empirical assessments and conceptual refinements. In M. P. Zanna (Ed.), *Advances in experimental social psychology* (Vol. 29, pp. 61–139). San Diego: Academic Press.

Gregory, T. (2002, September 15). Venere in brodo di giuggiole. *Il Sole-24 Ore*, No. 252, p. 33.

Handel, S. (1989). *Listening: An introduction to the perception of auditory events*. Cambridge, MA: MIT Press.

Hirschmann, J. R., & Munter, C. H. (1988). *Overcoming overeating*. New York: Fawcett Columbine.

Hollander, A. (1994). *Sex and suits*. New York: Knopf.

Horney, K. (1945). *Our inner conflicts: A constructive theory of neurosis*. New York: Norton.

Jones, E. E. (1964). *Ingratiation: A social psychological analysis*. New York: Appleton-Century-Crofts.

Kesten, D. (1997). *Feeding the body, nourishing the soul*. Berkeley, CA: Conari Press.

Levine, J. M., & McBurney, D. H. (1986). The role of olfaction in social perception and behavior. In C. P. Herman, M. P. Zanna, & E. T. Higgins (Eds.), *Physical appearance, stigma, and social behavior: The Ontario Symposium* (Vol. 3, pp. 179–217). Hillsdale, NJ: Erlbaum.

Locke, J. L. (1998). *Why we don't talk to each other anymore: The de-voicing of society*. New York: Touchstone.

McClelland, D. C., Atkinson, J. W., Clark, R. A., & Lowell, E. L. (1953). *The achievement motive*. New York: Appleton-Century-Crofts.

McKenna, K. Y. A., & Bargh, J. A. (2000). Plan 9 from cyberspace: The implications of the Internet for personality and social psychology. *Personality and Social Psychology Review, 4*, 57–75.

Olson, G. M., & Sherman, T. (1983). Attention, learning, and memory in infants. In P. H. Mussen (Ed.), *Handbook of child psychology* (Vol. 2, pp. 1001–1080). New York: Wiley.

Paolini, D. (2002, February 10). Amore in un boccone. *Il Sole-24 Ore*, No. 39, p. 44.

Piombo, M. (2001, May 27). A scuola lezioni di gusto. *Il Giornale*.

Pyszczynski, T., Solomon, S., Greenberg, J., & Stewart-Fouts, M. (1995). The liberating and constraining aspects of self: Why the freed bird finds a new cage. In A. Oosterwegel & R. A. Wicklund (Eds.), *The self in European and North American culture: Development and processes* (pp. 357–373). Dordrecht, The Netherlands: Kluwer Academic.

Rheingold, H.. (1993). *The virtual community: Homesteading on the electronic frontier.* New York: Harper.

Schachter, S. (1959). *The psychology of affiliation.* Stanford, CA: Stanford University Press.

Shaffer, D. R. (1993). *Developmental psychology: Childhood and adolescence.* Pacific Grove, CA: Brooks/Cole.

Smith, J. C. (1999). *Understanding childhood obesity.* Jackson, MS: University Press of Mississippi.

Snyder, M. (1987). *Public appearances/private realities.* New York: Freeman.

Solomon, S., Greenberg, J., & Pyszczynski, T. (1991). A terror management theory of social behavior: The psychological functions of self-esteem and cultural worldviews. In M. Zanna (Ed.), *Advances in experimental social psychology* (Vol. 24, pp. 93–159). San Diego: Academic Press.

Sontag, S. (2002, July 13). Il grande mistero della bellezza. *La Repubblica*, No. 162, p. 1.

Stearns, P. N. (1997). *Fat history.* New York: New York University Press.

Steins, G., & Wicklund, R. A. (1996). Perspective-taking, conflict, and press: Drawing an E on your forehead. *Basic and Applied Social Psychology, 18*, 319–346.

Thibaut, J. W., & Kelley, H. H. (1959). *The social psychology of groups.* New York: Wiley.

Tronick, E. Z. (1989). Emotions and emotional communications in infants. *American Psychologist, 44*, 112–119.

Veblen, T. (1899). *The theory of the leisure class.* New York: Macmillan.

Wicklund, R. A., & Gollwitzer, P. M. (1982). *Symbolic self-completion.* Hillsdale, NJ: Erlbaum.

Wicklund, R. A., & Steins, G. (1996). Person perception under pressure: When motivation brings about egocentrism. In P. M. Gollwitzer & J. A. Bargh (Eds.), *The psychology of action: Linking cognition to behavior* (pp. 511–528). New York: Guilford Press.

Wicklund, R. A., & Vandekerckhove, M. M. P. (1999). Conspicuous consumption. In P. E. Earl & S. Kemp (Eds.), *The Elgar companion to consumer research and economic psychology* (pp. 106–111). Cheltenham: Edward Elgar.

Wicklund, R. A., & Vida-Grim, R. (2001). Il ruolo della bellezza nella società: Funzione strumentale o apertura? In G. Pantaleo & R. A. Wicklund (Eds.), *Prospettive multiple nella vita sociale* (pp. 123–148). Padova/Bologna: Decibel/Zanichelli.

Wicklund, R. A., & Vida-Grim, R. (2002). Bellezza: Das Offerieren von Schönheit und Hässlichkeit im sozialen Umgang. In H. Reuter & M. A. Stadler (Eds.), *Lebenswelt und Erleben: Beiträge zur Erfahrungs psychologie* (pp. 273–297). Lengerich and Berlin: Pabst Science.

Part V

Freedom and the Will

Chapter 24

Being Here Now

Is Consciousness Necessary for Human Freedom?

JOHN A. BARGH

I do not think, therefore I am.
—JEAN COCTEAU

Although Socrates claimed that the unexamined life was not worth living, the examined life isn't any picnic either. Facing our mortality and the reality and meaning of our existence head on is not something that we generally enjoy doing. To the contrary, we are all quite resourceful in finding ways to avoid any thoughts about such topics (e.g., Becker, 1973; Solomon, Greenberg, & Pyszczynski, 1991, Chapter 2, this volume). And with good reason: Being more honest about the reality of one's life situation is linked to a greater likelihood of depression and suicide (e.g., Alloy & Abramson, 1979; Taylor, 1989). The honestly examined life, therefore, tends to be a pretty scary place.

It is somewhat paradoxical that among all of the earth's creatures, humans are superior both in the ability to recognize and ponder our own mortality and in the capability for mentally transforming our worlds to avoid thinking about it. The ability to detach oneself from the direct control and influences of one's current environment depends crucially on our capacity for mentally transforming and construing that environment (e.g., Mischel, 1973; Mischel, Cantor, & Feldman, 1996). These cognitive transformations enable us both to act when the current situation is unsupportive of that action (such as through a newfound belief in efficacy and agency within that situation; Bandura, 1986; Yalom, 1980) and to not act in the presence of "hot" situational triggers to action (such as when we delay immediate gratification in the service of more substantial and important long-term goals; Metcalfe & Mischel, 1999). Living thus a layer or two detached from the realities of our present situation also permits the operation of comforting "positive illusions" as to the true state of affairs (Murray, Holmes, & Griffin, 1996; Taylor, 1989) so that, like the children of Lake Wobegon, we can all be "better than average" on every dimension.

One such positive illusion—the feeling of control, of personal ownership or responsibility for one's own actions and their consequences (e.g., Langer, 1975)—has powerful social benefits as well. As Prinz (1997) and Bargh (1999) have argued, even if volitional states are determined, people behaving *as if* they have free will and are personally accountable for their actions is of tremendous, even essential, value for the functioning of modern societies. The personal belief in one's own agency has the consequence of infusing one's behavioral options with the normative expectations and guidelines of society at large. The knowledge (or threat) that one will be held accountable by others causes those norms to become very real constraints on one's actions.

The ability to detach our conscious mind from the mundane concerns of the present brings other tremendous advantages to the individual, such as the contemplation at leisure of past events so as to better understand their meaning, causes, and consequences (as Socrates had recommended), as well as the anticipation of and planning for future events (see Gollwitzer, 1999). Heidegger (1927/1962) emphasized this "time-traveling" quality of conscious experience; for him, existence or "Being" was, paradoxically, permeated by non-Being: "the no-longer (Past) and the not-yet (Future) that hold such power and influence over our thoughts and concerns and emotions" (Barrett, 1958, p. 226). A half-century later, Ram Dass (1971) famously urged us to "Be here now," precisely because we usually are not.

However, while we are away time traveling, somebody had better be home minding the store. Regardless of where in time and space our conscious mind is currently focused, we are stuck living in the present, with the strong and continuous need to respond adaptively and sensibly to those present circumstances (see Bargh, 1997). To free the conscious mind to reminisce about the past and to plan for the future, the nonconscious self-regulatory processes to be described in this chapter must be capable of handling the demands of the present. This strongly suggests that deliberate, conscious choice processes are not a necessary element of mundane functioning in the here and now.

CONSCIOUSNESS AND NONCONSCIOUSNESS IN EXISTENTIAL THOUGHT

However, existential philosophers have reified (some might even say deified) the role of deliberate, conscious choice in everyday life as the *sine qua non* of existence—the choices we make, or fail to make, are said to give life its meaning and define who we are as individuals. For Sartre (e.g., 1944), consciousness and freedom were one and the same thing (Barrett, 1958, p. 256). Existential philosophy has had a tremendous impact on contemporary psychology, especially through the humanist tradition which placed conscious choice as central and necessary to nearly all human behavior and judgment (see Bandura, 1986; Mischel et al., 1996; review in Bargh & Ferguson, 2000). In this approach, human freedom is pitted against direct environmental causes or influences on one's behavior such as external coercion and force (whether implied or actual), and gratifying short-term pleasures such as tasty desserts or cigarettes, the consumption of which defeat one's long-term goals. The emphasis on transcending or overcoming environmental control can also be seen as a reaction to the dominance of behaviorism—especially radical behaviorism—within experimental psychology for much of the 20th century (see Bargh & Ferguson, 2000), because behaviorism stressed the role of environmental causes to the exclusion of all others.

Because it equated freedom with conscious choice, existential philosophy was in fact antagonistic toward any conception of human nature in which people were said to be controlled by nonconscious forces. Thus, Sartre (for one) was strongly opposed to the idea of a hypothetical (Freudian) unconscious calling the shots (Barrett, 1958, pp. 254–255), just as he was to the Skinnerian notion of complete environmental hegemony. Sartre and other existential writers (such as Otto Rank) recoiled against any deterministic approach to the human mind, because they felt it let people off the hook too easily regarding the consequences of their actions.

One should keep in mind, however, that all three of these models of human nature—behaviorist, Freudian, and existential/humanist—take rather extreme positions by positing a single dominant cause of human behavior and higher mental processes to the exclusion of any others. The behaviorist stresses the role of the immediate environment, the Freudian the person's unconscious drives and wishes, the humanist the individual's conscious intentions and choice. When, half a century ago, the existentialists/humanists championed the causal importance of conscious choice (Kelly, 1955, Maslow, 1962; Rotter, 1954), they were reacting to the then-dominant behaviorist and psychodynamic conceptions of man. Given this context it is understandable that they pushed their own causal model as hard as they could, in order to best emphasize the importance of conscious choice as opposed to determining unconscious forces or environmental stimuli.

Historically, however, staked-out philosophical stances such as these have had two different, and often conflicting purposes, which need to be carefully distinguished. Both of these purposes in fact date back to the early Greek philosophers. One is a practical or utilitarian form, a "philosophy of life" that provides guidelines and rules for conduct and right living; the classic examples of this were the Stoics and Epicureans (Gottlieb, 2000). Barrett (1958) argued that prior to the advent of academic philosophy, philosophers lived their own lives fully in accord with their deeply held beliefs. Kierkegaard, for example, eschewed a happy domestic life with his beloved because it would interfere with his quest to find God. Sartre's insistence on personal freedom and responsibility is the modern exemplar of this kind of philosophy. Accordingly, existentialism lends itself quite readily to use as a therapeutic method, exhorting individuals against fatalistic acceptance of their lot in life and motivating them to take action to change it if necessary (Rank, 1930/1998; Yalom, 1980).

The other historical purpose of philosophy is to use logic and reason to better understand the universe and how it works, including of course the underlying mechanisms of human judgment and action. More than anyone else, Aristotle is associated with this "scientific" vein of philosophy. It is the stream of philosophical inquiry out of which every modern scientific discipline developed (Gottlieb, 2000)—including, most recently, psychology.

It is notable therefore that the more scientific and empirical of the existential writers, such as Jung (e.g., 1919), gave greater emphasis to the role of unconscious influences in everyday life than did the more practically and phenomenologically oriented existentialists such as Sartre. Let us say then that whereas existential psychology as a whole recognizes the reality of unconscious psychological processes, it chooses to emphasize conscious and intentional processes for the sake of the greater social good.

The modern notion of unconscious psychological phenomena—as in mental processes operating outside conscious awareness and often without conscious intent—has more in common with the mechanistic approach of the behaviorists than the dynamic approach of the Freudians. Today's unconscious is no longer only a hypothetical Freudian construct but an empirically established reality embedded in mainstream cognitive psychological theory (e.g., Hassin, Uleman, & Bargh, 2004; Kihlstrom, 1987). Mainly because of its roots in artificial intelligence research (among others), in which it was not possible or even plausible to posit intervening deliberate conscious choice processes, cognitive psychology is entirely comfortable with the idea of nonconscious mental and behavioral processes (e.g., Barsalou, 1992). And if the process could not be instigated by acts of free will or conscious choice in these models, then the cause had to be external to the individual (i.e., in his or her environment).

The positing of such environmental causation, however, harkens back to the stimulus–response (S-R) psychology of the behaviorists, which failed as an exclusive and all-encompassing account of human behavior (see Chomsky, 1959; Skinner, 1957). The contemporary theoretical solution to this difficulty has been to permit (as the behaviorists adamantly did not) these external causes to operate in combination with internal psychological mechanisms, such as perceptual, motivational, and behavioral constructs. The external situation or setting activates and puts into motion these internal psychological processes, which then operate in complex interaction with events and stimuli in the outside world—often over extended periods of time, unlike the old S-R psychology. Once activated, these systems operate outside conscious awareness and guidance. This model of human judgment and behavior, in which aware and intentional conscious choice is not a necessary component, has been found to have considerable predictive and explanatory power (Bargh & Ferguson, 2000; Ouellette & Wood, 1998).

CONSCIOUS CHOICE IS NOT ESSENTIAL TO EVERYDAY LIFE

With time and experience, behaviors and decisions that once required a good deal of conscious thought and monitoring no longer do so; they become more efficient in their use of limited attention, and more routinized so that we no longer have to make choices and decisions every step of the way (Bargh & Chartrand, 1999). As William James (1890) put it, consciousness tends to drop out of any process where it is no longer needed. As long as we make the same decisions and choices given the same circumstances, the choice itself becomes redundant with the circumstances, and so those choices start becoming "made for us" in the sense that we behave and react directly, based on what is going on in the environment. All skills develop in this way, gradually receding from the need for conscious control and so being capable of operating nonconsciously (Bargh & Chartrand, 1999).

This principle applies regardless of whether we intend for the skill or process to become automatic. For instance, we may want to become more proficient at driving a car or playing chess, and so we practice these skills, hoping to free our limited conscious attention and thought from details for which it is not really needed—leaving it instead free to plan ahead (looking for potential trouble spots on the road ahead, plotting game strategy) and to be ready for any unforeseen difficulties. But if we always make the same judgment or evaluation of a given object or event, that evaluation eventually becomes automatically associated with the object/event's mental representation, so that it becomes activated (made for us) upon the mere presence of that object/event in one's environment (e.g., Bargh, Chaiken, Govender, & Pratto, 1992; Fazio, Sanbonmatsu, Powell, & Kardes, 1986). One negative consequence of this phenomenon can be the automatic association of stereotypical beliefs and expectations about a social group, on the one hand, with the defining features (e.g., racial or ethnic, gender related, and age related) of that group, on the other hand, so that those stereotypical assumptions become automatically activated on just the presence of a group member in one's environment (e.g., Brewer, 1988; Devine, 1989).

Similarly for our frequently and consistently pursued goals: if in a given situation we tend to choose the same goal, the representation of that goal becomes more and more strongly associated with the mental representation of that situation (Bargh, 1990). Thus, eventually that goal comes to be activated automatically when one enters that situation and then operates to guide one's behavior toward the goal—without one consciously choosing or intending to pursue that goal at that moment, and even without the person aware of the real reasons for his or her behavior in that situation (Bargh & Gollwitzer, 1994; Bargh, Gollwitzer, Lee-Chai, Barndollar, & Troetschel, 2001; Chartrand & Bargh, 1996). A wide variety of goals have been demonstrated to become active and operate automatically in this manner, such as goals to judge and form an impression of someone, to achieve high performance on a task, to cooperate with another person, or to protect one's self-esteem (by derogating minority groups) following a failure experience (Spencer, Fein, Wolfe, Fong, & Dunn, 1998).

Such nonconscious motivational effects on one's behavior are likely to be quite common in the "real world" outside the laboratory, as their triggers are the frequently experienced and thought-about social features of one's life—for example, the people we are closest to. Fitzsimons and Bargh (2003) found in several studies that merely thinking about those with whom we have close relationships (e.g., mother and spouse) automatically activates the goals that we pursue when with them—even in situations in which that significant other is not physically present. Like the other nonconscious influences described in this chapter, people are not aware and, in fact, highly skeptical of the reality of such effects on their behavior when informed of them. Because our close relationships are such an important and frequently thought-about part of our phenomenal lives, nonconscious goal operation is more likely the rule in daily life than an exception to it.

In all these experiments, the goal under study is activated in a subtle and often subliminal manner (through what are termed "priming" techniques; see Bargh & Chartrand, 2000), and the participants during careful questioning after the experiment show no awareness of that activation—nor even of the operation of the goal to guide their behavior over extended periods. To give one example, participants primed with the goal of cooperation (so that it was operating nonconsciously) did cooperate in a commons-dilemma game more than did a control group, just as did another group of participants who were explicitly instructed by the experimenters to cooperate. After the "commons" task was completed, all participants gave estimates of how strongly they had been committed to the goal of cooperating with their game partner. In the conscious (explicit) goal group, these estimates correlated significantly with their actual amounts of cooperation shown in the task, indicating that these participants were aware of and could accurately report on their degree of cooperation. Not so for the nonconscious (primed) goal group; their subsequent self-ratings of how much they had just cooperated were unrelated (zero correlations) to their actual amount of cooperation. Thus, not only did these participants not choose or intend to cooperate, they were unaware of the motivation to cooperate that guided their behavior on the task (Bargh et al., 2001, Experiment 2).

In fact, such nonconscious goal pursuit shows all the same qualities as have been found over the years for conscious goal pursuit, including the tendency to resume and complete interrupted goals, and mood effects (happiness vs. dejection) of "succeeding" versus "failing" at a (nonconscious) goal one is not even aware of having (see review in Chartrand & Bargh, 2002).

A final domain of nonconsciously produced social behavior is less motivated and more perceptually or cognitively produced: that driven by the "perception–behavior link" (see Dijksterhuis & Bargh, 2001, for a review). In harmony with very recent findings in cognitive neuroscience of strong associative connections (in the premotor cortex) between the mental representations used for producing a certain type of action oneself and those used to perceive that same action when performed by someone else, social cognition research has shown that merely perceiving a type of action (e.g., aggressiveness and slowness) in another person makes it more likely one will engage in the same behavior. This "chameleon effect" (so-called because one tends to change his or her behavior to match that of whomever one is interacting with) extends from physical, motor behavior (such as body posture, hand and foot movements; Chartrand & Bargh, 1999) to abstract trait-like behavior (aggressiveness, intelligence, slowness; see Bargh, Chen, & Burrows, 1996; Dijksterhuis & van Knippenberg, 1998).

In all of these nonconscious phenomena, the experimental participant did not consciously choose to think, judge, or behave in the manipulated manner, yet nevertheless did so in much the same manner as when people are explicitly asked to do the same things. By subtle and unobtrusive activation of the mental representations (of objects, situations, goals, another person's behavior, etc.) involved—thus mimicking the effects of those situational features in the natural environment—complex judgments and social behaviors across many content domains were produced without the need for conscious intention and choice or even guidance of the process to completion. And in the automatic motivation research most clearly, the operation of the unconscious process extended over time and involved selective attention and use of environmental information, so that behavior in pursuit of a particular goal was adapted to the specific unfolding environmental events—and so goes far beyond simple, direct S-R control of single concrete behaviors (see Bargh, 2004).

Because this accumulating evidence is clearly against the necessity of conscious intention and choice in a wide variety of complex human activities, so existential philosophers such as Kierkegaard and Sartre likely were off target in highlighting consciously made choices as the quintessential human characteristic. Moreover, instead of being seen as antagonistic, competing centers of causal power, the individual's environment and his or her unconscious mental processes—in interaction with the goals, beliefs, values of the individual—are better considered as supportive and even essential contributors to successful adaptation and self-fulfillment. And, finally, given that the historical purpose of existential philosophy is not the defense and maintenance of a particular answer to the meaning of human life (namely, the uniqueness of conscious choice) but instead the rigorous and objective pursuit of the truth of the matter, whatever that might be, it becomes paramount for existential philosophy and psychology to reexamine the hypothesized central role of conscious choice. Indeed, one important contribution that an experimental existential psychology could make to existential philosophy more generally would be to provide the best scientific answers possible about the true causal role of human consciousness in producing one's daily life.

REASON VERSUS CHOICE AS THE ESSENTIAL
HUMAN CHARACTERISTIC

Traditionally, philosophers from Aristotle onward have looked for what it means to be human by focusing on the important or key differences between humans and other animals. For Aristotle, the "final cause" or purpose of a thing was what it naturally does, that other things do not do—its "distinctive function" (Gottlieb, 2000, p. 266). For example, the function of the eye is to see and the function of a chair is to be sat on. The distinctive function of humans, according to Aristotle (*Nicomachean Ethics*, X, p. 7), is the use and application of reason and intelligence in daily life. Therefore the path to fulfillment and complete expression of his or her inner essence is for the individual to regularly engage in rational and intelligent thought and action.

Aristotle's emphasis on pure thought and reason as the core of existence was greatly influential during the Renaissance and Enlightenment; exemplified by the *Cogito ergo sum* of

Descartes, which equated Being with consciousness. Still, it culminated in the writings of Kant, who subjected important philosophical concepts and categories to rigorous, rational analysis. This included the concept of existence, which Kant concluded was an empty and rather meaningless concept because saying that an object exists tells us nothing new about it (see Barrett, 1958, p. 162).

Starting with Kierkegaard, however, existentialist writers took issue with the validity of Kant's analysis, arguing that existence was not merely an abstract mental concept but a reality of every person's life. They did not see thought or reason as an abstract process detached from the realities of life one's own life, as did Plato with his ideal Forms, but more as Aristotle did, as being fully involved with planning, making choices, and performing intentional actions (Gottlieb, 2000, p. 267). For instance, Kierkegaard emphasized the "either/or" of (conscious) choice as giving life its meaning; he held that "any man who chooses or is forced to choose decisively . . . experiences his own existence as something beyond the mirror of thought. He encounters the Self that he is, not in the *detachment* of thought, but in the *involvement* and pathos of choice" (Barrett, 1958, p. 163).

It is interesting that both Kant and Kierkegaard followed Aristotle's lead in equating the meaning of existence with the intellect and reason yet emphasized separate and distinct aspects of intellectual activity—Kant the abstract, pure reasoning aspect and Kierkegaard the choice and planning aspect. Although both are forms of human mental life that presumably distinguish us from other animals, they are not the *same* form. Kierkegaard, in fact, distinguished between the two as the *esthetic* and the *ethical* modes of existence; the former corresponding to the abstract, pure domain of thought and perceptual experience, and the latter to the mundane, down-to-earth choices of action one has to make in the course of living one's life. He argued that life is actually lived at the ethical, not the detached, esthetic level (Barrett, 1958, p. 167).

"I CHOOSE, THEREFORE I AM"

Sartre (1944) also equated Being with conscious choices, strongly denying even the existence of an unconscious or nonconscious mind. In this way, Sartre's philosophy was very much a direct descendant of Cartesianism—the identification of mind with consciousness:

> A Cartesian subjectivity (which is what Sartre's is) *cannot* admit the existence of the unconscious because the unconscious is the Other in oneself, and the glance of the Other, in Sartre, is always like the stare of Medusa, fearful and petrifying[1] . . . In fact, Sartre denies the existence of an unconscious mind altogether; wherever the mind manifests itself, he holds, it is conscious. A human personality or human life is not to be understood in terms of some hypothetical unconscious at work behind the scenes and pulling all the wires that manipulate the puppet of consciousness. (Barrett, 1958, pp. 254–257)

Sartre's notion of human freedom developed out of extreme and exceptional circumstances: his experiences in the French Resistance during World War II. Existence and being were demonstrated by the conscious choice of "saying no" to the oppressing Nazi occupation forces. But as this was an exceptional circumstance, what then about the normal, usual, everyday conditions in which a human being fulfills his or her existence? Because Sartre's philosophy (like Descartes') acknowledges only conscious thought, it is limited or undermined to the extent that automatic or nonconscious mental processes are found to guide and govern everyday life.

Yet as a philosophy of and guide to life—as opposed to a rigorous and unflinching attempt at getting at the truth of existence—the reality of conscious choice may not matter. Sartre did, after all, "advance his view as a basis for humanitarian and democratic social action" (Barrett, 1958, p. 244). But if we are unconcerned about the truth of existence, why not go all the way back to Descartes and the pre-Enlightenment days and posit God or some other supernatural entity as the causal force? If we are bravely facing the realities of our existence, in all their apparent absurdity (*pace* Camus) then we need to face this one as well. Nietzsche announced that God was dead, Sartre fulfilled Nietzsche's prophecy by replacing God with man, and the capacity of man that inspired Sartre to do so was conscious choice. However, if conscious choice is an illusion, what then are we left with? Perhaps, as Barrett (1958, p. 244) suggested, we are back "in that anguish of nothingness in which Descartes floated [in his skepticism] before the miraculous light of God shone to lead him out of it."

DON'T TRUST THE FEELING OF WILL

One might argue that Sartre and others were being quite sincere and objective when they concluded, based on their subjective experiences, that conscious choice is the source of human freedom (and uniqueness). Following this phenomenological approach, one can easily come to believe in the power and causal efficacy of conscious choice in one's life—yet here is a case of subjective experience being suspect. When Descartes took on the ruthlessly skeptical stance that ultimately produced the *Cogito*, he rejected the certain validity of all of his subjective experience *except* for his own conscious thought. But Wegner's (2002) recent empirical research on the experience of choice and free will now gives us more reason than mere skepticism not to trust our subjective experience as a guide to truth in this matter.

Wegner has demonstrated that we do not experience the causal role of choice and will directly, as Descartes claimed, but only as the result of an inference, or causal attribution, based on the covariation of our thoughts and our actions. Most critically, Wegner's research has shown that manipulation of the factors presumed to underlie these attributions does produce subjective feelings of conscious choice and free will where they actually played no role in the outcome. Whether or not Wegner is ultimately found to be fully correct that the experience of conscious will is an illusion, his demonstrations on this point show at the very least that even the presumed phenomenological bedrock of the *Cogito* cannot be trusted. It too, is suspect, or at least potentially misleading, as a source of evidence.

This is part of a larger, more abstract problem with using subjective experience, including thought experiments, as the evidentiary basis for conclusions about human nature. For one thing, Beauregard and Dunning (1998), Wilson (2001), Pronin, Lin, and Ross (2002), and others have presented considerable evidence that we really do not know ourselves very well—mainly because all sorts of motivational biases and other hindrances get in the way of the accuracy of causal statements about ourselves (but not, so much, about others). Therefore, introspective evidence can be useful, suggestive, and even highly compelling (as it was to Descartes), but it should not be granted the status of direct and self-evident proof.

It could also be argued that Kierkegaard and Sartre were referring specifically to extreme conditions and circumstances—saying no to the dictator and his army, saying no to the corrupt and venal authority of the Church—and not to the typical daily life of individuals. Such a retreat raises other problems, however. The most obvious is that it leaves the "final cause"—the defining function or purpose—of human beings in the odd status of not existing under normal conditions. Another difficulty is the possibility that even under extreme circumstances there is no real conscious choice made. Wegner's research makes us wonder about the true causal role of any phenomenal experience of choice, for important and consequential decisions as well as for relatively innocuous responses in laboratory experiments (cf. Kuhl & Koole, Chapter 26, this volume). My suspicion is that there may be less actual choice involved in the extreme and pivotal moments emphasized by Kierkegaard and Sartre than in relatively trivial and mundane matters. One needs only to consider Martin Luther's famous words, when called to defend his life in front of the Church at the height of its power: "Here I stand; I can do nothing else." Why did he have this strong feeling, at the most crucial moment of his life, of actually having no choice at all? Luther was, I think, expressing his belief that his dramatic and incredibly consequential choice had been determined already for him by his beliefs, values, and past public statements and behaviors.

Perhaps, then, we should take Luther's words at face value. Pelham, Mirenberg, and Jones (2002) have recently shown that the sharing of seemingly superficial and trivial features, such as the letters in one's name, with those of potential occupations and places to live, significantly influences those major life decisions. Several studies examining census data, telephone directories, and social security records showed that, among other things, people were more likely to move to states and cities with names similar to their own names than other possible places to live. For example, there are disproportionately more Carols in Carolina, Phils in Philadelphia, and Kens in Kentucky than in other cities and states of comparable sizes. But people do not accept that these similarities played any role in their choice of where best to live, work, and raise a family, because they did not—at any conscious level, that is.

THEN WHAT *DOES* IT MEAN TO BE HUMAN?

An argument can be made that the human capacity for learning and using language (and at such an early age with very minimal experience of it) is part and parcel of another, more fundamental difference—the ability to absorb and acquire culture (e.g., Baumeister, 2004; Donald, 2001). No other animal accumulates learning and passes it along to subsequent generations at a level even approaching that of humans. As a result, none of us has to acquire local wisdom and knowledge by our own experience alone, repeating the mistakes and missing the same opportunities as did our ancestors. Instead, we stand on the tall shoulders of thousands of generations of predecessors.

This is a wonderfully flexible and adaptive arrangement, through which we soak up the local guidelines for behavior as well as the local knowledge of the environment—for example, every human being is born with the ability to learn and speak any language and absorb as second nature any human cultural system, depending on where in the world he or she happens to be born and raised (Donald, 2001). Here is one major clue that—far from being designed by nature as a way to oppose or countermand the influences of one's environment—the human mind allows us to uniquely adapt to and modify our behavior patterns effectively within that environment.

BEING HERE NOW

Recent evidence in the domain of comparative brain evolution strongly supports this idea. Whereas there is, overall, a high degree of overlap and similarity in brain structure and function between *homo sapiens* and our nearest primate relatives, one of the clear differences is in the capacity for building new, nonconscious skills. This involves a connection or pathway between the cerebellum (which compiles and stores the learned procedures) and the frontal lobes (which "load" and operate those procedures in the current environmental context), which, as Donald (2001) stresses, is *16 times* the proportional size in humans compared to the next closest primate. In other words, instead of possessing only a fixed set of rigid, innate predispositions or task-specific "demons" as do other animals (which determine for them what to attend to, how to behave, etc.), we build and develop them ourselves to fit our particular local environments and the goals and purposes we pursue within them. These not only reflect our own personal, local behavioral contingencies—based on our own particular cultural mores, norms, and reward structure—but also our own personal, idiosyncratic desires and goals (Bargh, 1990). Out of our idiosyncratic history of experience, then, develop ever more complex and abstract mental representations that come to guide our functioning on a moment-to-moment basis. Again, this frees our mind from much of present concerns, enabling it to plan for the future or consider the past.

Social cognition research too shows that our social knowledge structures—our expectancies and predictive models of social situations—naturally and automatically adapt to reflect both the long-term frequencies of events and the short-term, current situation (Higgins & Bargh, 1987). Moreover, those structures that reflect the contingencies of the current situation (including those representing our own current goals and needs) dominate the effect of the long-term expectancies when the two are in conflict (e.g., Bargh, Lombardi, & Higgins, 1988). In this fundamental, mechanistic, and nonconscious way, the human mind adapts flexibly to the realities and contingencies of the current environment.

Unlike the humanists' and existentialists' view, then, the human mind is not constantly in a struggle with the environment over control of our behavior. Instead, it adapts to and integrates itself with that environment with an exquisite degree of sophistication. Situational features activate and put into motion our own idiosyncratic chronic goal pursuits within that situation (Bargh, 1990), and we can even delegate future control over our behavior to the environment, setting up temporary contingencies in advance ("When X happens, I will do Y") to unfold automatically at the later appointed time (Gollwitzer, 1999). In these ways we strategically *use* the fact of environmental control championed by Skinner (e.g., 1957) to our own advantage.

CONCLUSIONS

Existential questions such as the role of consciousness and the extent of human freedom are no longer solely the domain of philosophy; they have finally become tractable through scientific methods. All the sciences spun off from philosophy once empirical methods and tools had been developed to enable the central issues to be investigated empirically (Gottlieb, 2000); it is only very recently that we have been able to do so in the case of free will and the functions of consciousness.

So, then, what does this new scientific study of free will tell us? First, that concurrent with the historical development of a conscious mind that is capable of transcending the present environment was the development of "backup" or default nonconscious capacities for dealing with that present (Bargh, 1997). Basic evaluative, comprehensional, motivational, and behavioral systems have been found to operate without the need for conscious choice or guidance—independently of conscious concerns but dependent on appropriate environmental circumstances and features. In essence, these automatic response systems keep the individual appropriately grounded in the present, so that the conscious mind can more safely examine one's past (via memory) and plan for one's future.

These nonconscious support systems also buffer one's conscious, phenomenal experience from the moment-to-moment mundane realities of one's present existence, providing layers of protection from the direct appreciation of and awareness of those realities. This helps the great majority of us avoid the pitfalls of depressive realism.

But if we are not consciously in control of our behavior on a moment-to-moment basis, and if conscious choice processes do not play a causal role in our mundane and possibly even important life decisions, then they cannot be the human *raison d'être*. Perhaps it is not so important for us after all to overcome or countermand the influence and forces of our environment, as many existential and humanist thinkers have it, but instead to adapt ourselves to that environment so completely and implicitly that we become its master. Knowing our local worlds so well that we anticipate its events and contingencies well before they occur, and having developed skills and behavioral repertoires that can take advantage of those events quickly and efficiently in the service of our important goals and needs, keeps us many steps ahead of the game. We create and compile these sophisticated nonconscious goal-pursuit skills through our conscious experience (Bargh & Chartrand, 1999; Donald, 2001). Thus, compared to existential philosophy, experimental existential psychology suggests a different approach to the question of the meaning of existence: Why try to beat the world, when it appears we were made to join it?

ACKNOWLEDGMENTS

Preparation of this chapter was supported by fellowships from the Guggenheim Foundation and the Center for Advanced Study in the Behavioral Sciences, Stanford, California, and by Grant No. MH60767 from the National Institute of Mental Health. Thanks to Frances Kamm, Daniel Wegner, and Dennis Phillips for helpful discussions of these issues, and to Sander Koole for extensive feedback on a previous draft.

NOTE

1. There is a long historical tradition of treating nonconscious influences on behavior as somehow non-human; in fact prior to Freud's location of the source of irrational or counternormative behavior in the unconscious, such behavior was widely believed to be the result of demonic possession (Bargh & Barndollar, 1996). Anything, it would seem, but to accept it as a natural and even essential part of existence.

REFERENCES

Alloy, L. B., & Abramson, L. Y. (1979). Judgement of contingency in depressed and non-depressed students: Sadder but wiser? *Journal of Experimental Psychology, 108,* 441–485.

Bandura, A. (1986). *Social foundations of thought and action: A social cognitive theory.* Englewood Cliffs, NJ: Prentice-Hall.

Bargh, J. A. (1990). Auto-motives: Preconscious determinants of social interaction. In E. T. Higgins & R. M. Sorrentino (Eds.), *Handbook of motivation and cognition* (Vol. 2, pp. 93–130). New York: Guilford Press.

Bargh, J. A. (1997). The automaticity of everyday life. In R. S. Wyer, Jr. (Ed.), *Advances in social cognition* (Vol. 10, pp. 1–63). Mahwah, NJ: Erlbaum.

Bargh, J. A. (1999). The cognitive monster: The case against controllability of automatic stereotype effects. In S. Chaiken & Y. Trope (Eds.), *Dual process theories in social psychology* (pp. 361–382). New York: Guilford Press.

Bargh, J. A. (2004). Bypassing the will: Towards demystifying the nonconscious control of social behavior. In R. Hassin, J. Uleman, & J. Bargh (Eds.), *The new unconscious*. New York: Oxford University Press.

Bargh, J. A., & Barndollar, K. (1996). Automaticity in action: The unconscious as repository of chronic goals and motives. In P. M. Gollwitzer & J. A. Bargh (Eds.), *The psychology of action* (pp. 457–471). New York: Guilford Press.

Bargh, J. A., Chaiken, S., Govender, R., & Pratto, F. (1992). The generality of the automatic attitude activation effect. *Journal of Personality and Social Psychology, 62,* 893–912.

Bargh, J. A., & Chartrand, T. (1999). The unbearable automaticity of being. *American Psychologist, 54,* 462–479.

Bargh, J. A., & Chartrand, T. L. (2000). The mind in the middle: A practical guide to priming and automaticity research. In H. T. Reis & C. M. Judd (Eds.), *Handbook of research methods in social and personality psychology* (pp. 253–285). New York: Cambridge University Press.

Bargh, J. A., Chen, M., & Burrows, L. (1996). Automaticity of social behavior: Direct effects of trait construct and stereotype priming on action. *Journal of Personality and Social Psychology, 71,* 230–244.

Bargh, J. A., & Ferguson, M. L. (2000). Beyond behaviorism: On the automaticity of higher mental processes. *Psychological Bulletin, 126,* 925–945.

Bargh, J. A., & Gollwitzer, P. M. (1994). Environmental control over goal-directed action. *Nebraska Symposium on Motivation, 41,* 71–124.

Bargh, J. A., Gollwitzer, P. M., Lee-Chai, A. Y., Barndollar, K., & Troetschel, R. (2001). The automated will: Nonconscious activation and pursuit of behavioral goals. *Journal of Personality and Social Psychology, 81,* 1014–1027.

Bargh, J. A., Lombardi, W. J., & Higgins, E. T. (1988). Automaticity in Person x Situation effects on person perception: It's just a matter of time. *Journal of Personality and Social Psychology, 55,* 599–605.

Barrett, W. (1958). *Irrational man: A study in existential philosophy.* New York: Random House.

Barsalou, L. W. (1992). *Cognitive psychology: An overview for cognitive scientists.* Hillsdale, NJ: Erlbaum.

Baumeister, R. F. (2004). *The cultural animal: Human nature, meaning, and social life.* New York: Oxford University Press.

Beauregard, K. S., & Dunning, D. (1998). Turning up the contrast: Self-enhancement motives prompt egocentric contrast effects in social judgments. *Journal of Personality and Social Psychology, 74,* 606–621.

Becker, E. (1973). *The denial of death.* New York: Free Press.

Brewer, M. B. (1988). A dual process model of impression formation. In T. K. Srull & R. S. Wyer (Eds.), *Advances in social cognition* (Vol. 1, pp. 1–36). Hillsdale, NJ: Erlbaum.

Chartrand, T. L., & Bargh, J. A. (1996). Automatic activation of impression formation and memorization goals: Nonconscious goal priming reproduces effects of explicit task instructions. *Journal of Personality and Social Psychology, 71,* 464–478.

Chartrand, T. L., & Bargh, J. A. (1999). The chameleon effect: The perception-behavior link and social interaction. *Journal of Personality and Social Psychology, 76,* 893–910.

Chartrand, T. L., & Bargh, J. A. (2002). Nonconscious motivations: Their activation, operation, and consequences. In A. Tesser, D. A. Stapel, & J. V. Wood (Eds.), *Self and motivation: Emerging psychological perspectives* (pp. 13–41). Washington, DC: American Psychological Association.

Chomsky, N. (1959). Review of *Verbal Behavior* by B. F. Skinner. *Language, 35,* 26–58.

Dass, R. (1971). *Be here now.* New York: Crown.

Devine, P. G. (1989). Stereotypes and prejudice: Their automatic and controlled components. *Journal of Personality and Social Psychology, 56,* 680–690.

Dijksterhuis, A., & Bargh, J. A. (2001). The perception-behavior expressway: Automatic effects of social perception on social behavior. In M. P. Zanna (Ed.), *Advances in experimental social psychology* (Vol. 33, pp. 1–40). San Diego: Academic Press.

Dijksterhuis, A., & van Knippenberg, A. (1998). The relation between perception and behavior, or how to win a game of Trivial Pursuit. *Journal of Personality and Social Psychology, 74,* 865–877.

Donald, M. (2001). *A mind so rare.* New York: Simon & Schuster.

Fazio, R. H., Sanbonmatsu, D. M., Powell, M. C., & Kardes, F. R. (1986). On the automatic activation of attitudes. *Journal of Personality and Social Psychology, 50,* 229–238.

Fitzsimons, G. M., & Bargh, J. A. (2003). Thinking of you: Nonconscious pursuit of interpersonal goals associated with relationship partners. *Journal of Personality and Social Psychology, 84,* 148–164.

Gollwitzer, P. M. (1999). Implementation intentions: Strong effects of simple plans. *American Psychologist, 54,* 493–503.

Gottlieb, A. (2000). *The dream of reason: A history of philosophy from the Greeks to the Renaissance.* New York: Norton.

Hassin, R., Uleman, J., & Bargh, J. (Eds.). (2004). *The new unconscious.* New York: Oxford University Press.

Heidegger, M. (1962). *Being and time* (J. Macquarrie & E. Robinson, Trans.). London: Blackwell. (Original work published 1927)

Higgins, E. T., & Bargh, J. A. (1987). Social perception and social cognition. *Annual Review of Psychology, 38,* 369–425.

James, W. (1890). *Principles of psychology.* New York: Holt.

Jung, C. G. (1919). Instinct and the unconscious. *British Journal of Psychology (General), 10,* 15–26.

Kelly, G. A. (1955). *The psychology of personal constructs.* New York: Norton.

Kihlstrom, J. F. (1987). The cognitive unconscious. *Science, 237,* 1445–1452.

Langer, E. J. (1975). The illusion of control. *Journal of Personality and Social Psychology, 32,* 311–328.

Maslow, A. (1962). *Toward a psychology of being.* New York: Van Nostrand.

Metcalfe, J., & Mischel, W. (1999). A hot/cool-system analysis of delay of gratification: Dynamics of willpower. *Psychological Review, 106,* 3–19.

Mischel, W. (1973). Toward a cognitive social learning reconceptualization of personality. *Psychological Review, 80,* 252–283.

Mischel, W., Cantor, N., & Feldman, S. (1996). Goal-directed self-regulation. In E. T. Higgins & A. W. Kruglanski (Eds.), *Social psychology: Handbook of basic principles* (pp. 329–360). New York: Guilford Press.

Murray, S. T., Holmes, J. G., & Griffin, D. W. (1996). The benefits of positive illusions: Idealization and the construction of satisfaction in close relationships. *Journal of Personality and Social Psychology, 70,* 79–98.

Ouellette, J., & Wood, W. (1998). Habit and intention in everyday life: The multiple processes by which past behavior predicts future behavior. *Psychological Bulletin, 124,* 54–74.

Pelham, B. W., Mirenberg, M. C., & Jones, J. T. (2002). Why Susie sells seashells by the seashore: Implicit egotism and major life decisions. *Journal of Personality and Social Psychology, 82,* 469–487.

Prinz, W. (1997). Explaining voluntary action: The role of mental content. In M. Carrier & P. Mechamer (Eds.), *Mindscapes: Philosophy, science, and the mind* (pp. 153–175). Konstanz, Germany: Universitaetsverlag.

Pronin, E., Lin., D. Y., & Ross L. (2002). The bias blind spot: Perceptions of bias in self versus others. *Personality and Social Psychology Bulletin, 28,* 369–381.

Rank, O. (1998). *Psychology and the soul.* Baltimore: Johns Hopkins University Press. (Original work published 1930)

Rotter, J. B. (1954). *Social learning and clinical psychology.* Englewood Cliffs, NJ: Prentice-Hall.

Sartre, J.-P. (1944). *Being and nothingness.*

Skinner, B. F. (1957). *Verbal behavior.* New York: Appleton-Century-Crofts.

Solomon, S., Greenberg, J., & Pyszczynski, T. (1991). A terror management theory of social behavior: The psychological functions of self-esteem and cultural worldviews. In M. Zanna (Ed.), *Advances in experimental social psychology* (Vol. 24, pp. 104–159). Orlando, FL: Academic Press.

Spencer, S. J., Fein, S., Wolfe, C. T., Fong, C., & Dunn, M. A. (1998). Automatic activation of stereotypes: The role of self-image threat. *Personality and Social Psychology Bulletin, 24,* 1139–1152.

Taylor, S. E. (1989). *Positive illusions.* New York: Basic Books.

Wegner, D. M. (2002). *The illusion of conscious will.* Cambridge, MA: MIT Press.

Wilson, T. D. (2001). *Strangers to ourselves.* Cambridge, MA: Harvard University Press.

Yalom, I. (1980). *Existential psychotherapy.* New York: Basic Books.

Chapter 25

Ego Depletion, Self-Control, and Choice

KATHLEEN D. VOHS
ROY F. BAUMEISTER

Existential psychology has long remarked on the central importance of choice and control for understanding the human condition. Heidegger's (1954/1968) analyses featured the ongoing process of realizing some alternatives while letting others fall away, and Sartre (1943/1956) placed special emphasis on free choice as the defining feature of human existence. In psychology, self-regulation or self-control has been considered a vital human ability (e.g., Baumeister, 1998; Carver & Scheier, 1998; Higgins, 1996) because it enables people to override their impulses, thereby freeing humans from control by the immediate stimulus environment—a crucial aspect of freedom that was central to Kant's (1797/1967) discussions of human freedom.

Our laboratory research has shown that self-regulation draws on a common psychological resource, one that operates like a strength or an energy supply. When people resist temptation, override natural or overlearned tendencies, or regulate their responses, they seem to deplete this common resource, and subsequently the psyche is in a weakened state and exhibits impaired regulatory functioning. We have demonstrated this effect with numerous laboratory procedures, including regulating emotions, suppressing thoughts, persisting in the face of failure, agreeing to perform counterattitudinal behaviors, regulating the impulse to spend money, resisting temptation, overriding attentional lures, and passive responding. This wide variety of phenomena suggest that one part of the psyche is a generalized resource that is used to control cognitive, behavioral, attention, emotional, and impulsive responses.

The resource model has recently been extended to include the notion of decision making as another process that taps into, and hence taxes, self-resources. Research reviewed in this area includes demonstrations that self-control is impaired after making choices and choice making (here, in the form of intelligent and logical decisions) is less effective after engaging in self-control.

The last area we cover involves the subjective experience of time after self-regulation. This research demonstrates that people misperceive the flow or passage of time during and after they have engaged in self-regulation, an effect that is presumably related to low self-regulatory resources. Specifically, people who have self-regulated and who are therefore low in self-regulatory resources believe that much more time has passed than it has. This type of misperception of time, consequently, has negative implications for ensuing self-regulation efforts, with diminished self-control resulting from overly long-duration perceptions.

NATURE, CULTURE, AND THE EXECUTIVE FUNCTION

The broader existential context of this work must take into account the importance of choice and self-regulation in human functioning. Baumeister (in press) has proposed that the key to understanding the operation of the human psyche is that is designed by nature (through evolution) for the purpose of facilitating participation in culture. Culture is thus a step beyond being a merely social animal. Although culture offers human beings immense advantages which can be measured in the biological terms of survival and reproduction (among other ways), it makes much more extensive demands on the psyche than other ways of living. Culture accumulates knowledge in the collective and produces progress across generations, but to make use of these opportunities the psyche must be capable of language, lifelong learning, flexibility (free will), and the ability to alter present actions based on past and future events. Likewise, culture organizes behavior such as by extensive division of labor, allowing immense gains in efficiency and productivity, but for people to carry that off they must also have cooperation, theory of mind, and perhaps intentional teaching along with other inner mechanisms.

Although coming at the idea from a slightly different perspective, terror management theorists (e.g., Greenberg, Pyszczynski, & Solomon, 1986) also stress the role of culture in the human experience. From this approach, the beliefs, principles, and procedures of a given culture are endorsed by its people not because they are inherently good but rather because adherence to cultural values serve to buffer people from the psychological blow that accompanies awareness of one's own mortality. Our approach differs from the mortality salience approach in that our perspective stresses the similarities of cultures—such as being a part of a integrated network and accumulating knowledge—as providing immense reproductive and survival benefits to humans.

According to our view, culture greatly increases the complexity of life and the frequency of multidimensional decisions (i.e., decisions in which there are different options that vary along multiple dimensions). Moreover, nature could not possibly anticipate all the choices that people will face and therefore could not hard-wire the solutions and responses. Instead, it was necessary to give people a much more powerful choice-making apparatus. Put more simply, instead of programming people as to how to act in culture, nature had to give them the capacity to program and reprogram themselves. This idea was anticipated in interesting ways by Becker (1962), in his writings about how culture released humans from being organisms that merely reacted to environmental stimuli and who could instead choose for themselves how to behave.

The capacity for choice would constitute what would popularly be known as free will. Recent philosophical and psychological treatments of free will (e.g., Wegner, 2002) have tended to require that it consist of making utterly random decisions that are unaffected by any prior or external event, but the capacity for making such choices would seem to be fairly useless in evolutionary terms, and there is no reason to expect that natural selection would instill a capacity for such random and irrelevant decisions. However, the capacity to appraise alternatives meaningfully, evaluate them in terms of potential costs and benefits (including those distant in time), and then implement action based on the results of those comparisons would be highly adaptive. Indeed, the very concept of rationality presupposes some kind of free will, because there is no use to being able to use reason and logic to decide the optimal course of action if the person cannot also overcome impulses so as to pursue that course of action (Searle, 2002). We think that that is what people mean by free will and that that capacity might well have been cultivated by natural selection.

The complexity of cultural demands would also require that people need self-regulation, much more than other animals would. A person who always acted on his or her first impulse would make a very poor and unwelcome member of most social groups. Self-regulation allows people to override their initial impulses and responses, so that the person can substitute an action that would be more appropriate to the situation.

We think that to make the human being able to cope with the rising demands and opportunities of cultural life, nature instilled in the human psyche a capacity for self-regulation and active choice. This capacity is costly and is therefore rather limited, which is why the resource gets depleted when it is used. Still, it is far more extensive than what other species have, and people do make considerable use of it, to their considerable benefit.

One of the most obvious benefits concerns time. Humans far surpass other species in their ability to use future, anticipated events and outcomes to inform what they do in the present. The inner animal is always in danger of slipping back into the present orientation, in which one does what seems most appealing right now, but restraining such impulses for the sake of long-term benefits is highly adaptive. As just one example, agriculture would have been impossible without a future orientation, because farmers must plant their seeds instead of eating them now, and planting requires an understanding that a few seeds can produce much more food many months from now. The adaptive benefits of being able to delay gratification could in theory be alone sufficient to explain why natural selection produced the human capacity for self-regulation.

Thus, evolution seems to have created the human psyche with a powerful and adaptive capacity for making choices and controlling its responses. Still, this capacity depends on a limited resource that operates like a stock of energy. When this capacity is depleted, many functions of the self will be degraded: People will control themselves less effectively, such as becoming more impulsive, as well as more passive. The civilized being that is considerate to others, plans for the future, and restrains its antisocial impulses will give way to a creature more resembling its evolutionary ancestor: disregarding the feelings of others, living in the present and disregarding the future, and yielding to temptation.

Another line of research has suggested that humans' evolved capacity for self-regulation may be linked to the expectation of rewards in the form of belongingness. Using self-control is an expensive ticket to participation in culture, requiring the person to renounce immediate gratification in exchange for reaping the benefits of belonging to the culture. If the rewards of belongingness are not anticipated, then the sacrifices of self-control are no longer worthwhile. Sure enough, laboratory experiments have confirmed that when people are excluded from social groups, they cease to control and regulate their behavior properly: They become more aggressive and antisocial, more impulsive, more oriented toward the present instead of the future, but also more self-defeating in the sense that they choose short-term gains or risky options without sufficient regard for the risks and costs that may attend their choices

(Baumeister, Twenge, & Nuss, 2002; Twenge, Baumeister, Tice, & Stucke, 2001; Twenge, Cantonese, & Baumeister, 2002).

Moreover, and also to this point, a series of studies by Vohs and colleagues (e.g., Vohs, Ciarocco, & Baumeister, 2003; see Vohs & Ciarocco, 2004, for a review) has shown that self-regulation and interpersonal functioning are intimately tied. That is, these studies demonstrate that the capacity to regulate the self's intrapsychic responses is compromised after people have engaged in difficult, demanding, or novel interpersonal tasks. For instance, after having to act in a counternormative manner (e.g., having women present themselves as being highly competent and having men present themselves as being especially socially skilled), people are less able to override the impulse to quit doing an aversive physical task. In parallel, having to perform basic regulatory processes impairs successful interpersonal functioning. For example, after people have concentrated their attentions for a period of time, they become overly self-aggrandizing and narcissistic on subsequent tasks, a state that is accompanied by a decreased concern with what others think of them. In sum, research in our lab is triangulating on the idea that interpersonal ties and self-regulation are integrally related. They are related because the cultural animal relies on self-regulation to participate successfully in society.

Thus, we propose that the self's executive function is the product of a special line of evolutionary development, helping to make the human psyche capable of exploiting the value and power of culture (Baumeister, in press). Human beings might well periodically bewail the limits of their own self-control, and probably everyone would be better off if we had 10 times as much capacity for self-control as we actually have. But evolution only works incrementally, and the immense success of the human species is attributable in part to the fact that we do have much more self-control than our biological ancestors. Free will and self-control enable people to live together in a society organized by culture.

SELF-REGULATORY CAPACITY AS A RESTRICTED RESOURCE

The research and interpretations of findings in this chapter are derived from a self-regulatory resource model and thus an explanation of the model's tenets and parameters is in order. Based on a review of the self-regulation and behavioral change literatures, Baumeister, Heatherton, and Tice (1994; see also Baumeister & Heatherton, 1996) proposed that very different self-regulation tasks all draw on a single common resource, that can be depleted by exertion, thereby impairing performance subsequently on even seemingly unrelated tasks. For instance, personal coaches (e.g., for weight loss) often advise their clients not to attempt more than one behavioral change goal (e.g., also quit smoking), because such simultaneous attempts make the person less likely to succeed at reaching either goal. Likewise, the practice of making a "to do" list of self-control acts on New Year's Eve and then getting up on the morning of January 1 (or maybe January 2) with hopes of achieving all of them typically flops. Thus, it occurred to us that perhaps self-control abilities across a range of responses came from a global supply of energy.

We started testing this notion in the laboratory using a two-task paradigm in which (in the crucial conditions) self-control is first performed on one task, and then a second self-control performance is required immediately thereafter. We reasoned that if self-regulatory abilities function like a schema, then self-control would increase from Task 1 to Task 2 because the initial act of self-control would prime the schema, thereby facilitating subsequent self-control. If self-control is a skill, then there should be little or no change from one task to another, given that skills take repeated trials and practice across time to master. If self-control comes from a shared resource, however, then self-control should diminish from Task 1 to Task 2. In over 15 published studies, we have obtained evidence of the last pattern: Self-regulation is impaired if an earlier task has also required self-regulation.

TESTS OF THE RESOURCE MODEL

Our approach has been to examine self-control abilities in the laboratory, focusing largely on the causes and consequences of poor self-control. The studies described here center mainly on tests of the basic tenets of the model, such as investigations of the generalizability of the resource and studies on the role of individual differences in transforming situational features into resource-depleting elements. Two extensions of the model are described hereafter, demonstrating that decision making and choice also pull from the shared resource and that time perception is an integral part of self-regulatory endeavors.

Some of the most basic and fundamental self-control abilities involve controlling the content of thoughts and modifying the valence and intensity of emotions. If controlling emotions or thoughts depletes this precious resource, then this depletion should produce decrements in the ability to perform self-regulation in a subsequent task. This is precisely what was found in two studies. In Baumeister, Bratslavsky, Muraven, and Tice (1998, Study 3), participants were asked either to suppress their emotions or not to control their emotions while watching an emotional film. Participants either watched a comedic or a sad film. Later, they were asked to solve a series of anagrams. The results showed that participants who had controlled their emotions—regardless of the type of film—solved fewer anagrams during the second task.

Complementary findings were reported in Muraven, Tice, and Baumeister (1998, Study 3). In this study, participant were asked to suppress thoughts of a white bear or they were asked to complete simplistic math problems, with the former task requiring more regulatory resources. Success at the dependent measure meant showing no amusement when watching during a comedic film with the instructions not to show any amusement. Controlling one's thoughts did indeed have a negative impact on participants' ability to control their emotional expressions during a comical film. In another study, suppressing forbidden thoughts, as compared to not controlling thoughts and compared to exaggerating one's thoughts, led to a subsequent tendency to give up quickly on unsolvable anagrams. (The two control conditions were not different from each other.) One alternate explanation of these data is suggested by studies by Wegner and colleagues, which have shown that a rebound effect occurs after a mental control episode. Applied to these findings, it may have been that interfering thoughts about white bears may have led to participants' early termination of the anagram task and may possibly have made the funny film seem less funny. When combined with the other studies on controlling one's emotions and forcing oneself to eat radishes instead of chocolate (Baumeister et al., 1998), we think that the data point to a crippled capacity to self-regulate (i.e., resource depletion) is the cause of later self-control failure.

Although the studies reviewed thus far provide tantalizing evidence that depletion affects a variety of regulatory acts, it is unclear how depletion operates in other contexts in which already-ingrained inhibitions coincide with situational forces to affect self-regulation. We conducted a series of studies showing that the "main effects" of depletion can be exaggerated by individual differences in chronic inhibitions. Vohs and Heatherton (2000) reasoned that not all features of the situation would be equally depleting for all individuals and that this effect would depend crucially on whether the person was trying to regulate with respect to a certain situational aspect. Chronic dieters were used as the example of people who chronically restrain their caloric intake. Indeed, eating may be an especially interesting case of self-regulation because although people do choose to regulate their eating patterns, they cannot exit the regulatory loop entirely by simply refraining from engaging in the behavior (as they can from, say, smoking or imbibing alcohol). Dieters, but not nondieters, were found to be situationally depleted by having to resist the temptation of alluring candies and they subsequently were less able to control their eating (Study 1) and were less persistent (Study 2). In a third study, dieters who had to change and modify their emotional reactions to a sad movie were less able to control their eating. Thus, eating regulation both affected and was affected by the availability of self-regulatory resources—but only among people for whom caloric regimens were highly important and thus demanded much regulation.

These studies were conceptually replicated in a series of studies pertaining to impulsive spending. Vohs and Faber (in press) conducted three studies. Participants were depleted either from attentional or behavioral demands. Participants who were depleted, compared to those with full regulatory resources, responded in a manner that conformed to impulsive spending patterns: They endorsed more impulsive spending statements and were willing to pay more money for a set of high-priced products. A third study found that these effects were moderated by trait impulsive spending scores, and actual spending was used as the dependent measure. Specifically, the spending behaviors of people who chronically attempt to limit their spending were most affected by the (unrelated) situational manipulations of regulatory resources. Their spending was the highest of all groups, although the usual main effect of depletion condition was still seen. Thus, a proclivity to inhibit one's impulsive spending behaviors interacted with situational manipulations to amplify the depletion effect.

Thus far, we have focused on studies of self-regulation. These show that one common resource appears to be used for many different kinds and spheres of self-regulation, including regulation of thoughts, emotions, task performance, and impulses. The fact that this single resource is used for many different acts would qualify it as one of the most important components of the self.

ACTIVE CHOICE MAKING USES REGULATORY RESOURCES

The notion of choice has a long and rich history in existential discussions. Sartre (1943/1956) noted that life is marked with a never-ending stream of choices, given that there is at least one alternate option available for every response. In our analysis of choice as a form of self-regulation, we are specifically interested in active choice and decision making, without referring automatic or nonconscious responses that humans may emit, which may or may not be a function of choice (e.g., Bargh, 1989). We mean the term "choice" as referring to the psychological contemplation of possible options and the ultimate selection among them.

Although the energy resource that is used in self-regulation must already be regarded as highly important, its importance would be even greater if it had applications beyond self-regulation. Baumeister (1998) proposed that self-regulation is one part of the self's executive function, alongside choice, responsible decision making, and active (instead of passive) responding. That link made plausible a conceptual leap: Would the energy resource used for self-regulation also be used in those other executive function activities?

The first study to explore that possible link borrowed manipulations of choice from the long tradition of research on cognitive dissonance. One of the core ideas behind dissonance is that the act of choosing one option changes one's evaluations and feelings about both options (typically, so that the chosen option is more valued than the unchosen option). This approach to choice making is similar to Heidegger's (1954/1968) belief that choice making is problematic in part because it necessitates that one option go unchosen. According to Heidegger, selecting one option entails losing the unselected option. In self-regulatory resource terms, choosing one option over another is said to deplete some of the self's resources due to heightened degrees of evaluation, active decision making, and eventual commitment that is inherent in the process of choosing.

In the dissonance–depletion experiment (Baumeister et al., 1998), there were four experimental treatment conditions regarding the type of essay written and the method by which participants came to write the essay. In the counterattitudinal choice condition, participants were induced to make a choice to write an essay favoring tuition increases; in the counterattitudinal no-choice condition, participants were simply ordered to write the same protuition increase essay, with a small apology that the experimenter could not offer them any choice; in the proattitudinal choice condition, participants wrote an antituition essay by their own choice, and there was a control condition in which attitudes were assessed without any speech or essay. The dependent measure was persistence at tracing lines on an unsolvable puzzle, which requires self-regulation to overcome one's frustration and disappointment in order to make oneself keep trying. The results showed that both the counterattitudinal and the proattitudinal choice conditions differed significantly from both the control and counterattitudinal no-choice conditions. The two choice conditions did not differ significantly from each other, meaning that high choice was related to lower persistence, even when it was a proattitudinal essay. A priori, we had expected the two high-choice conditions to be significantly different from each other, but this finding that they are not prompted our later work on the act of choice making as being a central role of the self that requires regulatory resources (see the section on choice). Again, it may be that the process of decision making entails subprocesses such as comparison, evaluation, and commitment that deplete the self of its regulatory resources.

In sum, this research showed that making a meaningful personal choice to perform attitude-discrepant behavior brought about a decrement regulatory persistence. Put more simply, making the choice depleted some resource, leaving the person less able to self-regulate performance.

Active responding is another job of the self's executive function, and thus passive responding would require less expenditure of those same resources. In fact, many failures of self-control come from simple passivity, with common examples of the no-action response including failing to take one's medications and neglecting to exercise. In another experiment (Baumeister et al., 1998, Study 4), we examined whether an initial act of self-regulation (presumably causing ego depletion) would make people more passive in a subsequent context. Participants having to either cross off all the "e"s on a piece of a paper with this as the only instruction or in a more difficult manner with several rules (e.g., should only cross off an *e* if it was not adjacent to another vowel). The more difficult version was considered to require self-regulation, because the participant would have to break the habit acquired in the first trial (in which all instances of the letter "e" would be crossed off). Participants were shown a very boring movie and for some participants, quitting watching the movie was passive, whereas for others quitting required an active response. Participants who had to remember and enact several rules in order to complete the "e" task were more likely to take the passive option and continue watching the boring movie. Even when the outcome is aversively boring, people were more likely to endure it passively when they were depleted.

Through choice, people determine the outcome of a given situation and thus may exert control over their environment. However, choice is not always desirable. Research by Iyengar and Lepper (2000) revealed that people who faced 24 response options, as opposed to 6, were less satisfied and performed worse. Research by Burger (1989) suggests that for some people some of the time, the option of having control is rejected and choice is an undesirable outcome. Our research suggests that choosing may deplete the self of valuable resources that would otherwise be used to regulate the self actively.

In five studies, we have found evidence that choice and decision making render the self less able to regulate subsequently due to a reduction in regulatory resources (Vohs, Twenge, Baumeister, Schmeichel, & Tice, 2003). In a prototypical experiment (i.e., Study 1), participants were randomly assigned to either make a series of binary choices between two similar options (e.g., "Do I like the yellow candle or the blue candle?"), or they were asked to rate the same items when reviewing, for example, how frequently they had used the product. Later, all participants were asked to drink as many 1-ounce cups as they could of a concoction of Kool Aid and vinegar. The concoction is actually healthy to drink, but it tastes quite bad, and thus drinking it requires self-regulation not unlike the discipline needed to make someone consume a bitter medicine. Participants who had made the binary choices drank less of the bad-tasting drink than did the ratings-condition participants. In a subsequent study, a similar manipulation was used but participants were later asked to hold their hand in extremely cold water for as long as possible. Again, choice-condition participants were less able to keep their hand immersed in the frigid water. These findings suggest that making the series of choices depleted the self's resources. These data are intriguing and suggestive of depleted resource effects, but other explanations exist. For instance, it could have been that participants in the choice conditions were primed with a choice-making schema and thus were more willing to refuse to drink ill-tasting beverages or to keep their hands in frigid water.

To further test the idea of choice making and to get around alternate explanations concerning priming, we sought out evidence for the choice-making effect in a more naturalistic setting. In this study, participants were shoppers at a retail mall who completed a questionnaire on the degree to which they had made active choices in their shopping excursion thus far. They were then asked to complete as many 3-digit + 3-digit addition problems as they could (when faced with a set of 120 problems). Shoppers who said they had made many active choices that day completed fewer math problems and spent less time on the task.

DEPLETION LEADS TO POORER INTELLECTUAL PERFORMANCE

A set of studies that revealed the detrimental cognitive consequences of depleting self-regulatory resources (Schmeichel, Vohs, & Baumeister, 2003a) provides the complement to the studies on active choice making. In these studies, participants were asked to engage in a traditional act of self-control, such as managing emotions or attention control. Later, participants' cognitive abilities were tested. In three studies, we found that people who were depleted were less intelligent and less able to perform high-level mental operations. Namely, these participants performed more poorly when responding to difficult reading comprehension questions taking from the Graduate Record Examination (GRE) and when decoding complex analytic items (also from the GRE). Resource depletion did not, however, affect performance on lower-level cognitive tasks such as rote memorization and reproducing crystallized facts. From these data, it appears that regulatory resources are recruited when people attempt to execute higher-order mental operations.

Together, these results suggest that choice, decision making, and self-regulation are vitally intertwined. Specifically, making choices is costly to the psychological system and can result in ensuing cognitive performance decrements. One can imagine situations in which there is a high degree of exacting and difficult decisions and also a need for steady, unwavering self-control. Alternately, one can imagine situations consisting of heavy self-regulation demands as well as important high-level, intellectual solutions. We suggest that it is in precisely these situations, where consequences of self-regulation failure may be the gravest, that they are also the most likely.

SELF-AFFIRMATION SEEMS TO REBUILD THE RESOURCE

One way people cope with anxiety (existential or otherwise) is to defend against ego-threatening information actively. Behavior that contradicts one's attitudes, information that suggests one is at risk for disease, and evaluations of poor performance may provoke anxiety because they suggest the self is inconsistent, unhealthy, or simply less able than others. However, people frequently minimize negative implications for the self by discrediting the source of ego-threatening information or by minimizing the negativity of unwelcome feedback. These reactions can sustain positive self-views and limit anxiety without directly confronting the less desirable aspects of the self.

Vigilant ego defense may be minimized, however, by activating or affirming central aspects of self-worth (Arndt, Schimel, Greenberg, & Pyszczynski, 2002; Schimel, Arndt, Pyszczynski, & Greenberg, 2001; Steele, 1988). When the self has been affirmed, precious self-resources need not be used to defend the self from threat and instead may be directed toward other challenges. For example, self-affirmation helped ruminators control their intrusive thoughts more effectively (Koole, Smeets, van Knippenberg, & Dijksterhuis, 1999). We explored other self-regulatory benefits of self-affirmation in a series of studies that combined self-affirmation and ego depletion. If self-affirmation temporarily frees self-resources from ego defense, then those resources should be more readily applied to other self-regulatory challenges.

In one study, we assessed self-regulated persistence at difficult anagrams after a demanding mental control task. Participants who had been provided an opportunity to think and write about a highly important value before the mental control task were able to overcome the effects of ego depletion. Self-affirmed participants persisted longer at the difficult anagrams than participants who had not been self-affirmed (Schmeichel, Vohs, & Baumeister, 2003b).

In a second study, we found that ego depletion did not impair performance on a test of executive functioning when people had affirmed an important aspect of themselves. After thinking and writing about core values, participants who performed a resource-demanding version of the Stroop color–word interference task performed well on a subsequent test of higher-order cognitive processing, the Tower of Hanoi task. Depleted participants who had not been affirmed, however, performed quite poorly. Presumably, the self-affirmation liberated self-regulatory resources from ego-defensive concerns, and those resources were then more available for effective executive functioning and high-level cognition.

A third study demonstrated that the effects of self-affirmation on self-regulated performance were not due to positive affect. Again, depleted participants performed better on a self-regulated task when they had affirmed central aspects of self-worth. In a comparison group, a positive mood induction did not affect self-regulated performance. This pattern of results suggests that simply putting people into a good mood is not enough to counter the deleterious effects of ego depletion. Instead, we believe that self-affirmation, by temporarily sating ego defensiveness, facilitates self-regulated responding in other domains.

THE SUBJECTIVE EXPERIENCE OF TIME IS ALTERED BY SELF-REGULATION

We last discuss research centering on the concept of time, which also features prominently in existential writings. The idea that human life is not limitless and thus people are mortal beings who will cease to exist some day amounts to a psychological burden, one that is uniquely held by humans. Humans may be better able to grasp the physical and psychological reality of mortality in part because humans have a sense of past and future time periods. Nonhuman animals, conversely, live only in the immediate present and consequently do not recognize past experiences or future possibilities (see Roberts, 2002). Thus, the concept of time progression is specific to humans and thus may also be related to other, human-only capacities such as self-regulation (i.e., animals do not appear to have self-regulation abilities; see Roberts, 2002). In an existential context, Becker (1962) suggested that the understanding of time is centrally important for humans because it provides a milieu in which goals and goal-related movements can exist. In our studies on time, we sought to investigate the link between self-regulation and the subjective experience of time in a series of recent studies (Vohs & Schmeichel, 2003).

We began with the idea that engaging in self-regulation and the experience of time moving very slowly (i.e., that more time has passed in a given period than has actually gone by, such as thinking that an hour has passed when it has only been 10 minutes) have some common properties. At their core, longer-duration estimates and self-regulation both involve difficult mental operations that occur with some frequency during a specific period. There is some evidence that periods in which many cognitive operations take place lead to longer time estimates. Furthermore, a central property of self-regulation may involve being cognizant of time, which results in longer-duration estimates (Block & Zakay, 1997). Thus, we hypothesized that being in a state of resource depletion after engaging in self-control would lead to longer estimates of duration, such that depleted people would experience time as moving much more slowly than nondepleted people.

Furthermore, we postulated that self-regulation and the ensuing state of low regulatory resources would render the person transfixed in the present, such that immediate stimuli, impulses, and desires would be most prominent and the idea of abstract, high-level goals would be distant. We called this experience the "extended-now" state and hypothesized that being in an extended-now state (i.e., operationalized by longer-duration estimates and thus thinking that more time has passed than it actually has) would lead to poorer self-regulation.

The results of five studies provided evidence in support of these hypotheses (Vohs & Schmeichel, 2003). We found that participants who had depleted their regulatory resources, by controlling emotions, thoughts, or behavior experienced time as moving much more slowly (as indicated by their estimates of experimentally controlled time intervals) than participants who did not engage in self-control. Depleted participants also gave up sooner than nondepleted participants on later acts of self-control (replicating the classic depletion effect). Last, time perceptions statistically mediated the effect of being resource depleted on subsequent self-regulation performance.

In sum, research on time perception and self-regulation reveals that they are bidirectionally related: when people engage in an act of self-control, they deplete their resources and experience time as moving slowly, suggesting that they enter into a state of extended now in which they are attuned to the present and less aware of the future. Being in such a state and feeling that subjective durations are overly long leads to subsequent impairments in self-control endeavors. Thus, depleted people are bogged down in the present and seem to be less aware of the future consequences of their current behavior. Experiencing time in this way is detrimental to self-control capacities.

CONCLUSION

We have reviewed five different lines of research that relate self-regulatory abilities and regulatory resources to existential concerns such as time perception, choice, self-affirmation, rational thought, and self-defense. The idea that people are motivated to exert effort to control themselves and their world is not new, but it continues to impel philosophers, theoreticians, and researchers alike to understand the causes and consequences of such motives. We believe that at self-regulation lies at the heart of the control motive and our approach has been to study the operations of the regulatory system in terms of a limited resource that can be drained with use but that seems to be renewable over time.

Our research program started by examining the costs of engaging in self-regulation, focusing on repercussions for future acts of self-control (e.g., Baumeister et al., 1998; Muraven et al., 1998) and then investigated the internal state of the depleted person, such as in the work on subjective time perceptions (Vohs & Schmeichel, 2003). We have expanded the model to include the role of individual differences and regulatory resources (see Faber & Vohs, 2004, for a review; also Vohs & Heatherton, 2000) and incorporate processes underlying choice-making (Vohs et al., 2003) and intelligent thought (Schmeichel et al., 2003a). Last, we have begun to see how the resources can be repleted, and we have seized on self-affirmation as one likely route (Schmeichel et al., 2003b). In total, this research program has gone beyond the mechanistic notion of self-regulation as an open-ended feedback loop to larger, abstract, and more complex notions of control, humanity, existence, and meanings of life.

There are many avenues that still need exploring and perhaps the biggest and most interesting avenue concerns understanding what the resource is. Some scientists we have spoken with suggest looking neuroscientifically to see if the brain regions that are devoted to planning (e.g., prefrontal cortex) house this resource. We are tackling this question in another way, by linking regulatory resources to other self-related phenomena such as self-affirmation, rational choice, and free will, as a way to test the range of effects touched by the resources. Finding what is and is not affected by self-regulatory resources will help us further define what we think the resources are, a search that will most likely lead us down new and exciting paths in the process. We encourage fellow self-regulation researchers to also broaden their perspective on self-regulation and hope that the architects of existential discussions will make room for self-regulation at the table.

REFERENCES

Arndt, J., Schimel, J., Greenberg, J., & Pyszczynski, T. (2002). The intrinsic self and defensiveness: Evidence that activating the intrinsic self reduces self-handicapping and conformity. *Personality and Social Psychology Bulletin, 28,* 671–683.

Bargh, J. A. (1989). Conditional automaticity: Varieties of automatic influence in social perception and cognition. In J. S. Uleman & J. A. Bargh (Eds.), *Unintended thought* (pp. 3–51). New York: Guilford Press.

Baumeister, R. F. (1998). The self. In D. T. Gilbert, S. T. Fiske, & G. Lindzey (Eds.), *Handbook of social psychology* (4th ed., pp. 680–740). New York: McGraw-Hill.

Baumeister, R. F. (in press). *The cultural animal: Human nature, meaning, and social life.* New York: Oxford University Press.

Baumeister, R. F., Bratslavsky, E., Muraven, M., & Tice, D. M. (1998). Ego depletion: Is the active self a limited resource? *Journal of Personality and Social Psychology, 74,* 1252–1265.

Baumeister, R. F., & Heatherton, T. F. (1996). Self-regulation failure: An overview. *Psychological Inquiry, 7,* 1–15.

Baumeister, R. F., Heatherton, T. F., & Tice, D. M. (1994). *Losing control: How and why people fail at self-regulation.* San Diego: Academic Press.

Baumeister, R. F., Twenge, J. M., & Nuss, C. K. (2002). Effects of social exclusion on cognitive processes: Anticipated aloneness reduces intelligent thought. *Journal of Personality and Social Psychology, 83,* 817–827.

Baumeister, R. F., & Vohs, K. D. (2003). Self-regulation and the executive function of the self. In M. R. Leary, & J. P. Tangney (Eds.), *Handbook of self and identity* (pp. 197–217). New York: Guilford Press.

Becker, E. (1962). *The birth and death of meaning: A perspective in psychiatry and anthropology.* New York: Free Press.

Block, R. A., & Zakay, D. (1997). Prospective and retrospective duration judgments: A meta-analytic review. *Psychonomic Bulletin and Review, 4,* 184–197.

Burger, J. M. (1989). Negative reactions to increases in perceived personal control. *Journal of Personality and Social Psychology, 56,* 246–256.

Carver, C. S., & Scheier, M. F. (1998). *On the self-regulation of behavior.* New York: Cambridge University Press.

Faber, R., & Vohs, K. D. (2004). To buy or not to buy?: Self-control and self-regulatory failure in purchase behavior. In R. F. Baumeister & K. D. Vohs (Eds.), *Handbook of self-regulation: Research, theory, and applications* (pp. 509–524). New York: Guilford Press.

Greenberg, J., Pyszczynski, T., & Solomon, S. (1986). The causes and consequences of the need for self-esteem: A terror management theory. In R. F. Baumeister (Ed.), *Public self and private self* (pp. 189—212). New York: Springer-Verlag.

Heatherton, T. F., & Baumeister, R. F. (1996). Self-regulation failure: Past, present, and future. *Psychological Inquiry, 7,* 90–98.

Heidegger, M. (1968). *What is called thinking?* (J. G. Gray, Trans.) New York: Harper & Row. (Original work published 1954)

Higgins, E. T. (1996). Knowledge and activation: Accessibility, applicability, and salience. In E. T. Higgins & A. W. Kruglanski (Eds.) *Social psychology: Handbook of basic principles* (pp 133–168). New York: Guilford Press.

Iyengar, S. S., & Lepper, M. R. (2000). When choice is demotivating: Can one desire too much of a good thing? *Journal of Personality and Social Psychology, 79,* 996–1006.

Kant, I. (1967) *Kritik der praktischen Vernunft* [Critique of practical reason]. Hamburg, Germany: Felix Meiner Verlag. (Original work published 1797)

Koole, S. L., Smeets, K., van Knippenberg, A., & Dijksterhuis, A. (1999). The cessation of rumination through self-affirmation. *Journal of Personality and Social Psychology, 77,* 111–125.

Muraven, M., Tice, D. M., & Baumeister, R. F. (1998). Self-control as limited resource: Regulatory depletion patterns. *Journal of Personality and Social Psychology, 74,* 774–789.

Roberts, W. A. (2002). Are animals stuck in time? *Psychological Bulletin, 128,* 473–489.

Sartre, J. P. (1956). *Being and nothingness* (H. E. Barnes, Trans.). Secaucus, NJ: Citadel Press. (Original work published in 1943)

Schimel, J., Arndt, J., Pyszczynski, T., & Greenberg, J. (2001). Being accepted for who we are: Evidence that social validation of the intrinsic self reduces general defensiveness. *Journal of Personality and Social Psychology, 80,* 35–52.

Schmeichel, B. J., Vohs, K. D., & Baumeister, R. F. (2003a). Ego depletion and intelligent performance: Role of the self in intelligent thought and other information processing. *Journal of Personality and Social Psychology, 85,* 33–46.

Schmeichel, B. J., Vohs, K. D., & Baumeister, R. F. (2003b). *Self-affirmation prevents ego depletion.* Manuscript in progress, Florida State University, Tallahassee, FL.

Steele, C. M. (1988). The psychology of self-affirmation: Sustaining the integrity of the self. In L. Berkowitz (Ed.), *Advances in experimental social psychology* (Vol. 21, pp. 261–302). New York: Academic Press.

Twenge, J. M., Baumeister, R. F., Tice, D. M., & Stucke, T. S. (2001). If you can't join them, beat them: Effects of social exclusion on aggressive behavior. *Journal of Personality and Social Psychology, 81,* 1058–1069.

Twenge, J. M., Cantonese, K. R., & Baumeister, R. F. (2002). Social exclusion causes self-defeating behavior. *Journal of Personality and Social Psychology, 83,* 606–615.

Vohs, K. D., & Ciarocco, N. J. (2004). Self-regulation requires interpersonal functioning. In R. F. Baumeister & K. D. Vohs, (Eds.), *Handbook of self-regulation* (pp. 392–407). New York: Guilford Press.

Vohs, K. D., Ciarocco, N., & Baumeister, R. F. (2003). *Self-regulation and self-presentation: Regulatory resource depletion impairs management and effortful self-presentation depletes regulatory resource.* Manuscript under review.

Vohs, K. D., & Heatherton, T. F. (2000). Self-regulatory failure: A resource-depletion approach. *Psychological Science, 11,* 249–254.

Vohs, K. D., & Schmeichel, B. J. (2003). Self-regulation and the extended now: Controlling the self alters the subjective experience of time. *Journal of Personality and Social Psychology, 85,* 217–230.

Vohs, K. D., Twenge, J. M., Baumeister, R. F., Schmeichel, B. J., & Tice, D. M. (2003). *Decision fatigue: Making multiple personal decisions depletes the self's resources.* Unpublished manuscript, University of Utah.

Wegner, D. M. (2002). *The illusion of conscious will.* Cambridge, MA: MIT Press.

Chapter 26

Workings of the Will

A Functional Approach

JULIUS KUHL
SANDER L. KOOLE

It is often said that people like being in control of things (Alloy & Abramson, 1979; Vohs & Baumeister, Chapter 25, this volume; Langer, 1975). Viewed from this perspective, having willful control over one's own actions is highly desirable. However, willfulness also has some deeply unsettling existential implications. When someone has the power to willfully decide what he or she does, this person is fully responsible for his or her own actions. Willfulness thus eliminates any excuses or mitigating circumstances that might explain one's personal weaknesses and wrongdoings. As existential thinkers such as Heidegger and Sartre have pointed out, the mere realization of this responsibility can be terrifying. Indeed, many modern individuals seem eager to flee from the "tyranny of choice" (Schwartz, 2000), avoiding or even outright denying their ability to take charge of events. Unfortunately, the denial of personal responsibility ultimately keeps people from living their lives as they truly want. One of the major goals of existential psychotherapy has thus been to liberate people from their responsibility defenses, allowing them to regain volitional control over their own actions (Yalom, 1980).

Much as modern individuals have struggled with the existential burdens of the will, experimental psychologists have struggled with the conceptual role of the will in human functioning. At the beginning of the 20th century, the experimental study of the will made a promising start (Ach, 1910; Lewin, 1926; Lindworsky, 1923). However, this period was followed by the rise of behaviorism, which emphatically refused to accord a scientific status to the will (Skinner, 1971; Watson, 1913). After the cognitive revolution, experimental psychologists were once again at liberty to theorize about volitional processes such as self-regulation (Carver & Scheier, 1981), executive functioning (Vohs & Baumeister, Chapter 25, this volume; Norman & Shallice, 1986), autonomy (Deci & Ryan, 2000), delay of gratification (Metcalfe & Mischel, 1999), and action control (Kuhl & Beckmann,

1985). Yet, in spite of the substantial progress that has been made in these areas, the will continues to be a highly controversial topic, and attempts to deny the will its independent conceptual status have not ceased (Bargh, Chapter 24, this volume; Libet, 1985; Wegner & Wheatley, 1999).

In this chapter, we focus on the will as a central theme in experimental existential psychology. Specifically, we argue that the will represents an independent psychological concept that lends itself to rigorous scientific analysis. In the following section, we begin by considering some of the most important theoretical objections that previously have been raised against the scientific status of the will. As we show, none of these objections constitutes a compelling argument against a scientific analysis of the will. Next, we discuss a functional approach to the will, an approach that may be useful in guiding the experimental analysis of the will. Finally, we consider some of the existential–psychological implications of our perspective on the workings of the will.

IN DEFENSE OF THE WILL

One of the most fundamental objections against the scientific status of the will has been concerned with the absolute freedom from causality that the notion of willfulness seems to imply. If willful behavior would be completely free from objective determination, then any scientific attempt to analyze the workings of the will would indeed be pointless. However, upon closer consideration, this argument of indeterminism is based on a confounding between subjective and objective determination. When we perceive a person's behavior as "willed" we typically mean that this behavior is self-determined, in the sense of being free from control by forces that are external to the self. Such "external" forces can be truly external (e.g., a mugger forcing me to give him my wallet), but they can also be "internal," as long as they are external to the self system. For example, when I stick to a good-paying job even though I hate it, my behavior is controlled by the monetary *incentive*, an internal motivational factor that is not integrated in the self. Subjectively speaking, self-congruent willful behavior tends to be experienced as free by the person him- or herself (Deci & Ryan, 2000). However, this does not mean that the self-system that controls the behavior is itself free from objective determination. Subjective freedom thus does not imply freedom of objective determination (nor does the former exclude the latter).

The distinction between subjective and objective determination can also be approached from a neuropsychological perspective. Neuropsychological research has identified several parts of the brain that mediate volitional processes, such as the frontal lobes (Fuster, 1989; Lezak, 1983; Luria, 1978) and the anterior cingulate cortex (Pardo, Pardo, Janer, & Raichle, 1990; Posner & Petersen, 1990). These brain structures greatly increase the flexibility of behavior, for instance, by facilitating shifting between cognitive sets and overriding habitual responses. For example, Luria (1978) described how a patient suffering from a lesion of the prefrontal cortex became distracted from his intention to leave the ward and buy cigarettes by external cues eliciting some routine behavior (e.g., he automatically followed a group of people walking down the hallway although he could still remember his intention to buy cigarettes). In this sense, the brain structures involved in volitional control of behavior can be said to "liberate" the person from the rigid type of behavior control that is characteristic of routine behavior. At the same time, the very brain structures that give rise to volitional behavior are themselves subject to a host of causal influences, including electrochemical inputs from other brain areas, changes in blood sugar levels, hormonal changes, and so on (LeDoux, 1995). Thus, at the level of brain processes, we again see how actions that are free and willful from a personal perspective can be objectively determined at the same time.

If the causal status of neurobiological influences on willful action is undebatable, then one might argue that psychologists could suffice with studying these objective causal influences instead of the more slippery volitional processes that can only be studied on a psychological level. After all, it could be argued that objective causal influences such as electrochemical events operate on a more basic level of analysis. However, this kind of reductionism is unlikely to shed much light on the workings of the will. Even if one would assume that all events in the universe, even mental events, are, in the final analysis, determined by the law of physics, predictability is very limited. The dissociation between determinism and predictability has even been shown for simple systems involving just two variables. To the extent that these variables affect each other in a reciprocal and nonlinear fashion, that is, when the nonlinear effect of one variable on the other is fed back to the first variable, the system can behave according to an unpredictable ("chaotic") but fully deterministic way (Gleick, 1990; Haken, 1981; Kuhl, 1986). Indeed, recent developments in dynamical systems theory have shown that fully determined complex systems have emergent properties, so that the behavior of the whole system cannot be reduced in a straightforward manner to the behavior of its constituent elements (Vallacher, Read, & Nowak, 2002). Accordingly, higher-order, system-level constructs such as willfulness and self-regulation provide the most parsimonious way to describe and explain the behavior of complex systems. Notably, the concept of will as we use it in this chapter cannot be reduced to the emergent properties of nonlinear interactions among systems determining behavior. Rather, the will is conceived as a superordinate system that coordinates many processes much like an executive board of a large company or the government of a country.

Whereas the foregoing arguments were strictly theoretical, some recent work has proposed empirical arguments against the causal role of the will. For instance, research by Libet (1985) has shown that people's awareness of their intention to move one of their fingers is preceded by brain-readiness potentials that presumably initiate the finger movement. These findings have been interpreted as evidence that behavior was not caused by a conscious intention because the intention to move one's behavior seemed to occur *after* the brain had initiated activities that typically precede motor behavior. In a related vein, a series of clever experiments by Wegner, Wheatley, and associates demonstrated that people can be tricked into believing that they voluntarily chose to perform certain actions (e.g., moving a mouse across a computer screen), even when these actions were objectively caused by an external event (Wegner & Wheatley, 1999). From the present perspective, these lines of research offer intriguing insights into the relation between conscious experience and volitional action. However, we do not think that this research provides any compelling argument against the causal role of the will in action control.

First, even if one would accept the previous findings as instances of volitional illusions, they do not prove that volition can *never* be a cause of behavior. Indeed, the particular actions that were investigated in these studies (i.e., simple motor movements) were hardly representative of the entire universe of actions that are generally considered volitional. Second, experimental research has shown that many actions that on the surface appear to be volitional are in reality performed because individuals feel pressured to do so (Deci & Ryan, 2000; Kuhl & Kazén, 1994). Similar pressures may well have been operating in the experiments by Libet (1985) and Wegner and Wheatley (1999). For instance, participants in

Libet's (1985) experiments were explicitly instructed to move their finger at a self-chosen time. These explicit instructions could have undermined participants' sense of personal freedom, thereby inhibiting the operation of volitional processes. Indeed, recent experiments have shown that some individuals (so-called state-oriented individuals) are likely to mistake external assignments for self-chosen commitments (Baumann & Kuhl, 2003; Kuhl & Kazén, 1994; Kazén, Baumann, & Kuhl, 2003). This judgmental error appears to indicate impaired volitional functioning, given that state-oriented individuals frequently experience difficulties when it comes to executing intended actions (Kuhl & Helle, 1986). These and related findings suggest that the suppression of willful processes through explicit instructions is a common phenomenon which may even occur outside awareness (Baumann & Kuhl, 2003; Kuhl & Kazén, 1994; Kazén et al., 2003).

Finally, the research by Libet (1985) and Wegner and Wheatley (1999) only speaks to the validity of people's conscious experience of the will. It thus remains an open question to which extent unconscious volitional processes are a causal force in human behavior. Libet (1999), who briefly entertained the notion of unconscious will, eventually considered it "unacceptable." In contrast, we believe that unconscious volition is a viable theoretical possibility. As we explain, this position follows naturally from a functional approach to the workings of the will.

A FUNCTIONAL APPROACH TO THE WILL

When psychologists are theorizing about the nature of the will, it is important to keep in mind that the will is more than just an abstract psychological construct. As Wegner and Wheatley (1999) noted, "We all have the sense that we do things, that we cause our acts, that we are agents." Indeed, for most people, willfulness constitutes a very compelling subjective experience. Consequently, it becomes tempting to equate the experience of willing with the actual functioning of the will. Though this confounding is understandable, we believe that it stands in the way of a genuine understanding of how the will operates. Notably, we do not dispute that the actual functioning of the will has important phenomenal correlates. Indeed, numerous studies have documented that many important aspects of willful behavior can be assessed through self-reporting (e.g., Deci & Ryan, 2000). Moreover, our own work on individual differences in action orientation suggests that even unconscious volitional functions may be tapped by self-report instruments, presumably because people can learn about unconscious volitional functions indirectly, by observing the consequences of these functions in their own actions (Kuhl & Fuhrman, 1998).

Although some aspects of willing may become consciously represented, conscious experience cannot fully reveal how the will operates. First of all, there are important limitations to people's ability to accurately report on their own mental processes (Nisbett & Wilson, 1977). Indeed, the aforementioned experiments by Wegner and Wheatley (1999) and Kuhl and Kazén (1994) highlight just how easily the conscious mind can be misled about the workings of the will. Second, people's self-reports are contaminated by a variety of factors, such as social desirability and cultural preconceptions about the will (Young & Morris, Chapter 14, this volume). Third, many volitional processes may be *in principle* inaccessible to conscious experience. Although the notion of unconscious volition has been scarcely considered by experimental psychologists, some existential psychologists have recognized that some acts of will appear to operate on "subterranean," unconscious levels (Farber, 1966; Jung, 1964; Yalom, 1980). For instance, Farber (1966) suggested that the important choices one makes in life are not consciously experienced as choices but can only be inferred after the fact. We believe that a similar conclusion can be derived from the commonly held conception of the will as a *central executive system*. According to this conception, willful processes are responsible for filtering, organizing, and integrating the vast array of different feelings, thoughts, needs, motivations, goals, norms, expectations, and so on, that collectively make up the person. Because the conscious mind has only a very limited processing capacity, it is unlikely that all these different self-aspects can be simultaneously represented in conscious awareness. As such, the will can only perform its central executive functions if it operates at least in part (most likely, in large part) on unconscious levels.

If conscious experience cannot reveal the whole story about the will, then how can psychologists obtain a deeper understanding of the workings of the will? We think this can be achieved by adopting a *functional approach* to the will. The functional approach tries to uncover the various subsystems that underlie volitional functioning. Whereas everyday, subjective accounts attribute all forms of willfulness to the whole person, the functional approach breaks down willful phenomena into the *subpersonal* mechanisms that mediate these phenomena (see also Greve, 2001). This kind of approach is commonplace in cognitive psychology, which has successfully analyzed the functional components of psychological phenomena with low levels of internal organization, such as the perception of isolated objects or simple motor actions. We believe that a similar approach can be fruitful in studying more complex psychological phenomena, such as motivation (Kuhl, 1984; 2000), authenticity (Koole & Kuhl, 2003) and the will. It should be noted that our functional approach to the will is not reductionistic because it treats volitional phenomena at a separate level of functioning. Thus, volitional mechanisms are considered as functionally independent, and hence irreducible to lower-level mechanisms, such as stimulus–response (S-R) associations, arousal, or affect.

Within personality psychology, a functional approach to high-level phenomena is not new. Indeed, Freud's classic model of id, ego, and superego can be seen as an initial attempt toward a functional analysis of motivational and volitional behavior. One familiar objection against these kinds of models has been that they were often very difficult to test empirically, and hence may degenerate into overly abstract, metaphorical accounts. However, this objection only applies to implementations of the functional approach that are too vague to permit empirical testing. The risk of creating merely metaphorical accounts can be overcome by explicating functional mechanisms in such a way that these mechanisms can be rigorously tested. The functional approach therefore is useful only when the relevant functional mechanisms are formulated with maximal explicitness and precision. At times, however, the functional approach may postulate mechanisms for which no empirical instruments are available, even though such instruments could be designed in principle. In such cases, the functional approach challenges researchers to develop measures that can reliably discriminate between the theorized functional mechanisms. Our own efforts to establish a functional account of the will have been guided by personality systems interactions (PSI) theory (Kuhl, 2000a, 2000b, 2001), which we present in the following section.

PERSONALITY SYSTEMS INTERACTION THEORY

PSI theory is an integrative framework that seeks to explain human personality functioning in terms of its underlying functional mechanisms (Kuhl, 2000a, 2000b, 2001). As a broad theoretical perspective, PSI theory addresses a wide range of personality phenomena, including creativity (Biebrich & Kuhl, 2002; Koole & Coenen, 2003), intuition (Baumann & Kuhl, 2002), the self (Koole & Kuhl, 2003), and depression (Kuhl & Helle, 1986). Originally, however, PSI theory was developed out of a conceptual analysis of volitional action control (Kuhl, 1984; Kuhl & Beckmann, 1994a). As such, the will continues to occupy a central place within PSI theory.

In agreement with other approaches (e.g., Vohs & Baumeister, Chapter 25, this volume; Metcalfe & Mischel, 1999), PSI theory conceives of the will as a set of central executive processes that regulate the person's thoughts, feelings, and actions in a top-down manner. PSI theory further distinguishes between two fundamental forms of willing or *volitional modes*. The first form of willing is responsible for inhibiting impulsive actions and maintaining a single-minded focus on goals that are activated in memory. This volitional mode is referred to as *self-control*. By contrast, the second form of willing directs the person's functioning toward activities that are either intrinsically appealing or congruent with a multitude of the person's inner values and autobiographical experiences. This second volitional mode is referred to as *self-maintenance*.[1]. Self-control and self-maintenance represent functionally opposite ways of volitional action control. Indeed, the brain systems that presumably underlie self-control and self-maintenance are assumed to be mutually inhibitory. Accordingly, the person cannot engage both volitional functions simultaneously. However, by switching between modes, it is possible to coordinate two volitional modes with each other (Fuhrmann & Kuhl, 1998). Indeed, the functional dissociation between self-maintenance and self-control is often hard to notice in well-balanced, effectively functioning individuals. Even so, it remains important to distinguish between self-control and self-maintenance on a conceptual level, because the two volitional modes are responsible for qualitatively different forms of action control.

SELF-CONTROL

Self-control is an immensely useful form of action control. Among other things, it enables people to acquire healthy eating habits (Fuhrman & Kuhl, 1998; Verplanken & Faes, 1999), meet important deadlines (Gollwitzer & Brandstätter, 1997; Koole & van 't Spijker, 2000), inhibit prejudiced reactions (Devine, 1989; Fiske, 1989), and engage in prosocial, self-sacrificial actions (Koole, Jager, Hofstee, & van den Berg, 2001; Van Lange et al., 1997). Self-control tends to be conscious and effortful and is thus in line with traditional psychological conceptions of the will as an explicit, conscious phenomenon. Metaphorically, self-control may be likened to an "inner dictatorship" (Fuhrman & Kuhl, 1998), during which a "narrow-minded" central executive imposes one dominant goal or perception on the system and suppresses opposing needs, feelings, and other self-aspects. A prototypical example of self-control is a student who attempts to enact her intention to study by inhibiting all thoughts related to attractive alternatives such as talking with friends or going to the movies (Metcalfe & Mischel, 1999; Wegner, 1994).

According to PSI theory, self-control can be further broken down into two separate functional systems. The first system that supports self-control is *intention memory*. Intention memory becomes activated when immediate enactment is not possible or undesirable. For instance, intention memory may become activated when people are undecided about where and how to act (Gollwitzer, 1999), when an action plan contains multiple steps (Goschke & Kuhl, 1993), or when immediate responding needs to be delayed (Metcalfe & Mischel, 1999). In these kinds of situations, it is useful to maintain an explicit memory representation of an intended action until the action can be performed. Intention memory is thus responsible for (1) maintaining abstract-symbolic representations of intended actions in working memory (Goschke & Kuhl, 1993; Kuhl & Helle, 1986), and (2) inhibiting the pathway between such intentions and intuitive behavior control systems, to prevent premature action (Kuhl & Kazén, 1999). According to PSI theory, intention memory is connected to a larger network of subsystems that support analytical thinking, verbal processing, and other functions that support planning (Shallice, 1988). Neuroanatomically, the operation of intention memory may be attributed to left-hemispheric (prefrontal) processing (Knight & Grabowecky, 1995). The organization of the left hemisphere consists of a large number of small neuronal networks that function like an ensemble of highly specialized "experts" (Scheibel et al., 1985). This combination of high specialization and low integration is highly conducive to analytical thinking, which is characterized by high competition between alternatives: Things are either true or false, good or bad, useful or useless.

Specifically, PSI theory assumes that self-control is also supported by lower-order cognitive processes, in the form of an *object recognition* system. Object recognition is a primarily perceptual system that focuses on explicit identification and recognition of elementary sensations (e.g., a visual object, a sequence of tones, an emotion, and a semantic category). Characteristic for object recognition (especially in connection with negative mood) is a focus on discrepancies. The system is especially focused on sensations that diverge from previously held expectations, standards, or wishes. Object recognition thus performs the discrepancy-detecting monitoring function that is part of cybernetic models of self-regulation (Carver & Scheier, 1981; Miller, Galanter, & Pibram, 1960). Object recognition can also act as a warning system, which alerts the person to potentially dangerous situations by highlighting unexpected or undesirable events.

Several lines of research have shown that it is possible to obtain separate measures of the self-control functions. For instance, Goschke and Kuhl (1993) investigated the operation of intention memory in a prospective memory paradigm. In this paradigm, participants were asked to memorize pairs of behavioral scripts (e.g., cleaning up one's desk), some of which were to be executed later on. The results indicated that recognition memory for the to-be-executed script was especially efficient, an effect that was termed the "intention-superiority effect" (ISE). The ISE can be regarded as a marker of intention memory activation, because it indicates the degree to which intentional structures are activated in working memory (for alternative measures of intention memory, see Förster & Liberman, 2002; Koole, Smeets, van Knippenberg, & Dijksterhuis, 1999; Shah, Friedman, & Kruglanski, 2002). In a related vein, Kuhl and Kazén (1999) used the classic Stroop color-naming task to study the inhibitory link between intention memory and intuitive behavior control. In this research, even brief exposures (< 1 s) to positively charged words were able to remove the inhibition between intention memory and intuitive behavior control, such that the classic Stroop interference effect was effectively eliminated. Object recognition can similarly be studied in various ways. Beckmann (1989) used a perceptually based indicator of object recognition (i.e., recognition accuracy of tachistoscopically presented words). Notably, object recognition may also facilitate the perception of internal "objects" (i.e., thoughts or sensations). Indeed, Kuhl and Baumann (2000) have argued that uncontrollable ruminations can indicate excessive operation of object recognition, especially when these take the form of negative intrusions. Ruminations become uncontrollable when superordinate systems are inhibited (e.g., through negative affect) to the extent that they cannot filter out unwanted productions of the object recognition system.

SELF-MAINTENANCE

Even a casual glance at human behavior reveals that the conscious, self-controlled conception of the will cannot account for the full spectrum of willful phenomena. Indeed, some of the most powerful forms of willing are accompanied by experiences of "flow" (Csikszentmihalyi, 1990), "self-congruence" (Kasser & Sheldon, Chapter 29, this volume), or "self-determination" (Deci & Ryan, 2000). Apparently, some forms of willing are enjoyable, congruent with multiple needs and self-aspects, and autonomous. This self-determined willing is closely related to Rank's (1945) "creative will," willing that does not involve suppression and has access to the individual's deepest emotions and desires. In line with these notions, PSI theory assumes that there exists a form of willing that is fundamentally different from self-control. This second mode of volition is "self-maintenance." Metaphorically, self-maintenance resembles an inner democracy, during which the central executive "listens to many voices," that is, pursues goals that simultaneously satisfy multiple self-aspects. Applied to the student who wants to study and hang out with her friends, this means that she would be sensitive to all her needs, emotions, and thoughts and find a way to take care of them simultaneously (e.g., by studying together with friends) or successively (e.g., study for a while, then go out with friends), or find even more creative ways to integrate her diverse inclinations.

Like the self-control mode, the self-maintenance mode can be further broken down into two functional systems. The first functional system that supports self-maintenance is "extension memory." Extension memory is a central executive system that consists of extended cognitive–affective networks. Extension memory supports an intelligent, high-inferential form of intuition (Baumann & Kuhl, 2002), which is capable of integrating multiple inputs from both cognitive and affective subsystems through parallel-processing mechanisms (Rumelhart, McClelland, & The PDP Research Group, 1986). Extension memory is typically invoked when the person confronts seemingly contradictory aspects of an object, person, or situation. In these situations, it is highly adaptive to engage in holistic processing, which integrates vast amounts of information at speeds that are much greater than can be handled by logical-analytical thinking (i.e., intention memory). Extension memory also forms the basis for "implicit self-representations," integrated representations of internal states such as needs, motives, emotions, somatic feelings (e.g., muscle tensions), motives, values, and autobiographical experiences that involve the self (Koole & Pelham, 2003; McClelland, Koestner, & Weinberger, 1989; Wheeler, Stuss, & Tulving, 1997). On a neuroanatomical level, the operation of extension memory is attributed to right-hemispheric (prefrontal) processing. The organization of the right hemisphere is much like a global network that integrates information from a vast variety of input systems. As such, the right hemisphere is ideally suited for integrative information processing (Beeman et al., 1994; Rotenberg, 1993).

Self-maintenance is further supported by a lower-order behavior control system, "intuitive behavior control." Intuitive behavior control consists of a multitude of highly contextualized behavioral programs that guide the automatic execution of concrete actions and intuitive responses to objects or events. Intuitive behavior control refers to behavior-regulating mechanisms that are purposeful but lacking in explicit intentionality. One of the earliest forms of intuitive behavior control can be observed in newborn children, who already display emotional contagion and imitation of the emotional expressions of their caretakers (Meltzoff & Moore, 1994). Some of these intuitive behaviors persist into adulthood (Chartrand & Bargh, 1999; Van Baaren, Maddux, Chartrand, de Bouter, & van

Knippenberg, 2003), whereas additional intuitive behaviors may be acquired later in life. Intuitive behavior programs are especially important for conducting positively toned, spontaneous social interactions (Papousek & Papousek, 1982). Finally, intuitive behavior control is "promotion-oriented" (cf. Higgins, 1998), being geared toward maximization of positive affect, rewards, or need satisfactions.

A number of methodologies have been found useful in assessing the self-maintenance functions. Extension memory activation is often accompanied by experiential correlates, which include feelings of freedom (Yalom, 1980), mastery (Dweck, 1986), and self-determination (Deci & Ryan, 2000). According to PSI theory, it is possible to interpret these subjective experiences in functional terms. Behavior that is controlled by extension memory has much more flexibility than rigid S-R behavior control, because the parallel processing networks of extension memory can process vast numbers of behavioral options, including even options that are highly unusual or removed from the immediate action context. The subjective experience of freedom that often accompanies this kind of behavior control may thus be based on an intuitive sense of the vast number of behavioral options that individuals have at their disposal. In a related vein, feelings of mastery may be based on an intuitive computation of the vast networks of experiences that the individual can tap in order to solve a particular problem. Finally, the experience of self-determination may arise through an intuitive sense that one's activities are congruent with all the extended networks of personal needs, motives, self-aspects, and autobiographical experiences that have been recruited through extension memory.

The cognitive structures of extension memory are too extended to be completely accessible to conscious experience. As such, it remains crucial to develop measures of extension memory that do not rely on introspection. The information-processing functions of extension memory can be assessed using various indicators of integrative processing, such as summation priming (Beeman et al., 1994; cf. Bolte, 1999), coherence judgments (Baumann & Kuhl, 2002), and measures of creative thinking (Biebrich & Kuhl, 2001; Koole & Coenen, 2003). The activation of implicit self-representations in extension memory may be tapped through measures of self-accessibility (Koole & Jostmann, 2003) or other measures of implicit self-concept (Greenwald & Banaji, 1995; Koole, in press; Koole & Pelham, 2003). Finally, access to the self's choices may be assessed through the self-discrimination paradigm (Kuhl & Kazén, 1994). In the latter paradigm, participants and the experimenter select an equal number of activities from a list, which are to be executed by the participants later on. After a distracter task, participants are again presented with the entire list and indicate for each activity whether it was self-chosen. A self-discrimination index can be constructed by taking the number of assigned activities that participants erroneously designate as self-chosen. Various experiments have supported the validity of the self-discrimination measure. For instance, research has established that state-oriented individuals are much more likely to display self-discrimination errors (Kuhl & Kazén, 1994), especially when it comes to unattractive activities (Kazén et al., 2003) and when negative affect is high (Baumann & Kuhl, 2003). Accordingly, self-discrimination errors occur especially under conditions that theoretically are characterized by reduced access to extension memory (i.e., the combination of state orientation and negative affect).

Activation of intuitive behavior control is best assessed through implicit measures because intuitive behavior control operates primarily at the level of subsymbolic motor movements. Kuhl (2001, p. 330) has listed various information processing characteristics that may be used to develop objective measures of intuitive behavior control. These characteristics include multimodal sensations, orientation toward the immediate present, egocentric perception, context specificity, reciprocity between sensation and motor movements, implicit knowledge, impressionistic processing, and a focus on concrete instances (prototypes). Useful experimental methods for the assessment of intuitive behavior control include the performance of well-practiced motor skills (Heckhausen & Strang, 1988; Kuhl & Koch, 1984), signal detection methods (i.e., the maximization of hits; see Higgins, 1998), seating distance (Wisman & Koole, 2003), and social mimicry (Chartrand & Bargh, 1999).

INTERACTIONS BETWEEN VOLITIONAL SYSTEMS: THE MEDIATING ROLE OF AFFECT

Self-control and self-maintenance are mutually exclusive forms of volitional action control. Thus, at any given point in time, it is impossible for the person to be at once self-controlling and self-maintaining. Given that both self-control and self-maintenance are highly adaptive forms of executive control, a vexing self-regulatory dilemma is created. If the person emphasizes self-control, he or she runs the risk of becoming overly analytical and inhibited (due to chronic activation of intention memory) and may suffer from uncontrollable negative ruminations and periods of alienation (Kuhl & Beckmann, 1994b) due to chronic activation of object recognition and suppression of the self and other parts of extension memory. Conversely, if the person chooses to emphasize self-maintenance, he or she runs the risk of becoming overly impulsive (due to chronic activation of intuitive behavior control) and insensitive to genuine threats to well-being (due to chronic activation of extension memory suppressing unexpected or unwanted perceptions). Clearly, neither of these alternatives qualifies as adaptive self-regulation. How can people resolve this problem?

According to PSI theory, the solution lies in switching between self-control and self-maintenance in a flexible and dynamic manner. Even though self-control and self-maintenance cannot be performed simultaneously, the person may alternate between self-control and self-maintenance from moment to moment. For instance, a person may first construct a complex action plan (using intention memory) and then proceed by putting this plan into action (using intuitive behavior control; cf. Kuhl & Kazén, 1999). Thus alternating between intention memory and intuitive behavior control is highly beneficial for forming and subsequently enacting intentions (or *volitional efficiency*; Kuhl, 2000b; Oettingen, Pak, & Schnetter, 2001). In a related vein, alternating between object recognition and extension memory is vital for *personal growth* (Kuhl, 2000a). Specifically, the person may first notice a new, self-alien experience (using object recognition) and then integrate this experience into the larger scheme of his or her personal motives, needs, and autobiographical experiences (using extension memory). In short, to function optimally (i.e., to attain high volitional efficiency and personal growth), dynamic alternations between self-control and self-maintenance functions are necessary.

The ability to alternate between different volitional functions requires additional coordination. According to PSI theory, this coordination mechanism is provided by the *affective systems* (Kuhl, 1983a). Specifically, affect acts as an internal signal that modulates the dynamic energy flow between volitional systems (see Martin, 1999, for a related view). Notably, this modulating function of affect is assumed to occur over and above the hedonic functions of affect (i.e., motivating the person to maximize pleasure and to minimize pain). The underlying idea here is that affective changes inform the self-regulatory system that a different approach to the situation is needed (see also Clore, Schwarz, & Conway, 1994, for related mood-as-information models). Our perspective is also consistent with the view that affect may be aroused from both cognitive (e.g., appraisal) or purely affective (e.g., visceral) sources, and that changes in affect may or not be consciously perceived by the person (LeDoux, 1995). PSI theory further argues that positive and negative affect (though often negatively correlated) has distinct functional roles, in addition to the ones illustrated by previous research, such as facilitation of behavior and creative performance (Ashby, Isen, & Turken, 1999; Isen, 1984). Positive affect modulates the information flow between intention memory and intuitive behavior control. Decreases in positive affect signal that important needs are not being met, because some obstacle has to be overcome, and hence lead to activation of intention memory. Conversely, increases in positive affect signal that need satisfaction is no longer problematic and hence lead to activation of intuitive behavior control. Negative affect modulates the energy flow between object recognition and extension memory. Increases in negative affect signal the possible presence of an immediate, unpredictable danger and hence cause an increase in the activation of object recognition. Conversely, decreases in negative affect indicate that the situation is relatively safe and predictable and hence cause extension memory to become activated. On the basis of its extended experiential networks, extension memory is highly suited for sensing the underlying predictability of large numbers of complex events.

Because of the modulatory role of affect, circumstances that influence the person's affective states have profound implications for volitional behavior. For instance, being in a friendly emotional climate and a predictable environment will lead most individuals to adopt the self-maintenance mode. Conversely, a hostile emotional climate in a highly unpredictable environment will cause most individuals to revert to the self-control mode. In addition to these external factors, enduring personality dispositions may exert an important influence on the person's affective states and, hence, on volitional functioning. For instance, a predisposition to neuroticism may lead individuals to have frequently elevated levels of negative affect, which leads to frequent activation of object recognition accompanied by suppression of extension memory. Likewise, a predisposition to extraversion may lead individuals to have frequently elevated levels of positive affect, which leads to frequent activation of intuitive behavior control accompanied by suppression of intention memory. The dispositional factors that influence sensitivity for positive and negative affect may be innate or learned.

VOLITIONAL AFFECT REGULATION

People are not just passive observers of their own feelings. Indeed, the emotion literature indicates that people continually monitor and regulate their own affective states (Gross, 1999). PSI theory provides a theoretical explanation for these intense affect regulation efforts. Because affective change has important consequences for volitional functioning, the ability to maintain certain affective states is vital to effective action control. Some affect regulation mechanisms occur on early, relatively primitive levels of information processing. Examples are the perceptual blocking ("repression") of negative affect (Bruner & Postman, 1948; Dawson & Schell, 1982; Greenwald, 1988; Hock, Krohne & Kaiser, 1996; Langens & Mörth, 2003) or the instinctive urge to affiliate with others in times of distress (Schachter, 1959; Wisman & Koole, 2003). However, affect regulation may also occur on higher, more sophisticated levels of information processing of the kind that is supported by prefrontal brain regions. When such high-level processes are involved in affect regulation, PSI theory speaks of *volitional affect regulation*. Volitional affect regulation is possible when the volitional functions (i.e., intention memory and extension memory) have developed links with the affective systems. Accordingly, volitional affect regulation skills are fostered by an environment that encourages individuals to use volitional processes to down-regulate unwanted affect (see Kuhl, 2000a, for a more formal model).

PSI theory further distinguishes between volitional affect regulation by means of intention memory and volitional affect regulation by means of extension memory. Affect regulation by means of intention memory operates through conscious, deliberative processing. Recent work by Gross (2002) and associates has studied two kinds of deliberative affect regulation. First, individuals may use emotional suppression to inhibit the expression of their aversive affective states. Suppression strategies tend to be ineffective (Gross, 2002) and may even add to the unwanted affect (Wegner, 1994). Second, individuals may down-regulate negative affect by changing one's conscious reappraisals of events (for instance, people may adopt a neutral perspective when they are experiencing something negative). Although reappraisal is more effective than suppression, it can only be implemented before the unwanted affect has been triggered. Once an affect has become fully processed, reappraisal is no longer viable. According to PSI theory, a considerably more flexible and efficient control over one's affective states can be achieved through extension memory. Extension memory is closely connected with the affective systems (Dawson & Schell, 1982; Wittling, 1990). As such, extension memory seems especially suited to regulate the person's affective states. Moreover, due to its parallel processing characteristics, extension memory is capable of responding much more quickly and efficiently to affective change than the sequential operators of intention memory.

Kuhl (1981, 1994) has developed a measure to assess individual differences in affect regulation through extension memory. Because this kind of affect regulation is a central component of effective action control, individuals who are highly skilled at coping through extension memory are referred to as action-oriented individuals. Theoretically, action-oriented individuals are presumed to be capable of highly efficient and context-sensitive affect regulation, leading to smooth execution of intended actions, even in the face of stressful circumstances. By contrast, individuals low on action orientation are presumably lacking in such powerful affect regulation skills, causing them to be more vulnerable to aversive affect and unwanted ruminations. Because the latter individuals are easily preoccupied by their own aversive states, they are referred to as state-oriented individuals. Converging lines of research have supported the validity of the distinction between action- and state-oriented coping styles in terms of self-regulation of affect on explicit affect (Brunstein & Olbrich, 1985; Kuhl, 1981, 1983b; Rholes, Michas, & Schroff, 1985) and implicit affective processes (Heckhausen & Strang, 1988; Koole & Jostmann, 2003; Rosahl, Tennigkeit, Kuhl, & Haschke, 1993). For instance, Koole (2003) found evidence that stress inductions cause action-oriented individuals to display reversed affective priming for negative affect, a pattern indicative of volitional inhibition of negative affect. No such findings emerged among state-oriented individuals. Moreover, and consistent with the notion that action orientation is an acquired skill, clinical studies indicate that action orientation can be boosted through psychotherapy (Kaschel & Kuhl, 2004; Schulte, Hartung, & Wilke, 1997).

According to PSI theory, self-regulation of affect is not confined to the maintenance or restoration of pleasant mood and its implications for subjective well-being and health. Instead, self-regulation of affect also modulates the interaction among the four mental systems that is needed for switching among mental systems according to situational requirements, for putting the will into effect, and for developing a creative and wise self-system (Figure 26.1). Accordingly, PSI theory predicts that action orientation should be a key moderator of the entire range

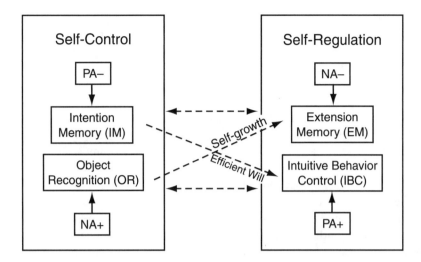

FIGURE 26.1. Cognitive systems of PSI theory and their modulation by high (+) versus low (–) positive (PA) or negative (NA) affect. Dashed arrows indicate antagonisms between cooperating systems that can only be overcome through an affective change.

of volitional functions. Consistent with this prediction, research has found reliable effects of action orientation on various indicators of intention memory, object recognition, extension memory, and intuitive behavior control (Kuhl, 2000a, 2001). In line with the generality of the action orientation construct, the effects of action orientation have been obtained across a broad range of content domains, ranging from cognitive performance (Goschke & Kuhl, 1993) to physiological functioning (Walschburger, 1994), social perception (Baumann & Kuhl, 2002) and work performance (Diefendorff, Hall, Lord, & Strean, 2000). Across these diverse domains, action-oriented individuals consistently display optimal volitional performance, whereas state-oriented individuals have displayed a variety of volitional deficits. However, this asymmetry between action- and state-oriented individuals only emerges under stressful conditions. Under relaxing conditions, when self-regulation of affect is not needed, state-oriented individuals may even outperform action-oriented individuals[2] (Kuhl & Beckmann, 1994a; Menec, 1995). From a functional perspective, however, the volitional deficits observed among state-oriented individuals under stressful conditions are often most informative, because such deficits may reveal dissociations between volitional functions that are smoothly coordinated in action-oriented individuals. As such, the study of individual differences in action orientation has contributed valuable insights to the functional analysis of the will.

CONCLUSIONS AND FUTURE DIRECTIONS

In this chapter, we have argued that the will deserves to be taken seriously as a scientific construct. The will has had a highly controversial history in psychology. Accordingly, we began the chapter by addressing some of the most frequently heard objections against the will. As it turned out, none of these objections constitutes a compelling argument against the independent conceptual status of the will. We then discussed PSI theory, a functional account that explains the workings of the will in terms of dynamical interactions between cognitive and affective systems. The analysis that PSI theory offers is not reductionistic, because it assumes separate mechanisms to account for willful functioning instead of reducing the will to lower-level phenomena such as S-R associations. At the same time, PSI theory is undeniably deterministic, by specifying volitional systems and processes that can be empirically assessed and tested. The tension that has existed between deterministic and reductionistic approaches to the will has thus been resolved by PSI theory.

Doubtless, future scientific developments will continue to contribute to the functional analysis of the will. New knowledge about brain functioning, dynamical systems theory, behavioral genetics, and personality and social psychology will almost certainly enrich our thinking about the will. Consequently, we anticipate that the field's knowledge of volitional processes will expand dramatically over the next few decades. One of the main challenges for researchers is to keep up with all the new discoveries that are made on the workings of the will. The development of broad, integrative theories are needed to organize this ever-growing body of findings and to keep its major findings accessible. In this regard, PSI theory may serve a useful function, as a theoretical framework that spans a broad range of volitional phenomena.

But what about the deeper existential issues that are connected with the will? Can a functional analysis such as PSI theory speak to persistent problems of the will such as responsibility avoidance, alienation, and existential guilt? Although this challenge is daunting, we believe that the functional approach has at least the potential to help individuals who are struggling with these existential concerns. First, the functional approach offers a precise scientific language for existential concepts such as the will, self, and intuition. As Jung (1957) noted, "scientific knowledge . . ., in the eyes of modern man, counts as the only intellectual and spiritual authority." Thus, a rigorous scientific approach to existential issues is increasingly needed to overcome modern individuals' discomfort with the metaphorical models that have traditionally been espoused by existential approaches. Second, the measures that are developed within the functional approach may be useful in uncovering the functional causes of people's existential concerns. A major advantage of the objective measures of the functional approach is that they can provide information on *implicit* volitional processes. As noted by Yalom (1980), implicit volitional processes often provide the key to the deeper existential problems with which individuals are struggling. At the University of Osnabrück, we have been collaborating with psychotherapists in order to capitalize on the applied significance of the functional approach. In so doing, we have found that our experimental techniques can be turned into sensitive diagnostic instruments for assessing specific volitional malfunctions (Kaschel & Kuhl, 2004). Finally, by offering a wealth of new conceptual and empirical tools, the functional approach may contribute to the development of particular methods of helping individuals to overcome volitional and existential problems in everyday life as well as in organizational contexts (Kuhl & Henseler, 2003).

We are not arguing, however, that the functional approach provides a simple formula to rid people once and for all from all their existential concerns about responsibility, willing, and decision making. Rather, the functional approach acknowledges the complexity that is inherent in the workings of the will and thus highlights the many ways in which healthy forms of willing can be frustrated. Instead of helping people to avoid existential problems altogether, the functional approach is designed to help people to confront their existential concerns without getting stuck. Indeed, when people manage to overcome these existential concerns, even the most troubling feelings of guilt, anxiety, or alienation may be transformed into opportunities for psychological growth.

ACKNOWLEDGMENTS

This chapter was facilitated by an Innovation Grant from the Netherlands Organization for Scientific Research (NWO) awarded to Sander L. Koole and by a stay of Sander L. Koole at the Peter Wall Institute for Interdisciplinary Studies at the University of British Columbia, Vancouver, Canada.

NOTES

1. In earlier publications, we also referred to self-maintenance by the term "self-regulation" (e.g., Kuhl, 2000a). We now prefer to use the latter term in a more general sense, as encompassing the two modes of volition.
2. The performance advantage for state-oriented individuals under relaxing conditions might seem counterintuitive and hence require some further explanation. PSI theory has related this pattern to the workings of the hippocampus (Kuhl, 2001). The hippocampus is most efficient at moderate levels of stress. Thus, very low levels of stress and very high levels of stress lead to inferior performance. Now, state-oriented people may reach this optimum much quicker than action-oriented people, so that the optimal performance for both groups is reached at different levels of stress. If this reasoning is correct, the performance advantage for state-oriented individuals under relaxing conditions should emerge primarily for tasks that involve the hippocampal system (e.g., spatial orienting tasks). This implication could be tested in future research.

REFERENCES

Ach, N. (1910). *Über den Willensakt und das Temperament [On the act of will and temperament]*. Leipzig: Quelle & Meyer.

Alloy, L. B., & Abramson, L. Y. (1979). Judgment of contingency in depressed and nondepressed students: Sadder but wiser? *Journal of Experimental Psychology: General, 108,* 441–485.

Ashby, F. G., Isen, A. M., & Turken, A. U. (1999). A neuropsychological theory of positive affect and ist influence on cognition. *Psychological Review, 106,* 529–550.

Baumann, N., & Kuhl, J. (2002). Intuition, affect and personality: Unconscious coherence judgments and self-regulation of negative affect. *Journal of Personality and Social Psychology, 83,* 1213–1223.

Baumann, N., & Kuhl, J. (2003). Self-infiltration: Confusing assigned tasks as self-selected in memory. *Personality and Social Psychology Bulletin, 29,* 487–497.

Beckmann, J. (1989). Erhöhte Leistung bei unzureichender Motivationskontrolle [Facilitated performance as a function of insufficient self-motivation]. *Zeitschrift für Experimentelle und Angewandte Psychologie, 36,* 1–15.

Beeman, M., Friedman, R. B., Grafman, J., Perez, E., Diamond, S., & Lindsay, M. B. (1994). Summation priming and coarse coding in the right hemisphere. *Journal of Cognitive Neuroscience, 6,* 26–45.

Biebrich, R., & Kuhl, J. (2002). Neurotizismus und Kreativität: Wie kann die Selbst steuerung bei der Problembewältigung helfen? [Neuroticism and creativity: How can self-regulation improve problem-solving?]. *Zeitschrift für Differentielle und Diagnostische Psychologie, 23,* 171–190.

Bolte, A. (1999). *Intuition und Emotion: Einflüsse von Stimmungen auf semantische Aktivierung und implizite Urteilsprozesse [Intuition and emotion: Influences of mood on semantic activation and implicit judgment]*. Unpublished dissertation, Universität Osnabrück.

Bruner, J. S., & Postman, L. (1948). Symbolic value as an organizing factor in perception. *Journal of Social Psychology, 27,* 203–208.

Brunstein, J. C., & Olbrich, E. (1985). Personal helplessness and action control: An analysis of achievement-related cognitions, self-assessments, and performance. *Journal of Personality and Social Psychology, 48,* 1540–1551.

Carver, C. S., & Scheier, M. F. (1981). *Attention and self-regulation: A control-theory approach to human behavior.* New York: Springer-Verlag.

Chartrand, T. L., & Bargh, J. A. (1999). The chameleon effect: The perception–behavior link and social interaction. *Journal of Personality and Social Psychology, 76,* 893–910.

Clore, G. L., Schwarz, N., & Conway, M. (1994). Affective causes and consequences of social information processing. In R. S. Wyer & T. K. Srull, *Handbook of social cognition* (Vol. 1, pp. 323–417). Hillsdale, NJ: Erlbaum.

Csikszentmihalyi, M. (1990). *Flow: The psychology of optimal experience.* New York: Harper Perennial.

Dawson, M. E., & Schell, A. M. (1982). Electrodermal responses to attended and nonattended significant stimuli during dichotic listening. *Journal of Experimental Psychology: Human Perception and Performance, 8,* 315–324.

Deci, E. L., & Ryan, R. M. (2000). The "what" and "why" of goal pursuits: Human needs and the self-determination perspective. *Psychological Inquiry, 11,* 227–268.

Devine, P. G. (1989). Sterotypes and prejudice: Their automatic and controlled components. *Journal of Personality and Social Psychology, 56,* 5–18.

Diefendorff, J. M., Hall, R. J., Lord, R. G., & Strean, M. L. (2000). Action-state orientation: Construct validity of a revised measure and its relationship to work-related variables. *Journal of Personality and Social Psychology, 85,* 250–263.

Dweck, C. S. (1986). Motivational processes affecting learning. *American Psychologist, 41,* 1040–1048.

Farber, L. (1966). *The ways of the will.* New York: Basic Books.

Fiske, S. T. (1989). Examining the role of intent: Toward understanding its role in stereotyping and prejudice. In J. S. Uleman & J. A. Bargh (Eds.), *Unintended thought* (pp. 253–283). New York: Guilford Press.

Förster, J., & Liberman, N. (2002, June 26–29). *Introducing a motivational priming model.* Presentation at the 13th general meeting of the European Association of Experimental Social Psychology, San Sebastian, Spain.

Fuhrman, A., & Kuhl, J. (1998). Maintaining a healthy diet: Effects of personality and self-reward versus self-punishment on commitment to and enactment of self-chosen and assigned goals. *Psychology and Health, 13,* 651–686.

Fuster, J. M. (1989). *The prefrontal cortex.* New York: Raven Press.

Gleick, J. (1990). *Chaos—Making a new science.* New York: Penguin.

Gollwitzer, P. M. (1999). Implementation intentions: Strong effects of simple plans. *American Psychologist, 54,* 493–503.

Gollwitzer, P. M., & Brandstätter, V. (1997). Implementation intentions and effective goal pursuit. *Journal of Personality and Social Psychology, 73,* 186–199.

Goschke, T., & Kuhl, J. (1993). The representation of intentions: Persisting activation in memory. *Journal of Experimental Psychology: Learning, Memory, and Cognition, 19,* 1211–1226.

Greenwald, A. G. (1988). Self-knowledge and self-deception. In J. S. Lockard & D. L. Paulhus (Eds.), *Self-deception: An adaptive mechanism?* (pp. 113–131). Englewood Cliffs, NJ: Prentice-Hall.

Greenwald, A. G., & Banaji, M. R. (1995). Implicit social cognition: Attitudes, self-esteem, and stereotypes. *Psychological Review, 102,* 4–27.

Greve, W. (2001). Traps and gaps in action explanation: Theoretical problems of a psychology of human action. *Psychological Review, 108,* 435–451.

Gross, J. J. (1999). Emotion regulation: Past, present, future. *Cognition and Emotion, 13,* 551–573.

Gross, J. J. (2002). Emotion regulation: Affective, cognitive, and social consequences. *American Psychologist, 39,* 281–291.

Haken, H. (1981). *Synergetics: An introduction.* Heidelberg, Germany: Springer-Verlag.

Heckhausen, H., & Strang, H. (1988). Efficiency under record performance demands: Exertion control-an individual difference variable? *Journal of Personality and Social Psychology, 55,* 489–498.

Higgins, E. T. (1998). Promotion and prevention focus as a motivational principle. In M. P. Zanna (Ed.), *Advances in experimental social psychology* (Vol. 30, pp. 1–46). San Diego: Academic Press.

Hock, M., Krohne, H. W., & Kaiser, J. (1996). Coping dispositions and the processing of ambiguous stimuli. *Journal of Personality and Social Psychology, 70*, 1052–1066.

Isen, A. M. (1984). Toward understanding the role of affect in cognition. In R. S. Wyer, Jr. & T. K. Srull (Eds.), *Handbook of social cognition* (Vol. 3, pp. 179–236). Hillsdale, NJ: Erlbaum.

Jung, C. G. (1957). *The undiscovered self.* Boston: Bay-Back Books.

Jung, C. G. (1964). *Man and his symbols.* New York: Dell.

Kaschel, R., & Kuhl, J. (2004). Motivational counseling in an extended functional context: Personality systems interaction theory and assessment. In W. M. Cox & E. Klinger (Eds.), *Motivational counseling: Motivating people for change* (pp. 99–119). Sussex, UK: Wiley.

Kazén, M., Baumann, N., & Kuhl, J. (2003). Self-infiltration vs. self-compatibility checking in dealing with unattractive tasks: The moderating effect of state vs. action orientation. *Motivation and Emotion, 27,* 157–197.

Knight, R. T., & Grabowecky, M. (1995). Escape from linear time: Prefrontal cortex and conscious experience. In M. S. Gazzaniga (Ed.), *The cognitive neurosciences* (pp. 1357–1371). Cambridge, MA: MIT Press.

Koole, S. L. (in press). Defending the self through willpower: Effects of action orientation and external demand on autonomy-related implicit self-evaluations. *Social Cognition.*

Koole, S. L. (2003). *Volitional regulation of automatic affect: Action orientation can reverse affective priming effects.* Manuscript in preparation, Free University, Amsterdam.

Koole, S. L., & Coenen, L. (2003). *Volition and creativity.* Unpublished data, Free University, Amsterdam.

Koole, S. L., Jager, W., Hofstee, W. K. B., & van den Berg, A. E. (2001). On the social nature of personality: The influence of extraversion and agreeableness and feedback about collective resource use on cooperation in a resource dilemma. *Personality and Social Psychology Bulletin, 27,* 289–301.

Koole, S. L., & Jostmann, N. (2003). *Getting a grip on your feelings: Effects of action orientation and social demand on intuitive affect regulation.* Manuscript submitted for publication, Free University, Amsterdam.

Koole, S. L., & Kuhl, J. (2003). In search of the real self: A functional perspective on optimal self-esteem and authenticity. *Psychological Inquiry.*

Koole, S. L., & Pelham, B. W. (2003). On the nature of implicit self-esteem: The case of the name letter effect. In S. Spencer & M. P. Zanna (Eds.), *Motivated social perception: The ninth Ontario symposium.* Hillsdale, NJ: Erlbaum.

Koole, S. L., Smeets, K., Van Knippenberg, A., & Dijksterhuis, A. (1999). The cessation of rumination through self-affirmation. *Journal of Personality and Social Psychology, 77,* 111–125.

Koole, S. L., & van 't Spijker, M. (2000). Overcoming the planning fallacy through willpower: Effects of implementation intentions on actual and predicted task completion times. *European Journal of Social Psychology, 30,* 873–888.

Kuhl, J. (1981). Motivational and functional helplessness: The moderating effect of state vs. action orientation. *Journal of Personality and Social Psychology, 40,* 155–170.

Kuhl, J. (1983a). Emotion, Kognition und Motivation: II. Die funktionale Bedeutung der Emotionen für das problemlösende Denken und für das konkrete Handeln [Emotion, cognition, and motivation II: The functional significance of emotionas for problem-solving and for action control]. *Sprache und Kognition, 4,* 228–253.

Kuhl, J. (1983b). Motivationstheoretische Aspekte der Depressionsgenese: Der Einfluß der Lageorientierung auf Schmerzempfinden, Medikamentenkonsum und Handlungskontrolle [Pain perception, medication, and action control as a function of state orientation]. In W. Wolfersdorf, R. Straub & G. Hole (Eds.), *Der depressive Kranke in der psychatrischen Klinik: Theorie und Praxis der Diagnostik und Therapie* (pp. 411–424). Regensburg, Germany: Roderer.

Kuhl, J. (1984). Volitional aspects of achievement motivation and learned helplessness: Toward a comprehensive theory of action-control. In B. A. Maher (Ed.), *Progress in experimental personality research* (vol. 13, pp. 99–171). New York: Academic Press.

Kuhl, J. (1986). Motivational chaos: A simple model. In D. R. Brown & J. Veroff (Eds.), *Frontiers of motivational psychology* (pp. 54–71). Heidelberg/New York: Springer-Verlag.

Kuhl, J. (1994). Action versus state orientation: Psychometric properties of the Action Control Scale (ACS-90) (S. 47–59). In J. Kuhl & J. Beckmann (Eds.), *Action control: From cognition to behavior*. Göttingen/Toronto: Hogrefe.

Kuhl, J. (2000a). A functional-design approach to motivation and volition: The dynamics of personality systems interactions. In M. Boekaerts, P. R. Pintrich & M. Zeidner (Eds.), *Self-regulation: Directions and challenges for future research* (pp. 111–169). New York: Academic Press.

Kuhl, J. (2000b). The volitional basis of personality systems interaction theory: Applications in learning and treatment context. *International Journal of Educational Research, 33*, 665–703.

Kuhl, J. (2001). *Motivation und Persönlichkeit: Interaktionen psychischer Systeme* [Motivation and personality: Personality systems interactions]. Göttingen, Germany: Hogrefe.

Kuhl, J., & Baumann, N. (2000). Self-regulation and rumination: Negative affect and impaired self-accessibility. In W. Perrig & A. Grob (Eds.), *Control of human behavior mental processes and consciousness: Essays in honor of the 60th birthday of August Flammer* (pp. 283–305). New York: Wiley.

Kuhl, J., & Beckmann, J. (1985). (Eds.). *Action control: From cognition to behavior*. Heidelberg/New York: Springer-Verlag.

Kuhl, J., & Beckmann, J. (1994a). *Volition and personality: Action versus state orientation*. Göttingen/Seattle: Hogrefe.

Kuhl, J., & Beckmann, J. (1994b). Alienation: Ignoring one's preferences. In J. Kuhl & J. Beckmann (Eds.), *Volition and personality: Action versus state orientation* (pp. 375–390). Göttingen/Seattle: Hogrefe.

Kuhl, J., & Fuhrmann, A. (1998). Decomposing self-regulation and self-control: The volitional components checklist. In J. Heckhausen & C. Dweck (Eds.), *Life span perspectives on motivation and control* (pp. 15–49). Mahwah, NJ: Erlbaum.

Kuhl, J., & Helle, P. (1986). Motivational and volitional determinants of depression: The degenerated-intention hypothesis. *Journal of Abnormal Psychology, 95*, 247–251.

Kuhl, J., & Henseler, W. (2003). Entwicklungsorientiertes Scanning (EOS) [Evolvement-oriented Scanning (EOS)]. In L. von Rosenstiel & J. Erpenbeck (Eds.), *Handbuch der Kompetenzmessung* [Handbook of competence assessment]. Heidelberg, Germany: Spektrum Akademischer Verlag.

Kuhl, J., & Kazén, M. (1994). Self-discrimination and memory: State orientation and false self-ascription of assigned activities. *Journal of Personality and Social Psychology, 66*, 1103–115.

Kuhl, J., & Kazén, M. (1999). Volitional facilitation of difficult intentions: Joint activation of intention memory and positive affect removes stroop interference. *Journal of Experimental Psychology: General, 128*, 382–399.

Kuhl, J., & Koch, B. (1984). Motivational determinants of motor performance: The hidden second task. *Psychological Research, 46*, 143–153.

Langens, T. A., & Mörth, S. (2003). Repressive coping and the use of passive and active coping strategies. *Personality and Individual Differences, 35*, 461–473.

Langer, E. (1975). The illusion of control. *Journal of Personality and Social Psychology, 32*, 311–328.

LeDoux, J. E. (1995). Emotion: Clues from the brain. *Annual Review of Psychology, 46*, 209–235.

Lewin, K. (1926). Untersuchungen zur Handlungs- und Affekt-Psychologie. II. Vorsatz, Wille und Bedürfnis. [Investigations into action and affect psychology. II. Intention, will, and need] *Psychologische Forschung, 7*, 330–385.

Lezak, M. D. (1983). *Neuropsychological assessment*. New York: Oxford University Press.

Libet, B. (1985). Unconscious cerebral initiative and the role of conscious will in voluntary action. *Behavioral and Brain Sciences, 2*, 529–566.

Libet, B. (1999). Do we have free will? *Journal of Consciousness Studies, 6*, 47–57.

Lindworsky, J. (1923). *Der Wille. Seine Erscheinung und Beherrschung nach den Ergebnissen der experimentellen Forschung* [The will. Its manifestation and control after the results of experimental research]. Leipzig, Germany: Barth.

Luria, A. (1978). *The working brain: An introduction to neuropsychology*. Harmondsworth, UK: Penguin.

Martin, L. L. (1999). I-D compensation theory: Some implications of trying to satisfy immediate-return needs in a delayed culture. *Psychological Inquiry, 10*, 195–208.

McClelland, D. C., Koestner, R., & Weinberger, J. (1989). How do self-attributed and implicit motives differ? *Psychological Review, 96*, 690–702.

Meltzoff, A. N., & Moore, M. K. (1994). Imitation, memory, and the representation of persons. *Infant Behavior, 17*, 83–100.

Menec, V. H. (1995). *Volition and motivation: The effect of distracting learning conditions on students differing in action control and perceived control.* Doctoral dissertation, University of Manitoba.

Metcalfe, J., & Mischel, W. (1999). A hot/cool-system analysis of delay of gratification: Dynamics of willpower. *Psychological Review, 106*, 3–19.

Miller, G. A., Galanter, E., & Pribram, K. H. (1960). *Plans and the structure of behavior.* New York: Holt, Rinehart & Winston.

Nisbett, R. E., & Wilson, T. D. (1977). Telling more than we can know: Verbal reports on mental processes. *Psychological Review, 84*, 231–259.

Norman, D. A., & Shallice, T. (1986). Attention to action: willed and automatic control of behavior. In R. J. Davidson, G. E. Schwartz & D. Shapiro (Eds.), *Consciousness and self-regulation: Advances in research* (Vol. 4, pp. 1–18). New York: Plenum Press.

Oettingen, G., Pak, H. J. & Schnetter, K. (2001). Self-regulation of goal-setting: Turning free fantasies about the future into binding goals. *Journal of Personality and Social Psychology, 80*, 736–753.

Papousek, H., & Papousek, M. (1982). Integration into the social world: Survey of research. In P. Stratton (Ed.), *Psychobiology of the human newborn* (pp. 367–390). New York: Wiley.

Pardo, J. V., Pardo, P. J., Janer, K. W., & Raichle, M. E. (1990). The anterior-cingulate cortex mediates processing selection in the Stroop attentional conflict paradigm. *Proceedings of the National Academy of Sciences, 87*, 256–259.

Posner, M. I., & Petersen, S. E. (1990). The attention system of the human brain. *Annual Review of Neuroscience, 13*, 25–42.

Rank, O. (1945). *Will therapy and truth and reality.* New York: Knopf.

Rholes, W. S., Michas, L., & Schroff, J. (1985). Action control as a vulnerability factor in dysphoria. *Cognitive Therapy and Research, 13*, 263–274.

Rosahl, S. K., Tennigkeit, M., Kuhl, J., & Haschke, R. (1993). Handlungskontrolle und langsame Hirnpotentiale: Untersuchungen zum Einfluß subjektiv kritischer Wörter (Erste Ergebnisse) [Action control and slow potential shifts: The impact of words reminding of stressful life-events]. *Zeitschrift für Medizinische Psychologie, 2*, 1–8.

Rotenberg, V. (1993). Richness against freedom: Two hemispheric functions and the problem of creativity. *European Journal for High Ability, 4*, 11–19.

Rumelhart, D. E., McClelland, J. L., & The PDP Research Group (1986). *Parallel distributed processing: Explorations in the microstructure of cognition* (Vol. 1). Cambridge, MA: MIT Press.

Schachter, S. (1959). *The psychology of affiliation.* Stanford, CA: Stanford University Press.

Scheibel, A. B., Freid, I., Paul, L., Forsythe, A., Tomiyasu, U., Wechsler, A., et al. (1985). Differentiating characteristics of the human speech cortex: A quantitative Golgi study. In D. F. Benson & E. Zaidel (Eds.), *The dual brain* (pp. 65–74). New York: Guilford Press.

Schulte, D., Hartung, J., & Wilke, F. (1997). Handlungskontrolle der Angstbewältigung: Was macht Reizkonfrontationsverfahren so effektiv? [Action control in treatment of anxiety disorders: What makes exposure so effective?]. *Zeitschrift für Klinische Psychologie, 26*, 118–128.

Schwartz, B. (2000). Self-determination: The tyranny of freedom. *American Psychologist, 55*, 79–88.

Shah, J. Y., Friedman, R., & Kruglanski, A. W. (2002). *Forgetting all else: On the antecedents and consequences of goal shielding.* Madison: University of Wisconsin Press.

Shallice, T. (1988). *From neuropsychology to mental structure.* Cambridge, UK: Cambridge University Press.

Skinner, B. F. (1971). *Beyond freedom and dignity.* New York: Knopf.

Vallacher, R. R., Read, S. J., & Nowak, A. (2002). The dynamical perspective in personality and social psychology. *Personality and Social Psychology Review, 6*, 264–273.

Van Baaren, R. B., Maddux, W. W., Chartrand, T. L., de Bouter, C., & van Knippenberg, A. (2003). It takes two to mimic: Behavioral consequences of self-construals. *Journal of Personality and Social Psychology, 84*, 1093–1102.

Van Lange, P. A. M., Rusbult, C. E., Drigotas, S. M., Arriaga, X. B., Witcher, B. S., & Cox, C. L. (1997). Willingness to sacrifice in close relationships. *Journal of Personality and Social Psychology, 72*, 1373–1395.

Verplanken, B., & Faes, S. (1999). Good intentions, bad habits, and effects of forming implementation intentions on healthy eating. *European Journal of Social Psychology, 29*, 591–604.

Walschburger, P. (1994). Action control and excessive demand: Effects of situational and personality factors on psychological and physiological functions during stressful transactions. In J. Kuhl & J. Beckmann (Eds.), *Volition and personality: Action versus state orientation* (pp. 233–266). Göttingen, Germany: Hogrefe.

Watson, J. B. (1913). Psychology as the behaviorist views it. *Psychological Review, 20*, 158–177.

Wegner, D. M. (1994). Ironic processes of mental control. *Journal of Personality and Social Psychology, 101*, 34–52.

Wegner, D. M., & Wheatley, T. (1999). Apparent mental causation: Sources of the experience of will. *American Psychologist, 54*, 480–492.

Wheeler, M. A., Stuss, D. T., & Tulving, E. (1997). Toward a theory of episodic memory: The frontal lobes and autonoetic consciousness. *Psychological Bulletin, 121*, 331–354.

Wisman, A., & Koole, S. L. (2003). Hiding in the crowd: Can mortality salience promote affiliation with others who oppose one's worldviews? *Journal of Personality and Social Psychology, 184*, 511–526.

Wittling, W. (1990). Psychophysiological correlates of human brain asymmetry: Blood pressure changes during lateralized presentation of an emotionally laden film. *Neuropsychologia, 28*, 457–470.

Yalom, I. D. (1980). *Existential psychotherapy*. New York: Basic Books.

Chapter 27

The Roar of Awakening

*Mortality Acknowledgment
as a Call to Authentic Living*

LEONARD L. MARTIN
W. KEITH CAMPBELL
CHRISTOPHER D. HENRY

> The certain prospect of death could sweeten every life with a precious
> and fragrant drop of levity—and now you strange apothecary souls have
> turned it into an ill-tasting drop of poison that makes the whole of life
> repulsive.
> —FRIEDRICH NIETZSCHE, *The Wanderer and His Shadow* (1880/
> 1967, p. 185)

The first thing that comes to mind for many people when they think of existentialism is doom and gloom. For these people, an interest in existentialism is synonymous with an interest in topics such as death, depression, and anxiety. This is certainly true in the popular culture, but it also seems to be true among a number of serious researchers. In this chapter, we try to move beyond a doom-and-gloom conception of existentialism by emphasizing some of the broader, more optimistic implications of existentialist thought. Specifically, we explore the possibility that acknowledgment of the uncertainty and impermanence of one's existence can operate as a wakeup call. It can lead individuals to guide their lives by passionately chosen personal values rather than by passively internalized cultural values. This possibility was captured forcefully by Kuhl (2002) based on his work with terminally ill patients. He suggested that a confrontation with mortality "serves as a roar of awakening. . . . It ends the routine and indifference. . . . Because they know that they cannot escape death, they embrace life—their own life. The 'prescription' of how to live given by family, culture, profession, religion, or friends loses its grasp. Perhaps, in this way, knowing that you have a terminal illness is of value" (p. 227).

In making the case that acknowledgment of life's uncertainty and impermanence can fa-cilitate more authentic living, we discuss the range of possible reactions that, according to several prominent existential philosophers, individuals might display when they come to re-alize their death is certain and the universe contains no objective, universally applicable, log-ically defensible standards of value. Then, we look for evidence of these possible reactions in the attitudinal and behavioral aftereffects observed in individuals who have had a close brush with death in the real world. We also consider some psychological mechanisms that could account for these aftereffects. After that, we synthesize the preceding strands of thought into a theoretical framework, and we report on three experiments that tested some implications of that framework. Finally, we explore the relation between our research and research suggesting that mortality salience leads to defensiveness and simple cognitive processing (e.g., Solomon, Greenberg, & Pyszczynski, Chapter 2, this volume).

EXISTENTIALISM: WHAT SHOULD I DO
AND WHY SHOULD I DO IT?

Although it is difficult to provide a concise, generally agreed-on definition of existentialism, it is possible to summarize some of the area's general features (Grene, 1984; MacDonald, 2001). Perhaps the most useful feature to keep in mind is that existentialism is essentially a philosophy of values. Its primary focus is on the difficulties individuals face as they try to make moral and ethical choices in the absence of a system of values that can be shown in some objective way (e.g., logic or science) to be valid for each and every individual. The em-phasis existentialists place on individual values over absolute, universal values is based in large part on the existentialists' assumption that "there is no single essence of humanity to which we may logically turn as a standard or model for making ourselves thus or so" (Grene, 1984, p. 41). In other words, we are not provided with a fixed, ready-made, individ-ual nature from birth. Instead, we develop our individual nature as we make choices over the course of our lifetime.

To consider a concrete example, an individual is not born a theist or an atheist, an omnivore or a vegetarian, a liberal or a conservative. An individual may choose one of the values at some point in his or her life, but he or she may also choose the alternate value at a different point in life. These different choices are possible because, from an existentialist per-spective, individuals have the "freedom to *put out of play* all those factors which would have given you good 'cause' to do just this and *not otherwise*" (MacDonald, 2001, p. 39). As Ortega y Gasset (1936) described it, "To be free means to be lacking in constitutive iden-tity, not to have subscribed to a determined being, to be able to be other than what one was, to be unable to install oneself once and for all in any given being" (p. 303). In short, from the existentialist perspective, the essence of human nature is that it has no fixed essence, at least not at the level of individual choices and values.

When considered in this light, it becomes clear that the existentialist description of life as meaningless does not imply that there is no reason to live. It implies that there is no in-variant, objectively defensible reason to live. Individuals are free to act on the basis of the values that feel valid for them in the specific context in which they find themselves. Thus, far from being a call for individuals to give up on life, existentialism is a call for individuals to live passionately out of their own personal values.

Of course, guiding one's life on the basis of personal values is no more defensible in the logical sense than guiding it on the basis of externally defined values. The former, however, does allow individuals to develop their unique essence. This is important to existentialists because if individuals do not develop an essence for themselves, they will have their essence defined for them by outside forces (e.g., their culture). When this happens, individuals may live in accordance with values that are not personally valid for them and thus fail to reach their unique, individual potential. The result would be a life filled with anxiety, banality, and missed opportunities.

The strong emphasis existentialists place on developing one's unique essence led Grene (1984) to propose that in existentialism the ultimate value is not freedom but honesty. As she put it, "We are free in any case; from that fact, glorious and fearful, there is no escape as long as we live at all. But it is a fact that we may or may not face honestly. Good for the individual resides in the integrity with which he recognizes his freedom and acts while so recognizing it. Evil, conversely, is the lie of fraudulent objectivity, the denial of freedom" (p. 143). The existential call, therefore, is for each of us to individuate ourselves from the ostensibly valid, ready-made value systems (e.g., our culture) into which we have been born and to guide our life on the basis of freely chosen personal values.

There is one final implication of existentialist thought we should mention as relevant to the ideas we discuss in this chapter. If there really is no objective, universally valid system of values, there can be no logically justifiable way to reward or punish an individual for choosing one direction in life as opposed to another. It is possible, therefore, to question the existence of even an ultimate payoff (e.g., heaven and hell). Although one may choose, through faith, to believe in such an eventuality, even religious existentialists (e.g., Kierkegaard and Tillich) agree that there can be no logically justifiable reason for believing.

Not surprisingly, some individuals react with denial or anxiety when confronted with the existential conception of the universe. From an existentialist perspective, however, this reaction is not inevitable. After all, if humans have no built-in value system, and if there is no logically defensible, objective value system, then each individual is free to choose how he or she reacts to a universe in which death is certain but important values are not. Individuals may find such a universe to be overwhelming and depressing, or they may find it to be liberating and exhilarating.

In our opinion, these speculations about the different reactions individuals could display when confronting death and value uncertainty are among the more provocative implications of existential philosophy for empirical research. We believe these speculations could provide the basis for a number of interesting research questions. For example, can individuals really acknowledge the lack of objective certainty in important values as well as the certainty of death yet still live a vital, fulfilling life? To what extent can individuals free themselves from internalized cultural values to live a more self-directed life? Because we consider these speculations to be among the more provocative ones in existentialism, we discuss them in more detail later by highlighting some of the relevant points made by two of the most prominent existentialist thinkers: Kierkegaard and Heidegger.

Kierkegaard

Like most existentialists, Kierkegaard (1961, 1983) began with the assumption that there is no universally valid, objectively defensible system of values, and, therefore, that there is no logically defensible basis for any given life choice (e.g., profession, ethics, and mate). Kierkegaard argued, however, that despite the absence of a logically or objectively defensible basis, individuals still need to make choices, and they should do so by taking a *leap of faith*. In much the way that individuals may believe in a supreme being or an afterlife without any objective support for their belief, so too can they make other choices in their life. Specifically, they can make passionate, committed choices even while being fully aware that they can never know with objective certainty that they are doing the right thing. In Kierkegaard's (1961) terms, "An objective uncertainty held fast in an appropriation process of the most passionate inwardness, [is] the highest truth attainable for an *existing individual*" (p. 182).

Individuals who take a leap of faith become fully immersed in life while maintaining an attitude of nonattachment toward the details of this life. Thus, they are able to "live joyfully and happily . . . every moment on the strength of the absurd . . . to find not repose in the pain of resignation, but joy on the strength of the absurd" (Kierkegaard, 1983, p. 79). Individuals who have not taken a leap of faith, on the other hand, act within the world in a completely different manner. They lose themselves in their daily business and worldly affairs and fail to define their essence for themselves. They end up making their life choices on the basis of widely shared cultural values that may not be valid for them as unique individuals. As a result, these individuals fail to become the unique individuals they are capable of becoming.

Individuals who have not taken a leap of faith are also likely to experience a form of anxiety Kierkegaard referred to as dread. Dread is a general feeling that signals to the individual that something is generally not right with his or her life. According to Kierkegaard, dread can be interpreted as God's way of prompting individuals to adopt a personally valid way of life. Unfortunately, though, individuals may misinterpret their dread and end up trying to ignore or repress it. In doing this, they miss the call to more passionate living.

In sum, for Kierkegaard, the meaning of life is revealed not through objective, logical inquiries but in the concrete actions individuals freely choose as they define their individual essence. An individual's choices should be made passionately on the basis of values that are subjectively valid for them even if the values are at odds with the cultural norms and even if there is no way to prove the values objectively valid. Adoption of this committed lifestyle involves a leap of faith, and this leap, in turn, may be facilitated by a correct interpretation of one's dread as a call to active, self-directed living.

Heidegger

Like Kierkegaard, Heidegger (1927/1982) distinguished between a life of active choosing and a life in which individuals allowed their essence to be defined by values external to themselves. He referred to the former as an authentic life and the latter as an inauthentic life, and he provided detail on the role one's society could play in influencing which of these modes of life an individual adopted. Specifically, Heidegger noted that individuals are born into a world of preformed values (i.e., a culture), and that, as they develop, individuals internalize many of these values, even without intending to do so. To live an authentic life, therefore, individuals need to shed any cultural values they may have internalized that are not personally valid for them and make choices based on personally valid (i.e., authentic) values.

Heidegger believed, as did Kierkegaard, that individuals could be helped along the road to a personally valid mode of life by a form of anxiety. Specifically, Heidegger believed that individuals not living authentically might come to experience a form of anxiety he called angst. This unpleasant feeling arises from the individuals' realization that the cultural values on which they have been basing their choices may not be valid for them as individuals. With this realization, the stage is set for the individual to live an authentic life.

Unfortunately, individuals may rarely arrive at this realization. This is because society can provide individuals with an everyday life that is so distracting that individuals get immersed in the details of their life and lose contact with their angst and their personally valid values. When this happens, individuals fail to create their essence through their own choices but instead fall back into their culture and allow their choices to be determined for them by the cultural norms.

Ironically, the one factor that can set an individual reliably on the path to authentic living is a full acknowledgment of his or her personal death. According to Heidegger, full realization that "*I* am going to die. Not anyone else, but I, alone, as an individual" arouses in individuals a primordial sense of certainty that shocks them into identifying themselves as an individual apart from their culture. It is as though an individual's unique personal existence stands out most sharply when contrasted with the individual's unique personal nonexistence. If *I* die, then *I* must live. With a genuine acknowledgment of his or her personal death, individuals develop the insight to individuate themselves from their culture and the motivation to choose their own goals and pursue them passionately.

Commonalities

Obviously, we have not reviewed all of existential philosophy, nor have we addressed all the important ideas put forth by the two philosophers we highlighted. We have, however, outlined some points we consider central to an empirical study of existentialism. These points can be summarized as follows:

1. There is no value system that can be shown logically to be valid for each and every individual.
2. Each of us is born into a world awash in preformed values (i.e., our culture), and we inevitably internalize many of these values even without intending to do so.
3. We need to realize that our cultural values are not logically defensible and that some of these values might not be subjectively valid for us.
4. Some forms of anxiety can facilitate this realization, but only if we interpret the anxiety for what it is, a sign that we are not guiding our lives on the basis of personally meaningful values.
5. The most powerful inducement for us to adopt a personally valid, self-directed life is the acknowledgment of our personal death. This acknowledgment provides us with both the insight and the urgency we need to define our essence through active choices based on passionately chosen personal values rather than inappropriately internalized cultural values.

In short, existentialism suggests that each of us is in the ironic position of having the very experiences we may be trying to avoid (anxiety, uncertainty, death) be precisely what we need to acknowledge in order to live more authentically.

THE EFFECTS OF REAL-LIFE CONFRONTATIONS WITH MORTALITY

It is clear from our brief summary that although most existentialists do address doom-and-gloom topics such as death, anxiety, and meaninglessness, they typically do so in a way that allows us to go beyond doom and gloom. For example, the two philosophers we discussed (see also Frankl, Jaspers, May, Nietzsche, and Yalom) agreed that it is possible for individuals to live a rich, fulfilling life even while acknowledging that their death is inevitable and their value judgments are not logically defensible. In fact, they agreed that it is only by acknowledging the certainty of death and the uncertainty of values that individuals can live a rich, fulfilling life.

Of course, finding that a number of philosophers agree on a certain conclusion does not necessarily make that conclusion valid. After all, the philosophers could have used faulty reasoning or they could have gone beyond their reasoning to speculate on psychological reactions (e.g., anxiety). We could have more confidence in their conclusions, therefore, if we could find some converging evidence. Interestingly, such evidence exists. It can be seen in the changes in attitudes and behavior often displayed by individuals who have had close brushes with death (e.g., Grey, 1985; Kinnier, Tribbensee, Rose, & Vaugh, 2001; Noyes, 1982–1983; Ring, 1984).

Relative to individuals who have not had a close brush with death, those who have tend to be more serene, more self-assertive, and more confident. They are also less concerned with the opinions of others, less easily intimidated, and less concerned with materialism, fame, and money. They may also report a sense of liberation, of being able to choose not to do what they do not want to do. Although they report some regret, they report little or no remorse. They consider the former to be a part of life but the latter to be a waste of time and energy. They also display a greater appreciation for nature and the ordinary things in life (e.g., a sunset and hugging a child). Clearly, individuals who have acknowledged their death are not sentenced to a life of anxiety, depression, and meaninglessness.

This conclusion should not be particularly surprising when one considers that aspects of growth have been observed after a variety of traumatic experiences (e.g., Collins, Taylor, & Skokan, 1990; Davis, Nolen-Hoeksema, & Larson, 1998; Lehman et al., 1993; Ellard, 1993; Park, Cohen, & Murch, 1996; Tedeschi & Calhoun, 2004). In fact, it appears not only that traumatic experiences can produce positive as well as negative aftereffects but that the two are related. Calhoun and Tedeschi (1999), for example, found that individuals who acknowledged the unpleasant aspects of their traumatic experience were more likely to show growth than individuals who did not acknowledge those aspects. Thus, a close brush with death can be profoundly upsetting, but it can also set the stage for growth.

If the existentialists are correct, however, then not only might we see growth in some generic sense after a close brush with death, but we might see specific kinds of growth. Specifically, we should find that survivors of a close brush with death experience less fear of death, less reliance on cultural values, greater reliance on personally valid values, and greater appreciation of life moment to moment. We consider each of these possibilities in turn.

Lower Fear of Death

One of the most common aftereffects of a close brush with death is a decrease in the survivor's fear of death and dying (Greyson, 1992; Noyes, 1982–1983). Individuals who believe their death is imminent (or who thought they had in fact died) often report that the approach to death felt more like a letting go than an annihilation. This is true even when the close brush with death did not increase the survivor's belief in an afterlife. In fact, the fear of death decreases even if the survivors have no clear interpretation of their experience. As one survivor put it, "I can't tell what happened to me because I don't know, but something happened and I've never been the same since. People describe me as being high on life, and they are right" (Ring, 1984, p. 99). Another said, "I find I no longer have any fear of death, even though I have no more knowledge than I had before about whether [I am] going to reincarnate, or survive death in some nonmaterial form, or simply come to an end as far as time is concerned" (Wren-Lewis, 1988, p. 117).

What is responsible for the decreased fear? Two factors, at least, seem crucial. One is the survivor's certain belief that death is imminent. The more intensely survivors experience this thought, the more positive aftereffects they experience (Greyson & Stevenson, 1980; Roberts & Owen, 1988). The other is an attitude of acceptance. Individuals who struggled to stay alive during their close brush with death displayed fewer signs of growth than individuals who were open to the possibility of their death (Noyes, 1980). Together, these findings suggest that fear of death decreases when individuals look death in the eye and think, "This is it. This is where it ends. Right here, right now, like this. And it's OK." This conclusion fits perfectly with the existential assumption that honest acknowledgment of the certainty of our death can produce positive outcomes, including a decrease in our fear of death.

Shedding of Cultural Values in Favor of Self-Values

Another common aftereffect in individuals who have survived a close brush with death is a decreased concern with extrinsic, cultural values and an increased commitment to intrinsic, personal values (Flynn, 1984; Ring, 1984; Sutherland, 1990). An individual dying from AIDS put it this way:

When you're dying, you're stripped of everything that's important to society—money, image—so all you have left is that honesty. It takes so much energy to pretend when you can use that energy for other things . . . all that crap just flies off of you; it just sort of comes off you like layers of skin. All of a sudden, you're starting from scratch, like when you were born. . . . I believe in myself now. I never had that before. And I am not afraid of being who I am. (in Kuhl, 2002, p. 230)

A woman dealing with terminal cancer expressed the same insight this way:

There's less fear in my life because I'm not in the loop of stress that most of us get into from working and worrying about money and the kids, rather than just being with what is. It's about acceptance rather than still struggling to make it your way. All the ego stuff, all the future fear—"God, did I gain weight? Am I turning gray?" Most of those things aren't important any more. It's like really downsizing to the essence. It wasn't things that I wanted. It was a way of life. And so I systematically set out to live it. A lot of the programming from my youth was still there before the illness, like "You need to be successful." You're in this prison. I've switched to what's important. (in Branfman, 1996)

Not only do these reports fit with general existentialist thinking, but the reasons survivors give for their change also seem to fit. As the AIDS patient discussed previously put it, "I realized when I was dying that I was going to die alone, that no one was coming with me; I was going alone. Then I realized that each person's journey is truly one of aloneness and that whatever happens in your life it's only you, it's always going to be only you" (in Kuhl, 2002, p. 228).

In sum, after individuals have acknowledged the certainty of their death, they tend to pay more attention to who and what they are as unique individuals and they rely less on culturally conditioned standards. With less pressure to meet the cultural standards, the survivors experience a feeling of freedom and forgiveness. As one survivor put it, "When I came back from that, I really understood. I had a real feeling of understanding that I was a good person and all I had to do was be me" (in Ring, 1984, p. 107).

Greater Immersion in Life

So far, we have seen reports suggesting that survivors of a close brush with death experience less fear of death, less concern with preconditioned cultural values, and greater attention to their personal values. One obvious next question might be, "What is life like for these people?" The existentialists lead us to believe that such a life could be rich and meaningful. The data suggest that they are right.

Survivors of a close brush with death treat life as a gift and they try not to waste it. They trivialize the trivial and emphasize what seems important and valid for them (Noyes, 1982–1983; Yalom, 1980). This attitude toward life was captured dramatically by a woman following her diagnosis of terminal cancer: "Before I lived nice cotton—clean, cool, healthy. But now I live velvet—beautiful, purple, magic carpet velvet. I call this my "Year of Ecstasy." . . . Even though my previous life was good, it was not the bliss, the splendor, the ecstasy of how I live now" (Branfman, 1996).

These kinds of reports make it clear that individuals can live a positive life after acknowledging their mortality. It is important, however, to interpret correctly the nature of the positivity. Survivors of a close brush with death do not typically become shortsighted hedonists who have difficulty attaining long-term goals. To the contrary, they typically become more engaged in life, and they successfully pursue long-term personal goals. They do so, however, while staying mindful of their moment-to-moment experience. A good example of this shift in orientation can be seen in the reactions of former senator and presidential candidate Paul Tsongas following his repeated bouts with cancer. He noted that he lost his ego-enhancing ambition but not his desire to help (Shapiro, 1993). In short, survivors of a close brush with death do not live for the present. They live in the present.

Consistent with this mindfulness of moment-to-moment experience, survivors also tend to become more appreciative of the simple things in life such as a growing plant, a flying bird, or even the texture of the sidewalk. As one survivor put it, "You know you've seen them before but they meant nothing; you see them afterward and they mean everything" (Kuhl, 2001, p. 265). Another noted, "After my first cancer, even the smallest joys in life took on a special meaning—watching a beautiful sunset, a hug from my child, a laugh with Dorothy. That feeling has not diminished with time. After my second and third cancers, the simple joys of life are everywhere and are boundless, as I cherish my family and friends and contemplate the rest of my life, a life I certainly do not take for granted" (Jordon, 2000, p. 216).

It seems that without the burden of extrinsic, cultural expectations, survivors of a close brush with death can take life on its own terms. They experience each moment as complete in itself. This sentiment was captured perfectly by Wren-Lewis (1988) describing his own orientation to the world following his close brush with death: "I feel I know exactly why the Bible says that God looked upon the creation and saw that it was good" (p. 115).

ARE THE AFTEREFFECTS REAL?

As much as we might like to believe these positive reports from survivors of a close brush with death, we have to admit that it is possible to be cynical. After all, how do we know the aftereffects are real? Is it not more likely that the aftereffects reflect the operation of some sort of defense mechanism? Perhaps the survivors are engaging in self-deception or self-presentation. Although it is difficult to rule out these interpretations definitively, there are reasons to question them.

For example, many of the aftereffects have been verified by close others. Specifically, in some studies (Groth-Marnat & Summers, 1998; Park et al., 1996; Weiss, 2002), when investigators asked the survivors to rate themselves in terms of a number of attitudinal and behavioral items indicative of growth, they also asked spouses, children, and friends of the survivors to rate the survivors on the same items. The two sets of ratings have been found to correlate significantly, and to reveal positive changes in a number of areas. Thus, if the survivors are faking it, they are being very convincing over long periods of time (e.g., years) in the presence of those who know them best and with whom they spend the most time.

Another reason for believing the survivors' reports is that these reports are not correlated with the motivation to report in a socially desirable way. Specifically, there is no correlation between the positive aftereffects survivors report and their score on the Marlowe-Crowne social desirability scale (e.g., Greyson, 1983; Tedeschi & Calhoun, 1996). Moreover, as we noted earlier, individuals actually display more growth if they acknowledge the negative aspects of their experience than if they do not. Together, these findings suggest that the survivors' reports reflect a complex, integrated view of the world and not a shallow Pollyana view of the world.

The conclusion that a traumatic event can lead to growth might be a little easier to accept if one moves beyond a simple happy–unhappy view of adjustment (e.g., Waterman, 1993). Survivors of a close brush with death are not necessarily happier than individuals who have not had a close brush with death (Greyson, 1992, 1996). On the other hand, they tend to report greater purpose in life, a greater sense of fulfillment or self-actualization, and greater wisdom (Noyes, 1982–1983).

It is reasonable to believe, therefore, that the aftereffects of a close brush with death reflect genuine responses to a real life wakeup call. This belief is made even more reasonable by the existence of theoretical mechanisms that could account for posttraumatic growth. Specifically, a number of researchers have begun to explore the psychological processes that can lead individuals to experience positive effects following a traumatic experience (e.g., Carver, 1998).

THE ROLE OF SHATTERED ASSUMPTIONS

One promising model of posttraumatic growth was proposed by Tedeschi and Calhoun (2004; Tedeschi, Park, & Calhoun, 1998). They began with the assumption that as individuals go through life, they build up sets of beliefs about who they are and how the world works. Tedeschi and Calhoun refer to this set of beliefs as an assumptive world (see also Janoff-Bulman, 1992; Janoff-Bulman & Yopyk, Chapter 8, this volume; Parkes, 1971). One's assumptive world might include beliefs such as "The world is just," "The U.S. mainland is safe from terrorist attacks," and "Heart trouble only affects people older than me." The problem, of course, is that events in the real world can challenge such beliefs.

When the challenge is great enough, individuals may be forced to drop their beliefs and develop new ones. It is in this context that growth can occur. As Janoff-Bulman (1998) put it, "It is not simply that some trauma survivors cope well and perceive benefits in spite of their losses, but rather that the creation of value and meaning occurs because of their losses, particularly the loss of deeply held illusions" (p. 35). Subsequent to the trauma, individuals may rebuild their assumptions in ways that map more closely onto the world as it is for them now, and this, in turn, may facilitate future coping. Individuals may also be provided with opportunities they did not see before (e.g., new careers and new relationships). In these ways, and others, it is possible for individuals to experience some growth along side of, and because of, the loss and pain associated with the trauma.

This challenge–rebuilding process could plausibly account for at least some of the after-effects of a close brush with death. Consider, for example, that each of us presumably believes we are going to die. We may tend to conceptualize our death, however, as something that happens to someone else (e.g., an older me) in another place at another time (e.g., years from now when I am ready to go). A close brush with death can challenge that conceptualization, however. For example, after receiving her diagnosis of terminal cancer, one survivor put it this way, "Like most people, I thought, 'This is something I'll only have to consider when I'm 84. But getting a terminal diagnosis was, 'You've got a limited amount of time. Now, really, what do you want to do? How do you want to be?' It hit me right here, in my heart" (in Branfman, 1996). Individuals may also have long-term plans (e.g., to have a family) or they may be engaging in immediate effort for a long-term payoff (e.g., saving for retirement). A close brush with death can cause individuals to reassess their plans and priorities (Yalom, 1980). In short, when individuals acknowledge their mortality, they may examine their guiding assumptions and open up to the possibility of adopting new assumptions.

This possibility was addressed explicitly by Furn (1987; Clark, 1987) when she proposed that the aftereffects of a close brush with death may be viewed as a form of culture shock. In both phenomena, she suggested, individuals experience a basic change in their worldview. "To the extent that a widely shared value system is synonymous with 'culture,' it may be said that NDErs [near death experiencers] have philosophically and behaviorally adopted a new culture. . . . The NDErs conception of self, of others, of nature, of the nature of life, and of time may be significantly altered during a generally extended period following the NDE" (Furn, 1987, p. 11).

PULLING ONESELF TOGETHER VERSUS LETTING ONESELF GO

Although a close brush with death and other traumatic events may induce individuals to revise their worldviews, the events may differ in the kinds of revisions they induce. As we noted earlier, individuals who struggled to stay alive during their close brush with death showed less growth than did individuals who accepted the possibility of their death (Noyes, 1980). Drawing on these findings, as well as on his own close brush with death, Wren-Lewis (2004) suggested that most traumas shatter benign or optimistic world assumptions (e.g., the world is a fairly safe, predictable, and controllable place), whereas a close encounter with death generally challenges more negative assumptions (e.g., I am not worthy, life is a vale of tears, and it's every man for himself). Wren-Lewis reported that his own close brush with death provided him with the

> mind-boggling discovery of oneness with an essentially benign inner reality underlying a world which had hitherto been superficially perceived as hostile, competitive and "red in tooth and claw." Far from being a sense of "dauntless human spirit," . . . the post-NDE [near death experience] feeling is of being able to relax into everlasting arms at the core of existence. (p. 92)

This difference may explain why the reactions seen after a close brush with death reflect more of a letting go than a pulling together, more of a feeling of coming home than of character building. Wren-Lewis (2004) described his own feeling as

> much more like that of having been suddenly and instantaneously cured of something akin to a brain cataract which had obscured my perceptions for as long as I can remember. Far from seeming like a new and more spiritual stage in my personal development, the deepened consciousness felt more natural, almost more ordinary and obvious, than the life-awareness I'd previously taken for granted for over half a century. (p. 91)

He added that the real wonder is not that individuals who have had a close brush with death see the world this way, but that the rest of us do not, for this is simply the way it is (Wren-Lewis, 1994).

A THEORETICAL SYNTHESIS

Taken together, these various lines of investigation suggest the following: As individuals make their way through the world, they develop beliefs about who they are and how the world works. Some of these beliefs arise from personal experience, whereas others are internalized indirectly from the individual's culture. In some cases, the cultural values will be congruent with the individuals' personal values. In other cases, they will be incongruent with these values. Moreover, some of the beliefs will have positive implications (e.g., the world is just), whereas some will have negative implications (e.g., no one will like you if you are overweight).

As long as these beliefs allow individuals to function more or less effectively in the world, individuals have no reason to question the beliefs. Sometimes, though, events occur that force individuals to question and revise their beliefs. Although this questioning and revising can be unpleasant, it can also set the stage for growth. It can motivate individuals to open up to new beliefs which, in turn, may allow them to function more effectively in the world as it is.

Although a variety of experiences, including positive ones, may lead individuals to revise their worldview (Calhoun & Tedeschi, 1999), acknowledgment of one's mortality may be a particularly effective and ubiquitous inducer of such revision. It may also have other unique features. For example, acknowledgment of one's mortality may cause individuals to focus their revising primarily on the beliefs they have internalized from their culture that do not fit with their personal values. It may also cause individuals to question beliefs with negative implications (e.g., contingent self-esteem) moreso than those with positive implications (e.g., you are inherently worthwhile)—presumably because the former are more likely to have been a function of imposed cultural standards.

In short, acknowledgment of one's death can cause individuals to realize that their life is their own whether it ends with death or there is a subsequent judgment and afterlife. Either way, the individual goes alone. This realization gives individuals the freedom to relax back into themselves. As a result, they may decrease their reliance on general prior knowledge (e.g., culture), increase their open, online evaluative processing, base their choices more closely on their self-knowledge, and place more emphasis on the pursuit of personal over culturally derived goals. We conducted three studies to assess these possibilities.

EMPIRICAL EVIDENCE

Online Bottom-Up Processing

If the preceding synthesis is correct, then when individuals give serious consideration to their death they are likely to adopt a more online, bottom-up form of processing. To test this hypothesis, we had participants write about their death or about television (e.g., Greenberg, Pyszczynski, & Solomon, 1990) and then evaluate the suitability of a target person for a job. We presented all participants with the same set of mixed valence information about the target person. For some participants, the positive information (e.g., works well with co-workers) came first, whereas for others the negative information (e.g., had some difficulties on a recent business trip) came first.

By definition, primacy effects occur when the initial information in a sequence exerts a disproportionate influence on participants' evaluations, whereas recency effects occur when the later information in the sequence exerts a disproportionate influence. Thus, primacy effects are thought to occur when individuals close off their processing prior to a full consideration of the information (i.e., the later information). Because of this premature closure, individuals may be less aware of plausible alternative hypotheses and/or inconsistent bits of evidence later in the sequence (Kruglanski, Ramat-Aviv, & Freund, 1983; Newston & Rindner, 1979). This characterization fits with the findings that primacy effects are more likely when participants are instructed to make global evaluations or make their evaluations under time pressure, whereas recency effects are more likely when participants are instructed to make differentiated judgments or believe it would be costly for them not to process the information fully (e.g., Freund, Kruglanski, & Shpitzajzen, 1985; Kruglanski et al., 1983; Newston & Rindner, 1979).

From these findings we can hypothesize generally that individuals processing in a more routine, top-down fashion will show primacy effects, whereas individuals processing in a more open, online evaluative mode will show recency effects. We predicted, therefore, that participants who wrote about watching television would show primacy effects, whereas individuals who wrote about their death would show recency effects.

The data supported these predictions. Specifically, among participants who wrote about television, evaluations of the job candidate were more favorable when the positive information came first than when the negative information came first. Among those who wrote about their death, however, evaluations of the job candidate were more favorable when the negative information first than when the positive information came first. This crossover pattern is consistent with the hypothesis that individuals who wrote about their death maintained a more open, online evaluative set (Freund et al., 1985; Kruglanski et al., 1983; Newston & Rindner, 1979).

Choices Directed by Self-Knowledge

According to the existentialists and the reports from survivors of a close brush with death, individuals who have acknowledged their death make evaluations more in accordance with their personal values. We tested this hypothesis using a procedure developed by Setterlund and Niedenthal (1993). These authors had participants rate the extent to which a series of trait adjectives (e.g., sociable and intelligent) were descriptive of themselves. Then, they had participants rate the extent to which they would like to eat at various restaurants. The restaurants were described in terms of the traits of the people who ate there. Restaurant H, for example, was described by the traits unconventional, intelligent, friendly, and spontaneous. Restaurant K was described by the traits sophisticated, well-mannered, sociable, and witty.

Presumably, the more the traits associated with a restaurant overlap with those participants considered to be self-descriptive, the more participants would like to eat at that restaurant. This would be true, however, only to the extent that participants were in touch with their personal values. Consistent with this hypothesis, Setterlund and Niedenthal found a stronger relation between the self-descriptive traits and liking for the restaurants when participants had clear self-concepts than when they did not.

If a consideration of their death puts participants in touch with their personal values, then there should be a stronger relation between the participants' self-ratings and their liking for the restaurants when participants have thought about their death than when they have not. To assess this prediction, we had participants rate the extent to which they considered various traits to be descriptive of themselves. Then, we had participants write either about their death or about television. Finally, we had them rate their desire to eat at various restaurants described in terms of various trait adjectives.

Consistent with expectations, there was a greater connection between participants' self-ratings and their liking for the restaurants among participants who wrote about their death than among participants who wrote about television. The results suggest that following a confrontation with one's death, individuals move away from routine, generic processing toward individuated, online processing based on their personal values.

Switch from Cultural to Personal Goals

According to the existentialists and survivors of a close brush with death, acknowledgment of one's mortality can lead an individual to rely more on the self than the cultural values in making evaluations. To test this hypothesis, we had participants write about their ideal life while either considering their death or not. Then, we had them rate the extent to which they wished to pursue a variety of goals. Some of these goals reflected personal values such as growth and acceptance, whereas others reflected culturally derived values such as fame and appearance (Kasser & Ryan, 1996). Thus, we predicted that participants would show relatively less interest in the culturally derived goals after having thought about their death.

Some participants were asked to write about their ideal life, but no mention was made of their death. Other participants were asked to write about the life they ideally would like to live if they had only 1 year to live. Then, participants in both groups were provided with eight index cards with each card having printed on it a short description of a personal goal (e.g., growth) or a culturally derived goal (e.g., appearance). Participants were also given 100 poker chips and asked to distribute the poker chips over the eight cards to reflect how much of themselves they wished to invest in each of the goals. As predicted, participants who had written about their ideal life with only 1 year to live distributed proportionately less chips on the cultural values and proportionately more on the personal values compared to participants who wrote about their ideal life without considering their death.

Taken together, our findings are consistent with the suggestions of a number of existential philosophers and the reports of individuals who have survived a close brush with death. They have suggested that when individuals think about their death, the individuals open up to a more online, evaluative mode of processing guided by their self-knowledge, and this results in a shift away from the pursuit of culturally derived goals toward the pursuit of personal ones.

WAKEUP VERSUS DEFENSIVENESS

Following mainstream existential thought (e.g., Kierkegaard and Heidegger), we raised the possibility that in acknowledging their mortality individuals can gain the insight and motivation they need to question the preformed value system into which they were born (e.g., their culture) and to engage in more open, evaluative processing guided by their personally chosen values. The results of our three studies were consistent with this possibility. A quite different view of the effects of thinking about one's mortality, however, has been proposed in the context of terror management theory (Solomon et al., Chapter 2, this volume). That theory, derived from Becker (1973), has suggested that mortality salience leads individuals to engage in a strong defense of their cultural worldview and to simplified cognitive processing. Evidence consistent with this hypothesis has also been obtained.

The existence of evidence consistent with two seemingly opposing hypotheses raises at least three logical possibilities. The defensiveness hypothesis is entirely correct and can explain our findings, the wakeup hypothesis is entirely correct and can explain the defensiveness findings, or both hypotheses have some validity but operate under different conditions. We address the third possibility.

Whether thoughts of one's mortality leads to defensiveness or growth may depend on the way in which the thoughts were brought to mind. Effects have been observed when mortality has been brought to mind through subliminal presentation of death-related words (Arndt, Greenberg, & Pyszczynski, 1997), by having participants interviewed in front of a funeral home (Jonas, Schimel, & Greenberg, 2002), after individuals have experienced a life-threatening accident (Noyes, 1982–1983), and after individuals have received a terminal diagnosis (Kuhl, 2002). Obviously, these situations differ in terms of their blatancy and intensity, but they may also differ in the psychological processes they induce.

It is reasonable to believe, for example, that receipt of a terminal diagnosis is much more threatening than subliminal presentation of words related to death. One might expect, therefore, that the former would induce greater defensiveness than the latter. Presumably, the greater is the threat to one's life, the greater the defensiveness. One problem with this hypothesis, though, is that the opposite hypothesis seems just as plausible. Highly threatening experiences may be precisely the kind needed to challenge an individual's worldview and thus provide the openness needed for growth. It seems likely, therefore, that there is an additional variable that moderates the effects of blatancy and intensity.

Greenberg, Arndt, and Simon (2000) proposed that one's reaction to mortality salience may depend on when that reaction is measured. Specifically, they suggested that individuals may repress thoughts of mortality immediately following mortality salience. With the passage of time, however, the thoughts may drop out of focal awareness yet still be accessible. It is at this point that individuals defend their worldview. Although plausible, this time-course hypothesis seems incomplete.

As currently formulated, it provides no place for growth. Individuals either defend themselves through repression or they defend themselves by bolstering their worldview. Nowhere in the sequence do individuals question their worldview and open up to alternative beliefs. Moreover, there is evidence that posttraumatic growth does not follow a simple time course (Milam, 2004). Some survivors show immediate benefits that last for years, others show immediate distress that transforms into growth over time, and others show immediate positive effects that descend into difficulties over time (see also Downey, Silver, & Wortman, 1990).

Perhaps one way to find the moderating variable is to think about the difference between defensiveness and growth. In both cases, individuals experience a threat to their worldview. With defensiveness, however, individuals retreat from the threat, whereas with growth, individuals change to meet the threat. It is possible, therefore, that factors that foster trust and the tolerance of ambiguity would facilitate growth, whereas factors that foster fear and the intolerance of ambiguity would facilitate defensiveness. To use a music metaphor, individuals who have learned only to play note for note from a musical score will feel less comfortable when the score is removed than individuals who have learned how to improvise.

From a psychology perspective, we might see more growth among individuals who, for example, can tolerate ambiguity, have a secure attachment style, or were raised by authoritative parents. Growth might also be facilitated when the thoughts of mortality are made salient in a supporting, nonthreatening environment, as might be the case in existential therapy (Yalom, 1980) or in some forms of Buddhist training. More generally, we should see growth among individuals who trust in their own ability and who believe in the benign nature of the universe.

It is interesting, in this context, to note the parallels between growth from acknowledging one's mortality and the features of successful therapy (Raft & Andersen, 1986; Yalom, 1980). Both involve an alteration of the individual's assumptive world. In humanistic therapy, for example, therapists try to create an atmosphere in which their clients can explore their true feelings and motivations in a nonevaluative context. In this encouraging, supportive environment, clients can recognize which of their values are truly representative of themselves as individuals and which reflect cultural values they have inappropriately internalized (i.e., conditions of worth). With this recognition, they may experience less anxiety and live more out of their personal values. Although much more directive, cognitive therapy seeks to do essentially the same thing. In this case, the therapist attempts quite forcefully to get the client to question his or her beliefs and replace them with new ones. The common denominator of these therapies and a close brushes with death is a dropping of the individuals' current beliefs and an opening up to new ones that allow the individuals to direct their lives more from their own values than from extrinsic values.

It is also interesting in this context to consider the therapeutic recommendations derived from terror management theory. Proponents of terror management (e.g., Simon, Greenberg, Harmon-Jones, Solomon, & Pyszczynski, 1996; Solomon, Greenberg, & Pyszczynski, 1991) have noted that, under the right conditions with the right clients, increasing mortality salience might improve psychological functioning. They suggested, for example, "carefully guiding mildly depressed individuals to contemplate their mortality may be a valuable tool for getting them to invest in their worldviews and to see them as meaningful, thereby making the goals and standards of their worldviews more apparent so that they can begin to find more effective ways to meet those standards" (Simon et al., 1996, p. 88). As can be seen, their suggestion that some forms of mortality salience can be beneficial is similar to ours, but the reason they give for the benefit is quite different from ours.

Following mainstream existentialism (e.g., Kierkegaard and Heidegger), we suggested that the benefit comes from inducing individuals to question their cultural worldview and follow their personal values. Following Becker, the terror management theorists have proposed that the benefit comes from inducing individuals to invest more strongly in their cultural worldview. The terror management theorists have emphasized the latter strategy for two reasons. First, they assume that "decay and death are inescapable physical evils that *we can only deal with via fragile symbolic social constructions*" (Solomon et al., 1991, p. 31; emphasis added). Second, they assume that "self-worth is inherently a cultural construction and thus must always be validated externally; otherwise it cannot be sustained. Thus, the client should not be focused on deriving self-esteem internally, but on adopting values, roles, and behaviors that provide compelling, consistent social validation of his or her self-worth" (p. 31).

In short, both positions agree that there can be some psychological benefit to having one's mortality made salient, under the right conditions with the right individuals. The terror management perspective, however, assumes that the fear of death is instinctual and so cannot be permanently put aside. It can only be buffered through symbolic cultural means. The wakeup view (e.g., Kierkegaard and Heidegger), on the other hand, assumes that the fear of death is a misinterpretation of the anxiety that arises when individuals fail to live in accordance with their personal values. It dissipates when individuals adopt an authentic life. Thus, we are again left with three possibilities. Either the defensive view is correct, the wakeup view is correct, or each has some validity under different conditions.

SUMMARY AND CONCLUSIONS

We have suggested that a genuine acknowledgment of one's mortality can be a powerful catalyst for personal growth. We think it is important when making this case, though, not to discount the painful and confusing aspects of such an acknowledgment. As we noted earlier, appropriate expression of negative feelings contributes to growth and an improved quality of life. In the words of Janoff-Bulman (1998), "In the end survivors often feel both more vulnerable and more appreciative, two states that are fundamentally linked. It is knowing the possibility of loss that promotes the gains of victimization, and that of disillusionment that creates a newfound commitment to living fully" (p. 35).

It may be most accurate, therefore, to conceptualize the acknowledgment of death as a *crisis* in the sense of the word revealed in the Chinese ideogram. The ideogram consists of two characters, one representing *danger* and one representing *opportunity*. The first aspect may spring more readily to mind when individuals acknowledge their death, but the second is still present, and it is that second, often overlooked, aspect we have emphasized in this chapter. Acknowledgment of death can be unpleasant, but it can also serve as a roar of awakening. We think it is time for experimental existentialists to help individuals find the roar rather than the doom and gloom.

REFERENCES

Arndt, J., Greenberg, J., & Pyszczynski, T. (1997). Subliminal exposure to death-related stimuli increases defense of the cultural worldview. *Psychological Science, 8,* 379–385.

Branfman, F. (1996). How terminal diagnosis saved Jackie McEntee's life. Retrieved July 9, 2003, from *http://www.salon.com/weekly/jackie960805.html.*

Becker, E. (1973). *The denial of death.* New York: Free Press.

Calhoun, L. G., & Tedeschi, R. G. (1999). *Facilitating posttraumatic growth: A clinician's guide.* Mahwah, NJ: Erlbaum.

Carver, C. S. (1998). Resilience and thriving: Issues, models, and linkages. *Journal of Social Issues, 54,* 245–266.

Clark, K. (1987). Response to "Adjustment and the near-death experience." *Journal of Near-Death Studies, 6,* 20–23.

Collins, R. L., Taylor, S. E., & Skokan, L. A. (1990). A better world or a shattered vision? Changes in life perspective following victimization. *Social cognition, 8,* 263–285.

Davis, C. G., Nolen-Hoeksema, S., & Larson, J. (1998). Making sense of loss and benefiting from the experience: Two construals of meaning. *Journal of Personality and Social Psychology, 75,* 561–574.

Downey, G., Silver, R. C., & Wortman, C. B. (1990). Reconsidering the attribution-adjustment relation following a major negative event: Coping with the loss of a child. *Journal of Personality and
Social Psychology, 59*, 925–940.

Flynn, C. P. (1984). Meanings and implications of near-death experiencer transformations. In B.
Greyson & C. P. Flynn (Eds.), *The near-death experience: Problems, prospects, perspectives* (pp.
278–289). Springfield, IL: Charles C Thomas.

Freund, T., Kruglanski, A. W., & Shpitzajzen, A. (1985). The freezing and unfreezing of impressional
primacy: Effects of the need for structure and the fear of invalidity. *Personality and Social Psychology Bulletin, 11*, 479–487.

Furn, B. G. (1987) Adjustment and the near-death experience: A conceptual and therapeutic model.
Journal of Near-Death Studies, 6, 4–19.

Greenberg, J., Arndt, J., & Simon, L. (2000). Proximal and distal defenses in response to reminders of
one's mortality: Evidence of a temporal sequence. *Personality and Social Psychology Bulletin, 26*,
91–99.

Greenberg J., Pyszczynski, T., & Solomon, S. (1990). Evidence for terror management theory II: The
effects of mortality salience on reactions to those who threaten or bolster the cultural worldview.
Journal of Personality and Social Psychology, 58, 308–318.

Grene, M. (1984). *Introduction to existentialism.* Chicago: University of Chicago Press.

Grey, M. (1985). *Return from death: An exploration of the near-death experience.* London: Arkana.

Greyson, B. (1983). Near-death experiences and personal values, *American Journal of Psychiatry, 140*,
618–620.

Greyson, B. (1992). Reduced death threat in near-death experiencers. *Death Studies, 16*, 523–536.

Greyson, B. (1996). "NDEs and satisfaction with life": Reply. *Journal of Near-Death Studies, 14*,
218–219.

Greyson B., & Stevenson, I. (1980). The phenomenology of near-death experiences. *American Journal
of Psychiatry, 137*, 1193–1196.

Groth-Marnat, G., & Summers, R. (1998). Altered beliefs, attitudes, and behaviors following
near-death experiences. *Journal of Humanistic Psychology, 38*, 110–125.

Heidegger, M. (1982). *Being and time* (J. Macquarrie and E. Robinson, Trans.). New York: Harper &
Row. (Original work published 1927)

Janoff-Bulman, R. (1992). *Shattered assumptions: Towards a new psychology of trauma.* New York:
Free Press.

Janoff-Bulman, R. (1998). Disillusionment and the creation of value: From traumatic losses to existential gains. In J. H. Harvey (Ed.), *Perspectives on loss: A sourcebook. Death, dying, and bereavement* (pp. 35–47). Philadelphia, PA: Brunner/Mazel.

Jonas, E., Schimel, J., & Greenberg, J. (2002). The Scrooge effect: Evidence that mortality salience increases prosocial attitudes and behavior. *Personality and Social Psychology Bulletin, 28*, 1342–
1353.

Jordon, H. (2000). *No such thing as a bad day: A memoir.* Atlanta, Ga: Longstreet Press.

Kasser, T., & Ryan, R. M. (1996). Further examining the American dream: Differential correlates of
intrinsic and extrinsic goals. *Personality and Social Psychology Bulletin, 22*, 280–287.

Kierkegaard, S. (1961). *Concluding unscientific postscript* (D. Swenson & W. Lawrie, Trans.). Princeton, NJ: Princeton University Press.

Kierkegaard, S. (1983). *Fear and trembling* (H. V. Hong & E. H. Hong, Trans.). Princeton, NJ: Princeton University Press.

Kinnier, R. R., Tribbensee, N. E., Rose, C. A., & Vaugh, S. M. (2001). In the final analysis: More wisdom from people who have faced death. *Journal of Counseling and Development, 79*, 171–177.

Kruglanski, A. W., & Ramat-Aviv, I., & Freund, T. (1983). The freezing and unfreezing of lay-infer-
ences: Effects on impressional primacy, ethnic stereotyping, and numerical anchoring. *Journal of
Experimental Social Psychology, 19*, 448–468.

Kuhl, D. (2002). *What dying people want: Practical wisdom for the end of life.* New York: Public Affairs.

Lehman, D. R., Davis, C. G., DeLongis, A., Wortman, C. B. Bluck, S., Mandel, D. R., et al. (1993).
Positive and negative life changes following bereavement and their relations to adjustment. *Journal of Social and Clinical Psychology, 12*, 90–112.

MacDonald, P. S. (Ed.). (2001). *The existentialist reader: An anthology of key texts*. New York: Routledge.

Milam, J. E. (2004). Posttraumatic growth among HIV/AIDS patients. *Journal of Applied Social Psychology*.

Newston, D., & Rindner, R. J. (1979). Variation in behavior perception and ability attribution. *Journal of Personality and Social Psychology, 37*, 1847–1858.

Nietzsche, F. (1967). The wanderer and his shadow. In W. Kaufmann (Ed.), *On the genealogy of morals and Ecce Homo* (pp. 179–186). New York: Vintage Books.

Noyes, R. (1980). Attitude change following near-death experiences. *Psychiatry, 43*, 234–242.

Noyes, R., Jr. (1982–1983). The human experience of death, or what can we learn from near-death experiences? *Omega, 13*, 251–259.

Ortega y Gasset, J. (1936). History as a system (W. C. Atkinson, Trans.). In R. Klibanshy & H. J. Paton (Eds.), *Philosophy and history* (pp. 283–322). Oxford, UK: Oxford Press.

Park, C. L., Cohen, L. H., & Murch, R. L. (1996). Assessment and prediction of stress-related growth. *Journal of Personality, 64*, 71–105.

Parkes, C. M. (1971). Psycho-social transitions: A field for study. *Social Science and Medicine, 5*, 101–115.

Pyszczynski, T., & Greenberg, J. (1992). *Hanging on and letting go: Understanding the onset, progression, and remission of depression*. New York: Springer-Verlag.

Raft, D., & Andersen, J. J. (1986). Transformations in self-understanding after near-death experiences. *Contemporary Psychoanalysis, 22*, 319–346.

Ring, K. (1984). *Heading toward Omega: In search of the meaning of near death experience*. New York: Morrow.

Roberts, G. A., & Owen, J. H. (1988). The near-death experience. *British Journal of Psychiatry, 153*, 607–617.

Setterlund, M. B., & Niedenthal, P. M. (1993)."Who am I? Why am I here?" Self-esteem, self-clarity, and prototype matching. *Journal of Personality and Social Psychology, 65*, 769–780.

Shaprio, N. (1993). [Executive producer]. (1993, April 13). *Dateline*. New York: National Broadcasting Company.

Simon, L., Greenberg, J., Harmon-Jones, E., Solomon, S., & Pyszczynski, T. (1996). Mild depression, mortality salience, and defense of the worldview: Evidence of intensified terror management in the mildly depressed. *Personality and Social Psychology Bulletin, 22*, 81–90.

Solomon, S., Greenberg, J., & Pyszczynski, T. (1991). Terror management theory of self-esteem. In C. R. Snyder & Forsyth, D. R. (Eds). *Handbook of social and clinical psychology: The health perspective* (pp. 21–40). New York: Pergamon Press.

Sutherland, C. (1990). Changes in religious beliefs, attitudes, and practices following near-death experiences: An Australian study. *Journal of Near-Death Studies, 9*, 21–31.

Tedeschi, R. G., & Calhoun, L. G. (1996). The Posttraumatic Growth Inventory: Measuring the positive legacy of trauma. *Journal of Traumatic Stress, 9*, 455–472.

Tedeschi, R. G., & Calhoun, L. G. (2004). Posttraumatic growth: Conceptual foundations and empirical evidence. *Psychological Inquiry, 15*, 1–18.

Tedeschi, R. G., Park, C. L., & Calhoun, L. G. (1998). *Posttraumatic growth: Positive changes in the aftermath of crisis*. Mahwah, NJ: Erlbaum.

Waterman, A. S. (1993). Two conceptions of happiness: Contrasts of personal expressiveness (Eudamonia) and hedonic enjoyment. *Journal of Personality and Social Psychology, 64*, 678–691.

Weiss, T. (2002). Posttraumatic growth in women with breast cancer and their husbands: An intersubjective validation study. *Journal of Psychosocial Oncology, 20*, 65–80.

Wren-Lewis, J. (1988). The darkness of God: A personal report on consciousness transformation through an encounter with death. *Journal of Humanistic Psychology, 28*, 105–122.

Wren-Lewis, J. (1994). Aftereffects of near-death experiences: A survival mechanism hypothesis. *Journal of Transpersonal Psychology, 26*, 107–115.

Wren-Lewis, J. (2004). The implications of near-death experiences (NDES) for understanding posttraumatic growth. *Psychological Inquiry, 15*, 90–92.

Yalom, I. D. (1980). *Existential psychotherapy*. New York: Basic Books.

Chapter 28

Autonomy Is No Illusion

Self-Determination Theory and the Empirical Study of Authenticity, Awareness, and Will

RICHARD M. RYAN
EDWARD L. DECI

Existentialism is often regarded as a pessimistic philosophy rather than the philosophy of liberation and engagement that it more truly represents. As Warnock (1970) suggested, existentialism's central mission is evangelical. It is intended to bring to its audience the "good news" of freedom—the news that we are each at the center of our existence, responsible for what we do. However, one dimension of pessimism that may be warranted concerns the extent to which people are not actually willing or able to engage that freedom and live authentically. Nietzsche and Kierkegaard, the harbingers of the movement, were among the most pessimistic, believing that few people have the courage to engage their inherent capacities for freedom.

Self-determination theory (SDT; Deci & Ryan, 1985; Ryan & Deci, 2000b) is an empirical approach to motivation, development, and personality that is deeply concerned with the dynamics of autonomy, with regulation by the self. Our interest not only has been in understanding the nature and consequences of autonomy; it has also been in detailing how autonomy can be either diminished or facilitated by specific biological, developmental, and social conditions. In this sense, SDT has examined the conditions that make it more or less possible to be autonomous or volitional and has shown how differences in the degree of autonomy affect human functioning and experience. That is, our interest is in the interplay between the vulnerabilities for being controlled and the possibilities for vital, authentic living.

The concepts of autonomy and authenticity, and the sense of will and responsibility associated with them, are seen by some as problematic for a scientific psychology. Bandura (1989), for example, defined autonomy as behavior that is completely "independent" of any environmental influences, so he declared it a nonsensical construct, a conclusion that we fully agree follows from his definition. More recently, however, several theorists have used cognitive and neuropsychological evidence to suggest that freedom and will may be illusions. Bargh and Ferguson (2000) reviewed evidence that people's intentions are often, if not always, influenced by processes of which they are unaware, a fact with which any theory of autonomy must be grapple. Wegner (2002) defined will as behavior whose original impetus lies in a conscious thought. He then showed that people are often mistaken about the causes of their behavior or intentions, suggesting therefore that the whole issue of will may be illusory. These concerns are interesting, and we address them at length. However, we agree that if one defines will or autonomy as a disembodied prime mover, as an infallible sensibility, or as an original impetus that arises *ex nihilio* in conscious thought, there can be little case for the existence of will or autonomy.

In contrast, we argue that the concept of autonomy as used within SDT, as well as in most existentialist thought, is not incompatible with determinism, nor does it require an immaterial prime mover. In fact, autonomy is a critical form of human functioning that, not surprisingly, like all human functioning, requires a brain and a body and, moreover, a context of influences and opportunities for action. Autonomy concerns how various urges, pushes, desires, primes, habits, goals, and needs from the brain, the body, and the context are orchestrated within the individual. To the degree that one's behavior is organized in accord with abiding values and interests, rather than being controlled or entrained by forces alien to them, it is experienced as autonomous. Autonomy thus concerns the difference between behavioral engagement that is congruent and fitting with one's values, interests, and needs (i.e., with one's self) versus alienated, passively compliant, or reactively defiant.

Differences between autonomous and heteronomous action are manifold, both in terms of physiological processes and functional outcomes and in terms of performance and experience (Ryan, Kuhl, & Deci, 1997). Autonomous functioning requires a brain, and especially the integrative processes that are particularly, but not exclusively, dependent on the prefrontal cortex and its afferent and efferent connections. Extensive evidence shows that self-regulated persistence and judgments of volition can be disrupted by specific types of neurological damage (Spence & Frith, 1999), which is instructive concerning the mechanisms through which autonomy works. But social and interpersonal events can also damage or thwart autonomy and are much more salient in their everyday influence. Social controls, evaluative pressures, rewards, and punishments can constrain behavior or direct people away from more integrated regulation. Thus, both biological and social factors can, in different ways, disrupt autonomous functioning. Such disruptions or "pathologies" of autonomy are among the most common of clinical and behavioral problems (Ryan, Deci, & Grolnick, 1995; Shapiro, 1981), suggesting that the issue of autonomy is indeed more than an irrelevant illusion. Further, an absence of autonomy in work, school, health care, or any other domain where commitment matters can be associated with huge costs in efficiency and quality of experience (La Guardia & Ryan, 2000; Ryan & Deci, 2000b). Finally, autonomy is a relevant issue in every developmental epoch and every culture, because universally humans are faced with norms and demands that they are more or less able to adopt and assimilate as legitimate and meaningful, and thus to abidingly enact.

This in no way contradicts the fact that humans frequently misattribute the causes of their behavior or intentions, sometimes out of ignorance of the processes and influences underlying them and sometimes out of defensive motives. In fact, the need to defensively disown intentions, to project personal causation under conditions of ambiguity, to behave reactively in overtly controlling situations, or to deny or hide from one's own motives are all phenomena that suggest the compelling importance, rather than irrelevance, of autonomy.

Such phenomena confirm what we, and existentialists alike, have long argued—namely, that autonomy is a human potential rather than a given.

In this chapter we focus on the issues of human autonomy and self-determination. In line with classic existentialist thought, we argue that people vary considerably both in the degree to which they experience autonomy or authenticity and in the degree to which they attempt to act in accord with, or run from, authentic motives. Moreover, these variations predict more or less optimal functioning in every domain and in every society. People who are "unfree," who either feel pressured or compelled to act against their interests and values or have "merely swallowed" the rules of the societies around them, are less well both individually and socially. Further, those who stay mindless of their own motives and needs and of the pressures and possibilities that surround them are less likely to self-regulate effectively. When lacking autonomy, not only is experience less optimal but so also is performance, persistence, and the quality of engagement. The evidence, derived largely from SDT, suggests that variations in autonomy have functional import and that knowledge concerning autonomy is practical—it can be used to promote (or diminish) the expression of human potentials and psychological well-being. Indeed, the evidence could not be clearer that autonomy is not a mere illusion.

We specifically address the philosophical status of autonomy and its viability as a scientific construct. We begin by tracing the historical connections between existential and phenomenological thought and the central concepts of SDT. We then provide a necessarily cursory review of the evidence concerning the importance of human autonomy for optimal functioning. Following this we address current controversies concerning autonomy, including the recent claims that will is illusory, that the self is a ghost, that awareness is irrelevant, and that autonomy is neither causally potent nor a universal concern.

THE RELATIONS OF EXISTENTIAL–PHENOMENOLOGICAL THOUGHT TO SDT

Despite the contemporary nature of the debates about self-determination or autonomy, consideration of the self as the center of synthesis and initiation has deep historical roots within phenomenological traditions of philosophy, dating particularly to Kant. The term "autonomy" is especially relevant to this tradition. Autonomy literally means "self-governing" and implies, therefore, the experience of regulation by the self. Its opposite, "heteronomy," refers to regulation from outside the self, by alien or external forces, be they in the brain, the mind, or the world around. Comprehension of the phenomenal nature of autonomy versus heteronomy is therefore relevant to understanding its functional consequences.

Pfander (1908/1967) provided one of the earliest analyses of the phenomenology of autonomy. Using methods drawn from Brentano and Husserl, Pfander sought to distinguish between self-determined acts—those that reflect one's *will*—and other forms of striving, effort, or motivation. For Pfander, acts of will are distinguished because they are experienced "precisely not as an occurrence caused by a different agent but as an initial act of the ego-center itself" (p. 20). For him, then, although inner urges or extant external pressures may supply the "grounds" or impetus for willing, the act of will or self-determination is essentially characterized by an *endorsement* of the behavior by the self or "ego center." In contrast, insofar as one's actions are perceived to be compelled by forces outside the self (or ego center) that one does not endorse, autonomy is not in evidence.

Ricoeur (1966) further examined the complexities of will and self-determination in his classic work *Freedom and Nature*. Like Pfander, he pointed out that will refers to acts that are fully endorsed by the self. Thus actions in accord with values and interests are autonomous. But Ricoeur elaborated that this need not imply a literal absence of external pressures, grounds, or even mandates to act in a certain way. We could be autonomous even under such pressures, provided that we concur with them. Insofar as the circumstances and our evaluation of them also *engender in us* reasons for obeying the outer or inner pressures, we do not necessarily lose our sense of will or autonomy when acting in accord with the pressures. Thus self-determination can be used to connote independent choices, but it can also describe acts of volitionally consenting to inputs such as obligations, inducements, urges, pressures, or rising desires.

As an example, consider a man who has fully assimilated and embraced collectivist cultural norms and practices. In a moment when he is pressured or tempted to act individualistically, he is likely to either implicitly or explicitly experience discrepancy and conflict. To be autonomous, he would have to find a meaningful way to coordinate the individualistic aim with his prior beliefs or revise either the aim or the prior beliefs. Anything less would represent less than full endorsement by the self and lack of integrity in behavior.

More existentially oriented theorists distinguish between *authentic* and *inauthentic* actions in a similar manner. Kierkegaard provided perhaps the most forceful voice in this literature of freedom and authenticity, and his definitions are inexorably connected to his conception of self. In his view the self is not a thing but a continual activity of synthesis. As he puts it in a famous passage, the "self is a relation which relates itself to its own self . . . in short it is a synthesis" (1849/1954, p. 146). Yet Kierkegaard abhorred the idea that this synthesis was an automatic process, an idea he felt was emphasized in the dominant German philosophies of his time (Olafson, 1967; Mullen, 1981) and, as we have argued, has also been too readily assumed in some organismic psychologies (Ryan, 1995). Rather, for Kierkegaard, to achieve a self is to be committed to relating the self to the self, of taking responsibility for ever reevaluating what one believes, and then acting in accord with that best synthesis. In this view, a genuine human being is "infinitely interested in his existence," and what one does is the current best synthesis of all that one truly believes, knows, and feels. To the extent that synthesis is complete and one is not duplicitous or self-deceptive then one will "will one thing" (1846/1948) and thus experience an (always relative) integration. To fail or balk at this task of selfhood is to be inauthentic (to be in despair). Thus the degree to which the self authors actions is, for Kierkegaard, a measure of one's integration and, ultimately, one's humanity.

Kierkegaard (1849/1954) also described authenticity as an ongoing achievement that entails considering not only possibilities but also the realities or necessities with which one must contend. The instantiation of human selfhood is thus not a matter of making fantastic choices but rather a struggle to realize one's potential in this world, within this culture. The synthetic work of the self is that of creating a synthesis of *possibility* and *necessity*. Too much weight given to either of these dialectical poles represented for Kierkegaard a fall into despair. A life emphasizing possibility over necessity is a life of dreaming and imagination, a despair of infinitude. Conversely, a life driven by necessity (a despair of finitude) would have us denying both our actual freedom and responsibility to live according to abiding values.

Wild (1965) instructively highlighted these ideas by discussing the two primary dictionary meanings of the term "authenticity." The first is its definition as "really proceeding from it reputed source or author." Authentic actions are those that one identifies as one's own and for which one takes responsibility. But a second meaning is also relevant. Authentic also means something that is real and actual (as opposed to pretended). An authentic action ideally fits with both definitions—it is characterized by a sense of authorship and it apprehends and deals with actuality as opposed to fantasy, pretense, or "as if" experiences.

These existential–phenomenological analyses specify that for an act to be autonomous or authentic it must be "endorsed" by the self or experienced as one's own doing. This of course applies to behaviors that are easily chosen (playing tennis might typically be autonomous, being fun and intrinsically motivated), as well as to those representing more difficult choices (working on an arduous but valued task). In the latter case, behavior is experienced as self-endorsed because of its fittingness with values and personal commitments. These analyses also underscore that there must be some relative unity underlying one's actions if they are to be experienced as autonomous; they must be endorsed by the whole self; they must feel congruent. Finally, they also convey that autonomy is defined *not* by the presence or absence of external influences but rather by one's consent or assent to such influences. Often this consent or assent is reflective and conscious; sometimes it need not be. In short, autonomy is in no meaningful sense equivalent to "independence" (Ryan, 1993). Finally, by no means do the constructs of authenticity and autonomy stand in contradiction to the facts of necessity. Neither concept implies infinite choice in the sense that we can choose to do what is unrealistic, to ignore what is, or to become "anything we want." Instead, autonomy and authenticity involve a synthesis of the actual and the possible.

Dworkin (1988) offered an analytical approach to the concept of autonomy and arrived at conclusions quite similar to those of existential phenomenologists. First, Dworkin underscored that autonomy does not require behaving without or against constraints or demands. Clearly one can assent to certain constraints and, in so assenting, be autonomous. For example, one might feel constrained in stopping for a particular red light, but if one assents to the value of traffic laws as useful in insuring safety, one could willingly consent to them and in doing so lose no autonomy. Indeed, one can enact autonomy through this higher-order, reflective commitment. As Dworkin described it, autonomy entails endorsement of one's actions at the *highest order of reflection*. Thus, people could reflect on motives that emerge for them, and they would be autonomous to the degree that they act in accord with the reflected appraisal of those motives. They might in turn evaluate their autonomy with regard to acting on that appraisal by again reflecting on it from yet a higher-order perspective. This is not an infinitely regressive process, however, because, practically, there are very few actions for which more than a few levels of reflection are possible. More important, at some level people will find a relatively full degree of endorsement and, therefore, autonomy, all things considered. Dworkin further underscored that autonomy does not definitionally entail "being subject to no external influences" as Bandura (1989) has defined it. No world is absent of influences. Rather, the issue of autonomy is whether the following of influences or inputs reflects mere obedience or coercion or, alternatively, a self-endorsed and reflective valuing of the direction or guidance that these inputs provide.

The process of *reflective appraisal from a higher order* to which Dworkin and others in more analytic philosophical traditions refer (e.g., Frankfurt, 1971; Hill, 1991; Wolff, 1990) is plainly similar to what Kierkegaard described as relating the self to the self. In our SDT view, this means taking interest in one's evaluations, choices, feelings, and actions and, in doing so, organizing and regulating them from the standpoint of the whole. This is an essential synthetic process that is implicitly (and sometimes explicitly) involved in what we describe as integrated self-regulation, and, although it is an evolved and natural process, it is also an act that, especially in times of distress, may require support. Indeed, relating or coordinating values, beliefs, and potential actions is a process that can be nurtured or undermined by social contexts.

We can take this one step further. We believe that an important element in the online, synthetic, or coordinating state of mind that promotes autonomy is interested attention (Deci & Ryan, 1985) or mindfulness (Brown & Ryan, 2003). Indeed, it is our perspective that a relaxed interest in or mindfulness of what is occurring promotes autonomy and self-regulation by allowing the individual to access to the largest extent the relative congruence of one's behavior and the consequences of it. As with autonomy, mindfulness is not some metaphysical concept or some immaterial cause. The process of mindfulness, in fact, requires a brain, as does all self-regulation (and many forms of non-self-regulation). This makes neither of them merely vacuous or epiphenomenal. Instead, mindfulness is a psychological state that allows for a fuller consideration of possibilities and, thus, a fuller endorsement of the actions in which one engages.

THE SELF IN CLINICAL PERSPECTIVES: ON THE NATURE OF THE "TRUE SELF"

Posing a construct of autonomy suggests, as we have seen, that humans can be either authentic or inauthentic, which means living or not living in accord with abiding values and sensibilities. This connects with the idea, central to a plethora of clinical theories, of a *true self* (Deci & Ryan, 1995, 2000). The concept of true self suggests that people often act in ways that are inconsistent, self-deceptive, or out of touch with central needs, motives, or values. Such incongruence, in turn, is associated with various forms of dysfunction (Rogers, 1963; Ryan et al., 1995). Within the existential tradition, incongruence is manifest as bad faith (Sartre, 1956), despair (Kierkegaard, 1849/1954), or fallenness (Heidegger, 1962).

Among the clinical theories that embrace this construct is that of Winnicott (1965), who argued that much of the psychopathology he encountered was the result of an inflation of the "false self" and the corresponding underdevelopment of a "true self." In Winnicott's view, people who are acting in accord with their true selves have a sense of feeling real and vital because they have access and sensitivity to their feelings, their bodies, and their needs. For Winnicott, this "in touchness" depends developmentally on a facilitating environment in which caretakers are responsive to and validating of the spontaneous strivings and needs of the child. This validation of inner experience aids the growth of self-awareness and the confidence and vitality associated with it. Conversely, an impinging or overly controlling caretaking environment forces the developing child to distort or ignore inner experience and results in a hypertrophy of a false self, an overresponsiveness to external contingencies, which serves to keep alive the dyadic connection. That is, the false self attempts to preserve relatedness at the price of autonomy. Winnicott further suggested that loss of connection with one's true self also diminishes people's creative nature, their ability to initiate freely, to be vital, and to enjoy life.

Horney (1950) articulated a similar construct that she labeled the *real self* and defined as the "*original* force toward individual growth and fulfillment" (p. 158). This real self is an "intrinsic potentiality" common to all human beings" (p. 17) that is the deep source of development. As for Winnicott, although the real self represents a developmental tendency, it requires favorable conditions for growth. Horney argued that these conditions included an atmosphere of warmth and support to provide both inner security and freedom that enable one to have access to and express feelings and thoughts. Conditions unresponsive to these needs produce a basic anxiety, which ultimately forestalls relating to others in a spontaneous and authentic manner. Following Kierkegaard, Horney believed that loss of (or failure to find) the real self results in despair. In her view, most neurotic phenomena represent one's being alienated with respect to this vital core of psychic life and effectively result in one's "abandoning of the reservoir of spontaneous energies" (p. 159) that true self-regulation affords.

In a number of other well-known theories within humanistic and existential traditions the construct of an authentic or true self figures centrally, including those of Rogers (1963), Jourard (1968), Fromm (1955), Laing (1960), and Moustakas (1995). Although each differs in nuances and specifics, common elements can be abstracted. First, the true self is typically viewed as a natural endowment. This true self is not merely a social product or implant but, rather, is a nascent sensibility that can be nurtured or thwarted, dulled or sharpened, by social conditions. Second, the true self is not a self-concept that must be defended, judged, or esteemed but, rather, a motivational force and synthetic tendency (Deci & Ryan, 1995). Theories from Horney to Winnicott ascribe to the true self energy that has direction—a direction variously described as directed toward the realization of one's potentials or expression of all that one is. The true self is thus deeply connected to the idea of *eudaimonia*, or the well-being that derives from the fulfillment of one's potentials (Ryan & Deci, 2001). Third, the true self is integrative in nature; it serves a synthetic function and represents a centering and health-promoting force in development. Finally, although development of the true self is an innate, natural, propensity, it is not the only motivational force at work, and it is a force that can be derailed or thwarted. As the fictional character Demian decried, "I only wanted to live in accord with the promptings of my true self. Why was that so difficult?" (Hesse, 1925, p 99).

Difficult indeed. A common theme of the clinical literature is that psychological ill health is the all too typical product of alienation from one's true self. Social forces of dissuasion are manifold. In early development they include lack of warmth and responsiveness and/or overcontrol from caregivers, which can lead individuals to ignore or distort their own inner signals and, thus, to disable self-regulation (Ryan, 1993). Throughout life, forces that can undermine autonomy continue, including the seductions of extrinsic rewards, contingent regard, and excessive challenges (Deci & Ryan, 1995). Indeed, according to SDT, contexts that thwart basic needs for autonomy, competence, or relatedness can lead to a loss of awareness and thus to a vulnerability to controlled regulation (Deci & Ryan, 2000). The social conditions that make the voice of the self so difficult to attend to present an intriguing puzzle for empirical study, a puzzle that has been a primary agenda of SDT for three decades.

Thus far we have reviewed a number of existential and clinical formulations that serve as a backdrop to our empirical inquiries. First, the sense of self phenomenologically relates to the experience of action or behavior that one actively and integratively endorses, or one is "wholeheartedly" behind. Autonomy also refers to actions that phenomenologically represent the unity of oneself as a person, or what one would endorse "at the highest order" of reflection. Finally, autonomy or self-regulation does not entail independence from external or internal influences. Rather, it concerns one's assent to do what one does, and it is this subjective assent or endorsement of actions or decisions that is the critical experiential issue.

FROM PHENOMENOLOGICAL TO EMPIRICAL ANALYSES: PERCEIVED LOCUS OF CAUSALITY

The phenomenological and clinical traditions we reviewed have historically been relatively divorced from empirical psychology. Yet these phenomenological ideas concerning will and autonomy made their entrance into mainstream psychology largely through the formulations by Heider (1958) and deCharms (1968) of "naive" psychology.

Heider (1958) was concerned with the nature of perceptions of common interpersonal events and how their construction plays a determinative role in behavior. His stated purpose in writing *The Psychology of Interpersonal Behavior*, a seminal foundation for all of attribution theory, was to articulate the naive psychology by which people make sense of their own and others' actions. He argued that it is this naive psychology that "we use to build up our picture of the social environment and which guides our reactions to it" (p. 5). Heider's interest in the phenomenal determinants of behavior is clear, and it is noteworthy that he was well trained in phenomenological thought, having been a student of Meinong, and conversant with Husserl's methods (Spiegelberg, 1972). More important, Heider understood that subjective variables such as motives, beliefs, and values shape action and behavior and thus are appropriate objects of scientific inquiry. As he stated: "motives and sentiments are psychological entities. They cannot be measured by a ruler, weighed by a scale, nor examined by a light meter. They are 'mentalistic concepts,' so-called intervening variables that bring order into the array of behavior. . . . " (p. 32).

Heider's perspective does not suggest that causal analyses of the neurological underpinnings of cognitions or motives are without scientific interest, but, rather, it maintains that such analyses do not supplant or preclude the importance of a phenomenal analysis. When the latter is simply reduced to the former, we lose an important and practical level of analysis.

Among the most central constructs within naive psychology is that of *personal causation*. Specifically, Heider argued that action and/or outcomes could be perceived either as personally caused or as a result of nonintentional or impersonal causes. The critical feature of personal causation was, according to Heider, *intentionality*, which implies both ability and effort toward some end. Heider detailed the circumstances that lend support to phenomenal judgements of effort (e.g., persistence and equifinality) and ability (e.g., perceived obstacles and talents). In contrast, *impersonal causation* is marked by an absence of control or initiation with regard to action or outcomes. An outcome perceived to be impersonally caused is thought not to be within the control of an individual to bring it about (or to prevent it).

DeCharms (1968) extended Heider's work in his classic book *Personal Causation*. He argued that intentional action is itself not always free or self-initiated. In fact, he pointed out how often we perform intentional actions precisely because we feel pressured or coerced to do so by external agents. A bully "makes" his victim do his bidding, and a boss demands that a worker take on an extra duty. Compliance with such demands is fully intentional but may not feel voluntary. To clarify this difference between freely performed and externally controlled intentional action deCharms proposed a further distinction within Heider's category of personally causation, namely that some intentional acts are characterized by an *internal perceived locus of causality* (IPLOC) and others by an *external perceived locus of causality* (EPLOC). The former concerns actions that are done willingly—one experiences oneself as having initiative and interest in the activity—whereas the latter represents intentional acts in which one feels like a *pawn* to external pressures or inducements.

These two types of intentional behavior are exemplified in everyday occurrences. Consider a woman who intentionally travels to work each morning. In one case she may disdain her job yet feel compelled by financial stress or social pressures to keep at it. In this case she lacks a full sense of volition; she is not self-determined in her work. Her feigned involvement bespeaks her inauthentic engagement. She experiences herself as a pawn in deCharms's use of the term. How different is the second case in which her sister "wants" to go to work, finds it fitting and meaningful, and considers it an expression of her true self. Here, the sister has an IPLOC; she is self-determined. Described here is the very real difference between alienated and unalienated labor which will affect not only job performance but also health and well-being.

DeCharms (1968) further claimed that people have a "primary motivational propensity" to be origins of behavior. In his view we are "constantly struggling against being confined and constrained by external forces—against being moved about like a pawn" (p. 273). For deCharms, however, the distinction between being an origin and a pawn was not an all-or-none matter but was (1) continuous, or a matter of degree, and (2) variable. He states: "A person feels more like an Origin under some circumstances and more like a Pawn under others" (p. 274).

Another conceptual point made by deCharms warrants emphasis. Unlike neobehaviorist applications of Heider's attribution theory (e.g., Bem, 1967), deCharms held the view that knowledge of one's volition is not exclusively derived by taking oneself as an object of social perception. Rather, one's volition is directly known, an aspect of personal knowledge (Polanyi, 1958). We do not always *infer* our motives from "post hoc" analyses of our behavior, although we may sometimes, under special circumstances, do that. Instead, we can *know* when we concur with our actions and when we have been coerced or pressured into them because we directly experience the organization and regulation of behavior. No doubt, attribution rules are useful for making inferences about others, and they can be useful in inferring our own internal states in times of confusion or ambiguity. But we can also access a direct source of knowledge concerning the degree of integrity in our own actions. Thus, when people behave, they have some internal information for judging whether the behavior is authentic or imposed, self-endorsed, or alien. When the capacity to sense this difference is impaired or neglected, behavioral regulation and mental health suffer accordingly (Ryan et al., 1995). Importantly, this view is supported by solid experimental evidence such as the findings that when motor areas of the cerebral cortex are stimulated to produce muscular contractions, patients typically know that they were not origins of those actions (Spence & Firth, 1999).

From the perspective of SDT, the construct of perceived locus of causality offered an operational route into the issue of autonomy or self-determination versus heteronomy or control. By instantiating conditions that add salience to external forces or reasons for acting, presumably the perceived locus of causality could be shifted from internal to external, thus facilitating the experience of being a pawn. Conversely, conditions that conduce toward an IPLOC should maximize the sense of self-determination and its consequences concerning the quality of behavior and experience.

Perceived Locus of Causality and Behavioral Regulation

One of the significant consequences that deCharms suggested would be associated with shifts in perceived locus of causality (PLOC) was a change in *intrinsic motivation*. He argued that intrinsic motivation is in evidence only when one experiences an IPLOC. Exploration, curiosity, creativity, and spontaneous interest are all characterized by feeling like an origin, and, in fact, deCharms believed that factors that detract from the perception that action is self-determined will diminish the occurrence of these type of behaviors. DeCharms' (1968) hypothesis concerning the relations between PLOC and intrinsic motivation has been widely tested, beginning with Deci's (1971) creation of the experimental "free-choice persistence" paradigm. The negative effect on intrinsic motivation of controlling extrinsic rewards, which conduce toward an EPLOC, has been widely sustained (see, Deci, Koestner, &

Ryan, 1999). Moreover, other events that have controlling significance such as surveillance, external evaluation, or threats of punishment also generally undermine intrinsic motivation (see Deci & Ryan, 1985, or Ryan & Deci, 2000a, for reviews).

Unfortunately, deCharms also argued that, in contradistinction to intrinsic motivation, extrinsically motivated behavior is invariantly characterized by an EPLOC. That is, he claimed that acts that are done "in order to" achieve outcomes separable from the action itself are always accompanied by the sense of being a "pawn" to external forces. It is perhaps because of this sharp division in which intrinsic motivation was viewed as self-determined whereas extrinsically oriented behavior was viewed as non-self-determined that most early experiments and scales pitted intrinsic motivation against extrinsic motivation as opposites (e.g., Harter, 1981). However, SDT has taken a different position regarding extrinsic motivation.

It is certainly the case that some extrinsically motivated behaviors are, as deCharms suggested, characterized by an EPLOC, or sense of being controlled. Indeed, the undermining of intrinsic motivation by most tangible reward contingencies attests to this. Further, examples such as a teenage boy who does a chore only because he expects to avoid his parents' wrath is engaging in a behavior for a perceived external cause. Such behavior requires no internalized value for the chore per se, and to the extent that the behavior is threat-regulated, he would not do it unless the punishment contingencies were in effect. However, one can also imagine another teenager who willingly does his chores "in order to" help out his parents, who are overworked and whom he wants to support. Here, his behavior will be experienced as more volitional. He feels self-initiating, and although he does it for extrinsic or instrumental reasons (to relieve his parents), he endorses and values that reason, so his actions are experienced as voluntary. Similarly a woman who does arduous volunteer work might be performing non-intrinsically satisfying actions with a full sense of volitional commitment.

Self-Determination Theory's Continuum of Autonomy

According to SDT, extrinsically motivated actions can vary from those that are heteronomous to those that are highly autonomous—that is from having a fully external PLOC to a highly internal PLOC. When one fully endorses the reasons for pursuing an extrinsic goal, or when one engages in extrinsic motivation as an outcome of well-integrated values, one can be fully autonomous. However, when one's engagement in uninteresting activities is wholly compelled by external contingencies and the value of the activities are not embraced, then alienation and heteronomy characterize one's behavior. Between these extremes lie extrinsically oriented activities that reflect merely partial internalization's of values or goals whose motivational basis is partly heteronomous and partly autonomous.

In short, extrinsically motivated behaviors fall along a continuum of relative autonomy that reflects the degree of internalization and integration to the self of non-intrinsically motivated action regulation (Ryan & Connell, 1989). Specifically, SDT classifies the most heteronomous forms of motivation as being *externally regulated*; those that reflect the partial assimilation of external controls as *introjected*; those that reflect a personal valuing of the actions as *identified*; and those that are both personally valued and well-synthesized with the totality of one's values and beliefs as *integrated* (Ryan & Deci, 2000b). These various types of extrinsic motivation have been psychometrically shown to fall along an underlying continuum of relative autonomy (Ryan & Connell, 1989; Vallerand, 1997). In turn, studies have shown that the greater the relative autonomy of behavior, the more consistent one's effort, the higher the quality of performance (at least at complex or creative tasks), and the more positive one's experience. Research demonstrates this across domains as diverse as religion, education, work, relationships, health behaviors, and sport, among others (Deci &

Ryan, 2000; Ryan & Deci, 2000b). In other words the relative autonomy of extrinsic motivation matters very much in our ongoing lives.

Despite SDT's historical linkage with the work of Heider and deCharms there are two issues with the terminology that were inherited from them that require clarification. First, the term "internal," as used in the phrase internal locus of causality, refers to the phenomenal self and not the person. This is a critical point insofar as there are intrapsychic pressures that can be experienced as alien or external to the self. For instance, we have shown how ego involvement, a self-controlling motivational state that we classify under the broader category of introjection, undermines intrinsic motivation, thereby attesting to the controlling character of this type of intrapersonal regulation (Ryan, 1982). The regulation is within the person but external to his or her sense of self. Second, the term "causality" refers not, in our view, to an ultimate initiating stimulus but, rather, to the extent to which the self concurs with and/or organizes the actions in which one is engaged. This later point is crucial because the original impetus to nearly all actions lies outside the phenomenal self, in one's environment, brain, or other parts of the organism. Some of the actions that follow from these prompts involve initiative and assent and thus have the phenomenal feel of events that the self has caused or is responsible for, whereas others do not. We return to this point in greater detail later in the chapter.

THE IMPACT OF AUTONOMY VERSUS HETERONOMY ON BEHAVIOR, PERFORMANCE, AND WELL-BEING

Literally hundreds of experiments within the tradition of SDT have examined the import of relative autonomy on human functioning. SDT's empirical strategy is multimethod. A primary strategy is to create experimental conditions conducive to either the experience of autonomy or heteronomy and look at their contrasting consequences. This has been done interpersonally, by computer presentations, and through primes. A second strategy is simply to ask people about their relative autonomy in different situations or for different goals and then to examine the correlates and consequences of those reports. Some such studies are correlational, others causal in the sense of looking at effects over time. Third is the strategy of searching out naturally occurring conditions that support or thwart autonomy and examining their effects. For instance one could look at the quality of experience and behavior in classrooms run by teachers who use controlling versus autonomy-supportive methods of motivation. Finally, there is the within-person strategy involving an examination of variations in felt autonomy from moment to moment or context to context and of the conditions and effects that covary with it. Using all these strategies and focusing on a wide array of moderators and outcomes, SDT provides a comprehensive picture of the importance of autonomy and the dangers of heteronomy not only for health, development, and well-being but also for productivity, creativity, and generativity. Rather than provide an extensive review of this research (see, e.g., Deci & Ryan, 2000; Ryan & Deci, 2000b), we highlight a few significant themes.

Intrinsic Motivation

SDT began with inquiries into the facilitation and undermining of intrinsic motivation. Although several factors are essential to intrinsic motivation, including perceived competence (Deci & Ryan, 1980a), the issue of autonomy is central. As already noted, experimental studies have manipulated external conditions of control (e.g., controlling rewards, imposed goals, surveillance, evaluations, threats of punishment) versus support for autonomy (e.g., informational rewards and feedback, opportunities for choice, nonevaluative supports, freedom from pressure and constraints) and reliably shown that the former undermine and the latter promote intrinsic motivation.

SDT further examines how these dynamics of external control are often mirrored in internal or intrapsychic controlling structures. For instance, Ryan (1982) put college students in an experimental condition in which their performance on a task was said to reflect their intelligence. It was reasoned that this linkage between performance and a self-esteem related trait would induce participants to become *ego-involved*, leading them to act in a self-controlling manner, pressuring themselves to achieve a good outcome. As predicted, participants in the ego-involving condition were subsequently less intrinsic motivated for the task relative to non-ego-involved counterparts due to the self-controlling nature of their motivation. A tradition of research has since looked at how introjects, in such forms as ego-involvement, objective self-awareness, and other self-controlling motives and orientations undermine intrinsic motivational processes (e.g., Plant & Ryan, 1985; Ryan, Koestner, & Deci, 1991).

Internalization

Despite the importance of intrinsic motivation as a prototype of optimal experience (Csikszentmihalyi, 1990; Deci & Ryan, 1985), most human behavior beyond early development is not intrinsically motivated. Most of our activities are not motivated by inherent satisfactions as much as by the desire to accomplish separable ends or goals, which is the formal definition of extrinsic motivation (Ryan & Deci, 2000a). As already stated, within SDT extrinsic motivation is considered to vary along a continuum of internalization that reflects relative degrees of autonomy, from behaviors done only because of external controls (external regulation) to behaviors that are done out of well-integrated values and beliefs (integrated regulation). Moreover, SDT-based research has shown repeatedly that the more autonomous the extrinsic motivation, the greater people's commitment, persistence, and performance and the more optimal their experience. Such evidence is not unique to the West, as some have claimed (e.g., Oishi, 2000) but, rather, has emerged in traditionally authoritarian and collectivistic cultural contexts as well as those characterized by democratic and individualistic cultures (e.g., Chirkov, Ryan, Kim, & Kaplan, 2003). Further, both experimental and field research has shown how controlling conditions undermine internalization or promote introjected forms of it (Deci, Eghrari, Patrick, & Leone, 1994) and can yield heavy costs in terms of behavioral outcomes and personal well-being.

Performance and Creativity

When autonomous motivations are undermined, whether that occurs by the thwarting of intrinsic motivation or integrated internalization, there have been well-documented costs in terms of human performance, especially performance that depends on flexible, heuristic, creative, or complex human capacities (see Amabile, 1983; Hennessy, 2000; Utman, 1997).

Quality of Relationships

Support for autonomy facilitates attachment, intimacy, and the outcomes associated with them. For instance Blais, Sabourin, Boucher, and Vallerand (1990) found that greater autonomy for being in a coupled relationship was associated with greater satisfaction, relationship stability, and well-being for both partners. La Guardia, Ryan, Couchman, and Deci (2000) used a within-person, multilevel modeling approach to show that people vary with different partners in their security of attachment, but moreover, that variation is to a significant degree a function of the degree to which the individual feels autonomous with that relational partner.

Well-Being

Autonomy is a central human need and thus its effects on well-being are robust and pervasive. Contexts that are controlling produce negative effects on well-being, whereas those that are autonomy supportive enhance it, a finding replicated across developmental epochs and varied cultures (Ryan & Deci, 2001). Moreover, individual differences in autonomy predict differences in well-being in a corresponding way (Deci & Ryan, 2000). Examination of many of the most common forms of psychopathology reveals disturbances of autonomy, and excessively controlling, pressuring, or contingently regarding social contexts play in etiological role in many mental illnesses (Ryan et al., 1995).

MORE EVIDENCE ON THE IMPORTANCE OF ENVIRONMENTS: THE SOCIAL PSYCHOLOGY OF AUTONOMY

Some existentialists like to make the provocative claim that we are always and in principle free—indeed we are condemned to freedom (e.g., Merleau-Ponty, 1964; Sartre, 1956). It is a polemical point, and it expresses the idea that even under adverse conditions we can take stock of ourselves and take responsibility. But in daily life, no matter what the abstract possibilities, we often feel we cannot be autonomous. Social controls, evaluative pressures, rewards, and punishments often constrain behavior, and when they do we feel less autonomous. These are the circumstances where our language shifts from "I will" or "I want" to "I should" or "I have to" in explaining why we do what we do.

Although direct coercion supplies an obvious example of circumstances conducive to heteronomy, there are even subtler and seemingly benign ways to undermine autonomy. As already noted, a common one is the controlling use of seductive rewards. Rewards can control behavior, a fact that operant psychology verified time and time again (Skinner, 1953). What operant psychology did not consider, however, was that regulation through external rewards (reinforcements) could supplant other regulators of behavior, including ones based in interests, values, and social concerns. When powerful rewards are dangled before people, those people can easily lose sight of other considerations. Rewards can reduce the scope of mindfulness and the healthy regulation that follows from it. In market economies the power of rewards to control behavior, even to the detriment of people's health and well-being, is amply documented. For instance, many people say that they are working too hard, and data support this perception (e.g., Schor, 1991). However, many experience no choice about the hours they work, feeling controlled by evaluations and the rewards tied to them. Further, the more people place priority on money and rewards, the more they report diminished autonomy, happiness, and quality of relationships (Kasser & Ryan, 1996; 2001).

Of course, money is only one form of control. In schools teachers have access to a variety of others, from evaluations and grades, to detentions, gold stars, and honor roles. They can as well use public praise and humiliation as a means of shaping behavior. Given the access to potent motivators such as these, the degree to which educators support autonomy versus control behavior is a powerful predictor of the motivation and interest their students exhibit for school activities. A large body of evidence derived from SDT shows the negative effects of controlling strategies not only on interest and self-motivation but also on educational persistence and the quality of learning outcomes (Ryan & La Guardia, 1999).

Similarly, we have recently been studying how controlling versus autonomy-supportive health care practitioners undermine versus facilitate autonomous engagement in health behavior change. Studies show that autonomy support leads to greater program involvement, adherence, and maintained change for behaviors such as smoking cessation, weight loss, glucose control, medication adherence, and exercise (Williams, 2002; Williams, Deci, & Ryan, 1998).

Perhaps the most pervasive and powerful force that controls behavior is contingent regard (Deci & Ryan, 1995). Because of the importance of the need for relatedness, people will do many things to be recognized or loved by others. In fact, socializing agents such as parents and teachers often make their affection or regard contingent upon the person's behaving in accord with their expectations. Recent research by Assor, Roth, and Deci (2004) found, for example, that parental use of conditional regard led their children to introject the regulation of expected behaviors, but it did so at significant personal and interpersonal costs. Children of parents who used more conditional regard displayed more fragile self-esteem, experienced more fleeting satisfaction following successes and more shame following failures, and felt more rejected by and resentment toward their parents.

The effects of social environments in fostering autonomy versus alienation and the consequences of these states have also been powerfully shown in a number of recent within-person studies. In diary work, Reis, Sheldon, Gable, Roscoe, and Ryan (1999) showed that people's daily well-being fluctuated in accord with whether they were in contexts and activities that they experienced as either autonomy supportive or controlling. In the relationship realm, La Guardia et al. (2000) found, at a within-person level of analysis, that the experience of autonomy support from others predicted security of attachment with those persons. Similarly, Ryan, La Guardia, Butzel, Chirkov, and Kim (2003) found that within-person variation in whom one turns to in emotionally charged times is largely a function of feelings of autonomy support versus control within that dyad. Clearly our performance and well-being within differing contexts and relationships are deeply affected by supports versus thwarts of our autonomy.

Given the pervasive effects found on human functioning of variations in both the experience of autonomy and the social conditions that either support or thwart it, it would seem undeniable that autonomy is indeed a central human concern. But as we argued at the outset of this chapter, autonomy continues to be a construct that many psychologists find problematic. Indeed, autonomy is castigated as too humanistic, too optimistic, too culturally specific, or not scientific enough. The fervor the issue seems to raise is surprising, particularly from critics who typically admit to the importance of the issue in their own daily lives, and who might be the first to resist heteronomous controls being placed on them at work, in their relationships, or by their governments. However, as we have investigated various suggestions that autonomy is an illusion, or a form of vitalism, we have found that many of the skeptics themselves embrace aspects of autonomy, often parenthetically. We now consider some current forms of skepticism.

PSYCHOLOGISTS ATTACK AUTONOMY: IS IT ILLUSORY?

Both in the popular and the professional literature there is no doubt that attacking cherished notions of human autonomy, choice, and free will has become a popular sport for psychologists and brain scientists. But the tactics vary. Some have a familiar ring, because they come from neobehaviorists who see the environment as, by definition, the ultimate cause of all behavior and who maintain that that fact closes the matter. Some new and novel attacks are forwarded from neuropsychologists, armed with techniques to track the activity of the brain during action sequences. In interpreting such data, some fall into what Pinker (2002) humorously labels "bad reductionism." Such reductionists, like their behaviorist counterparts, are focused on causes of behavior. Yet, whereas behaviorists tautologically located all causes in the external environment, contemporary reductionists have displaced ultimate causality inward: Definitionally they see all behaviors as caused by "the brain," which is somehow considered to logically preclude autonomous processes. Another set of critics has emerged from new and exciting work on implicit cognitive processes. Although the idea of nonconscious processes is by no means novel (Freud, 1909/1977), the new empirically based recognition of such processes has reraised the question whether there can be any autonomy or will when the causes of behavior are opaque to us. Finally, attacks on autonomy have also come from the distinct quarters of cross-cultural psychology. Some cultural relativists in particular view autonomy as a Western value and/or as merely a social construction. For them the concern is not causation but, rather, the idea of self as a potential referent for behavioral organization. To address these skeptical views concerning autonomy we briefly review each of them, discussing how their positions interface or coordinate with SDT's conceptual framework.

Bandura and Skinner: Autonomy as Independence from an Environment

Some psychological theorists have cast "straw man" definitions of autonomy that they then knock down as unscientific. Bandura (1989) in his social cognitive theory of "agency" supplied a striking example. He rendered the concept of autonomy meaningless by defining it as action that is "entirely independent" of the environment (p. 1175). If the environment has an influence on behavior, according to Bandura, there can be no autonomy. The issue of assent, consent, or volition with respect to an environment is thus expiated without serious—indeed, without even superficial—analysis. As we have shown, this is a philosophically problematic stance (Dworkin, 1988) because autonomy, both as analytically defined and as we define it within SDT, does not concern the locus of the impetus to action but rather its concordance and endorsement. Furthermore, no account we have ever found considers autonomous behavior to exist independent of supports, prompts, or initiating cues. By writing off the concept of autonomy altogether, Bandura's social-cognitive approach ultimately reduces agency to mere self-efficacy, the issue of being confident in one's ability to do or achieve something. Yet, the belief that one can obtain an outcome or successfully perform an action does not address whether one wants to do it or whether one values it—issues at the very the crux of human concerns about autonomy and true agency. A resentfully obedient, but competent, slave could be agentic by Bandura's definition, as long as he has a sense of efficacy in following all the alien and hated commands that beset him. Thus self-efficacy theory cannot distinguish between alienated and self-concordant actions, nor can it predict the consequences of this critical difference.

Skinner (1971) also wrote off autonomy by defining it as an ignorance of the actual factors that control behavior. As we shall see, this argument has a reprise in some of the newer neuroscience-based theses. Skinner argued that "if we do not know why a person acts as he does, we attribute his behavior to him" (p. 53). In his system of thought, the control over action was tautologically defined as residing in reinforcements that are external to the organism, so any unity or organization that appears in action is credited to the unity and organization of the reinforcement contingencies. Skinner's work provides another example of how the attempt to pit the idea of "the external" *against* the concept of autonomy leads to a premature evacuation of this construct that is so important for a practically valuable motivational psychology.

Although we have criticized Skinner's work on philosophical grounds, a few behaviorists have attempted to take on SDT on empirical grounds. Such debate is particularly illustrative, as it shows the power of SDT's predictive hypotheses to account for phenomena that behaviorism cannot because it fails to consider the dynamics of human autonomy. It also shows how ideological positions can lead to some erroneous results. The most highlighted aspect of this now three-decade-long exchange occurred in a "battle of the meta-analyses." In a prominent article about reward effects on intrinsic motivation Eisenberger and Cameron (1996) claimed "the null," arguing that rewards, regardless of whether they are controlling or informational as SDT classifies them, should have no negative effects on intrinsic motivation. Despite prior meta-analyses finding support for SDT's position, Eisenberger and Cameron identified no evidence for an undermining effect by rewards, a startling finding that contrasted with the empirical mainstream, and thus got big press for the *American Psychologist*. After repeatedly being denied an opportunity to respond in that venue, Deci et al. (1999) reanalyzed the data from the 128 experiments and presented some even more startling findings in *Psychological Bulletin*. Results detailed how Eisenberger and Cameron's analyses were plagued by miscalculations, inappropriate collapsing of conditions without doing moderation analyses, incorrect recording of effect sizes, misclassifications of conditions, and use of the wrong control groups. The errors and inappropriate procedures were so extensive that it was hardly surprising that when correctly analyzed, the results of reward effects on intrinsic motivation were perfectly fitting with the differentiated predictions of SDT concerning when rewards should undermine intrinsic motivation and when they should not. Eisenberger, Pierce, and Cameron's (1999) invited response did not dispute the primary findings of the Deci et al. meta-analysis.

The oddity of these debates is that, from the SDT perspective, we have never doubted the power of external rewards and reinforcements to control behavior. It is rather that because of their power to control, rewards can lead people away from their intrinsic inclinations, away from behaving authentically in accord with abiding values and interests. Arbitrary rewards, if compelling enough, can get people to do almost anything. Indeed, no one who looks at the reality of today's reward-based economies should doubt that powerful extrinsic rewards can lead people to forego autonomy, forget their values and needs, and neglect their loved ones and their health. That is precisely what alienation and unhealthy regulation is all about (Ryan & Deci, 2000d).

Does Autonomy Require a Brain?

As psychology seeks out the neurological underpinnings of behavior and experience, some interpret the new evidence as undermining ideas of autonomy or self-determination. Consider this passage from Pinker (2002), an accomplished leader in this field:

> [E]ach of us feels that there is a single "I" in control. But that is an illusion that the brain works hard to produce. . . . The brain does have supervisory systems in the prefrontal lobes and anterior cingulate cortex, which can push the buttons of behavior and override habits and urges. But these

systems are gadgets with specific quirks and limitations; they are not implementations of the rational free agent traditionally identified with the soul or the self. (p. 43)

In one fell swoop, the otherwise thoughtful Pinker evacuates the "I" as "illusion" and linguistically replaces it with a new intentional subject, "the brain," which pushes buttons and controls urges. The sense of self is just a postbehavior "spin," whereas the brain, reified as if it were an intentional agent, does the acting, deciding, and gadget activating. Such interpretations, found pervasively in today's popular neuropsychology, are fraught with philosophical confounds. First, the brain replaces the philosophical homunculus in this description. Second, the logic here is that if the brain is involved in action, it is therefore the ultimate and most relevant cause. No matter that the brain itself may be stimulated into action by social events, that the supervisory "gadgets" are mediated by people's psychological interpretations and construals, or that awareness and active reflection can alter those construals. For Pinker, and others, saying that the brain did it is apparently satisfying as an explanation. But locating causes exclusively or "ultimately" in the brain is as problematic as locating them exclusively or ultimately in the environment, as Skinner had done.

In fairness, Pinker's overall position leaves plenty of room for human deliberativeness and reflection to influence action, and we share with him an advocacy for consilience between levels of analysis. Our point is that consilience goes both ways. When Pinker (2002, p. 183) argued that society needs to influence behavior by "appealing to that inhibitory brain system" (i.e., the prefrontal cortex), we see a loss of perspective in terms of the multiple levels of analysis available across the varied disciplines of science. It is our inclination to appeal to people's motives, morals, and reflective capacities, which we presume would be associated with the stimulation of prefrontal–cortical activity.

Both autonomous self-regulation and controlled regulatory processes operate within an organism, and there can be no doubt that they have distinct biological supports (Ryan et al., 1997). The distinct regulatory processes also typically relate with, or follow from, different types of environments and cultural backdrops. They are also linked with divergent phenomenological experiences as well as different affective and behavioral consequences. In short, the antecedents, consequences, and functional underpinnings of autonomous versus controlled action are distinct. Grasping these facts at every level of analysis is particularly important for both scientific understanding and interventions.

As we discover in ever more detail the neurological processes that subserve, constrain, and sometimes direct action, some have suggested that this may eventually crowd out antiquated and ephemeral ideas of freedom and will (e.g., Bargh & Ferguson, 2000; Wegner, 2002). This speculation, however, rests on the view that autonomy or will is some non-brain-related force that intervenes in action, much like Descartes's soul tilted the Pineal gland to alter otherwise purely mechanical sequences of action. We know of no such force, and it is no wonder that will, so defined, recedes in the face of every new discovery in neuroscience, just as vitalism receded with new discoveries in genetics.

All events in the universe can (potentially) be described in material and efficient causal terms and can be described from molecular to molar levels of analysis and parsing of events. On one level of description we are interested in the most concrete and microscopic sequence of events entailed in actions. Consider a person who throws an object across a room. One appropriate causal account of the thrust can be found in the physical events inside the organism's brain that regulated the lifting, aiming, and release. Let us suppose we know these events in total detail, down to the molecular sequence of change. Has the person's behavior thus been "explained"? Of course at one level of analysis it has. But we submit that in most contexts an explanation of the sequence from stimulus conditions to brain cells to motor output would be highly unsatisfying, if not irrelevant and distracting. This is because the most meaningful and relevant level of analysis for the cause of this event lies in the interpretations and construals of events that gave rise to the molar behavior rather than in the brain processes that subserved it. It is likely to be more informative to know, for example, whether the person threw the object in anger or in sport. Explaining the reasons why a person acts as he or she does by measuring electrical potentials misses what will probably be the most critical issues. It is like responding to the question, "Why did he go to the store?" with a description of the cortical-readiness potential that preceded the movement of the legs.

The Regnant Level of Analysis for Any Problem

For every question asked about causation there is a level (or, in some cases, multiple interactive levels) of analysis that is most pertinent to addressing the problem posed. We label this the "regnant level" of explanation. It is the level that captures the most meaningful and molar organization of events, as well as the level where "intervention" in events would most likely and most effectively occur. In addition, because one purpose of science, as Bacon emphasized, is prediction and control, that purpose is often best served by attending to the regnant, rather than the *lowest*, level of analysis. Accordingly, the social circumstance, and its construal by the actor in our example of object throwing, is plausibly a more regnant cause than what cells in the brain activated the contraction of the hand muscles. To be sure, the later is a necessary and mediating event, but it is hardly explanatory. One could intervene in the object-throwing sequence by deadening the relevant brain pathways, but more likely we would want to stop it by helping the person better manage his or her anger or make better decisions about where to play sports. Similarly, why the stock market falls during a period of "war jitters" is better explained by people's expectations than by tracing the brain activity underpinning those expectations. This is because, if we want to intervene in stock buying behavior, we are unlikely to do so at the neurological level; instead, we would be more likely to do it at the level of beliefs and expectations, or at the level of economic issues that are giving rise to them. The mere fact that an explanation is at a lower level of analysis does not make it a better, fuller, or more definitive. Indeed, it can make it more irrelevant. Such causal explanations are not "wrong," they are just misplaced.

Sometimes a neurological/physiological explanation *is* the regnant level of explanation for behavior. This is particularly true for behavior that would fall under Heider's (1958) category of impersonal causation. Reflexive actions, such as an eye blink caused by a puff of air, are not typically experienced as intentional, as phenomenologists have specifically explicated (Ricoeur, 1966). However, even for certain nonreflexive behaviors that entail considerable coordination, there are mechanisms that appear to bypass all mediation by the reflective, evaluative capacities of the person, and when they occur people are unlikely to report feeling autonomy. Instead they typically say, "it happened to me," or "I couldn't help it." Understanding the mechanics of these events is extremely important for behavioral sciences.

In contrast to such events, and for many purposes of social design and intervention, behavior is explained most meaningfully by looking at molar social events and their construal. The very same proximal stimuli will engender different responses depending on their meaning or significance to the person. Social events have a *functional significance* (Deci & Ryan, 1985), which in turn shapes the organization of subsequent action. And where autonomy enters the picture is in this realm of meaning. As existentialists have argued, we act in accord with the meaning of events, and it is in the reflective construction of meanings that we can find our possibilities. When researchers look into the meanings of events and their predictive relations to what follows, they are not denying material causation or the necessity of a brain that undergirds these processes. However, they are also not getting lost in the twigs when trying to survey and manage the forest.

UNCONSCIOUS DETERMINATION

A less philosophical and more substantive concern stems from growing evidence that actions may be brought about or caused by factors of which people are unaware (Wilson, 2002). Bargh and Ferguson (2000), for example, cited studies in which people are implicitly or unconsciously primed to enact intentional behaviors and then attribute their actions to will or self-initiation. Such experiments call into question whether all acts are unconsciously determined, and whether our attributions of being self-motivated have any veracity.

Within the conceptual framework of SDT the issue of implicit and explicit motivation is orthogonal to the issue of autonomous versus heteronomous motivation (Deci & Ryan, 1980b). Implicit events may prompt either autonomous or controlled behaviors. And behaviors that are automatic—that are not consciously decided on—may be regulated by either autonomous or controlled processes. A woman who automatically shifts her car into fourth gear when the cue of engine noise nonconsciously prompts it may be acting fully autonomously. Were she to reflectively consider it, she would wholly endorse and stand behind the action. Conversely, some implicit motives drive heteronomous behavior. A man who has made a personal commitment to a diet for the sake of his health but after subliminal exposure to a junkfood ad finds himself mindlessly munching at the refrigerator, would be controlled in this action. Were he to reflectively consider it, he would agree that the behavior was inconsistent with his self-endorsed, overarching goal of health. If he did not reflect on the behavior, the marker of his heteronomy would be the guilt or shame that followed the munching. Explicit motives, too, may be heteronomous or autonomous, but this is more obvious. When someone explicitly decides to comply with a threat, the person may be aware of the decision but not feel any autonomy or willingness. On the other hand, explicit motives can be autonomous, as when someone openly considers an urge that has arisen and assents to its enactment. In that case, the choice "fits" with the person's central values. In short, the issue of automaticity versus conscious deliberateness does not inform us all that well concerning the autonomy of actions. Some habits and reactions are ones we would experience as autonomous; others seem alien, imposed, or unwanted.

In these examples what is clear is that autonomy lies not in people's power to have a conscious thought be the initial stimulus for their actions. Initial stimuli typically arise in the environment or the organism, so the impetus for many actions is not consciousness per se. In fact, we agree with Wegner (2002) that people are often wrong when they imagine that their own thoughts were the initial causes of their impulses or actions. However, the issue of people's autonomy lies in the regulatory process through which the behaviors, even if nonconsciously prompted, are governed. When people are (vs. are not) open to their experience, when they take interest in an urge or a prompt and consent to its enactment, their behavior can be autonomous and the brain processes involved in its regulation will be different from those involved if the behavior were controlled. This formulation is quite consistent with the experimental findings of Libet (1999), who showed that volitional action can be preceded by a readiness potential in the brain before any awareness of intention, but that consciousness has its function in approving (or vetoing) the commission of the act.

From the perspective of SDT, then, brain processes (and/or environmental cues that trigger them) can instigate behaviors that are regulated by either autonomous or controlled processes. In everyday life autonomy will be more likely when emitted behaviors, however instigated, accord with one's interests and values, and this is facilitated when one is mindful or nondefensively aware of both one's interests and needs as well as of the urges or intentions that arise. With such openness, consent for some behaviors will readily occur insofar as the urges or intentions are consistent with one's integrated sense of self, or self-concordant. But when they are contradictory, reflective attention to them has a functional value. Without the mindfulness, or open reflective attention, one's actions will often be controlled, and often costly.

Part of what is at issue in this discussion is one's definition of will and volition. Wegner and Wheatley (1999) specifically stated that "people experience conscious will when they interpret their own thought as the cause of their action" (p. 480). But as we outlined earlier, this is not the common definition of will in existential–phenomenological philosophies, nor is this the SDT definition of autonomy. Further, such a criterion for will—namely, one's conscious thoughts as the initial cause of behavior—seems designed to cast the concept of will into the intellectual trash bin. It is unlikely by any analysis that thoughts about initiating behavior, even reflective ones, come from nowhere or are disconnected from underlying brain processes or prior events. As Nietzsche (1949) noted, "a thought comes when it wishes and not when I wish, so that it is a falsification of the facts of the case the say that the subject 'I' is the condition of the predicate 'think' " (cf. Frattaroli, 2001, p. 192). This did not in any way contradict Nietzsche's (1949) insistence that one can observe these thoughts and engage some rather than others. Heidegger (1962) argued, in a related vein, that humans are embedded in a world of concerns, and these give rise to our goals and projects. If people's thoughts must be the ultimate impetus, rather than events in the world or the words of others, then this tautologically guarantees that will is a vacuous concept. We suggest instead that the exercise of will and autonomy is different from being an initial cause or stimulus to action. It rather concerns the capacity to effectively evaluate the meaning and fit of potential actions with one's overarching values, needs, and interests.

A quarter of a century ago, we argued for a distinction between automatic and automatized behaviors (Deci & Ryan, 1980b). Automatic behaviors are those that are pushed by controlled processes and whose occurrence is not consistent with one's choices or reflections and cannot easily be brought into the realm of active choice. Automatized behaviors, in contrast, are ones that, if reflected on, would fit with one's values or needs and could be readily changed when they no longer fit. Behavior becomes automatized because it is efficient and conserves resources, but it is not therefore heteronomous. Such a distinction between these two types of nonconsciously prompted behaviors is still needed.

Existentialists would have no problem with this. As Warnock (1970) argued, one reason existentialists wrote essays on freedom was to prompt, alert, and awaken people so they might more reflectively evaluate what they are doing. Kant, whose philosophy supplied the foundations for existentialist thought, similarly viewed autonomy as laying not in our being ultimate causes, but in acts of transcendence, of rising over what is occurring and taking stock of it.

Recent empirical studies bear directly on these points. Levesque and Pelletier (2003) provided evidence that under specific circumstances both implicit and explicit intrinsic motivation can predict persistence and affect. However, a further question is the degree to which explicit awareness could modify or override implicit motivation. In other words, can a person alter an implicit, automatic tendency? As Bargh (1997) noted, perhaps one way to gain control over an automatic process is to become aware of the automatic cognitions that trigger or prompt it. Accordingly, in a subsequent study Levesque and Brown (2003) examined whether mindfulness, or the tendency to be aware of what is occurring in the moment (Brown & Ryan, 2003), would moderate the power of implicit motives. They found that indeed it did—implicit motivation was a more potent predictor of behavior when mindfulness was low. This suggests that while implicit motives can control behavior, awareness is one possible antidote.

Mistaken Causality

Wegner (2002) raises the important fact that people also suffer illusions of control over outcomes. It is noteworthy that many of the best demonstrations of the "illusion" of a connection between one's intentional behavior and outcomes take place in ambiguous and strange situations—people using Ouija boards or dowsing for water. In addition, the illusions often concern one's actual control over outcomes rather than the autonomy of the acts themselves. As has been detailed elsewhere, there is no isomorphism between perceived locus of causality and one's locus of control over outcomes (Deci & Ryan, 1985). Hypothetically, at least, a person might autonomously divine for water, believing it to be a valuable activity, even though the person's capacity to find water may in actuality be completely unreliable. As well, one could heteronomously divine—for example, because others who believe in it pressure one to do it. Here the person is neither deluded nor autonomous. Despite the issue of terminology, Wegner's evidence shows that people are vulnerable to illusion and/or self-deception and that they can sometimes be tricked or fooled.

This idea—that people can be deluded or delude themselves—is not really problematic for a psychology of autonomy. Indeed, self-deception is, according to both existential thought and SDT, a vulnerability, a primary way in which people escape from the burdens of freedom and responsibility. What the evidence does not show, however, is that people typically cannot, with effort, courage, and interested reflection, tell the difference between autonomous and controlled actions or that they cannot, in nontrivial situations, reflectively evaluate behavioral possibilities and select those that are more congruent with, rather than contradictory to, their values and interests. That is the essence of autonomous self-regulation, and without it we would be nothing but a twitching mass of contradictory impulses, torn toward 100 directions at once.

Can people be fooled? Of course. The more ambiguous the context, the less certain the values, or the more salient the social pressures, the more easily this would be so. No one concerned with the dynamics of autonomy has ever argued that self-deception is not possible or that well-designed experiments might not deceive people as to their choices and needs. But this only shows the importance of a well functioning "self-compatibility" checker (Kuhl & Kazen, 1994)—in other words, a capacity for integrative awareness of one's sensibilities, values, and the consequences of possible actions (Deci & Ryan, 2000; Hodgins & Knee, 2002).

Interestingly and surprisingly, after many provocative statements about will being merely an illusion, Wegner states almost parenthetically that the experience of volition or will may be critical and important to human functioning. He describes will as an "authorship emotion" that is more or less present for any action and that supplies a useful guide to the selection and regulation of behavior. In other words, the sensibility concerning autonomy is informative and functional rather than simply illusory. Such an authorship emotion is, of course, no doubt an aspect of the sense of volition or of being an origin versus pawn that a long tradition in psychology from deCharms to SDT has had in focus.

Not only can people be mistaken about control over outcomes, they can sometimes be mistaken, or more actively self-deceptive, about the autonomy of their actions. For example, in the SDT framework, people experience a high degree of autonomy when they identify with certain activities and endorse their personal importance. But it is often the case that when these identifications are more reflectively considered, one finds them contradictory to other identifications in ways that were not previously considered. In fact we have specifically argued that some identifications are *compartmentalized*, and remain relatively unintegrated within the person. To the extent that compartmentalization is active, it represents a form of self-deception. One tries not to see how one value might conflict with another (Ryan & Deci, 2000c). Similarly, it is often the case in clinical work that what appears at first blush to be an identification is, when actively unpacked, an introject—the value or goal was not really assimilated as one's own. The classic example is the student who (tells himself that he) "wants" to be a doctor but who seems in reality to lack enthusiasm for his studies. Upon a reflective analysis, this "identification" turns out to be his parents' aspiration for him, not his own. To maintain relatedness, he swallows it whole, and has portrayed it as his own vocational wish. When such self-deception occurs, it can almost invariably be traced back to a conflict between needs—in this case between relatedness and autonomy.

For us, the importance of these recent critiques of freedom and will as illusory lies in their highlighting yet more sources of human vulnerability to nonautonomous regulation. As SDT has long argued, experiences of being coerced or seduced into actions can undermine people's autonomy for the actions and leave them more rigid and defensive (Deci & Ryan, 2000). In that state, people may, among other things, deceive themselves into thinking they have control over outcomes or autonomy concerning their behavior and they may adamantly and insistently proclaim as much. So, we agree that people often do not know what prompts or gives rise to a desire, impulse, or action tendency, and that they will at times claim to be the origins of such actions. Indeed, as clinicians we see this every day. We also agree, as Wilson (2002) pointed out, that people do not know how their inner machinery works. All the more reason to have a psychology of autonomy that would prompt people in turn to reflectively consider what they are doing and, from that basis, to regulate subsequent behavior.

AUTONOMY IS NOT ANTINATURALISTIC: A CONSIDERATION OF THE EVOLVED STRUCTURE OF SELF

The only basis for demarcating one living being from another, or from its inanimate surround, derives from the fact of its organized functioning (Mayr, 1982). The fundamental attribution of organization to living beings reflects a commitment on the part of philosophers and scientists to a belief in what Polanyi (1958) labeled "primordial centres of individuality" which is the foundation of all biological thought. Thus, there is no conceptual or ontological way of distinguishing an animate entity on the basis of physical–chemical constituents alone. Rather, observers witness an organizational process through which action is initiated in the service of maintaining a stability of constituents and which is related in an ordered way to the surround. Interestingly, this attribution of life-like qualities as a function of ordered patterns of behavior has been experimentally demonstrated by such thinkers as Michotte (1954) and Heider (e.g., Heider & Simmel, 1944). Our recognition of such ordering processes is, as Polanyi argued, a convivial passion, in which we appreciate patterned operations and attribute them to an active center. At all levels of life, organisms are engaged in "biotic performances" that betray an inner organization and in this we share a kinship (Maturana & Varela, 1992; Wilson, 1975).

At some point in the evolution of biotic forms, consciousness was certainly elaborated, probably in concert with the development of perceptual systems that extended and centralized the control of the organism as a whole with respect to its surround. It is also at this point, Polanyi argued that there emerged the "polarity" of subject and object with its fateful obligation to form expectations and to learn from experience. With this emergence "the first faint thrills of intellectual joy appeared in the emotional life of the animal" (Polanyi, 1958, p. 388). The human form of personhood certainly extended this already extant mental outreach program of life, insofar as the human invention of language and, along with it, appreciation of other centers of thought boost these intellectual joys of living action into stratospheric heights. But the point here is that the spectacle of evolutionary forms shows that there has been an emergence of a successive intensification of personal consciousness that can be best understood as evolving.

Organismic self-regulation, then, refers not to some brand-new package of selfhood handed down discontinuously from nature but to an attribute that has manifestations across manifold forms of life. It has its origins, or *deep structure*, in the principle that animate forms require an organizing or regulatory process. Yet, unlike other species, humans gain in the course of early development an awareness of themselves as an individual center of regulation and an appreciation of the individuality of other beings as subjective centers. This awareness is extended through language and symbolization. But this "awareness of" is a tool or instrument of the organismic center; it does not create it. It has its hazards, such as engendering the terror we face in becoming aware of our individual and impermanent existence (Pyszcynski, Greenberg, & Solomon, 1999). But it also has the advantage of being able, at times, to reflectively reevaluate what we are doing and to avoid being entrained, controlled, or knocked off course.

We can certainly, then, turn to evolutionary theory for some idea about the origins of the organization (i.e., self-regulation) function that coordinates action and is the fundamental aspect of the sense of self and autonomy. Evolutionary thinking provides an account of why self-organizational processes matter, relating them to the variety of adaptive outcomes yielded by coordinated behavior. Clearly, an organism that fails at the tasks of coordination of its parts and functions is in serious trouble in many contexts. An animal whose motives are divided or in conflict, and/or who fails to hierarchically coordinate its goals, will, quite simply, be less likely to survive, as when, for example, the animal fails to stop feeding when confronted by a predator or lets grooming take precedence over sleep. Equally hazardous would be an animal whose motivation was easily entrained or controlled by external forces. Further, organisms (particularly mammalian species whose adaptation is linked to developmental change) that do not initiate (e.g., that do not explore, assimilate new information, or manipulate novel objects) may find themselves less flexible in the face of change. Thus, such a functional account of self-regulation may find a friendly foundation within evolutionary thought (Deci & Ryan, 2000). Moreover, the clear connection between well-being and the experience of autonomy versus heteronomy suggests a strong evolved preference system that is not merely an invention of Western human beings. A basic tenet of evolutionary psychology is that preferences that promoted the fitness of our ancestors tend to endure. Given the strength of human tendencies to resist heteronomous control and to self-regulate when possible, it is hard to discard the hypothesis that autonomy is an evolved capacity.

Surprisingly, however, evolutionary psychologists, as opposed to theoretical biologists such as Jonas (1966) and Mayr (1982), have almost exclusively focused on the evolutionary basis of *drive-related* behaviors—particularly sex, dominance, and aggression—while nearly ignoring the evolution of the central organizing processes that serve to regulate such behaviors. Thus, by not placing the idea of organization at its center, one comes to think of evolution as a process through which we added thousands of compartmentalized but disparate and uncoordinated modules, each functioning independently of all others. Indeed, in principle, the framework of Tooby and Cosmides (1992), we have noted elsewhere (Deci & Ryan, 2000), eliminates all generalized coordinating functions from consideration as adaptations. Yet perhaps the most general and obvious bestowal of the history of life has been the existence within each of us of a regulatory capacity to coordinate not only these modules but also the drives, needs, goals, and wants associated with them. In humans we call this regulatory capacity autonomy. It too is an evolved process. If there is any discontinuity in the selfness of humanity from the rest of nature it is, from an organismic perspective, not in the having of a self (see Mitchell, 2003) but in the fact that we know more thoroughly that we have one. Nonetheless, as our review indicates, individuals in a stimulating world can readily lose sight of it and enact behavior that is unreflective and poorly integrated.

Thus, we attempt to place the idea of self back into biological perspective by acknowledging the continuity of our active phenomenal core with the coordinated and active nature of other entities with whom we share the condition of life (Maturana & Varela, 1992). We suggest that the phenomenal self has its roots in the very process from which organization unfolds. Although most animals lack awareness of individuality as such, they manifest an active organization of behavior. It is this organizational tendency that in evolutionary perspective represents the deep structure on which the sense of self and autonomy in humans is built.

AUTONOMY AS A CROSS-CULTURAL CONCEPT

The importance and universality of autonomy has also been disputed by another strand of contemporary psychologists, namely, postmodernists and cultural relativists. Cultural relativists see autonomy as merely a social construction rather than a necessary feature of a well-regulated organism. Perhaps the most prominent theorists in this regard are Markus and Kitayama (1991), who have argued that autonomy, individualism, and independence are Western values and thus would predict behavior and well-being only of individuals raised in accord with those Western values. Cultural relativism has perhaps reached its pitch with expectancy-valence theorists such as Oishi (2000), who maintains that autonomy has no relevance outside a few individualistic Western cultures. In this view, it would seem to follow that within some cultures it would not functionally matter whether one was coerced or invited to act—that is, whether one was heteronomously controlled or allowed volition. The approach implies that there would be no psychological reaction to enslavement, or to having behaviors or values imposed on one.

However, when looked into, Oishi and others are not talking about autonomy as herein defined—they are talking about independence and individualism. Oishi (2000), like Bandura (1989), defined autonomy as acting independently of external influences, which, as we have already argued, misses the issue of whether or not one endorses the influences upon one. Further, we do not dispute that cultures value independence differentially. Some value the individualistic pursuit of goals, whereas others emphasize following tradition and placing the group ahead of the individual. But the question is, if people truly valued and endorsed collectivism, would they not be volitional in behaving in accord with their collectivistic values? Conversely, if they act collectivistically only out of coercion, seduction, or introjection, would this not have psychological costs for them? To us, the answers seem clear.

In recent work we have challenged the cross-culturalists' marginalization of autonomy in several ways. First, where autonomy has been properly assessed it appears to function in the East as it does in the West. For example, Japanese researchers Yamauchi and Tanaka (1998) and Hayamizu (1997) both applied SDT assessments of autonomy to Japanese school children. The findings show that those children who lacked autonomy for school showed less motivation and interest, were more superficial in their approach to learning, and had lower well-being. Sheldon, Elliot, Kim, and Kasser (2001) did a multicountry study of what makes events satisfying and found striking similarities across East and West, with all cultures viewing autonomy as a core issue. Subsequently, Chirkov et al. (2003) asked people from four countries (Russia, the United States, Turkey, and South Korea) to describe the reasons why they would perform a variety of behaviors, some of which were collectivistic, some individualistic. Although there were reliable differences in the types of behaviors people saw as typical of their ambient cultures, more autonomous reasons for engaging in behavior were associated with greater well-being in all cultures; there was simply no moderation of this effect by culture. Similarly, Chirkov and Ryan (2001) studied adolescents' perceived autonomy support in Russia (where it has presumably not been a predominant value) and the United States (where, presumably, it has). Although Russian teens, as predicted, experienced less parent and teacher support for autonomy than did Americans, the impact of autonomy support was the same in both countries. Greater autonomy support predicted more internalized and autonomous regulation in school and better mental health.

AUTONOMY IN PROCESS: MINDFULNESS, AWARENESS, AND CONGRUENCE

To summarize, in all domains, at all ages, and in all cultures, the behaviors we emit are experienced as more or less autonomous, and that makes a difference to performance and well-being. This sense of autonomy is not simply a functionless construction, but rather it is a phenomenal state reflective of the quality of behavioral organization. Autonomy is salient when one's actions are truly self-regulated, meaning one's actions are self-endorsed and congruent with values, motives, and needs. Further, one's experience of autonomy is affected by the social context of behavioral regulation. When people experience others exerting pressure or offering reward contingencies for specific outcomes, they may come to feel less autonomous in what they do. Conversely, under conditions where people are provided with greater discretion and choice, and/or nonarbitrary and therefore self-endorsement-worthy reasons for acting, the sense of autonomy is likely to be facilitated.

Although social contexts can have a clear impact on autonomy, in an ultimate sense appropriate to this book on existentialism, autonomy is something one must also cultivate within oneself and have the courage to enact. That is, in every instance one can act autonomously, which requires that one act in accord with what is authentic and real. Accordingly, autonomy is fostered or undermined from within by the individual's scope of and exercise of awareness. People are most likely to be entrained by others into nonautonomous acts or to be fooled into believing they are autonomous when they are not, to the extent that their awareness of inner and outer events is constricted or clouded. Conversely, being as fully aware as possible of what is occurring supports volition and responsibility.

In exploring this connection between awareness and autonomy, we have recently turned our attention to the phenomena of *mindfulness*—the awareness of what is occurring in the present moment. In a series of studies, Brown and Ryan (2003) assessed both between-person and within-person differences in mindfulness. First, those higher in mindfulness had higher well-being, better need satisfaction, and a generally greater sense of being autonomous in their behavioral regulation. Then, within persons, being in a state of greater mindfulness led people to report more autonomy, and to make more reliable, satisfying, and valued or "good" behavioral decisions. That is, when mindful, people did a better job of self-regulation. It seems then that one way to improve self-regulation is to give more mindful attention to what is occurring both within and without. From this basis in awareness more self-concordant behaviors follow.

Awareness facilitates greater autonomy, but awareness is not a freedom from determinants. In fact, with awareness, people have a better grasp of what is going on, including what is determining or influencing their behavior. Brown and Ryan (2003) demonstrated this in a rather simple way. They assessed people's affective state or moods using both implicit (implicit association test) and explicit (self-report) measures. As much literature suggests, these two types of assessment show only modest relations to one another. However, people high in mindfulness showed a greater concordance between explicit and implicit measures. In a related research effort, Thrash and Elliot (2002) showed that implicit and explicit measures of achievement motives were more consistent for people who were high on a measure of self-determination which included a strong self-awareness factor.

Mindfulness, like self-regulation, is of course both a subjective experience and a state of the organism. Indeed, this organismic state can be cultivated and enhanced or neglected and allowed to diminish. Brown and Ryan (2003) showed that people who actively cultivated mindfulness through meditative practices had more of it and that people who increased in mindfulness showed increases in health and well-being variables. Of course, the whole history of wisdom, counseling, and active philosophy in the West tells us the same story. People become more capable of autonomy—or of enacting behaviors they can stand behind—the more they base decisions and behaviors in awareness of self and environment. This is one reason why counseling, when autonomy supportive, has produced more lasting and positive change (Deci & Ryan, 1985; Markland, Ryan, Tobin, & Rollnick, 2003; Williams, Grow, Freedman, Ryan, & Deci, 1996). Many techniques of therapy, from cognitive behavioral therapy's self-monitoring to Freud's free association to Gendlin's focusing, to motivational interviewing's reflective examination of discrepancies, are intended to foster conditions that support people's awareness of what concerns them in order to come to a clearer, more integrative, and thus autonomous resolution.

CONCLUSION: THERE IS GOOD NEWS AND THERE ARE PLENTY OF ILLUSIONS

In the context of a renewed vigor to claims that we possess no autonomy or capacity for will, SDT joins with existentialists in stressing the following: First, people are extremely vulnerable to being controlled and inauthentic. They are particularly vulnerable to the degree to which they either do not or cannot reflectively or mindfully consider feelings, motives, and needs. Reflective consideration, further, is not just a rational process; it concerns really allowing feelings, perceptions, beliefs, and agendas to come into awareness. Particularly important is the sense of ownership, congruence, and authenticity, which are the hallmarks of integrated action. Second, most people, most of the time, are not awake to what is occurring and are not mindfully or autonomously acting. This is because of the often distracting and seductive influences in life that diminish active awareness as well as of our defensive tendencies to avoid responsibility and its consequences. The power of nonconscious primes to instigate behavior one might not reflectively endorse has always been evident, but the capacity of our culture to harness and apply them is growing exponentially. This makes the engagement of autonomy all the more critical. Third, like our existential colleagues we see the inauthentic life as costly. It is not only functionally less adaptive in most contexts, it is also duller, less vital, and less eudaimonically fulfilling. Finally, we see no incompatibility between recognition of autonomy as a human potential and of a deterministic worldview. In fact, the very reason why existentialists wrote their provocative evangelical callings, and why in SDT we consult with organizations and invent clinical techniques to enhance self-regulation, is to awaken and refresh the possibility of autonomy. We are, in this sense, trying to provide inputs that will catalyze in our readers the capacity to self-regulate and the courage to be more fully human.

REFERENCES

Amabile, T. M. (1983). *The social psychology of creativity*. New York: Springer-Verlag.

Assor, A., Roth, G., & Deci, E. L. (2004). The emotional costs of parents' conditional regard: A self-determination theory analysis. *Journal of Personality, 72*, 47–88.

Bandura, A. (1989). Human agency in social cognitive theory. *American Psychologist, 44*, 1175–1184.

Bargh, J. (1997). The automaticity of everyday life. In R. S. Wyer Jr. (Ed.), *The automaticity of everyday life: Advances in social cognition* (Vol. 10, pp. 1–61). Mahwah, NJ: Erlbaum.

Bargh, J., & Ferguson, M. J. (2000). Beyond behaviorism: On the automaticity of higher mental processes. *Psychological Bulletin, 126*, 925–945.

Bem, D. J. (1967). Self-perception: An alternative interpretation of cognitive dissonance phenomena. *Psychological Review, 74*, 183–200.

Blais, M. R., Sabourin S., Boucher, C., & Vallerand, R. (1990). Toward a motivational model of couple happiness. *Journal of Personality and Social Psychology, 59*, 1021–1031.

Brown, K. W., & Ryan, R. M. (2003). The benefits of being present: Mindfulness and its role in psychological well-being. *Journal of Personality and Social Psychology, 84*, 822–848.

Chirkov, V., & Ryan, R. M. (2001). Parent and teacher autonomy-support in Russian and U.S. adolescents: Common effects on well-being and academic motivation. *Journal of Cross-Cultural Psychology, 32*, 618–635.

Chirkov, V., Ryan, R. M., Kim, Y., & Kaplan, U. (2003). Differentiating autonomy from individualism and independence: A self-determination theory perspective on the internalization of cultural orientations and well-being. *Journal of Personality and Social Psychology, 84*, 97–110.

Csikszentmihalyi, M. (1990). *Flow*. New York: Harper.

deCharms, R. (1968). *Personal causation: The internal affective determinants of behavior*. New York: Academic Press.

Deci, E. L. (1971). Effects of externally mediated rewards on intrinsic motivation. *Journal of Personality and Social Psychology, 18*, 105–115.

Deci, E. L., Eghrari, H., Patrick, B. C., & Leone, D. R. (1994). Facilitating internalization: The self-determination theory perspective. *Journal of Personality, 62*, 119–142.

Deci, E. L., Koestner, R., & Ryan, R. M. (1999). A meta-analytic review of experiments examining the effects of extrinsic rewards on intrinsic motivation. *Psychological Bulletin, 125,* 627–668.

Deci, E. L., & Ryan, R. M. (1980a). The empirical exploration of intrinsic motivational processes. In L. Berkowitz (Ed.), *Advances in experimental social psychology* (Vol. 13, pp. 39–80). New York: Academic Press.

Deci, E. L., & Ryan, R. M. (1980b). Self-determination theory: When mind mediates behavior. *Journal of Mind and Behavior, 1,* 33–43.

Deci, E. L., & Ryan, R. M. (1985). *Intrinsic motivation and self-determination in human behavior.* New York: Plenum Press.

Deci, E. L., & Ryan, R. M. (1995). Human autonomy: The basis for true self-esteem. In M. Kernis (Ed.), *Efficacy, agency, and self-esteem* (pp. 31–49). New York: Plenum Press.

Deci, E. L., & Ryan, R. M. (2000). The "what" and the "why" of goal pursuits: Human needs and the self-determination of behavior. *Psychological Inquiry, 11,* 227–268.

Dworkin, G. (1988). *The theory and practice of autonomy.* New York: Cambridge University Press.

Eisenberger, R., & Cameron, J. (1996). Detrimental effects of reward: Reality or myth? *American Psychologist, 51,* 1153–1166.

Eisenberger, R., Pierce, W. D., & Cameron, J. (1999). Effects of reward on intrinsic motivation—Negative, neutral, and positive: Comment on Deci, Koestner, and Ryan (1999). *Psychological Bulletin, 125,* 677–691.

Frankfurt, H. (1971) Freedom of the will and the concept of person. *Journal of Philosophy,* 68, 5–20

Frattaroli, E. (2001). *Healing the soul in the age of the brain.* New York: Penguin.

Freud, S. (1977) *Five lectures on psycho-analysis.* New York: Norton. (Original work published 1909)

Fromm, E. (1955). *The sane society.* New York: Fawcett.

Harter, S. (1981). A new self-report scale of intrinsic versus extrinsic orientation in the classroom: Motivational and informational components. *Developmental Psychology, 17,* 300–312.

Hayamizu, T. (1997). Between intrinsic and extrinsic motivation: Examination of reasons for academic study based on the theory of internalization. *Japanese Psychological Research, 39,* 98–108.

Heidegger, M. (1962). *Being and time.* New York: Harper & Row

Heider, F. (1958). *The psychology of interpersonal relations.* New York: Wiley.

Heider, F., & Simmel, M. (1944). An experimental study of apparent behavior. *American Journal of Psychology, 37,* 243–259.

Hennessey, B. A. (2000). Self-determination theory and the social psychology of creativity. *Psychological Inquiry, 11,* 293–297.

Hesse, H. (1925). *Demian.* New York: Harper & Row.

Hill, T. E. (1991). *Autonomy and self-respect.* New York: Cambridge University Press.

Hodgins, H. S., & Knee, C. R. (2002). The integrating self and conscious experience. In E. L. Deci & R. M. Ryan (Eds.), *Handbook of self-determination research* (pp. 87–100). Rochester, NY: University of Rochester Press.

Horney, K. (1950). *Neurosis and human growth.* New York: Norton.

Jonas, H. (1966). *The phenomenon of life: Toward a philosophical biology.* New York: Dell.

Jourard, S. M. (1968). *Disclosing man to himself.* Princeton, NJ: Van Nostrand.

Kasser, T., & Ryan, R. M. (1996). Further examining the American dream: Differential correlates of intrinsic and extrinsic goals. *Personality and Social Psychology Bulletin, 22,* 80–87.

Kasser, T., & Ryan, R. M. (2001). Be careful what you wish for: Optimal functioning and the relative attainment of intrinsic and extrinsic goals. In P. Schmuck & K. M. Sheldon (Eds.), *Life goals and well-being: Towards a positive psychology of human striving* (pp. 115–129). Goettingen, Germany: Hogrefe & Huber.

Kierkegaard, S. (1954). *Fear and trembling/Sickness unto death.* New York: Doubleday. (Original work published 1849)

Kierkegaard, S. (1948). *Purity of heart is to will one thing.* New York: Harper & Row. (Original work published 1846)

Kuhl, J., & Kazen, M. (1994). Self-discrimination and memory: State orientation and false self-ascription of assigned activities. *Journal of Personality and Social Psychology, 66,* 1103–1115.

La Guardia J. G., & Ryan, R. M. (2000). What is well-being and how does one attain it? A self-determination theory perspective on basic psychological needs. *Revue Québécoise de Psychologie, 21,* 281–304.

La Guardia J. G., Ryan, R. M., Couchman, C. E., & Deci, E. L. (2000). Within-person variation in security of attachment: A self-determination theory perspective on attachment, need fulfillment, and well-being. *Journal of Personality and Social Psychology, 79,* 367–384.

Laing, R. D. (1960). *The divided self.* Baltimore: Penguin.

Levesque, C. S., & Brown, K. W. (2003). *Mindful awareness as a moderator of the relation between implicit and explicit motives.* Unpublished manuscript, University of Southern Missouri.

Levesque, C. S., & Pelletier, L. (2003). On the investigation of primed and chronic autonomous and heteronomous motivational orientations. *Personality and Social Psychology Bulletin, 29,* 1570–1584.

Libet, B. (1999). Do we have free will? *Journal of Consciousness Studies, 6,* 47–57.

Markland, D., Ryan, R. M., Tobin, V., & Rollnick, S. (2003). *Motivational interviewing and self-determination theory.* Unpublished manuscript, University of Wales, Bangor.

Markus, H. R., & Kitayama, S. (1991). Culture and the self: Implications for cognition, emotion, and motivation. *Psychological Review, 92,* 224–253.

Maturana, H. R., & Varela, F. J. (1992). *The tree of knowledge: The biological roots of human understanding* (rev. ed.). Boston: Shambhala.

Mayr, E. (1982). *The growth of biological thought: Diversity, evolution, and inheritance.* Cambridge, MA: Harvard University Press.

Merleau-Ponty, M. (1964). *The primacy of perception.* Evanston, IL: Northwestern University Press.

Michotte, A. (1954). *The perception of causality.* New York: Basic Books.

Mitchell, R. W. (2003). Subjectivity and self-recognition in animals. In M. R. Leary & J. P. Tangney (Eds.), *Handbook of self and identity* (pp. 567–593). New York: Guilford Press.

Moustakas, C. (1995). *Being-in, being-for, being-with.* Northvale, NJ: Jason Aronson.

Mullen, J. D. (1981). *Kierkegaard's philosophy: Self-deception and cowardice in the present age.* New York: Mentor.

Nietzsche, F. (1949). *Beyond good and evil* (M. Cowan, Trans.). Chicago: Henry Regnery. (Original work published 1886)

Oishi, S. (2000). Goals as cornerstones of subjective well-being: Linking individuals and cultures. In E. Diener & E. M. Suh (Eds.), *Culture and subjective well-being* (pp. 87–112). Cambridge, MA: Bradford.

Olafson, F. A. (1967). *Principles and persons: An ethical interpretation of existentialism.* Baltimore: Johns Hopkins Press

Pfander, A. (1967). *Phenomenology of willing and motivation* (H. Spiegelberg, Trans.). Evanston, IL: Northwestern University Press. (Original work published 1908)

Pinker, S. (2002). *The blank slate: The modern denial of human nature.* New York: Viking.

Plant, R., & Ryan, R. M. (1985). Intrinsic motivation and the effects of self-consciousness, self-awareness, and ego-involvement: An investigation of internally controlling styles. *Journal of Personality, 53,* 435–449.

Polanyi, M. (1958). *Personal knowledge.* Chicago: University of Chicago Press.

Pyszczynski, T., Greenberg, J., & Solomon, S. (1999). A dual process model of defense against conscious and unconscious death-related thoughts: An extension of terror management theory. *Psychological Review, 106,* 835–845.

Reis, H. T., Sheldon, K. M., Gable, S. L., Roscoe, J., & Ryan, R. M. (2000). Daily well-being: The role of autonomy, competence, and relatedness. *Personality and Social Psychology Bulletin, 26,* 419–435.

Ricoeur, P. (1966). *Freedom and nature: The voluntary and the involuntary* (E. V. Kohak, Trans.). Evanston: Northwestern University Press

Rogers, C. (1963). The actualizing tendency in relation to "motives" and to consciousness. In M. R. Jones (Ed.), *Nebraska symposium on motivation* (Vol. 11, pp. 1–24). Lincoln: University of Nebraska Press.

Ryan, R. M. (1982). Control and information in the intrapersonal sphere: An extension of cognitive evaluation theory. *Journal of Personality and Social Psychology, 43,* 450–461.

Ryan, R. M. (1993). Agency and organization: Intrinsic motivation, autonomy and the self in psychological development. In J. Jacobs (Ed.), *Nebraska symposium on motivation: Developmental perspectives on motivation* (Vol. 40, pp. 1–56). Lincoln: University of Nebraska Press.

Ryan, R. M. (1995). Psychological needs and the facilitation of integrative processes. *Journal of Personality, 63,* 397–427.

Ryan, R. M., & Connell, J. P. (1989). Perceived locus of causality and internalization: Examining reasons for acting in two domains. *Journal of Personality and Social Psychology, 57,* 749–761.

Ryan, R. M., & Deci, E. L. (2000a). Intrinsic and extrinsic motivation: Classic definitions and new directions. *Contemporary Educational Psychology, 25,* 54–67.

Ryan, R. M., & Deci, E. L. (2000b) Self-determination theory and the facilitation of intrinsic motivation, social development and well-being. *American Psychologist, 55,* 68–78.

Ryan, R. M., & Deci, E. L. (2000c). The darker and brighter sides of human existence: Basic psychological needs as a unifying concept. *Psychological Inquiry, 11,* 319–338.

Ryan, R. M., & Deci, E. L. (2000d). When rewards compete with nature: The undermining of intrinsic motivation and self-regulation. In C. Sansone & J. M. Harackiewicz (Eds.), *Intrinsic and extrinsic motivation: The search for optimal motivation and performance* (pp. 13–54). New York: Academic Press.

Ryan, R. M., & Deci, E. L. (2001). On happiness and human potentials: A review of research on hedonic and eudaimonic well-being. *Annual Review of Psychology, 52,* 141–166.

Ryan, R. M., Deci, E. L., & Grolnick, W. S. (1995). Autonomy, relatedness, and the self: Their relation to development and psychopathology. In D. Cicchetti & D. J. Cohen (Eds.), *Developmental psychopathology: Vol. 1. Theory and methods* (pp. 618–655). New York: Wiley.

Ryan, R. M., Koestner, R., & Deci, E. L. (1991). Ego-involved persistence: When free-choice behavior is not intrinsically motivated. *Motivation and Emotion, 15,* 185–205.

Ryan, R. M., Kuhl, J., & Deci, E. L. (1997). Nature and autonomy: Organizational view of social and neurobiological aspects of self-regulation in behavior and development. *Development and Psychopathology, 9,* 701–728.

Ryan, R. M., & La Guardia, J. G. (1999). Achievement motivation within a pressured society: Intrinsic and extrinsic motivations to learn and the politics of school reform. In T. Urdan (Ed.), *Advances in motivation and achievement* (Vol. 11, pp. 45–85). Greenwich, CT: JAI Press.

Ryan, R. M., La Guardia, J. G. Butzel, J., Chirkov, V., & Kim Y. M. (2003). *On the interpersonal regulation of emotions: Emotional reliance across gender, relationships and cultures.* Unpublished manuscript, University of Rochester.

Sartre, J.-P. (1956). *Being and nothingness.* New York: Philosophical Library.

Schor, J. B. (1991). *The overworked American: The unexpected decline of leisure.* New York: Basic Books.

Shapiro, D. (1981). *Autonomy and rigid character.* New York: Basic Books.

Sheldon, K. M., Elliot, A. J., Kim, Y., & Kasser, T. (2001). What's satisfying about satisfying events? Comparing ten candidate psychological needs. *Journal of Personality and Social Psychology, 80,* 325–339.

Skinner, B. F. (1953). *Science and human behavior.* New York: Macmillan.

Skinner, B. F. (1971). *Beyond freedom and dignity.* New York: Knopf.

Spence, S. A., & Firth, C. D. (1999). Toward a functional anatomy of volition. *Journal of Consciousness Studies, 6,* 11–29.

Spiegelberg, H. (1972). *Phenomenology in psychology and psychiatry.* Evanston, IL: Northwestern University Press.

Thrash, T. M., & Elliot, A. J. (2002) Implicit and self-attributed achievement motives: Concordance and predictive validity. *Journal of Personality, 70,* 729–755.

Tooby, J., & Cosmides, L. (1992). The psychological foundations of culture. In J. H. Barkow, L. Cosmides, & J. Tooby (Eds.), *The adapted mind: Evolutionary psychology and the generation of culture* (pp. 19–136). New York: Oxford University Press.

Utman, C. H. (1997). Performance effects of motivational state: A meta-analysis. *Personality and Social Psychology Review, 1,* 170–182.

Vallerand, R. J. (1997). Toward a hierarchical model of intrinsic and extrinsic motivation. In M. P. Zanna (Ed.), *Advances in experimental social psychology* (Vol. 29, pp. 271–360). San Diego: Academic Press.

Warnock, M. (1970). *Existentialism.* London: Oxford University Press.

Wegner, D. (2002). *The illusion of conscious will.* Cambridge, MA: MIT Press.

Wegner, D. M., & Wheatley, T. (1999) Apparent mental causation: Sources of the experience of will. *American psychologist, 54,* 480–491.

Wild, J. (1965). Authentic existence: A new approach to "Value Theory." In J. M. Edie (Ed.), *An invitation to phenomenology: Studies in the philosophy of experience* (pp. 59–78). Chicago: Quadrangle.

Williams, G. C. (2002). Improving patient's health through supporting the autonomy of patients and providers. In E. L. Deci & R. M. Ryan (Eds.), *Handbook of self-determination research* (pp. 233–254). Rochester, NY: University of Rochester Press.

Williams, G. C., Deci, E. L., & Ryan, R. M. (1998). Building health-care partnerships by supporting autonomy: Promoting maintained behavior change and positive health outcomes. In P. Hinton-Walker, A. L. Suchman, & R. Botelho (Eds.) *Partnerships, power and process: Transforming health care delivery* (pp. 68–87). Rochester, NY: University of Rochester Press.

Williams, G. C., Grow, V. M., Freedman, Z., Ryan, R. M., & Deci, E. L. (1996). Motivational predictors of weight loss and weight-loss maintenance. *Journal of Personality and Social Psychology, 70,* 115–126.

Wilson, E. O. (1975) *Sociobiology: The new synthesis.* Cambridge, MA: Belknap Press.

Wilson, T. D. (2002). *Strangers to ourselves.* Cambridge, MA: Belknap Press.

Winnicott, D. W. (1965). *The maturational process and the facilitating environment.* New York: International Universities Press.

Wolff, S. (1990). *Freedom within reason.* New York: Oxford University Press.

Yamauchi, H., & Tanaka, K. (1998). Relations of autonomy, self-referenced beliefs and self-regulated learning among Japanese children. *Psychological Reports, 82,* 803–816.

Chapter 29

Nonbecoming, Alienated Becoming, and Authentic Becoming

A Goal-Based Approach

Tim Kasser
Kennon M. Sheldon

One of the fundamental conditions of human existence is the fact that we live in a world of time, in which the present develops from the past and becomes the future (Boss, 1963). As such, we humans must establish some type of relations with all three of these temporalities (May, 1983). For example, we might be burdened by past traumas or feel pleasant nostalgia for the past (see Sedikides, Wildschut, & Baden, Chapter 13, this volume); we might flee from the present or live with no concern for tomorrow. Although a person's relationships to the past and present are certainly important for understanding that individual, the future holds a special prominence in the writings of existentialists such as Heidegger (see Barrett, 1958), as it is the realm of temporality that holds not only the fact of the death or non-being that awaits each of us but also the potential for self-expression and self-development—in Kierkegaard's (1849/1941) words, the possibility of becoming "that self which one truly is" (p. 29).

Indeed, if there is a central proposition that diverse existential thinkers might agree with, it is that we humans have a special responsibility to try to fulfill our potentialities and possibilities, or to become who we really are. In this chapter, we distinguish this existentialist ideal, "authentic becoming," from more insalubrious possibilities of "non-becoming," in which individuals remain stuck in the past, and from "alienated becoming," in which people move into the future in ways that alienate them from their deepest desires and "true selves." We hope to demonstrate that non-becoming, alienated becoming, and authentic becoming are sound ideas that can be fruitfully understood and approached via contemporary empirical and theoretical work on people's personal goals and strivings. Our conviction that a goal-based approach is useful for understanding humans' relations with the future comes from the fact that goals and strivings represent people's proactive attempts to move from a current state to an improved or ideal future state (Emmons, 1989; Zaleski, 1994), which, as we try to show later, is part of the very nature of becoming.

We begin the chapter by describing how goals help people become and how problems with goals can explain non-becoming. Next we propose that whether becoming is authentic or alienated depends both on why people are pursuing their goals and what goals they are pursuing. We conclude with a discussion of the personal and social factors which support authentic becoming or which conduce toward non-becoming and alienated becoming.

At the outset, however, we want to make an important disclaimer: We are not trying to suggest that the only way to an ideal existence is through goal pursuit. The future is not everything about existence, and it is important for people's whole development that they are interacting with and learning from the past, as well as at times just "being here now" in the present; in other words, a balance of time experience probably helps adjustment. Further, there is much to be said for "letting things develop" and "going with the flow" as one moves into the future. If one's life is entirely structured by one's intentional goals, one may miss out on chance occurrences that happily help one move forward in life. Finally, as we discuss later in the chapter, sometimes goals direct people toward alienated becoming, in which case it is most sensible to abandon those goals. In short, we do not mean to say that goals are the be-all and end-all of a healthy existence but, rather, that they are an important facet of healthy becoming, and thus of healthy existence.

TO BECOME OR NOT TO BECOME: THAT IS THE QUESTION

As noted by many wags, change is the only constant, as something new is forever unfolding out of that which is. Time marches along ceaselessly, with the present receding into the past and becoming the future. This fact is part of what existentialists call the *umwelt*—the natural world of physical law (May, 1983). As beings-in-the-world, we therefore have to face and accommodate to this change.

One of the ways in which we try to change ourselves (and sometimes the world around us) is by setting goals—that is, by specifying some particular state in the future which we would like to reach and then mobilizing our inner and outer resources to bring that future state into existence. Carver and Scheier's (1981, 1990, 1998) control theory of action is especially useful for understanding how goal setting leads to becoming. According to this model, behavior is sequentially energized and regulated by peoples' cognitive control systems. Control systems are hierarchically organized, such that broader goals set the standard for and then regulate the operation of more concrete goals, which in turn set the standard for the operation of even more concrete goals, and so on down the line. In the process, individuals reduce discrepancies between current states and desired future states and move forward through time and become.

To take a somewhat prosaic example: when people are hungry, they typically form the goal of "eating something," which in turn initiates and regulates the pursuit of a series of lower-level goals: One forms the goal of getting up from one's chair to become a standing person rather than a sitting person; one walks to and opens the refrigerator to become a person looking at food rather than a person looking at a wall; one takes a slice of cold pizza out to become a person holding food rather than a person with an empty hand; one puts the pizza in one's mouth and chews to become a satiated person rather than a hungry person. In this way, becoming (i.e., changing state from hungry-in-the-chair person to satiated person) is mediated through a series of behavioral enactments organized by a series of behavioral goals.

The same analysis is also applicable at higher levels of the action system. For example, an undergraduate with the desired future goal of "becoming the chief executive officer (CEO) of a Fortune 500 company" may, at the present moment, be retrieving a book at the library, in order to complete a paper, in order to do well in a course, in order to achieve a high undergraduate grade point average, in order to be accepted to Harvard Business School, in order to achieve a managerial job at a large company—each of which is a goal that simultaneously serves his overarching career goal of becoming a CEO of a big company.

This general process in which more molecular behaviors are sequentially enacted in order to move the person, bit by bit, toward long-term goals is centrally relevant for any analysis of "becoming." But goals are also helpful in shedding light on people's *failure* to become and to move forward with the ever-changing flux and flow of existence. As described by Hall and Lindsey (1978), "To refuse to become is to lock oneself in a constricted and darkened room" (p. 331). Said differently, sometimes people relate to the future by not relating to it, by trying to avoid the possibilities it holds, or by inflexibly moving forward in a way that is unresponsive to changes in the world around. Next we discuss these three different ways in which people might fail to become from the perspective of theory and research on goals.

Catatonia

The cardinal feature of the subtype of schizophrenia known as catatonia is that the individual does not move; indeed, such individuals can be placed in unusual positions or pricked with pins but nonetheless remain fixed in space and time, seemingly unresponsive to the world (American Psychiatric Association, 1994). The person in this state of being does not seem to be moving forward into the future at all. Less extreme cases of stasis occur when people seem to have no goals for the future and no intentions to develop their potentials. Such persons are not necessarily content with who they are, but they are doing nothing to move forward. This state is notable in what Marcia (1993) refers to as identity diffusion. Diffused individuals have few commitments and do not seem to care where they are headed in life; instead, they just float around in a not-so-happy present, "going nowhere fast." They remain stagnant, while the rest of the world moves on.

The empirical literature on goals makes it reasonably clear that people who do not have goals indeed function more poorly and are less happy than those who do have goals. In other words, it is almost always worse to be in stasis or amotivated than to be moving into the future and motivated (Deci & Ryan, 1985). In support of this claim, Oyserman and Markus (1990) showed that delinquent adolescents who reported having salient possible self-images referring to any type of possible future (be it negative or positive) reformed and adapted better than did adolescents without such orienting self-goals. Industrial–organizational research similarly shows that employee performance is maximized when employees set goals, particularly when they set difficult, specific goals (Locke & Latham, 1990). In addition to merely having goals, it is also important to attach some personal importance to one's goals; those who do typically fare better than those who do not (Emmons, 1986).

Avoidance

A second type of non-becoming is an avoidant relationship to the future. People with this orientation are actually very interested in the future but their primary concern is to avoid a particular feared future, rather than to actively strive toward something new that is desired (Carver & Scheier, 1998). Although avoidance-oriented people are at least motivated, their focus is on stasis and their actions are aimed primarily at conserving a preferred state. For example, an insecurely attached woman may be constantly alert for signs that her lover's attention is fading, or a fearful student may try to anticipate every way in which he might make a mistake or displease the teacher, all in the service of lessening the likelihood that these negative outcomes might happen.

Unfortunately, the empirical literature indicates that people with strong avoidance orientations typically do not succeed very well in their goals and end up feeling worse about themselves (Elliot, Sheldon, & Church, 1997). In other words, the more people frame their goals in avoidance terms, the more poorly they do at attaining their goals, and the more problematic their goals are for their well-being. To return to our examples, the anxious woman's paranoia may wear thin and actually drive her lover away, and the apprehensive student's literalism may ultimately undermine his understanding and performance. Two noteworthy features of avoidance goals might explain this problem. First, it is more difficult to block all paths to a negative outcome than it is to find a single path to a positive outcome. In other words, the task of staying in one place, resisting the flux of the *umwelt*, is more difficult than we typically imagine. A second problem is that a continual focus on negative possibilities tends to produce a detrimental emotional tone and reduced cognitive expectancies, which can in turn contribute to poorer performance.

Obsession

A third type of non-becoming is being obsessed with goals that are inappropriate for the current situation. Here, rather than failing to set goals, or failing to set approach or change-promoting goals, the person may have failed to disengage from approach goals that are no longer (or were never) suitable. In other words, rather than being stuck in the past or present (like the catatonic or diffused person), an obsession leads a person to be stuck on the "wrong" future because of past decisions.

Consider the following example: I am walking to the kitchen in order to get myself something to eat when my child screams from his bedroom. Ideally, I am able to disengage from the first goal (i.e., getting food) and respond to what my environment has become (i.e., my child who was calm has become upset); thus, I change my path from the kitchen to the child's bedroom in order to adapt to a changing *umwelt*. What this example points to is that becoming, and the goal pursuit which acts in its service, is ideally a flexible enterprise in which the person responds to the changes that are occurring in both self and world and considers those as he or she continues to become at an individual level. Or, to return to our undergraduate who hopes to become an important CEO, he does not necessarily have to see the goal through to its very end if it turns out to be a poor choice. Signing up for microeconomics or even declaring a business major does not forever commit him to the higher-level goal; if it turns out that the undergraduate does not really have the aptitudes or interests that match with those required for managing an enormous company, or if a more interesting opportunity were to come his way, he would probably be best off to disengage from that goal and try something that brings more fulfillment.

Several theoreticians suggest that the failure to disengage from goals can lead to problems with depression (Carver & Scheier, 1990; Klinger, 1975; Pyszczynski & Greenberg, 1987), and Kuhl's (1981; see also Kuhl & Koole, Chapter 26, this volume) work on state-oriented individuals similarly suggests that people who have difficulty disengaging from inappropriate or failed goals are prone to negative affect. This work makes it clear that for optimal becoming to occur, people must be able to recognize that the past is past and that new or different goals may now be most adaptive. Unfortunately, however, many people attempt to relive the "glory days" and hold on to their youth (i.e., non-becoming) or just stay on the same treadworn path and thus continue to make the decisions that served them well (or even not so well) in the past.

ALIENATED AND AUTHENTIC BECOMING

The existentialists were among the first thinkers to deeply explore people's relationship to and movement into the future, but they also realized that mere becoming was not enough to ensure healthy becoming. Kierkegaard's injunction to "become that self which one truly is" implies that a person might become someone *other* than who one really is, or develop a *false self* which does not authentically represent the person. Thus, although people may successfully move into the future, pursuing personally important approach goals in a flexible manner, they may still fail to become who they really are. In other words, rather than becoming more authentic, they are becoming alienated from their deepest possibilities, their real needs, and their true self.

All of us at times pursue activities that do not fit with our interests, our needs, or our potentials. Such activities are annoying and irritating but, like death and gravity, are among the facts of existence to which we humans must adapt. From our goal-based perspective, the real problem occurs when individuals orient too much of their lives around goals that are not facilitative of authentic becoming and that instead serve to alienate the person. To return to our budding Fortune 500 CEO, suppose that since his early childhood his father has been pressuring him to make as much money as possible and to obtain a position of great power. Or, suppose that the culture in which this student lives glorifies profit seeking, acquisition, and wealth as primary signifiers of success and harbingers of happiness. Such interpersonal pressures and cultural encouragement might lead the student to ignore the facts that accounting, supply/demand curves, and the competition of the business world fit neither his aptitudes nor his interests, which seem to lie instead in the direction of carpentry. Although the student may nonetheless pursue the goal of being a CEO, it is actually in the service of becoming "a self that he is not."

Our early work (Sheldon & Kasser, 1995), based largely in self-determination theory (Deci & Ryan, 1985, 2000), attempted to understand these issues by examining the quality of people's personal goals as markers of personality integration, or what we called *congruence*. We suggested that the extent to which goals are integrated, congruent, or what we in this context would call authentic depends on two characteristics of the goals. First, goals are congruent and authentic when people pursue them for autonomous reasons of interest and identification rather than for controlled reasons of internal and external pressure. Second, goals are congruent when they are aimed toward intrinsic pursuits of personal growth, affiliation, and community feeling rather than extrinsic pursuits of financial success, image, and popularity. As we describe in more detail later, when people's goals are congruent, they move into the future in a way which supports authentic becoming, whereas when their goals are not congruent, individuals are less likely to become who they really are and instead move toward increased alienation.

The "Why" of Motivation and the Self-Concordance Construct

Existential thinkers such as Kierkegaard and Sartre placed great emphasis on the motivations behind people's actions (Barrett, 1958), as such inquiry helps to reveal whether or not one's behavior is authentic. Does one go to church and read the Bible from deep faith and commitment or to look good in the community and earn a few points in case there really is a God? Does one interact with one's neighbor to facilitate good community relations or because one wants to borrow his rototiller next Saturday? Asking these types of questions helps to clarify whether a person's behavior is an authentic expression of his or her real self or whether the behavior emanates from the self-serving desire to obtain rewards or to escape internal and social censure.

Substantial research supports the idea that the reasons people give for their behavior bear important relationships to both their motivation and their well-being (Deci & Ryan, 2000), and this is clearly also the case for personal goals (Sheldon, 2002). To investigate this issue, we have adopted self-determination theory's strategy of measuring people's "perceived locus of causality" (Ryan & Connell, 1989; Sheldon & Kasser, 1995, 1998, 2001), or what they experience as the reasons behind their behavior. Within this framework, people are considered to be acting authentically in their goal pursuit if they report "intrinsic" reasons for pursuing their goals, such as "for the fun or enjoyment the goal provides me," or "identified" reasons such as "because I personally value the goal." Feeling controlled (and thus alienated) is signaled when people report that they pursue their goals for "introjected" reasons such as "because I would feel ashamed, guilty, or bad about myself otherwise" or for "external" reasons such as "because of the praise or rewards I will get from others." A convenient summary variable, which Sheldon (2002) recently called self-concordance, can be computed by summing people's reported intrinsic and identified motivation and subtracting their external and introjected motivation (see Baumann & Kuhl, 2003, for another interesting way to assess alienation and authenticity in goals).

Past studies have found that people who rate their goals as more self-concordant (1) experience higher concurrent well-being (Sheldon & Kasser, 1995); (2) put more subsequent effort into their goals (Sheldon & Elliot, 1998, 1999); (3) better achieve their goals (Sheldon & Elliot, 1999; Sheldon & Houser-Marko, 2001); (4) derive more daily need satisfaction from their goal-based activity (Sheldon & Elliot, 1999); and (5) report greater gains in global well-being as a result of attaining their goals (Sheldon & Elliot, 1999; Sheldon & Kasser, 1998). Self-concordant individuals are also higher in a variety of positive personality traits, such as empathy, openness to experience, autonomy orientation, cognitive integration, and self-esteem (Sheldon & Kasser, 1995; see Sheldon, 2002, for a review).

Returning to our aspiring CEO, then, if he feels that the pursuit of his goal really is about keeping his father happy or living up to what he believes he "should" do in his particular capitalistic society, his becoming is alienated and taking him further from who he really is and what he really wants out of life. Consequently, he is likely to experience a number of decrements in his well-being and personal life. On the other hand, if he feels genuinely interested in the challenges involved and deeply committed and identified with his goal, his becoming is probably more authentic, and thus his general adaptation and happiness in life should be relatively high.

The What of "Motivation" and the Intrinsic–Extrinsic
Content Distinction

Existential thinkers questioned not only why people do what they do but also what they actually were doing. For example, May (1983) and Fromm (1976), as well as their humanistic cousins Maslow (1954) and Rogers (1964), insisted that understanding a person's authenticity also depends on asking questions such as the following: Has a person organized his life around money and status or around contributing to others and to society? What are the differences between a person who really wants the right "image" or "look" versus someone who really wants to become more accepting of who she really is? Framed in terms of Fromm's (1976) distinction, what is the difference between a lifestyle based on "having" and one based on "being"?

To conceptualize this aspect of alienated versus authentic becoming from a goal perspective, we have distinguished between goals that have "extrinsic" content and those that have "intrinsic" content (Kasser & Ryan, 1996). Extrinsic aspirations are typically focused on obtaining rewards or praise and are usually a means to some other end. Desires for money, image, and popularity are three typical extrinsic aspirations. Intrinsic goals, in contrast, are those that are assumed to be inherently satisfying to pursue, as they generally fulfill people's psychological needs. The three intrinsic aspirations we have studied are self-acceptance (knowing oneself), emotional affiliation (being connected to family and friends), and community feeling (helping the world).

Our research has typically used one of two methods for assessing people's intrinsic versus extrinsic goal orientation. First, with the Aspiration Index subjects rate the importance of a variety of different types of aspirations (Kasser & Ryan, 1993, 1996, 2001). In the second strategy, subjects generate their own goals and then rate how helpful each goal is in moving toward different intrinsic or extrinsic "possible futures" (Sheldon & Kasser, 1995, 1998, 2001). Both strategies provide a means of assessing the relative centrality (Rokeach, 1973) of intrinsic versus extrinsic goals within the person's goal system.

A growing body of research demonstrates that people who have relatively central intrinsic goals report higher well-being than do individuals oriented more toward extrinsic goals (see Kasser, 2002b, for a fuller review). Studies of teenagers, college students, and adults in various nations around the world have consistently demonstrated that when people place a relatively high value on money, image, and status, they report less happiness and greater distress on various indices of well-being. Evidence suggests that the strong pursuit of money, image, and status leads people into a style of life that poorly satisfies psychological needs, such as those for competence, relatedness, and autonomy (Deci & Ryan, 2000; Kasser, 2002a). For example, their sense of worth is continually hinged on their standing relative to others, their relationships with others are often insecure or objectifying, and they often feel pressures to do things they do not really want to do. In contrast, intrinsic aspirations appear to be more facilitative of need satisfaction, as they provide a healthy sense of esteem, bring people closer to each other, and promote feelings of authenticity and flow.

In thinking about our budding CEO, then, we may be especially worried about the course of his becoming if his strivings for wealth and status lead him to ignore his personal growth and interests, neglect social relationships, and do little to nothing to benefit the community around him. When a person's value system is unbalanced in this regard, the evidence suggests that the course of becoming is alienated. In contrast, authentic becoming might be possible if this student's pursuit of profit is balanced with the more intrinsic aims of life, and he recognizes that, like sweets and fats, money and power might taste good but can be unhealthy if ingested in large quantities.

THE DYNAMICS OF BECOMING

Having described some of the forms of becoming suggested by existential theory and contemporary goal research, we now discuss the factors that lead to variations in becoming. Why do some people remain stuck in the past or present, whereas others move forward into the future? Why do some people move toward futures that take them away from "who they really are," whereas others authentically become?

The Organismic Valuing Process

Sartre (1956) emphasized that humans have no choice but to take responsibility for creating themselves—we humans have no "essence" or inherent nature but must instead create a nature *ex nihilo*, from scratch. But are we completely adrift, with no way to tell what might actually be best for us? Although we agree with much of what existentialists have written about becoming, authenticity, and alienation, we are unable to agree with Sartre's view that people must create themselves with no guiding input from a "deeper self." Instead, we believe that all humans have a basic motive to self-actualize (Maslow, 1954; Rogers, 1961), individuate (Jung, 1951/1959), and/or integrate (Ryan, 1995), which helps guide and organize their lives.

In particular, we hold that all humans have an "organismic valuing process" (OVP; Rogers, 1964), which gives them potential access to subtle signals and deep internal information that can be used in decision making. Following Rogers, we conceive of the OVP as an emergent sense, hunch, intuition, or feeling that coalesces a good deal of information about the state of both the organism and its environment and then suggests the actions to undertake next in the service of the organism's overall health (Kasser, 2002b; Kuhl, 2000; Sheldon, Arndt, & Houser-Marko, 2003; see Kuhl & Koole, Chapter 26, this volume, for a similar discussion of what they call "extension memory"). As such, the OVP protects us from danger by telling us to spit out rotting food or to stay away from the one-eyed man with the machete. It is also, however, the part guiding us toward health, letting us know that the person we are sitting across from is the one we love and want to spend the rest of our life with, or even that we enjoy the challenge of writing chapters on experimental existential psychology.

Because the universal or species-typical OVP acts in the service of the organism's health and well-being, it should, on average and under normal circumstances, direct people toward becoming *and* authentic becoming, as both of these processes serve the organism's health. Although such human strengths or faculties are not widely appreciated or understood within psychology, some research on goals supports this positive assumption fairly well.

Speaking in terms of "becoming," most people do in fact have goals and view their goals as important. Subjects rarely have difficulty listing the 5 or even 10 goals that are typically required of most goal-assessment methodologies; similarly, a minority of people are identity diffused and thus lack goals to which they are committed (Marcia, 1993). Further, examination of the mean importance ratings placed on goals reveals that most people view their goals as being at least moderately important (Emmons, 1986; Kasser & Ryan, 1996). Finally, most people list more approach (i.e. becoming) goals than they list avoidance (i.e., non-becoming) goals (Elliot & Sheldon, 1996). These data show that people expend a good deal of psychic energy trying to move toward new and better circumstances and selves, and that, in general, they are reasonably good at it.

Speaking in terms of authentic becoming, research demonstrates that most people's goals are more congruent than noncongruent. First, examination of mean-level ratings of people's reasons for pursuing their strivings and projects shows that people generally feel more autonomous than controlled (Sheldon, 2002). Further, people across the globe rate intrinsic goals as more important than extrinsic goals (see Kasser, 2002b). Thus both features of congruent goals tend to be notable in the people surveyed in our research.

Lifespan data provide additional support for the idea that the OVP, operating over time, helps people to move into the future in an authentic way. For example, compared to younger individuals, older people report more self-concordant reasons for pursuing personal goals (Sheldon & Kasser, 2001), as well as for engaging in important social duties such as tax paying, voting, and gift giving (Sheldon, Kasser, Houser-Marko, Jones, & Turban, 2004). Similarly, older individuals are more likely to place high value on goals with intrinsic rather than extrinsic content (Kasser & Ryan, 1996; Sheldon & Kasser, 2001). Thus, maturity is associated with more congruent goal pursuit, and thus more authentic becoming, perhaps because it allows for more accumulated experience that helps the OVP suggest better and healthier pathways toward health and adaptation.

Even more convincing, longitudinal and experimental evidence for the OVP has recently been provided by Sheldon et al. (2003). This study focused on changes in peoples' goal choices and goal endorsements that occurred over time intervals ranging from 20 minutes to 6 weeks. When given the option, participants might not change their goals at all, but when they do change, which way do they go? Sheldon et al. reasoned that if there is no OVP, then when people change their goals they would be just as likely to shift their goal pursuit in directions detrimental to well-being as in directions supportive of well-being. On the other hand, if there is an OVP, then people should show a bias to shift primarily in directions which support their well-being (i.e., toward more congruent or authentic goal pursuit). As hypothesized, within-subject analyses revealed that when people changed their initial goal ratings choices, they were especially likely to shift toward more congruent goals. Notably, this finding held for both characteristics of authentic becoming (i.e., subjects were particularly likely to change toward both more self-concordant goals and goals with intrinsic rather than extrinsic content).

These various sources of data support the idea that we are not completely adrift when it comes to selecting healthy and beneficial goals for ourselves. Instead, under normal circumstances, people have the ability to perceive the direction most likely to lead them toward authentic becoming and greater well-being. As a result, they make appropriate choices concerning their goals to help them achieve this possibility.

When Becoming Goes Awry

Although we believe that goal pursuit is generally guided by the OVP and thus that people typically move toward health and authentic becoming, some individuals have experiences that lead them away from the OVP and teach them to ignore its suggestions. As a result, they are mired in non-becoming or alienated becoming. Research and theory suggest at least two dynamics that are at work in leading people away from becoming and from authentic becoming. First, people are sometimes exposed to environmental messages that suggest pathways to happiness that are at odds with the inner urgings of their OVP. As a result, people might take on beliefs and values that lead them toward alienated rather than authentic becoming. Second, people may experience environments in which they feel insecure, unloved, or highly controlled. Such qualities of environments often lead people to either give up on goal pursuit or to pursue noncongruent goals primarily concerned with gaining security or the approval of others. Next we briefly review some empirical evidence relevant to these claims.

Social Modeling

Parents, peers, teachers, and cultural institutions all tend to endorse and model certain types of goals, values, and behaviors as most optimal. This is the means by which different aspects of culture are maintained, for if the next generation failed to internalize beliefs and behaviors relevant to cultural institutions, those institutions would disappear for lack of followers. Problems in becoming occur when salient social models suggest to individuals that goals are either futile or worthless or that the paths to happiness are those that are actually at odds with the OVP. In the face of such conformity pressures, individuals sometimes ignore the advice of the OVP and instead succumb, to the detriment of their health and well-being.

Although most societies are goal oriented, sometimes individuals are exposed to subcultures and peer groups that suggest that, to quote the punk rock band the Sex Pistols, there is "No future for you." Those in a state of identity diffusion who are "going nowhere fast" often are embedded in a group of peers who share similar lifestyles and lack of motivation. Spending their time in hedonistic pleasures of the moment, without a care for tomorrow, certainly can be fun but rarely provides much of a ground for becoming to occur.

The larger, more notable problem, however, occurs when social institutions suggest beliefs, values, and goals that are at odds with the OVP and the person's real needs. Here we consider just two examples. First, we live in a culture in which the government and the corporate-controlled media continually suggest that the good life is the goods life, that success and happiness depend largely on one's wealth, status, and the possessions one has accumulated. This view is, of course, useful in maintaining the consumer-based hypercapitalistic economic system under which much of the world exists, but as demonstrated earlier, the internalization of such values actually leads people away from health and authentic becoming. A second type of message to which many people, particularly women, are exposed concerns the idea that one's body shape and sexuality are largely determinative of one's worth. To the extent that women and girls take on such messages, they often ignore their own inner desires to express themselves in other ways, to accept their imperfect bodies, and sometimes even to eat healthily (Kilbourne, 2004; see also Goldenberg & Roberts, Chapter 5, this volume).

Research indeed shows that when parents (the primary socializing agent of society) express strong extrinsic values, their children do the same (Kasser, Ryan, Zax, & Sameroff, 1995). Similar results are notable for other socializing forces, including peers and neighbors (Ahuvia & Wong, 1995). And, of course, we must not forget that other dominant socializer, the media. Research shows that people who watch a great deal of television, and are thus exposed to its many materialistic ads, are indeed more materialistic (Sirgy et al., 1998) and that women who are exposed to beautiful models in advertisements become less satisfied with themselves (Richins, 1991).

Relationship Quality

People are of course exposed to alienating messages to differing degrees, and this could be one reason why people sometimes take on paths of becoming that are relatively alienated. But we have also found that certain qualities of people's lives besides the models to which they are exposed can have important influences on the course of their becoming. Speaking broadly, those circumstances that make people feel insecure, unloved, or controlled by others are particularly likely to conduce toward non-becoming or alienated becoming. As described by Rogers (1961) and Maslow (1956), people in such circumstances give up on their desires for self-actualization and lose touch with the OVP; instead, they seek safety, security, and others' approval. As described by self-determination theory (Deci & Ryan, 1985), when they are controlled, people change their motivations from a desire to do things for reasons of sheer enjoyment and challenge to a desire to obtain rewards and praise. Through both sets of processes, they end up more alienated than authentic, as their OVP and deeper psychological needs are ignored. In short, to the extent that people have experienced many situations in life that scare them or threaten them with love withdrawal, we should find that they make whatever compromises are necessary to achieve security, rather than orienting toward what might help them grow.

Correlational evidence supports the idea that such qualities of experiences are associated with failures to become authentically. For example, people are more likely to become stuck in a diffused state of identity development, characterized by low commitment to goals and identity, when their parents are particularly distant (Marcia, 1993). Similarly, avoidance goals are more likely to predominate when parents threaten love withdrawal when their children do not achieve up to the parents' standards (Elliot & Thrash, in press). Furthermore, nonnurturant or cold parental styles are both cross-sectionally and longitudinally associated with more focus on extrinsic and less focus on intrinsic values (Cohen & Cohen, 1996; Kasser, Koestner, & Lekes, 2002; Kasser, et al., 1995; Williams, Cox, Hedberg, & Deci, 2000). Finally, new law students shift toward appearance values and away from community-contribution values during the first year of law school (Sheldon & Krieger, in press), presumably because of the strong insecurities promoted within the law school environment (Krieger, 1998).

Other experimental evidence shows that conditions that temporarily make people feel controlled or insecure are causally related to shifts toward less authentic becoming. A long history of research in the self-determination tradition, for example, documents that people move from autonomous to controlled motivations for their behaviors when they are exposed to salient controls such as rewards, contingent praise, deadlines, and ego involvement (see Deci & Ryan, 1985, for an overview). Although we are unaware of work that has applied these methods directly to people's self-reported goals, Baumann and Kuhl (2003) did find that inducing sadness in some subjects made them more susceptible to self-infiltration, which is similar in nature to controlled motivation. Other experimental research suggests that priming feelings of insecurity can make people focus more on extrinsic goals, particularly materialistic ones. For example, Kasser and Sheldon (2000) reported that, compared to a control group who wrote about music, students who wrote about their own death desired more money and luxury goods in the future (Study 1) and became greedier in a resource dilemma game (Study 2). Desires for materialism also rise when feelings of insecurity are primed in subjects who chronically feel self-doubt, and when feelings of normlessness are primed in subjects chronically high in anomie (Chang & Arkin, 2002).

CONCLUSION

To write this chapter, we formed a goal to express our view on existential concepts of becoming as they relate to what we know about goal pursuit. Through months of work, guided by our action systems, we engaged in a variety of subgoals to reach this end, including writing the subsections, editing for clarity, arguing with each other about the topics to be covered, the examples to be used, where to put a comma, and so on. But the chapter finally became something: It moved from an empty file on the computer (the modern equivalent of the blank page) to the words and ideas held within the two covers of this book. Becoming happened, as we moved from the past into the future. And although there were times when we questioned the importance of what we were saying, felt like we wanted to avoid the chapter, and even disengaged to pursue other writing (as well as other less academically productive activities), an end state was reached. How ideal it is will be determined by the editors, the publishers, and the readers.

And was it authentic, this particular becoming that you now read? Was our goal a congruent one? There were certainly times when we continued work on the chapter to fulfill our obligations to our friends the editors, and even perhaps hoped for a bit of recognition (i.e., citation) from our work; certainly money was not at issue, as most academics understand from the payment system of chapters. We do feel, however, that this chapter has been a challenge to write that has, at most moments, been fun. We also are sure that it expresses some ideas which we believe are important, not only for our own individual lives but also for psychology as a whole. And although we recognize that it is unlikely to bring us fame or riches, we do hope that it facilitates some movement forward (dare we say authentic becoming) in both our own personal lives and more broadly in the field of psychology.

REFERENCES

Ahuvia, A. C., & Wong, N. (1995). Materialism: Origins and implications for personal well-being. In F. Hansen (Ed.), *European advances in consumer research* (Vol. 2, pp. 172–178). Copenhagen, Denmark: Association for Consumer Research.

American Psychiatric Association. (1994). *Diagnostic and statistical manual of mental disorders* (4th ed.). Washington, DC: Author.

Barrett, W. (1958). *Irrational man: A study in existential philosophy.* New York: Doubleday.

Baumann, N., & Kuhl, J. (2003). Self-infiltration: Confusing assigned tasks as self-selected in memory. *Personality and Social Psychology Bulletin, 29,* 487–497.

Boss, M. (1963). *Psychoanalysis and Daseinsanalysis.* New York: Basic Books.

Carver, C., & Scheier, M. (1981). *Attention and self-regulation: A control-theory approach to human behavior.* New York: Springer-Verlag.

Carver, C., & Scheier, M. (1990). Origins and function of positive and negative affect: A control-process view. *Psychological Review, 97,* 19–35.

Carver, C., & Scheier, M. (1998). *On the self-regulation of behavior.* Cambridge, UK: Cambridge University Press.

Chang, L., & Arkin, R. M. (2002). Materialism as an attempt to cope with uncertainty. *Psychology and Marketing, 19,* 389–406.

Cohen, P., & Cohen, J. (1996). *Life values and adolescent mental health.* Mahwah, NJ: Erlbaum.

Deci, E. L., & Ryan, R. M. (1985). *Intrinsic motivation and self-determination in human behavior.* New York: Plenum Press.

Deci, E. L., & Ryan, R. M. (2000). The "what" and "why" of goal pursuits: Human needs and the self-determination of behavior. *Psychological Inquiry, 11,* 227–268.

Elliot, A. J., & Sheldon, K. M. (1996). Avoidance achievement motivation: A personal goals analysis. *Journal of Personality and Social Psychology, 73,* 171–185.

Elliot, A. J., Sheldon, K. M., & Church, M. A. (1997). Avoidance personal goals and subjective well-being. *Personality and Social Psychology Bulletin, 23,* 915–927.

Elliot, A. J., & Thrash, T. (in press). The intergenerational transmission of fear of failure. *Personality and Social Psychology Bulletin.*

Emmons, R. A. (1986). Personal strivings: An approach to personality and subjective well-being. *Journal of Personality and Social Psychology, 51,* 1058–1068.

Emmons, R. A. (1989). The personal striving approach to personality. In L. A. Pervin (Ed.), *Goal concepts in personality and social psychology* (pp. 87–126). Hillsdale, NJ: Erlbaum.

Fromm, E. (1976). *To have or to be?* New York: Harper & Row.

Hall, C. S., & Lindzey, G. (1978). *Theories of personality* (3rd ed.). New York: Wiley.

Jung, C. G. (1959). Aion. In *Collected Works* (Vol. 9). New York: Pantheon. (Original work published 1951)

Kasser, T. (2002a). *The high price of materialism.* Cambridge, MA: MIT Press.

Kasser, T. (2002b). Sketches for a self-determination theory of values. In E. L. Deci & R. M. Ryan (Eds.), *Handbook of self-determination research* (pp. 123–140). Rochester, NY: University of Rochester Press.

Kasser, T., Koestner, R., & Lekes, N. (2002). Early family experiences and adult values: A 26–year, prospective, longitudinal study. *Personality and Social Psychology Bulletin, 28,* 826–835.

Kasser, T., & Ryan, R. M. (1993). A dark side of the American dream: Correlates of financial success as a central life aspiration. *Journal of Personality and Social Psychology, 65,* 410–422.

Kasser, T., & Ryan, R. M. (1996). Further examining the American dream: Differential correlates of intrinsic and extrinsic goals. *Personality and Social Psychology Bulletin, 22,* 80–87.

Kasser, T., & Ryan, R. M. (2001). Be careful what you wish for: Optimal functioning and the relative attainment of intrinsic and extrinsic goals. In P. Schmuck & K. M. Sheldon (Eds.), *Life goals and well-being: Towards a positive psychology of human striving* (pp. 116–131). Goettingen, Germany: Hogrefe & Huber.

Kasser, T., Ryan, R. M., Zax, M., & Sameroff, A. J. (1995). The relations of maternal and social environments to late adolescents' materialistic and prosocial values. *Developmental Psychology, 31,* 907–914.

Kasser, T., & Sheldon, K. M. (2000). Of wealth and death: Materialism, mortality salience, and consumption behavior. *Psychological Science, 11,* 352–355.

Kierkegaard, S. (1941). *The sickness unto death.* Princeton, NJ: Princeton University Press. (Original work published 1849)

Kilbourne, J. (2004). "The more you subtract, the more you add": Cutting girls down to size. In T. Kasser & A. D. Kanner (Eds.), *Psychology and consumer culture: The struggle for a good life in a materialistic world* (pp. 251–270). Washington, DC: American Psychological Association.

Klinger, E. (1975). Consequences of commitment to and disengagement from incentives. *Psychological Review, 82,* 1–25.

Krieger, L. S. (1998). What we're not telling law students—and lawyers—that they really need to know: Some thoughts-in-acting toward revitalizing the profession from its roots. *Journal of Law and Health, 13,* 1–48.

Kuhl, J. (1981). Motivational and functional helplessness: The moderating effect of state versus action orientation. *Journal of Personality and Social Psychology, 40,* 155–170.

Kuhl, J. (2000). A functional-design approach to motivation and self-regulation: The dynamics of personality systems and interactions. In M. Boekaerts & P. R. Pintrich, (Eds.), *Handbook of self-regulation* (pp. 111–169). London: Academic Press.

Locke, E., & Latham, G. (1990). *A theory of goal setting and task performance.* Englewood Cliffs, NJ: Prentice-Hall.

Marcia, J. E. (1993). The status of the statuses: Research review. In J. E. Marcia, A. S. Waterman, D. R. Matteson, S. L. Archer, & J. L. Orlofsky (Eds.), *Ego identity: A handbook for psychosocial research* (pp. 22–41). New York: Springer-Verlag.

Maslow, A. H. (1954). *Motivation and personality.* New York: Harper & Row.

Maslow, A. H. (1956). Defense and growth. *Merrill–Palmer Quarterly, 3*, 36–47.

May, R. (1983). *The discovery of being.* New York: Norton.

Oyserman, D., & Markus, H. R. (1990). Possible selves and delinquency. *Journal of Personality and Social Psychology, 59*, 112–125.

Pyszczynski, T., & Greenberg, J. (1987). Self-regulatory perseveration and the depressive self-focusing style: A self-awareness theory of reactive depression. *Psychological Bulletin, 102*, 122–138.

Richins, M. L. (1991). Social comparison and the idealized images of advertising. *Journal of Consumer Research, 18*, 71–83.

Rogers, C. R. (1961). *On becoming a person.* Boston: Houghton Mifflin.

Rogers, C. R. (1964). Toward a modern approach to values: The valuing process in the mature person. *Journal of Abnormal and Social Psychology, 68*, 160–167.

Rokeach, M. (1973). *The nature of human values.* New York: Free Press.

Ryan, R. M. (1995). Psychological needs and the facilitation of integrative processes. *Journal of Personality, 63*, 397–427.

Ryan, R. M., & Connell, J. P. (1989). Perceived locus of causality and internalization: Examining reasons for acting in two domains. *Journal of Personality and Social Psychology, 57*, 749–761.

Sartre, J. P. (1956). *Being and nothingness.* New York: Philosophical Library.

Sheldon, K. M. (2002). The self-concordance model of healthy goal striving: When personal goals correctly represent the person. In E. L. Deci & R. M. Ryan (Eds.), *Handbook of self-determination research* (pp.65–86). Rochester, NY: University of Rochester Press.

Sheldon, K. M., Arndt, J., & Houser-Marko, L. (2003). In search of the organismic valuing process: The human tendency to move towards beneficial goal choices. *Journal of Personality, 71*, 835–869.

Sheldon, K. M., & Elliot, A. J. (1998). Not all personal goals are personal: Comparing autonomous and controlled reasons as predictors of effort and attainment. *Personality and Social Psychology Bulletin, 24,*546–557.

Sheldon, K. M., & Elliot, A. J. (1999). Goal striving, need-satisfaction, and longitudinal well-being: The self-concordance model. *Journal of Personality and Social Psychology, 76*, 482–497.

Sheldon, K. M., & Houser-Marko, L. (2001). Self-concordance, goal attainment, and the pursuit of happiness: Can there be an upward spiral? *Journal of Personality and Social Psychology, 80*, 152–165.

Sheldon, K. M., & Kasser, T. (1995). Coherence and congruence: Two aspects of personality integration. *Journal of Personality and Social Psychology, 68*, 531–543.

Sheldon, K. M., & Kasser, T. (1998). Pursuing personal goals: Skills enable progress but not all progress is beneficial. *Personality and Social Psychology Bulletin, 24*, 1319–1331.

Sheldon, K. M., & Kasser, T. (2001). Getting older, getting better? Personal strivings and psychological maturity across the life span. *Developmental Psychology, 37*, 491–501.

Sheldon, K. M., Kasser, T., Houser-Marko, L., Jones, T., & Turban, D. (2004). *Doing one's duty: Chronological age, felt autonomy, and subjective well-being.* Manuscript in preparation.

Sheldon, K. M., & Krieger, L. (in press). Does law school undermine law students? Examining changes in goals, values, and well-being. *Behavioral Sciences and the Law.*

Sirgy, M. J., Lee, D., Kosenko, R., Meadow, H. L., Rahtz, D., Cicic, M., et al. (1998). Does television viewership play a role in perception of quality of life? *Journal of Advertising, 27*, 125–142.

Williams, G. C., Cox, E. M., Hedberg, V. A., & Deci, E. L. (2000). Extrinsic life goals and health risk behaviors in adolescents. *Journal of Applied Social Psychology, 30*, 1756–1771.

Zaleski, Z. (1994). Toward a psychology of the personal future. In. Z. Zaleski (Ed.), *Psychology of future orientation* (pp. 10–20). Lublin, Poland: Towarzystwo Naukowe KUL.

Part VI

Postmortem

Chapter 30

The Best of Two Worlds

Experimental Existential Psychology
Now and in the Future

SANDER L. KOOLE
JEFF GREENBERG
TOM PYSZCZYNSKI

Questions about human nature and the meaning of existence have captured the imagination of poets, prophets, and philosophers across the millennia. Theoreticians in the brief history of psychology have also sometimes focused on these types of broad questions (e.g., Allport, Freud, James, Lifton, Rank, Rogers, Yalom). But over most of this history, existentially oriented questions have been considered outside the realm of empirical investigation. Indeed, experimental research and the existential perspective have traditionally been regarded as two irreconcilable approaches in psychology. The *Handbook of Experimental Existential Psychology* flies in the face of that tradition and signals the beginnings of a formal reconciliation. Experimental existential psychology is built on the brash assumption that psychologists can indeed use rigorous empirical methods such as laboratory experiments to study people's struggles to come to terms with the basic givens of existence. Experimental psychology and existential psychology no longer need to exist as separate disciplines; psychologists can now incorporate the best of these two worlds in their thinking.

As this *Handbook* testifies, experimental–existential approaches in psychology have blossomed in recent years. Experimental existential psychologists have addressed a large and still growing number of issues, including sexuality, human–nature relations, religion, morality, identity construction, nostalgia, culture, ideology, close relationships, group identifications, disgust, ostracism, communication, decision making, and goal striving. In light of these developments, it is clear that people's existential concerns can no longer be avoided or dismissed by experimental researchers. Instead, people's existential concerns are treated as a domain of inquiry that deserves careful consideration and systematic empirical attention.

Theoretical notions of existential psychology are increasingly sharpened by the input of experimental methodologies. Conversely, experimental methods are being extended, renewed, and revised to enable the investigation of complex existential–psychological phenomena. Though still a young scientific movement, experimental existential psychology is rapidly coming of age.

The present *Handbook* provides the most extensive overview to date of the first generation of experimental–existential research. In this last chapter, we draw on this growing body of knowledge to derive some general conclusions about the newly emerging experimental existential psychology. In the next paragraphs, we begin by examining the rationale for believing that people's existential problems can indeed be explored through rigorous empirical methods. After this, we examine what existential psychology has to offer to experimental psychology, and conversely, what experimental psychology has to offer to existential psychology. We end with some educated guesses regarding how experimental existential psychology might develop in the years to come.

THE ODD COUPLE OF EXISTENTIALISM AND EXPERIMENTALISM

Experimental existential psychology comprises a large number of different theoretical approaches, research topics, and paradigms. Yet underneath this apparent diversity, all experimental–existential psychologists subscribe to the basic notion that people's existential struggles are—at least, in principle—open to experimental scrutiny. At first glance, this notion seems anything but self-evident. Existentialists have traditionally been concerned with people's struggles with the really big questions of life, whereas experimentalists have been studying concrete human behavior in typically restricted and highly artificial laboratory settings. The approaches of existential psychology and experimental psychology thus would appear to be fundamentally incompatible.

On closer consideration, however, the incompatibility between existential psychology and experimental psychology may be more apparent than real. Existential questions might seem far removed from concrete behavior because most people do not confront them in the abstract terminology of existential psychology. Nevertheless, people's everyday lives are in fact replete with confrontations with the basic givens of existence. Take, for instance, the psychological confrontation with death. The problem of death is one of people's most fundamental existential concerns (e.g., Arndt, Cook, & Routledge, Chapter 3, this volume; Florian & Mikulincer, Chapter 4; Solomon, Greenberg, & Pyszczynski, Chapter 2; see also Yalom, 1980). Nevertheless, in the eyes of many, the problem of death might seem like a very remote concern, because most people spend only a fraction of their time consciously thinking about death. This line of reasoning, however, does not consider the more subtle and implicit ways in which people are confronted with death. As many experiments have shown, death concerns often become implicitly activated when people become aware of their own bodies (Goldenberg & Roberts, Chapter 5), when they encounter nature (Koole & Van den Berg, Chapter 6), when people are abandoned by close others (Mikulincer, Florian, & Hirschberger, Chapter 18), or when people are unable to identify with their own social group (Castano, Yzerbt, & Paladino, Chapter 19). The confrontation with death thus forms a ubiquitous aspect of everyday life, even though for many people this confrontation may take place primarily on unconscious, subterranean levels.

Research in experimental existential psychology suggests that other existential concerns are similarly widespread as the problem of death. The basic needs that people have for ultimate meanings may emerge most visibly during moments of religious elevation (Batson & Stocks, Chapter 9; Haidt & Algoe, Chapter 20) or in the aftermath of traumatic events (Janoff-Bulman & Yopyk, Chapter 8; Salzman & Halloran, Chapter 15). However, even during less dramatic moments, people's desire for meaning forms an integral part of the lay-epistemological process (Dechesne & Kruglanski, Chapter 16). Moreover, meaning becomes especially desirable as a function of common everyday concerns such as people's inner uncertainties (McGregor, Chapter 12), social injustice (Van den Bos, Chapter 11), or feelings of nostalgia (Sedikides, Wildschut, & Baden, Chapter 13). In an analogous manner, people may rarely become conscious of the full extent to which they are dependent on their psychological connections with other people. Nevertheless, people's existential needs for connectedness are felt throughout their everyday social interactions, as evidenced in people's attachments with close others (Mikulincer et al., Chapter 18; Wicklund & Vida-Grim, Chapter 23), people's fear of rejection (Case & Williams, Chapter 21), and in people's needs to communicate their deepest feelings to each other (Pinel, Long, Landau, & Pyszczynski, Chapter 22; Wicklund & Vida-Grim, Chapter 23). Finally, issues of free will and personal responsibility are not just abstract philosophical issues but are of immediate relevance to everyday practical matters such as decision making (Young & Morris, Chapter 14; Taubman - Ben-Ari, Chapter 7), self-control (Vohs & Baumeister, Chapter 25), emotion regulation (Kuhl & Koole, Chapter 26), and effective goal pursuits (Bargh, Chapter 24). Taken together, it becomes evident that existentialism is much more than a fancy discussion topic for people with a weak spot for Sartre and black turtleneck sweaters. Rather, the confrontation with existential concerns is a concrete reality in the everyday lives of ordinary people.

Once one accepts the idea that existential concerns are an urgent daily reality, it makes sense to study these concerns systematically and, whenever possible, experimentally. After all, if existential concerns are potentially relevant to almost everything that people do, it seems crucial for psychologists to find out as much as they can about how people cope with these concerns. Indeed, this volume documents how coping with existential concerns affects an extraordinarily wide range of important psychological phenomena, including risk-taking behavior (Taubman - Ben-Ari, Chapter 7; Young & Morris, Chapter 14), attitudes toward nature (Koole & Van den Berg, Chapter 6), morality (Tangney & Mashek, Chapter 10; Van den Bos, Chapter 11), intergroup behavior (Castano et al., Chapter 19; Dechesne & Kruglanski, Chapter 16), interpersonal behavior (Wicklund & Vida-Grim, Chapter 23; Mikulincer et al., Chapter 18; Pinel et al., Chapter 22), and authentic being (Kasser & Sheldon, Chapter 10; Martin, Campbell, & Henry, Chapter 27; Ryan & Deci, Chapter 28). If existential concerns influence so many different realms of human behavior, it seems reasonable to assume that these concerns can also influence behavior in the laboratory.

Laboratory experiments are a particularly powerful methodology because of their careful control of contaminating factors and their ability to probe into mediating mechanisms. For this reason, experiments provide a very useful tool for experimental–existential research. However, in the past, some scholars have objected that experiments may be unsuited to investigate the unique meanings of people's dealings with the givens of their own existence. Experimental existential psychology fully acknowledges that people may face their existential concerns in highly individualized and personal ways. At the same time, however, this does not rule out the existence of basic psychological principles which govern how people generally cope with existential concerns. If such principles operate at the level of underlying processes and mechanisms, general psychological principles might exist even when the contents of people's experiences are highly idiosyncratic and subjective. Experimental methods may thus be directed at the level of process rather than at the level of particular phenomenological contents. A nice illustration of this logic is provided by Pinel et al. (Chapter 22). In their work, Pinel et al. focus on the most subjective part of the self, the self that experiences, the "I" in Jamesian terms. By experimentally varying whether people feel that their I is shared with others, Pinel et al. have been able to explore the social functions of the I, even though Pinel et al. were not able to experimentally control the precise contents of their participants' I's. Accordingly, experimental research can be useful even to gain more insight into phenomena that are highly subjective and individualized.

Notably, experimental existential psychology does not regard the laboratory experiment as the only valid way of acquiring scientific knowledge. Many important phenomena in existential psychology, such as the person's religious beliefs (Batson & Stocks, Chapter 9), coping with traumatic events (Janoff-Bulman & Yopyk, Chapter 8), or near-death experiences (Martin et al., Chapter 27) can hardly be induced experimentally. Other relevant variables, such as personality characteristics (Dechesne & Kruglanski, Chapter 16; Florian & Mikulincer, Chapter 4; Kuhl & Koole, Chapter 26), are inherently determined by factors within the person rather than by the psychological investigator. When variables of these kinds are concerned, experimental existential psychologists have relied on careful measurement rather than manipulation of the variables of interest. Experimental existential psychology thus takes a pragmatic approach to the use of experimental method. Experimental existential psychology remains committed to maximally rigorous empirical research, while being sensitive the particular needs and constraints of a particular domain of investigation.

WHAT EXPERIMENTALISM CAN GAIN FROM EXISTENTIALISM

Experimental existential psychology builds on two venerable traditions within psychology. The first of these traditions, experimental psychology, has been dedicated to the experimental analysis of human functioning. The logic of the experimental method has become widespread throughout mainstream academic psychology, in areas such as cognitive psychology, social psychology, developmental psychology, and animal psychology. Across these different areas, researchers have developed a vast store of refined research techniques and meticulously documented empirical phenomena. Experimental psychology has thus gained considerable respectability and credibility as a scientific approach.

The main strength of experimental psychology has always been its emphasis on methodological rigor and precision. However, there is nothing inherent about the experimental method that suggests which problems in psychology are worth pursuing or which issues need to be resolved. Herein lies a potential weakness of traditional experimental psychology. Methodological rigor can become an end in itself, rather than a means for advancing psychological knowledge. When this occurs, researchers may conduct their research solely for the purpose of satisfying the demands of other researchers. This kind of purely method-driven research tends to become increasingly sterile and contrived, as it is not guided by a genuine curiosity about psychological questions. Moreover, because method-driven research is not deeply invested in its subject matter, this kind of research easily falls prey to momentary fads and fashions that are just as easily picked up as they are abandoned by researchers. To prevent this kind of intellectual regression, experimental psychology ultimately needs a meta-theoretical resource that allows it to tell which kinds of questions are worthy of intellectual pursuit. And this is where existential psychology comes in.

Existential thinking represents a broad meta-theoretical perspective that comprises questions that are of fundamental relevance to the entire human race. An infusion of existential thinking may thus keep experimental psychology from developing into a wholly self-absorbed, bloodless enterprise. After all, any science that can further our psychological understanding of these existential questions will not just cater to the interests of a small group of colleagues but, at least in principle, can benefit everyone. The present *Handbook* contains numerous examples of how existentialist ideas can be used to direct experimental methodologies toward profoundly meaningful sets of issues. For instance, a number of experimental–existential psychologists have recently adapted paradigms from implicit social cognition research to the study of existential issues. These include paradigms such as *construct accessibility research* (e.g., Bargh, Chapter 24; Solomon, Greenberg, & Pyszczynski, Chapter 2), *subliminal priming* (Arndt et al., Chapter 3; Bargh, Chapter 24; Dechesne & Kruglanski, Chapter 16; Koole & Van den Berg, Chapter 6), *word fragment completions* (Arndt et al., Chapter 3; Mikulincer et al., Chapter 18), the *Stroop task* (Kuhl & Koole, Chapter 26), and *the implicit association test* (McGregor, Chapter 12). Originally, these paradigms were developed to study basic (social-) cognitive processes, such as memory, cognitive control, and evaluative processing. In experimental existential psychology, however, these paradigms have been used and transformed to address questions about terror management, the will, morality, isolation, identity construction, and other fundamental existential issues. Experimental existential psychology can thus help researchers to discover new and meaningful ways in which experimental methodologies can be applied to theoretical problems.

Experimental psychology has long been plagued by fragmentation and a lack of theoretical integration. Without theoretical integration, experimental findings are little more than isolated facts that offer no deeper understanding into psychological questions. Accordingly, theoretical integration is vital to the long-term interests of experimental psychology. At this point, an infusion of existentialist thinking may again turn out to be extremely useful. By definition, existentialist thinking is focused on the big picture of human existence. Accordingly, existentialist ideas automatically direct people's attention to the larger context in which human behavior unfolds. The incorporation of such ideas into experimental research can thus be expected to promote integrative theorizing. Consistent with this view, this volume provides several examples of the commitment of experimental–existential psychologists to theoretical integration. Among these integrative perspectives are *terror management theory* (Solomon et al., Chapter 2), *attachment theory* (Mikulincer et al., Chapter 18), *personality systems interactions theory* (Kuhl & Koole, Chapter 26), and *self-determination theory* (Ryan & Deci, Chapter 28). These theories were developed for different purposes, by different researchers, and focus primarily on different substantive domains. Nevertheless, the theories are quite similar in pulling together many disparate literatures and phenomena in order to understand the deeper regularities that underlie human behavior. This focus on theoretical integration is strongly encouraged by experimental existential psychology.

WHAT EXISTENTIALISM CAN GAIN FROM EXPERIMENTALISM

Experimental existential psychology further builds on the tradition of existential psychology. The core business of existential psychology has been the analysis of how people cope with the deep concerns that characterize the human condition. Because the deep concerns of existential psychology coincide with the deep concerns of humanity, it seems understandable that existentialist ideas have attracted considerable popular attention and support, at least in Western society. Although mainstream experimental psychology has largely eschewed existentialist notions, existential psychology has had a major influence on psychotherapy, philosophy, theology, literature, and art (Pyszczynski, Greenberg, & Koole, Chapter 1; Yalom, 1980). Existentialist ideas have thus proven their utility in a wide variety of different contexts.

The freedom to think about the human condition in the broadest possible terms can be regarded as one the chief strengths of existential psychology. Like any freedom, however, the unique freedom of thinking in existential psychology entails certain risks. If existential psychology remains a purely abstract and theoretical enterprise, the contribution of ordinary, nonexpert individuals may be easily left out of the academic debate. Consequently, existential psychology may develop into an elitist enterprise, in which a handful of full-time experts can claim exclusive access to ultimate truths about the human condition. In this respect, the experimental method may complement existential psychology in an important way. The experimental method allows ordinary people to provide vital input (i.e., empirical data) that then serves as the basis for further discussion and interpretation by scholars. This means that the agenda of experimental existentialism can never be determined unilaterally by a particular group of scholars. Instead, an experimentally oriented existential psychology will necessarily involve a dialectic interchange between theoretical notions and the actual behavior of ordinary people.

A second set of advantages of experimental existentialism involves the greater level of precision that is afforded by the experimental method. By its own nature, existential psychology focuses on very broad and abstract issues. To make practical use of the insights of existential psychology, however, it is usually necessary to translate existentialist notions to a more concrete level. The experimental method forces researchers to be very concrete about their concepts, because these concepts must be translatable into actual research operations. Accordingly, an experimental–existential orientation fosters the development of theories that are midway between the highly abstract level of existentialism and the hyperconcrete level of experimentalism. In this volume, we see a number of examples of such midlevel theories, such as *female objectification theory* (Goldenberg & Roberts, Chapter 5), the *existential motives analysis of human–nature relations* (Koole & Van den Berg, Chapter 6), *uncertainty management theory* (Van den Bos, Chapter 11), *identity consolidation theory* (McGregor, Chapter 12), *lay epistemic theory* (Dechesne & Kruglanski, Chapter 16), *systems justifications theory* (Jost, Fitzsimons, & Kay, Chapter 17), *ostracism theory* (Case & Williams, Chapter 21), *social identity theory* (Castano et al., Chapter 19), *moral amplification theory* (Haidt & Algoe, Chapter 20), the *automotive model* (Bargh, Chapter 24), and *ego depletion theory* (Vohs & Baumeister, Chapter 25). These midlevel theories provide essential bridges between specific content domains (e.g., social justice, social cognition, and identity strivings) and broad existential issues (e.g., the problem of death). Experimental existential psychology is strongly committed to the development of such theoretical bridges, which help to spell out the implications of existentialism for everyday life.

A final advantage of experimental existentialism lies in the ability of the experimental method to support counterintuitive or controversial ideas. Theoretical claims that are based on logical argument alone can usually be dismissed rather easily by logical counterarguments. A combination of theoretical argument and matching empirical observation is generally much more compelling. Experimental existential psychology may thus help existential psychology to advance beyond self-evident truths. A striking example of this is terror management theory (TMT; Solomon et al., Chapter 2). Long before TMT was posited, existential thinkers had already argued for the importance of death anxiety in everyday life (e.g.,

Becker, 1973; Rank, 1941/1958; Kierkegaard, 1844/1957). However, this argument was met with a great deal of skepticism and had not really become widely accepted—that is, until TMT research was able to furnish strong experimental support for the pervasive importance of terror management processes. TMT research has further been able to show that fear of death primarily drives behavior on unconscious levels (Arndt et al., Chapter 3). This intriguing evidence might explain the lack of intuitive appeal of the notion of a ubiquitous fear of death, because theorizing about the unconscious is likely to be inherently more counterintuitive and hence more controversial. In this regard, it seems very fortunate that recent developments in experimental psychology have yielded compelling methods to establish the operation of unconscious processes (Arndt et al., Chapter 3; Bargh, Chapter 24; Kuhl & Koole, Chapter 26; see also Westen, 1998). Similar experimental methods should make it more feasible for existential thinkers of the future to persuade reluctant audiences of unexpected or unwelcome conclusions.

SUMMARY AND CONCLUSIONS

Experimental existential psychology challenges psychologists to use maximally rigorous empirical methods to study how people are coping with their most fundamental existential concerns. From the perspective of experimental psychology, an infusion of existentialist thinking promotes new applications of experimental paradigms and encourages the development of new experimental techniques in the study of existential issues. Moreover, an experimental–existential outlook is likely to promote theoretical integration across multiple domains of empirical inquiry. From the perspective of existential psychology, the experimental method acknowledges the importance of ordinary individuals in the debate on existentialist issues. In addition, the experimental method forces existentialists to formulate their ideas with greater precision and encourages midlevel theorizing that helps translate abstract existentialist ideas into concrete implications for everyday life. Finally, the experimental method permits existential psychology to develop theories on counterintuitive or controversial ideas, which experimental methods can back with solid empirical evidence.

In recent years, experimental–existential approaches have made considerable headway in psychology. As the present *Handbook* documents, researchers have created powerful new methods for studying existential issues. These new methodologies, in turn, have generated important insights and have established experimental existential psychology as a major hub of scientific activity. At the same time, researchers have come up with integrative theoretical perspectives and midlevel theories that afford greater precision in connecting existentialist ideas to psychological processes. Remarkably, the growth of experimental existential psychology has occurred in several places at once, without any kind of central coordination or professional organization. Experimental existential psychology has thus been able to achieve a tremendous amount of progress relatively quietly and almost overnight.

As a scientific enterprise, psychology has undergone quite a few trends and fashions that have come and gone over the years. Accordingly, the seasoned observer may wonder about the long-term impact of experimental existential psychology. Is experimental existential psychology a passing fad that will be forgotten in a few years time? Or will experimental existential psychology have an enduring impact? Although clearly, it is impossible to know what the future will bring, we see several grounds for believing that experimental existential psychology is here to stay. First, existential issues have been with humanity for as long as history can tell. It thus seems unlikely that the interest in existential issues will vanish shortly. Second, it seems probable that further technological developments will open up even more new venues for experimental existential psychology. Ironically, behaviorist psychologists once believed that experimental technology would eventually render existential psychology obsolete. In reality, the reverse has happened. As experimental methods have steadily become more sophisticated, the rigorous empirical study of existential issues has become increasingly feasible for psychologists. Thus, based on past experience, we can expect that further technological advances in experimentation will provide a further impetus to experimental existential psychology.

In thinking about future developments, it seems also relevant to ask how independent we should ideally want experimental existential psychology to be with respect to other areas of psychology. At present, experimental existential psychology is still largely grounded in social and personality psychology. It might be, however, that experimental existential psychology will eventually become better off by establishing its own independence. Our own view on this issue is that, for many years to come, experimental existential psychology will probably do best as a growing theme flowing through the many established branches in psychology. The ultimate aim of experimental existential psychology is to influence psychology at large, across its different branches and even across scientific and applied subdisciplines. This agenda implies clearly that experimental existential psychology should always be a force within mainstream psychology. Within the mainstream, however, experimental existential psychology should work hard to promote further the integration between psychological science and existentialist thinking. By achieving a level of visibility as a scientific movement, experimental existential psychology may stimulate other researchers to initiate experimental–existential approaches, even when their immediate colleagues might be skeptical.

Some 20 years ago, few people would have predicted that experimental psychology and existential psychology would ever join forces. As the *Handbook of Experimental Existential Psychology* makes clear, things have changed considerably since then. Experimental existential psychology has developed into a vibrant scientific discipline that uses the rigorous methods of experimental psychology to study people's deepest existential concerns. With the growing success of experimental–existential approaches, the time seems ripe to combine the best of the two worlds of existentialist thinking and experimental psychology.

REFERENCES

Becker, E. (1973). *The denial of death.* New York: Free Press.

Kierkegaard, S. (1957). *The concept of dread* (W. Lowrie, Trans.). Princeton, NJ: Princeton University Press. (Original work published 1844)

Rank, O. (1958). *Beyond psychology.* New York: Dover Books. (Original work published 1941)

Westen, D. (1998). The scientific legacy of Sigmund Freud: Toward a psychodynamically informed psychological science. *Psychological Bulletin, 124,* 333–371.

Yalom, I. (1980). *Existential psychotherapy.* New York: Basic Books.

Author Index

Subject Index

517